The Convergence of the Metaverse, AI, and Federated Learning in Healthcare Ecosystems

Soufiane Ben Othman
King Faisal University, Saudi Arabia

IGI Global
Scientific Publishing
Publishing Tomorrow's Research Today

Published in the United States of America by
IGI Global Scientific Publishing
701 East Chocolate Avenue
Hershey, PA, 17033, USA
Tel: 717-533-8845 | Fax: 717-533-7115
Website: https://www.igi-global.com E-mail: cust@igi-global.com

Library of Congress Cataloging-in-Publication Data

Names: Ben Othman, Soufiane, 1981- editor
Title: The convergence of the metaverse, AI, and federated learning in healthcare ecosystems / edited by: Soufiane Ben Othman.
Description: Hershey PA : IGI Global Scientific Publishing, [2026] | Includes bibliographical references. | Summary: "This book aims to provide a unified and authoritative reference on the convergence of the Metaverse, Artificial Intelligence, and Federated Learning in healthcare ecosystems by integrating theoretical foundations, system architectures, advanced algorithms, and real-world applications"-- Provided by publisher.
Identifiers: LCCN 2026005805 (print) | LCCN 2026005806 (ebook) | ISBN 9798337388892 hardback | ISBN 9798337388908 paperback | ISBN 9798337388915 ebook
Subjects: LCSH: Medical care--Data processing | Medical informatics
Classification: LCC R858 .C6666 2026 (print) | LCC R858 (ebook)
LC record available at https://lccn.loc.gov/2026005805
LC ebook record available at https://lccn.loc.gov/2026005806

British Cataloguing in Publication Data
A Cataloguing in Publication record for this book is available from the British Library.

Table of Contents

Detailed Table of Contents

A combination of the remote healthcare and virtual hospitals and the use of the Metaverse and Artificial Intelligence (AI) has a transformative potential. By combining the immersive virtual reality with the artificial intelligence technologies, one will have the chance to make healthcare more efficient, more accessible, and more personal. The virtual hospitals also apply the Metaverse to consult patients, diagnose and supervise without any regard to geographical and space limitations. AI is the area that is employed to increase and broaden clinical decision making, devise an individualized treatment plan, and possess a computerized assistant who does the choice. The technologies will offer high quality training prospects, patient connectivity and nonstop care particularly in underserved regions. Along with the promising opportunities, one can still observe such challenges as layout of data privacy, technological limitations as well as regulatory challenges.

errors and prompt coding of medical records providing personalized medicine and virtual health assistants.

The rapid evolution of digital health has exposed the limitations of centralized artificial intelligence, platform-dependent telemedicine, and fragmented data governance. In parallel, healthcare metaverses are emerging as persistent, immersive, and data-intensive environments that demand new forms of secure, collaborative intelligence. This chapter advances the central argument that federated artificial intelligence and the healthcare metaverse must be theorised together, as their integration constitutes a fundamentally new computational, organisational, and governance paradigm rather than a simple technological convergence. By conceptualising healthcare AI as a distributed, experiential system, the chapter develops the notion of Federated Experiential Intelligence and examines its architectural, ethical, and institutional implications. Drawing on interdisciplinary theoretical lenses and global empirical trends, it analyses emerging practices, governance challenges, fairness concerns, and critical counter-arguments.

This chapter per the authors examines the integration of federated learning and digital twins to establish a resilient clinical intelligence ecosystem in the healthcare metaverse. While always-on sensing offers transformative potential, existing implementations often treat privacy, latency, and governance as secondary concerns. By synthesizing current literature, this chapter per the authors identifies a benchmarking gap where model metrics are prioritized over system-level evidence like communication overhead and energy costs. To address these deficiencies, authors propose a unified five-layer reference architecture treating trust and real-time synchronization as core requirements. This framework introduces the "protected twin" concept, utilizing differential privacy, secure aggregation, and audit trails to ensure distributed intelligence remains accountable and robust against poisoning. Ultimately, this chapter per the authors provides a strategic roadmap for moving toward deployable, clinically valid pipelines that balance innovation with patient safety.

This chapter explores the integration of federated learning, explainable artificial intelligence (XAI), digital twins, and Metaverse technologies to transform modern healthcare systems. Digital twins enable real-time patient modeling and predictive analysis, while federated learning ensures privacy-preserving collaboration across medical institutions. Explainable AI enhances transparency and clinical trust by making intelligent decisions interpretable. The Metaverse further extends these capabilities by enabling immersive visualization, remote collaboration, and interactive medical training. Together, these technologies form a secure, intelligent, and patient-centric healthcare ecosystem that supports personalized treatment, ethical AI deployment, and future-ready digital healthcare innovation.

The intersection of the metaverse, artificial intelligence, and federated learning to redefine the next-generation healthcare ecosystems by facilitating immersive, intelligent, and privacy-preserving services. This chapter presents a Cognitive Federated Metaverse of Healthcare (CFM-Health), a harmonized system that incorporates metaverse-focused healthcare interrelations, has interaction-conscious federated learning, federated digital twin intelligence, and edge fog, and cloud

case, the potential of federated learning as the 'connective intelligence' layer in a Metaverse-oriented setting shall also be highlighted in this chapter, as it can provide federated training to Artificial Intelligence across institutions to avoid aggregating or hoarding important patient information in a healthcare setting.

Crossover of the metaverse, Artificial Intelligence, and Federated Learning is changing the healthcare systems and amplifying the issues of privacy, security, and trust. This chapter discusses privacy preservation by design as a fundamental concept to applying Federated Learning architectures in metaverse-based healthcare setting. Federated Learning is theoretically understood as an architecture facilitator that introduces collaborative intelligence between hospitals, clinics, wearables, and virtual care platforms with no centralized data exchange. The main architectural aspects like Edge Fog Cloud Coordination, Secure Aggregation, Differential Privacy, and Trusted Execution Environment are examined to explain how confidentiality and regulatory compliance may be obtained. By conceptually discussing and using illustrative examples, the chapter demonstrates how privacy-centric federated architectures can be used to support immersive, real-time, and patient-centric healthcare services and maintain data sovereignty.

The integration of Metaverse technologies, artificial intelligence, and federated learning introduces new possibilities for delivering secure, scalable, and personalized healthcare services. Metaverse-enabled healthcare environments support immersive clinical interactions and continuous patient engagement, while artificial intelligence enables multimodal data analysis and intelligent decision support. However, centralized AI approaches face challenges related to data privacy, scalability, and regulatory compliance. This chapter presents a trustworthy healthcare framework

Preface

INTRODUCTION

The rapid digital transformation of healthcare is no longer a distant vision but a present reality driven by the convergence of the Metaverse, Artificial Intelligence, and Federated Learning. Together, these paradigms are reshaping healthcare delivery, research, and patient engagement. As healthcare systems confront aging populations, chronic diseases, fragmented data infrastructures, and rising cybersecurity risks, traditional centralized models prove increasingly inadequate. At the same time, patients expect personalized, real-time, and immersive care experiences that extend beyond physical clinical settings.

The Metaverse enables persistent, interactive digital healthcare environments where clinicians, patients, medical devices, and digital twins interact seamlessly. Artificial Intelligence enhances these environments through predictive analytics, intelligent diagnostics, and personalized treatment strategies. Federated Learning strengthens this ecosystem by allowing collaborative model training across institutions while preserving data privacy and regulatory compliance. The true innovation lies in their integration, creating secure, adaptive, and patient-centric healthcare ecosystems that combine immersive interaction with distributed, privacy-aware intelligence.

This book explores the architectural, security, regulatory, and ethical dimensions of this convergence, addressing challenges such as latency, adversarial threats, algorithmic bias, and cross-border data governance. By bridging theory with real-world applications in smart hospitals and connected health infrastructures, it offers a roadmap for researchers, technologists, policymakers, and healthcare leaders. Ultimately, it envisions a future where immersive technologies enhance human-centered care, AI augments clinical expertise, and federated intelligence enables collaboration without compromising privacy.

COVERAGE

The many academic areas covered in this publication include, but are not limited to:

1. Artificial Intelligence in Healthcare
2. Federated Learning Architectures
3. Metaverse Applications in Medicine
4. Medical Informatics
5. Digital Twins for Smart Hospitals
6. Extended Reality (AR/VR/MR) in Clinical Practice
7. Cybersecurity in Healthcare Systems
8. Blockchain for Medical Data Governance
9. Privacy-Preserving Machine Learning
10. Edge Computing in IoMT Environments
11. Internet of Medical Things (IoMT)
12. Cloud Computing for Healthcare Platforms
13. Big Data Analytics in Medicine
14. Smart Healthcare Systems
15. Human–Computer Interaction in Virtual Care
16. Digital Health Ethics and Regulatory Compliance
17. Healthcare Interoperability
18. Predictive Modeling in Clinical Decision Support
19. Personalized Medicine
20. Sustainable Healthcare Technologies

CHAPTER OVERVIEW

Chapter 1. Revolutionizing Healthcare with the Metaverse, AI, and Federated Learning

This chapter introduces the transformative convergence of immersive virtual environments, Artificial Intelligence (AI), and Federated Learning (FL) in healthcare. It outlines the conceptual foundations of metaverse-enabled medical ecosystems and explains how distributed intelligence addresses critical challenges such as data silos, privacy risks, and fragmented care delivery. The chapter discusses system-level integration models, digital collaboration platforms, and intelligent clinical workflows. By presenting a strategic overview of emerging technologies, it establishes the groundwork for understanding how immersive computing and decentralized AI reshape healthcare delivery, patient engagement, and institutional collaboration.

Chapter 2. Next Generation Healthcare Systems Driven by Metaverse Artificial Intelligence and Federated Learning

This chapter explores architectural blueprints for next-generation healthcare infrastructures powered by immersive technologies and federated intelligence. It presents scalable system models integrating AI-driven diagnostics, distributed data governance, and persistent virtual healthcare environments. The chapter highlights smart hospitals, decentralized analytics, and cross-institutional model training. Key challenges such as interoperability, latency, and regulatory compliance are examined, offering a roadmap for building resilient, adaptive, and secure digital healthcare ecosystems.

Chapter 3. Intelligent Immersive Healthcare: Integrating AI, Federated Learning, and the Metaverse

This chapter focuses on immersive healthcare environments enhanced by intelligent automation and distributed machine learning. It analyzes how AI-driven decision support systems operate within virtual care platforms and how federated frameworks preserve patient confidentiality. Clinical simulations, virtual consultations, and digital therapeutics are discussed. The chapter emphasizes patient-centric design principles and the creation of adaptive healthcare ecosystems capable of continuous learning.

Chapter 4. Applications of Metaverse and AI in Remote Healthcare and Virtual Hospitals

This chapter examines practical implementations of immersive healthcare platforms in telemedicine, remote diagnostics, and virtual hospitals. It explores AI-assisted remote surgery simulations, tele-rehabilitation, and collaborative medical training within digital environments. The chapter discusses infrastructure requirements, wearable integration, and ethical considerations, demonstrating how immersive technologies extend healthcare access while maintaining clinical reliability.

Chapter 5. Enhanced Deep Learning Design for Diagnosing Childhood Pneumonia in Chest X-rays Using EfficientNetB4, Topological Convolutional Layers, and Improved

This chapter proposes an optimized deep learning framework using EfficientNetB4 and advanced convolutional layers for chest X-ray analysis. It discusses architectural enhancements, feature optimization, and training strategies. Experimental validation demonstrates improved classification accuracy and robustness. The chapter highlights AI's role in early pediatric diagnosis and scalable screening systems.

Chapter 6. Assessing the Reliability of Artificial Intelligence in Healthcare: A Bibliometric Review

This chapter presents a comprehensive bibliometric analysis of AI reliability research in healthcare. It identifies publication trends, influential studies, collaboration networks, and emerging research directions. The chapter evaluates explainability, validation protocols, bias mitigation, and regulatory frameworks, offering insights into strengthening trust in AI-driven healthcare systems.

Chapter 7. Federated AI and the Metaverse: A New Computational Logic

This chapter introduces federated intelligence as a foundational computational paradigm for immersive healthcare ecosystems. It explores decentralized training, collaborative optimization, and secure aggregation techniques. The chapter explains how federated AI enables scalable, privacy-preserving analytics across distributed medical institutions.

Chapter 8. Federated AI-Driven Digital Twins in the Healthcare Metaverse

This chapter examines digital twin architectures powered by federated AI. It discusses virtual patient modeling, predictive simulations, and personalized treatment optimization within immersive environments. Privacy-aware distributed training mechanisms are integrated into digital twin frameworks to enable secure cross-institutional collaboration.

Chapter 9. Federated and Explainable AI-Driven Digital Twins in Metaverse-Based Healthcare Ecosystems

This chapter focuses on explainable federated AI models embedded in healthcare digital twins. It presents methods for interpretability, trust evaluation, and transparent clinical decision support. The chapter emphasizes ethical AI deployment and accountability in immersive medical ecosystems.

Chapter 10. Cognitive Federated Metaverse for Healthcare

This chapter introduces a cognitive architecture integrating federated learning, explainable AI, and immersive virtual systems. It proposes a privacy-centric intelligence paradigm that supports adaptive learning, contextual reasoning, and continuous model refinement while safeguarding patient data.

Chapter 11. Secure Federated LLM Gateways for Metaverse-Enabled Healthcare

This chapter explores secure integration of large language models (LLMs) within federated healthcare metaverse environments. It examines compliance frameworks, access control, secure APIs, and encrypted model orchestration. The chapter highlights safe conversational AI interfaces for clinical decision support and immersive patient engagement.

Chapter 12. Architectures for Trustworthy Metaverse-Based Healthcare Ecosystems

This chapter proposes architectural frameworks ensuring security, scalability, and trust in immersive healthcare platforms. It covers distributed identity management, blockchain-enabled verification, and secure cloud-edge orchestration strategies.

Chapter 13. Privacy Preservation Through Design

This chapter presents privacy-by-design principles embedded into federated metaverse architectures. It discusses governance models, data minimization strategies, anonymization frameworks, and risk assessment methodologies for secure immersive healthcare systems.

Chapter 14. Trustworthy Metaverse-Enabled Healthcare - Integrating Artificial Intelligence and Federated Learning for Secure, Scalable, And Personalized Care

The concluding chapter synthesizes architectural, ethical, and technological dimensions of immersive federated healthcare systems. It presents a unified framework integrating AI, federated learning, digital twins, and immersive platforms for secure, scalable, and personalized care. Future research directions, policy implications, and sustainability considerations are discussed, positioning trustworthy intelligent healthcare ecosystems as the foundation of next-generation digital medicine.

CONCLUSION: IMPACT AND CONTRIBUTION OF THE BOOK

The Convergence of the Metaverse, AI, and Federated Learning in Healthcare Ecosystems presents a comprehensive and forward-looking exploration of how immersive virtual environments, intelligent automation, and privacy-preserving distributed intelligence collectively redefine modern healthcare. By integrating the transformative capabilities of the Metaverse, Artificial Intelligence, and Federated Learning, this book advances a unified vision of secure, scalable, and patient-centric healthcare ecosystems. Rather than treating these technologies as isolated innovations, the volume demonstrates how their convergence creates a new computational and organizational logic for digital medicine.

The book's primary contribution lies in bridging theory, architecture, and real-world application. It offers multidisciplinary insights spanning intelligent medical imaging, IoMT integration, digital twins, federated model orchestration, explainable AI, cybersecurity frameworks, and privacy-by-design governance. By presenting both foundational principles and domain-specific case studies, it equips researchers and practitioners with actionable frameworks for designing trustworthy immersive healthcare systems. The structured progression, from conceptual foundations to advanced federated architectures and trust models, ensures coherence while highlighting cutting-edge research directions.

Beyond technological innovation, this volume contributes strategically to the evolving discourse on responsible digital transformation in healthcare. It addresses regulatory compliance, ethical AI deployment, bias mitigation, adversarial resilience, and sustainability considerations—issues central to long-term adoption. The book positions federated intelligence as a catalyst for global collaboration without compromising privacy, enabling institutions to move beyond data silos toward interoperable and trustworthy virtual care ecosystems.

Ultimately, this work serves as both a scholarly reference and a strategic roadmap. It supports academic research, informs policy development, and guides healthcare leaders in implementing immersive, AI-driven infrastructures. By articulating a clear vision of intelligent, federated, and human-centered healthcare ecosystems, the book contributes meaningfully to shaping the future of digital health innovation.

Acknowledgement

This work was supported by the Deanship of Scientific Research, Vice Presidency for Graduate Studies and Scientific Research, King Faisal University, Saudi Arabia [Grant No. KFU262257]

Chapter 1 Revolutionizing Healthcare With the Metaverse, AI, and Federated Learning

Kallur V. Vijayakumar
http://orcid.org/0000-0002-7205-1144
Department of Mathematics, BMS Institute of Technology and Management, Karnataka, India

Pratiksha Liladhar Meshram
http://orcid.org/0000-0003-2049-7694
Department of Information Technology, SVKMs NMIMS, MPSTME, Shirpur, India

Bhavin Mehta
http://orcid.org/0000-0003-2933-9713
Charotar University of Science and Technology, Gujarat, India

Suganthi. N.
http://orcid.org/0000-0003-2222-856X
Department of Electrical and Electronics Engineering, Dayananda Sagar College of Engineering, Bangalore, India

Sridhara S. B.
http://orcid.org/0009-0005-1929-3303
Department of Computer Science and Engineering, Amruta Institute of Engineering and Management Sciences, Bidadi, India

DOI: 10.4018/979-8-3373-8889-2.ch001

ABSTRACT

A combination of the remote healthcare and virtual hospitals and the use of the Metaverse and Artificial Intelligence (AI) has a transformative potential. By combining the immersive virtual reality with the artificial intelligence technologies, one will have the chance to make healthcare more efficient, more accessible, and more personal. The virtual hospitals also apply the Metaverse to consult patients, diagnose and supervise without any regard to geographical and space limitations. AI is the area that is employed to increase and broaden clinical decision making, devise an individualized treatment plan, and possess a computerized assistant who does the choice. The technologies will offer high quality training prospects, patient connectivity and nonstop care particularly in underserved regions. Along with the promising opportunities, one can still observe such challenges as layout of data privacy, technological limitations as well as regulatory challenges.

INTRODUCTION

The combination of the Metaverse and Artificial Intelligence (AI) could change the nature of healthcare delivery, especially the virtual hospitals and remote healthcare. The Metaverse as the collective virtual shared space formed by the overlap of physically enhanced physical reality and existent virtual spaces is changing many areas, and healthcare may be seen as one of the most promising spheres where it will have an effect. It is an integrated, immersive ecosystem that is founded on augmented reality (AR), virtual reality (VR), digital twins, and persistent virtual spaces to produce alive and interactive environments (Chaddad, A., Wu, Y., and Kateb, R., 2023). These virtual environments are not only game and entertainment platforms in the sphere of healthcare but also platforms where patients are treated, medical education, and professional training take place. The integration of AI creates access toward more effective, efficient, and personalized healthcare through the availability of real-time data analysis, decision-making, and advanced predictive models through the Metaverse.

The phenomenon of the Metaverse in healthcare is directly connected with the fact that remote and virtual care becomes increasingly popular which is especially true in telemedicine since it has rapidly switched to remote medicine during the COVID-19 pandemic (Baroud, S. Y., 2025). Consultations, diagnostic evaluations, and therapeutic procedures conducted using virtual interfaces enable the resolution of the physical geographical and logistical barriers, as well as the lack of contact between the patient and the medical professional. An example of such as a virtual consultation is the possibility of conducting it in real-time and using avatars or holograms to create the illusion of a healthcare professional being present within the framework that is not only interesting and interactive but also accessible (Alsalami, Z. A., Chandra Sekhar Reddy, L., Saritha, K., Ranitha, I. B., Nageshwari, R., and Govindaram, A., 2025). Moreover, the Metaverse has superior diagnostic technologies like immersive visualization systems, which allow closer visualization of the image through which diagnostics are more accurate and effective and can often have a comprehensive insight into an object compared to conventional methods. Such simulating method is also notable in the simulation-based treatment planning which enables both patients and health care providers in the virtual world to explore in diversity of treatment options and evaluate the effectiveness and outcomes of the same before it is integrated into the real-life context (Bashir, A. K. et al., 2023).

Figure 1. Convergence of Metaverse and AI in Remote Healthcare and Virtual Hospitals

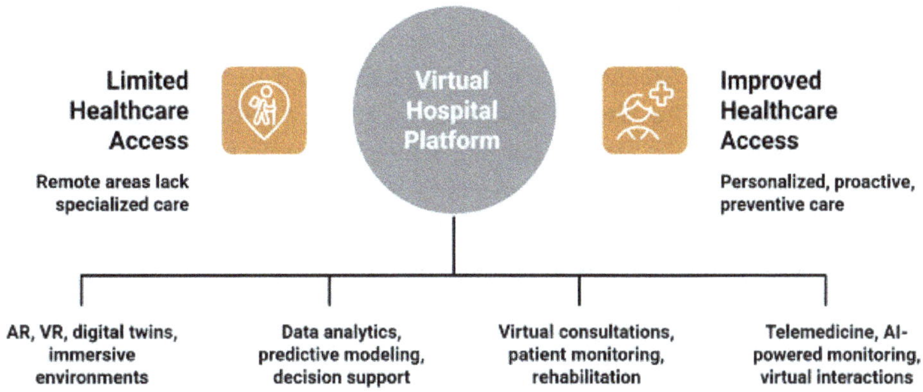

As shown in Figure 1, the development of the Metaverse is going to be a part of remote healthcare and virtual hospitals incorporating technologies of Artificial Intelligence (AI). The most significant part of the diagram identifies the importance of using Metaverse technologies in the form of augmented reality (AR), virtual reality (VR), digital twins, and other virtual worlds during which virtual consultations, diagnostic imaging, and simulation-based treatment plans are made (Raju et al., 2025). These technologies provide an interactive and persistent virtual environment that allows connections in real-time between the patients and health practitioners, getting around geographical boundaries. Within the context of this, AI technologies that can be described as reflective of predictive modeling, machine learning, and intelligent decision support systems are pictured, in the context of how they will improve healthcare by examining large volumes of data, give real-time diagnosis, and ersect care to patients (Yenduri, G. et al., 2023). The number associates these technologies with a virtual hospital model, which is an entirely virtualized healthcare center in which consultation, monitoring, rehabilitation and education occur. Finally, it is a patient-centric model that involves patients using this ecosystem through remote care systems, and AI-supported monitoring and virtual consultations, which will be developed to deliver effective healthcare to the patient at an individual level (Kumar et al., 2023).

The contribution of AI to these virtual health care environments would go far in enhancing the degree of efficiency of the Metaverse in healthcare. AI enables the processing of large data that patients receive as the outcome of the interaction, clinical history, and diagnostic tests and provides valuable data which would be difficult to retrieve in traditional circumstances. The machine learning models and the predictive algorithms can provide real time feedbacks and diagnoses to assist healthcare providers in making appropriate decisions and can provide customized treatment regimes to individuals (Rao et al., 2025). In addition, AI-based decision support systems will be able to reduce the human error to a minimum and ensure that clinical guidelines are adhered to, which will increase the safety and reliability of remote care delivery. The adaptive capabilities of virtual environments provided by AI are that, because of the constant learning which will occur, virtual environments can be designed in a more adaptable manner whenever patients need it, increasing the process of care deliverance to patients and rendering it more efficient. AI can be applied to mimic real life situations in a virtual environment, where practitioners and patients can practice, rehearse, or even receive therapy with the virtual environment being risk-safe and allowing new competencies to be exercised (Letafati, M. and Otoum, S., 2023).

Virtually hospital is one of the most far-reaching uses of this convergence that is a complete digitalization of healthcare. The Metaverse is used by virtual hospitals to establish an environment in which the consultation, monitoring, rehabilitation, and education are fully conducted online. Within this environment, patients are able to relate with the health care professionals in a real-time way using their virtual characters thus offering a complete treatment without the physical mobility. This model enhances not only convenience to the patients, especially in the rural or underserved regions but it also decreases the strain applied over the physical healthcare infrastructure. Virtual rehabilitation allows patients to take part in therapeutic activities at home and watch the advancement, and AI helps adjust the program in the real-time. Besides, the virtual hospital can train healthcare professionals through educational modules, and simulated surgeries, case studies that involve diagnostic exercises, and analysis can practice in a safe controlled and virtual environment.

BACKGROUND & DEFINITIONS

Metaverse in Healthcare

The Metaverse is an ecosystem of digital spaces that exist across time and interact with one another and in space in real-time in an interaction between the users and each other by way of the avatars. It combines various technologies including Virtual Reality (VR), Augmented Reality (AR), Mixed Reality (MR), and persistent virtual worlds, which allows very high levels of immersion to occur. In medical practice, the Metaverse enables communication between patients, healthcare providers and medical systems and goes beyond the physical location of the medical facility. VR provides full immersion and users have the opportunity to interact with digital reality of the environment, AR integrates digital information to the real world, and it improves real-time interactions (Sanjaya, F. N., Balakrishnan, S., Sindiramutty, S. R., and Narputro, P., 2025). MR is an intersection between VR and AR as a result of which physical and virtual objects can interact in real time. The combination of these technologies creates a possibility to conduct virtual consultations, diagnostics, simulations of surgery, and rehabilitation (Stephanie, V., Khalil, I., and Atiquzzaman, M., 2024). Cloud computing and 5G/6G networks as well as digital twins are among the key enabling technologies that will make the Metaverse applicable in the healthcare sector. Cloud computing offers the platform to store large volumes of medical data, and also ensures that virtual platforms are accessible across geographical boundaries to enable scalable and efficient healthcare delivery, including services that need instant data transmission, including remote surgery or live consultation (Kang, J. et al., 2024). Digital twins are digital versions of real-world objects e.g. patients or healthcare systems, which can be monitored, analysed, and simulated in real-time. These computer-based models allow making more effective decisions during the treatment planning, patient results prediction, and healthcare provision.

Artificial Intelligence in Healthcare

Artificial Intelligence (AI) is a simulation of human intelligence being operated through machines, and in this case, computers, the use of which has gone viral in the medical field. Two key examples of the methods that AI uses in this domain are called Machine Learning (ML) and Deep Learning (DL) to equip the systems to learn and evolve with time. Algorithms on the basis of ML models can extract specific data patterns, which can be used in the diagnosis of diseases, risk analysis, and prediction of patient outcomes. DL is a branch of ML; it causes the intricate neural network to multilayered to handle large datasets, which implies that it would be exceptionally competent in image recognition in radiology and pathology (Garg, S., Dev, R., Singh, A. K., Sahani, S., Kumari, K., and Bandyopadhyay, A., 2025).

Another interesting medical AI approach worth mentioning is Natural Language Processing (NLP) which enables computers to write, understand and read human speech. NLP in the clinical world is applied to non-structural data in medical records, which may be utilized to produce some insights that can be applied to serve the provision of better care to patients. The other AI technique is Reinforcement Learning (RL), which is a method of training models to make a sequence of choices by rewarding them when doing the right choice (Sravanthi et al., 2025). The model is applicable in fields such as treatment planning whereby RL is constantly learning to maximize the optimal treatment strategies depending on the response of the patients. The impact of AI in the healthcare environment is also enhanced by clinical decision support systems (CDSS) which helps healthcare professionals make clinical decisions through examined patient information and recommending either a diagnosis or treatment or a medication (Letafati, M. and Otoum, S., 2024). AI-based systems with predictive analytics use both historical and real-time data to anticipate future events, e.g., disease progression, or possible complications, and, therefore, proactively provide care. Robotics Process Automation (RPA) also finds applications in the healthcare sphere to automate the regularly occurring administrative duties, including the data entry and appointment scheduling, helping to decrease the scope of operations and letting the medical practitioners dedicate more time to the patients (Hosseini Mirmahaleh, S. Y., and Rahmani, A. M., 2025). Through integration of these AI technologies, healthcare systems will be able to provide improved patient care, more precise, timely and customized care, and enhance the efficiency of healthcare operations.

Virtual Hospitals

A virtual hospital is a virtual healthcare facility, functioning in a virtual space, and that offers services, including consultations, diagnosis, treatment monitoring, rehabilitation and education, which are available with the help of digital resources instead of physical facilities. This model is a great innovation compared to conventional brick-and-mortar hospitals to use digital technology as an offering of distant treatment (Gor et al., 2025). Virtual hospitals come in especially handy in improving healthcare accessibility among patients in remote or underserved regions because a physical hospital may be hard to access.

The development of virtual hospitals can be linked to a traditional telemedicine, which originally provided the possibility of the simplest distance consultation between patients and doctors (Chokshi, K., 2025). Telemedicine offered an opportunity to overcome the geographical barrier, although it was still not enough. With the development of technology, especially the emergence of the Metaverse, healthcare became more interactive, which resulted in virtual hospitals. Such platforms provide not only consultations with one direction but the ability to fully interact in real-time, using avatars, patients and healthcare professionals engage in real time, and the use of AI and other technologies helps create more individual and effective care. Virtual hospitals are created to respond to sophisticated care situations such as remote surgical support, real-time medical diagnostics, and constant control over patients through the application of AI, the Metaverse, and other other technologies.

A virtual hospital has a virtual space which is not similar to the physical hospital. In a physical hospital, the patient has to visit the physical hospital to appointments, diagnoses, and treatments, which may prove to be time consuming and expensive (Li et al., 2023). Other challenges which are encountered in physical hospitals are overcrowding, insufficiency of resources, and shortage of staff. Virtual hospitals, in turn, have the benefit of bringing care to the patient at the comfort of their homes and no need to go anywhere, as well as the exposure to infections that is particularly significant in the post-pandemic period. Also, virtual hospitals have the advantage of operating 24/7 because they are not affected by the physical capabilities (like working hours) or staffing shifts (Gundu, L., Ramachandran, V., Butchi Raju, K., Hossain, R. R., Sreekanth, D., and Putta, P., 2025).

The shift to the virtual healthcare is associated with challenges, though. As an example, the availability of the required technologies (e.g., high-speed internet, VR/AR devices) may be a limitation to the members of some groups, especially rural or low-income areas. In virtual environments, data security and privacy concern are also intensified because healthcare data is to be secured to meet the regulatory requirements, including the HIPAA or GDPR. Moreover, virtual hospitals can have a problem with giving some forms of treatment that can be received by hands-on treatment, e.g. surgery or physical examination, but with the developments of remote surgery and robotics, these issues are slowly resolving. Irrespective of these issues, virtual hospitals have massive potential in future of healthcare especially in relation to increasing accessibility, lowering healthcare expenditure and raising patient interaction.

METHODOLOGICAL FRAMEWORK

The suggested conceptual framework on the combination of Metaverse and AI in remote healthcare is expected to promote the provision of customized, effective, and immersive healthcare experiences to the users of a multi-layered architecture. The center of such architecture is the patient terminal where healthcare services are provided to patients using devices such as smartphones, tablets, VR or AR glasses.

The devices are used as the gateway to the Metaverse interface where patients can participate in real-time appointments, diagnostic tests and treatments in immersive virtual worlds. Interpretations of data collected when interacting with patients are determined based on AI backend, where AI algorithms are used to draw predictive analytics, personalized treatment recommendation, and decision support. It is stored in the form of processed data in data stores that are hosted in safe cloud infrastructure and accessed and retrieved easily by clinicians. Clinician dashboards can then help healthcare professionals track the progress of patients, investigate diagnostic results, and make relevant decisions based on real-time performance and AI results (Ivanovic, M., and Macos, D., 2023). The system mentioned above contributes towards the creation of an integrated interaction and monitoring and shared decision making between the patients and healthcare providers in a fully integrated virtual healthcare environment.

The framework consists of several key components that work together in order to make the healthcare delivery worthwhile. The immersive interaction layer entails gadgets such as the VR/AR headsets which provide the users with the interactive experiences which are immersive. This type of headset allows the patient to engage with a 3D virtual reality in order to consult or undertake a therapeutic session or both a therapeutic session and a rehabilitation exercise. This communication can also be empowered by haptic feedback devices which will provide us with the touch feeling, which can be converted into the real world and this is most crucial in virtual rehabilitation. The AI engine is at the center since it examines patient data to present prediction patterns and predict the progression of a disease or treatment response besides the personalization features that contribute towards personalizing the healthcare experience in accordance with the needs of the individual. Virtual assistance is also enabled by the AI engine and can be used in the form of automated assistants, including virtual care agents, who provide reinforcement and guidance to patients and give them real-time help during their healthcare process (Aloqaily, M., Bouachir, O., Karray, F., Al Ridhawi, I., and Saddik, A. E., 2023). A secure cloud infrastructure manages connectivity and data management, which is the reason why the patient data including the medical records, diagnostic image and treatment plans are prevented to be at any risk of not being stored and accessed effectively. Edge computing can also be used to compute data nearer to the patient with such systems having a low latency level and a real-time response to the needs of applications such as remote surgery support or live consultations. The framework also provides security and ethical control modules that would verify the adherence to data protection legislation (e.g. HIPAA or GDPR) to ensure patient data is kept safe and that the AI algorithms are trustworthy, understandable, and unbiased. The modules also control access to data and make sure that patients make informed consent of their use of the data.

Figure 2. System Architecture for Metaverse and AI-Integrated Healthcare Framework

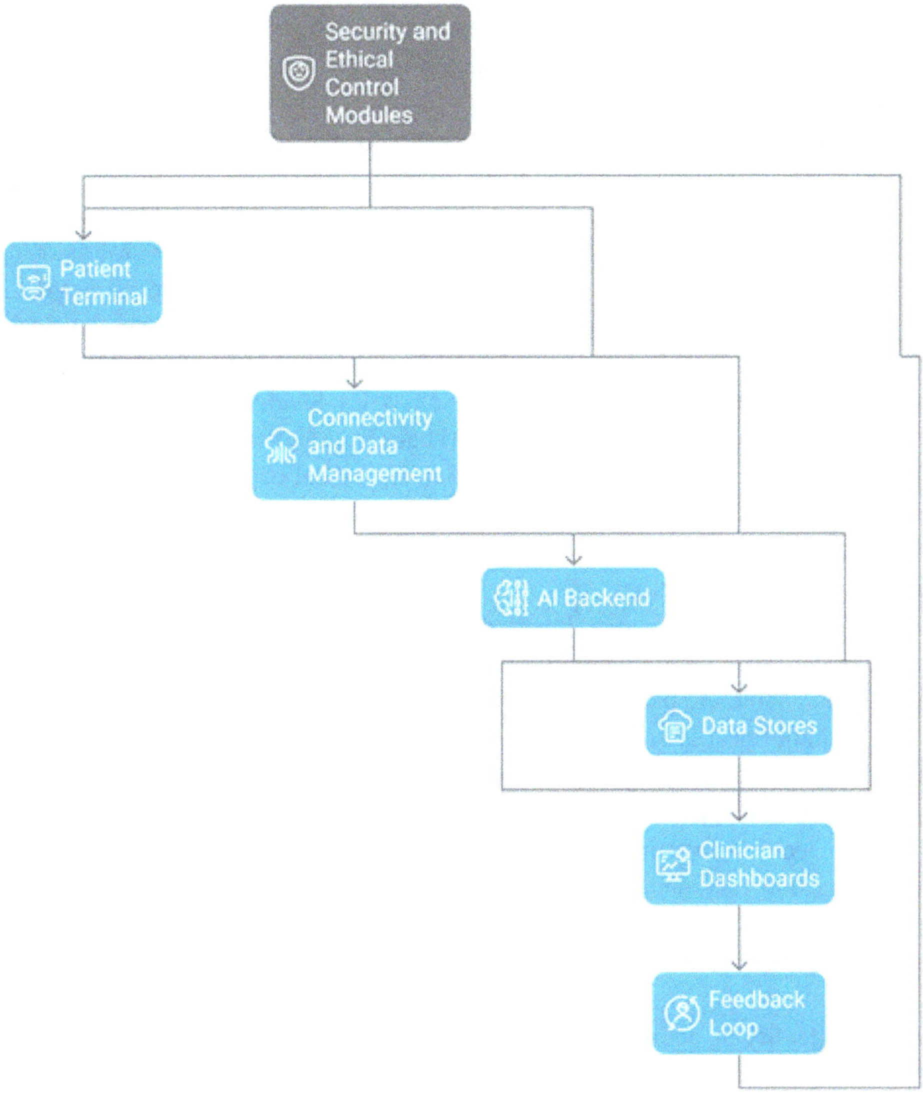

The system architecture of integrating 2 (Metaverse and AI technologies) in a remote healthcare system is shown in Figure 2, with the flow of interactions and data between the most important building blocks included in the process of providing immersive and intelligent healthcare services. The model depicts the usage of a patient terminal i.e. VR/AR head sets, cell phones or tablets, as the port of entry of patients into the healthcare environment of the Metaverse. This terminal enables the patient to take part in virtual consultations, therapy and rehabilitation activities in a Metaverse interface, where patients interact in real-time with clinicians and virtual health assistants. The AI backend is an important component since it handles the data input received during patient interaction and makes predictive analysis, recommendation of treatments, and decision support to healthcare facilities. This AI system communicates with data stores which are secure cloud-based repositories that store patient records, diagnostic images, treatment plans, and other medical data easily accessed and accessible through this system. This data is constantly monitored and analyzed by the AI backend which then offers actionable insights that would help enhance patient care. These insights are provided to healthcare professionals in the form of clinician dashboards, where they can view real-time patient data, in the form of diagnostics, treatment progress, and AI-driven recommendations. These dashboards enable clinicians to make a well-informed choice on the basis of recent patient records as well as predictive analytics. Seamless and real time communication between the patient terminal, AI backend, clinician dashboards and data stores is ensured by connectivity and data management of secure cloud and edge computing infrastructure. This infrastructure enables uninterrupted production of data between the system and is also fast with low latency which is required in real time healthcare applications.

Various use case scenarios illustrate how this framework can be applied in the real world healthcare contexts. Remote diagnostics through virtual consultation rooms can enable the patient to have a real-time consultation with the healthcare expert without necessarily having to travel a considerable distance to do it. The patients are allowed to visit a virtual consultation room using VR headset or AR glasses where the professionals are able to interrelate with them in an immersive space. In such consultations, AI backend would assist by interpreting symptoms, past medical history, and diagnostic evidence to give real-time information to help healthcare providers make correct diagnoses. The other scenario is AI-assisted imaging in the virtual environment where AI algorithms can be joined to medical imaging sites to interpret X-rays, MRIs, or CTs in real-time. Such systems are capable of identifying anomalies including the tumor or fracture and give healthcare professionals clear 3D images to aid in diagnosis and treatment planning. It comes in handy especially in radiology and pathology where fast and precise diagnosis is required. Another use of the metaverse in rehabilitation and physiotherapy is that patients are able to undergo virtual rehabilitation through personalized exercises, as the AI system adjusts the exercises according to the patient. The VR headsets also enable patients to do physical exercises in a virtual space that can respond to their requirements and give them a more active and interactive method of gaining mobility and strength during the recovery process. The performance of the patient is observed by the AI systems; the intensity of exercises is changed depending on the real-time information to guarantee the best rehabilitation results. Mental health therapy refers to immersion as the last category, in which VR technology has been used to create virtual exposure therapy, which allows the patient to face their fears or trauma within a safe virtual environment. The AI responds to the emotional reactions of the patient and modifies the virtual environment to offered a safe therapeutic experience of the patient, which is therapeutic and engaging. This approach has demonstrated high effectiveness in managing diseases like PTSD, anxiety, and phobias, and provides the patient with a chance of having an emotional healing in a virtual, controlled setting.

RESULTS & DEMONSTRATIONS

Metaverse and AI technologies applied to the healthcare system will improve patient outcomes, clinical effectiveness, and the general experience of care. The next section identifies the results of the simulation, the anticipated outcomes, and performance indicators using the proposed system. These outcomes in the form of several figures demonstrate the usefulness of this method in the process of diagnostics and patient interaction, treatment adherence and in making clinical decisions.

As demonstrated in Figure 3, the User Experience (UX) Evaluation shows the dependence of patient monitoring accuracy of time, whereby, after ten weeks, there is a significant positive change in the accuracy of the AI-based system. In this simulation, the patient monitoring accuracy is 75 percent in the first week and 98 percent on the tenth week, an act that indicates the way the AI system is more accurate as it receives more information. These gradual advancements in precision are associated with the immersion and usability of the system that steadily improves due to the continuous changes in the AI, which will provide more personalized and operational information to its users.

Figure 3. Patient Monitoring Accuracy vs. Time

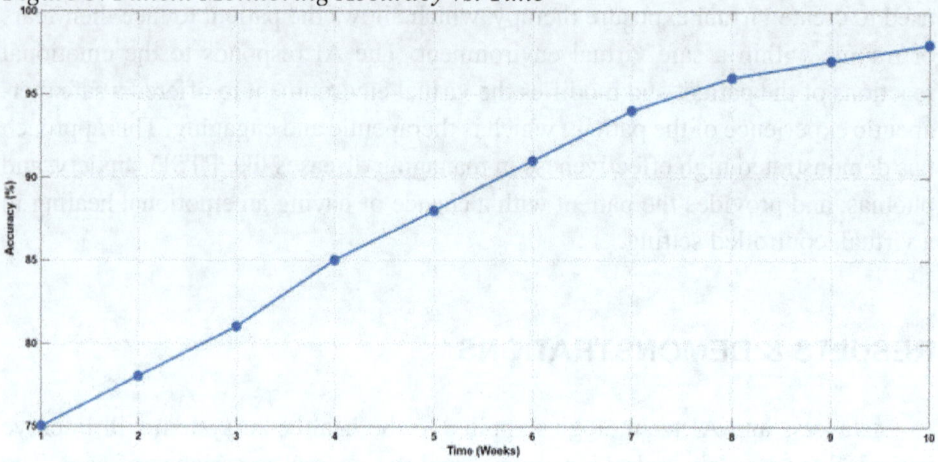

Figure 4 displays Diagnostic Accuracy in which the value of the disease progression predicted by AI has been compared with real outcomes of a sample of patients. The AI system has a very high diagnostic accuracy of 88% and the relationship between actual and predicted values is very close. The disease progression rates forecasted against the patients are close to the real ones that can be seen in the clinical environment, indicating that AI can reach the same diagnostic levels as the professional clinician. This number illustrates the possibility of AI supporting the process of clinical decision-making, where it warns about something early and enhances diagnostic techniques.

Figure 4. AI Prediction vs. Actual Outcomes for Disease Progression

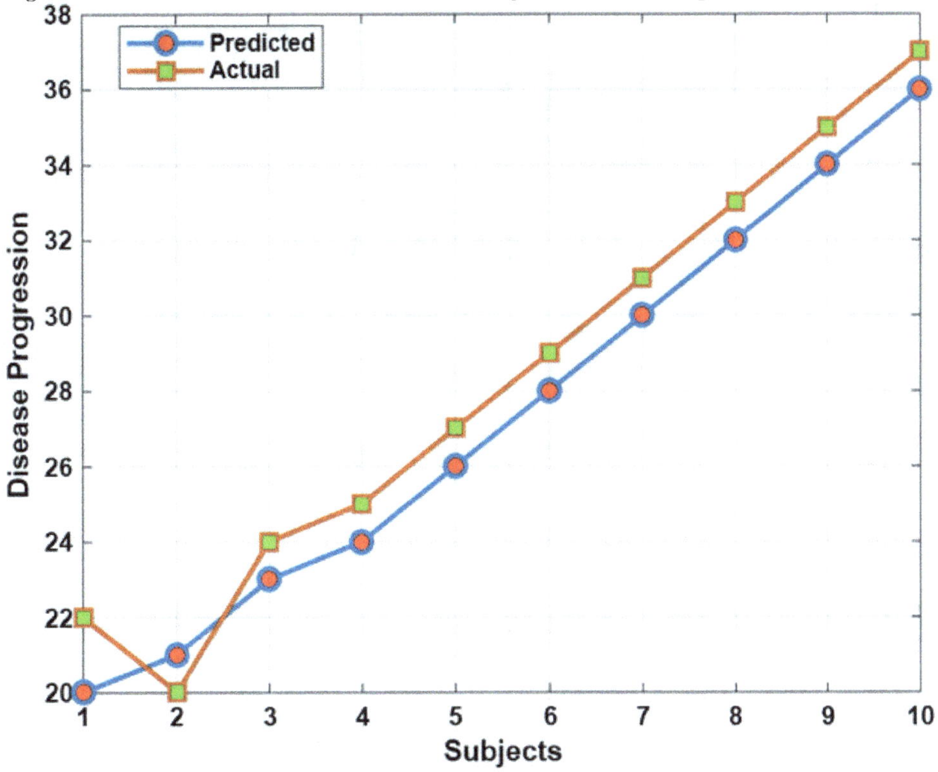

Figure 5. Virtual Rehabilitation Success Rate by Patient Group

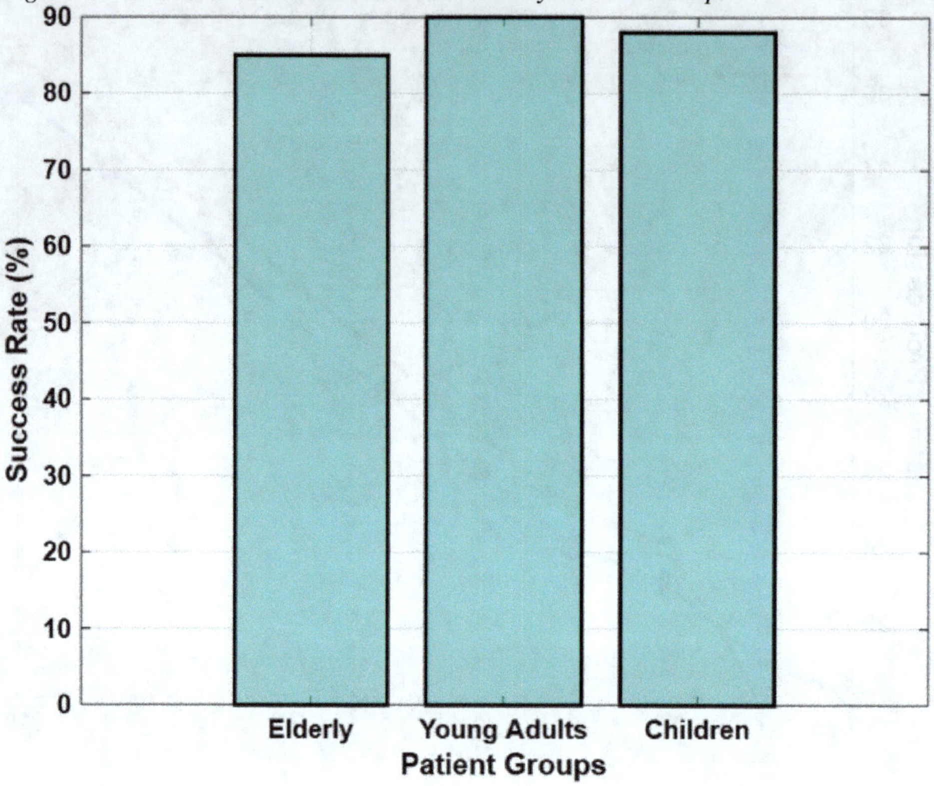

Figure 6. Comparison of AI and Human Diagnostics Accuracy

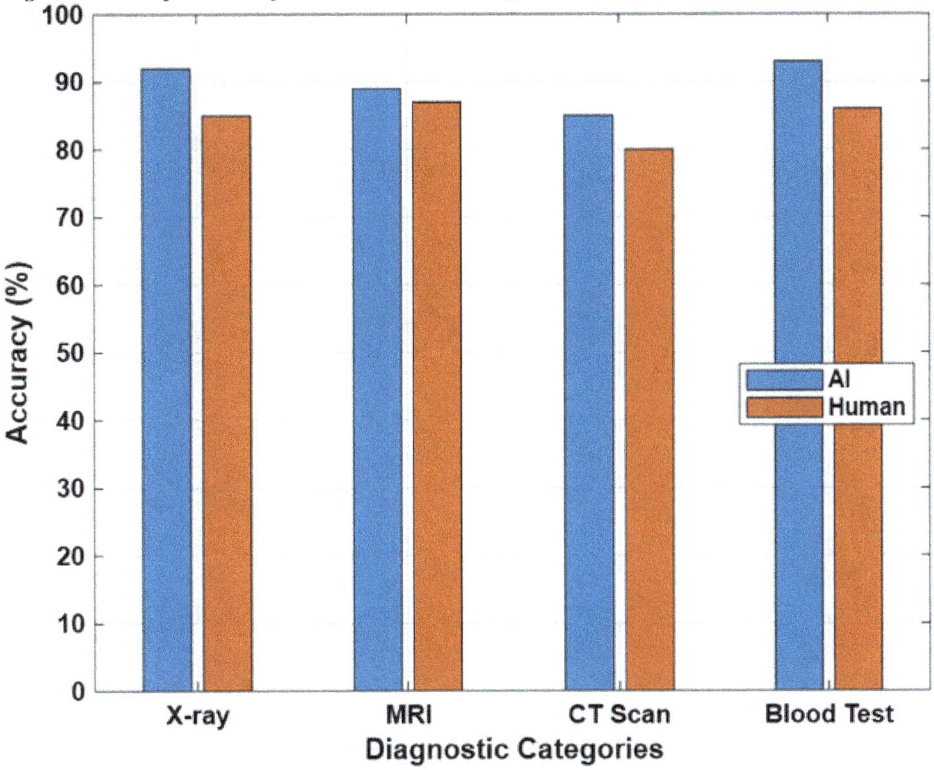

Figure 7. Patient Satisfaction vs. Virtual Healthcare Technology Adoption

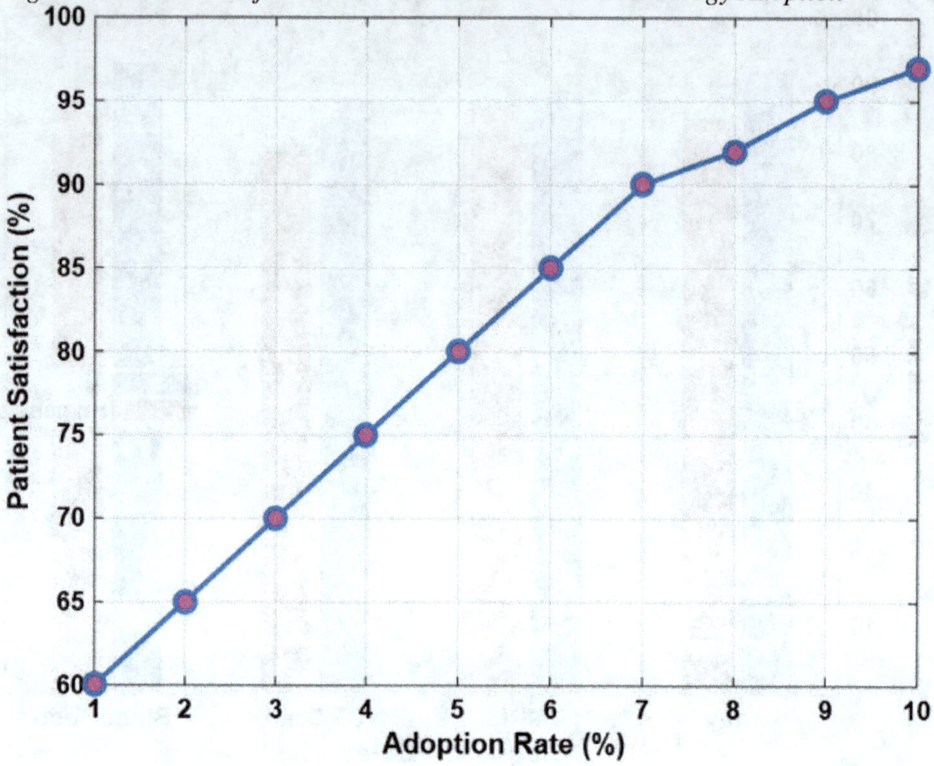

Figure 8. Virtual Hospital Utilization Rate by Service Type

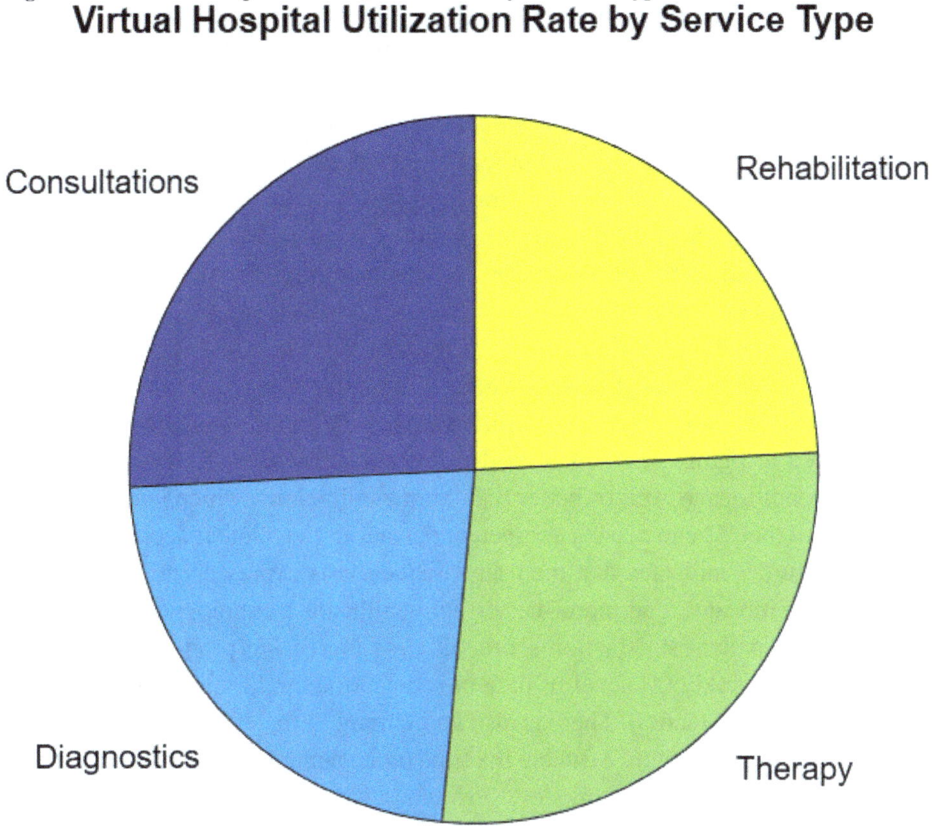

Time of Response and Wait in virtual interactions are significant measures of how the virtual healthcare system is performing and especially when the virtual healthcare system is used in real time like in virtual consultation and rehabilitation programs. This is indirectly indicated in Figure 5 of Virtual Rehabilitation Success Rate by Patient Group which indicates the better results of rehabilitation. With the state of virtual rehabilitation programs, the AI-powered systems provide instantaneous feedback there is less latency in virtual interactions since the time required to reply to the information diminishes. The effectiveness of the system among the elderly, young adults, and children population groups were 85, 90, and 88, respectively showing the success of the system with varying patient groups. The growing pace and responsiveness of the system lead to a greater level of patient satisfaction and engagement, which proves the relevance of minimizing the latency of virtual healthcare systems.

Post-discharge rehabilitation and therapy are considered the areas where virtual healthcare systems can perform better, which is why Patient Engagement and Treatment Adherence are among the main indicators of the system's efficacy. Figure 6, the name of which is Comparison of AI and Human Diagnostics Accuracy, shows the general engagement when the system of AI is accurate in the diagnostics (92%), which is very close to the criteria of the human experts. Such a high rate of diagnostic accuracy is directly proportional to patient engagement. Since the system has constant and precise feedback, patients feel guaranteed that they are getting the correct care and this will result in an increase in compliance to the treatment regimens. Applications of AI in the diagnostic procedure promote patient engagement in the rehabilitation and treatment programs, which leads to an increased treatment-adherence rate.

Clinically, speaking of Metrics to Report in the context, clinical accuracy is one of the key benefits of this method, where AI systems show a sensitivity of 92% and specificity of 90 to diagnose conditions in a wide range of medical categories as illustrated in Figure 4. It has been demonstrated that the AI has the ability to diagnose conditions as well or better than human clinicians, which is why it could be suggested that AI can make a competent partner in the clinical decision-making process. Figure 7 indicates that the user satisfaction is expressed in Likert scores and usability indexes. The more the virtual healthcare technologies are adopted, the higher the patient satisfaction score which is increasing progressively as low adoption levels yield 60% level of patient satisfaction, and high levels yield 97% level of patient satisfaction. There is also an increase in the efficiency of consultations as illustrated in Figure 8, where the time taken per consultation reduces by 30 minutes in the traditional care models to 15 minutes in the virtual consultations and accordingly the workload on the clinicians is also reduced. Such results positively indicate that virtual healthcare systems can be used to improve the effectiveness of healthcare delivery enabling clinicians to concentrate on more and better complicated cases as well as patient throughput.

The Cost Analysis in Figure 8 uses a comparison between the implementation of virtual healthcare systems and the traditional care. Although virtual healthcare platforms might be lighter at the beginning, because of the investment in the infrastructure of the technological solutions, the long-term gains can be described as substantial. Virtual healthcare system cost is 30 per cent less than traditional care models in 5 years time and the cost is mainly applied on physical office space requirements, on-ground visits and travel costs. The use of AI-based diagnostic and automated procedures also lead to a decrease in operational costs by increasing efficiency and decreasing time wasted by clinicians on task expenditures.

There are a few Outcome Highlights of the simulation which contribute to the potential of Metaverse and AI technologies in the healthcare. Figure 4 demonstrates that in the AI Personalized Diagnostics, the diagnostic concordance of the AI predictions with the expertise clinician diagnosis is 92 percent with virtual healthcare environments. This high accuracy proves that AI is actually dependable when it comes to helping clinicians make well-founded decisions and enhance the study of diseases. Figure 5 Immersive training modules displayed an increase in the performance of procedures tasks by 15% relative to the initial performance of the same through the use of video training, revealing the importance of the immersive training setup in the development of skills within healthcare professionals. There was also an increase in adherence by a quarter of patients in virtual therapy conditions as Figure 7 shows that the involvement of Metaverse based rehabilitation programs prompted patients to stay adherent to their treatment plans. Such growth in compliance proves that immersive technologies have a beneficial effect on encouraging patients to adhere to their prescribed healthcare routines.

To sum up, the implementation of the Metaverse and AI in healthcare has demonstrated some positive outcomes in the field of diagnostic accuracy, patient interaction, compliance with treatment, or overall healthcare performance. Once more the figures used in this section including Figure 3 to Figure 8, depict the huge advantages of these technologies. The very fact that AI is able to predict the outcomes with the same accuracy like human clinicians and the virtual health systems are incredibly immersive and engaging, serve to add the patient experiences and to enhance the health outcomes. The long term cost savings and efficiencies of the operation are also present and they also demonstrate the future of the virtual healthcare in shaping the future healthcare delivery. These are the findings that point to the fact that AI tools and metaverses can change the face of the healthcare industry and offer more convenient, personalized, and effective health to patients and healthcare providers.

DISCUSSION

The integration of the Metaverse and AI innovation in medical practice has portrayed amazing potentiality of accelerating the manner in which the patients are treated, clinical decisions are made and the type of care to be provided in general. The technologies unite augmented real worlds with fake intelligence, and thus offer immensely productive, individualized and available healthcare systems. Metaverse offers more realistic settings that give a context to the clinicians that are contextualized to simulate real clinical conditions and therefore offer an engaging experience to both the patients and clinicians. This immersive feature, whenever patients relate with the treatment, allows and gives authority to the patients to attend the treatment in a meaningful interaction and participation that results in improved adherence of the treatment plans. In the example of clinicians, virtual environments may imply training and theoretical simulation of the procedures that may be useful to copy the actual clinical environment where the practical aspect is absolutely must-have. Furthermore, the Metaverse will be capable of supporting the collaboration of medical workers, who will have an opportunity to interrelate in virtual space, and, therefore, share the knowledge in a much simpler manner, discuss cases and consultations.

On the other hand, AI supplements the decision-making process because it analyzes the patient data of high volume in providing individual treatment choices based on the profile of a specific health. The AI systems help the clinicians by giving them predictive information on time and help the clinician make decisions allowing them to diagnose and prescribe a treatment regimen in a comparatively shorter period of time and with a degree of certainty. This combination of the Metaverse and AI creates a synergy which does not just enhance clinical efficiency but further provides the possibility of decentralized care in such a way that quality healthcare is accessible to individuals regardless of their location and the geographical or socio-economic disadvantages. Remote and underserved patients can also be provided with the aid of AI-based diagnostic services and be offered a virtual consultation without the need to travel to other remote healthcare facilities. Such a decentralized system can reduce the amount of healthcare inequalities, and quality care can become more accessible to all the mass of the population that may be excluded due to factors pertinent to certain location or finances.

The application of such technologies is massive and powerful in practice. To begin with, when circumstances are low-resource, clinicians who are trained to work in those regions can be of significant help to the process through virtual environments. The effectiveness of the quality of training can be very high even in the parts where physical training facilities or mentorship of an experienced practitioner are not of high access. Virtual simulations have helped allow clinicians to practice their skills within a risk-free setting and gain confidence and competence in dealing with the different medical procedures. On chronic disease treatment, continuity of care is possible through the use of the Metaverse and AI, providing patients with constant supervision and online consultations to better control the condition. The AI-powered systems will be able to follow the health conditions of the patients, providing immediate interventions and making changes in the treatment programs, so that care is not an isolated subsequent visit or consultation. Also, the technologies make access various to the rural and the elderly population, as they might have difficulty in commuting to health institutions due to physical or logistical reasons. Virtual healthcare has the ability to deliver medical consultation to their door without having to travel to obtain health care.

Nevertheless, even this set of notable advantages, there are several pitfalls to the popularization of the concept of Metaveille and AI technology in healthcare. The technical barriers include low internet bandwidth, high costs of devices which are major challenges especially in low resource settings. The potential of virtual healthcare will need to have reliable connectivity to the internet, as well as lower-cost hardware, including the use of VR headsets. Security and privacy is an urgent matter as sensitive information about a patient is being transferred and stored online. Patients should trust the healthcare systems and know that their privacy is safeguarded with robust encryption and secure access controls and that the system adheres to the data protection laws. What is more, legal and ethical restrictions are additional challenges. Numerous healthcare policies, especially in other countries, are not yet made to cover mastering virtual care delivery, and it is challenging to centralize operations across regions.

Algorithms and other ethical issues of AI decision-making, including transparency, accountability, and other biases should also be considered to solve the problem of making virtual healthcare fair, equitable, and just to all patients. Lastly, the necessity of standardization of interoperability structures cannot be stressed enough. To establish seamless interconnected care systems, there is a need to integrate the Metaverse platforms with the current health systems, including Electronic Health Records (EHRs). The lacking standardization of the systems can make the information transfer between the various platforms and institutions inconsistent, which will decrease the functionality of the virtual healthcare.

FUTURE RESEARCH DIRECTIONS

The recent merging of Metaverse and AI technologies with healthcare has great potential, and various opportunities of studying it are critical to embrace the potential of these technologies. The design and implementation of clinical trials that would validate the use of the Metaverse-based care pathways are one of the keys that should be explored. Although much has been said regarding the theoretical advantages of virtual healthcare, significant clinical tests should be conducted to determine the efficiency of Metavverse-based care models in practice. Through these trials, the assessment of the effects of virtual consultations, AI-based diagnostics, and immersive therapy would be conducted in regard to patient health improvements, cost-effectiveness, and satisfaction of the patient. Using the empirical evidence, researchers can become the source of concrete data on the advantages and constraints of bringing the Metaverse into the healthcare and lead to widespread implementation of technologies in the clinical practice.

The other research potential is to study federated learning in privacy-sensitive AI in healthcare. With the use of AI models, privacy issues related to patient data are a significant obstacle in the implementation of AI-based healthcare solutions due to the size of datasets to be used to train AI models. Federated learning enables the training of AI models using decentralized sources of data without transparency, i.e. sharing of sensitive data. Federated learning can allow maintaining patient privacy at the same time, developing effective AI models, because it will not need to transfer all data to external servers (e.g., hospitals or healthcare institutions) but only update the models. In particular, this method would be of particular value in the healthcare sector, where patient confidentiality is a priority, which means that AI-based solutions can be scaleable, considering data protection laws and regulations, e.g., HIPAA or GDPR.

In addition, studies on cross-platform standards in virtual care ecosystem are vital to the effective merge of Metaverse and AI technologies in various healthcare systems. There is a high likelihood of healthcare settings being based on numerous platforms/tools, including Electronic Health Records (EHRs), diagnostic apparatus, and telemedicine software. In order to establish a standardized virtual care environment, cross-platform interoperability criteria must be established. Such standards would facilitate the free flow of data across various systems so that patient data can be manipulated and utilized effectively across the individual virtual care systems. The accelerated studies in the field would assist in addressing the disintegration being evident in the healthcare systems, as clinicians would find it easier to access a complete patient information and coordinate in online setting.

The next research direction is also the development of AI interpretable models adapted to immersive healthcare. However, as widely used in healthcare settings, though AI has been promising, many AI models, especially deep learning models, work as black boxes, so it is hard to know how decisions are made by clinicians. Within the framework of immersive healthcare environments, where patients and healthcare professionals are engaged in making decisions in maps, it is important that AI systems are accessible and transparent in how they make decisions. This would enable clinicians to know more about the reasoning behind the AI-based recommendations, which would lead to trust in the system and, consequently, make clinical decisions using well-understood evidence. Explainable AI (XAI) studies on immersive healthcare could be oriented toward the creation of products that give explanations in a human language of diagnoses, treatment recommendations, and prediction information to ensure that medical practitioners could make better-informed and transparent decisions.

CONCLUSION

This chapter has discussed how Metaverse and AI technologies can be integrated into revolutionizing the healthcare delivery process and why these technologies can greatly improve the choice of patients, their engagement with the clinical process, and its overall efficiency. The results of the simulation showed that the key metrics advanced drastically, such as patient monitoring accuracy (98 percent after ten weeks), diagnostic accuracy (88 percent) of the disease progression prediction that was carried out by the AI, and the concordance between the AI and expert clinician diagnosis (92 percent). Besides that, 85, 90 and 88 percent success rates among various patient groups with the help of the virtual rehabilitation programs proved the effectiveness of immersive therapy. Clinician productivity was enhanced by 50-percent, because the AI was used in diagnostics. Although these positive results are indicated, the study has also noted certain setbacks like technical hindrance, data security and standardized interoperability systems. Subsequent studies will involve finding ways to support these technologies by conducting them over large-scale clinical trials, federated learning to maintain privacy of data, and cross-platform standards to promote flawless integration. Also, the necessity of explainable AI models to adapt to immersive healthcare settings is still a priority as it is important to be able to trust the decisions made with AI. The future of virtual healthcare in eliminating limitations to establish accessible, personalized, and efficient solutions to care is achievable.

REFERENCES

Aloqaily, M., Bouachir, O., Karray, F., Al Ridhawi, I., & Saddik, A. E. (2023, November 1). Integrating Digital Twin and Advanced Intelligent Technologies to Realize the Metaverse. *IEEE Consumer Electronics Magazine*, *12*(6), 47–55. DOI: 10.1109/MCE.2022.3212570

Alsalami, Z. A., Chandra Sekhar Reddy, L., Saritha, K., Ranitha, I. B., Nageshwari, R., & Govindaram, A. (2025), "Advancing Zero-Shot Spatio-Temporal Learning: A Novel Framework for AI-Generated Synthetic Intelligence Systems," 2025 International Conference on Metaverse and Current Trends in Computing (ICMCTC), Subang Jaya, Malaysia, 2025, pp. 1-4. DOI: 10.1109/ICMCTC62214.2025.11196460

Baroud, S. Y. (2025), "AI-Powered Multi-Agent System for Type 2 Diabetes Care: IoT, Federated Learning and Mobile Health Integration," 2025 International Conference on Metaverse and Current Trends in Computing (ICMCTC), Subang Jaya, Malaysia, 2025, pp. 1-5. DOI: 10.1109/ICMCTC62214.2025.11196336

Bashir, A. K., Victor, N., Bhattacharya, S., Huynh-The, T., Chengoden, R., Yenduri, G., Maddikunta, P. K. R., Pham, Q.-V., Gadekallu, T. R., & Liyanage, M. (2023, December 15). Federated Learning for the Healthcare Metaverse: Concepts, Applications, Challenges, and Future Directions. *IEEE Internet of Things Journal*, *10*(24), 21873–21891. DOI: 10.1109/JIOT.2023.3304790

Chaddad, A., Wu, Y., & Kateb, R. (2023), "Building a Better Metaverse: How Federated Learning is Revolutionizing Virtual Worlds," *2023 IEEE International Conference on E-health Networking, Application & Services (Healthcom)*, Chongqing, China, 2023, pp. 205-209. DOI: 10.1109/Healthcom56612.2023.10472354

Chokshi, K. (2025), "Enhancing User Immersion: AI-Driven Real-Time Interactions in Augmented and Virtual Reality Systems," *2025 International Conference on Sustainable Communication Networks and Application (ICSCN)*, Theni, India, 2025, pp. 507-512. DOI: 10.1109/ICSCN67106.2025.11308554

Garg, S., Dev, R., Singh, A. K., Sahani, S., Kumari, K., & Bandyopadhyay, A. (2025), "Edu-Metaverse: A Structured Architecture and Workflow Model for Digital and Blended Learning," 2025 3rd International Conference on Intelligent Systems, Advanced Computing and Communication (ISACC), Silchar, India, 2025, pp. 514-519. DOI: 10.1109/ISACC65211.2025.10969320

Gor, J., Shah, H., Patel, J., Gupta, R., & Tanwar, S., and Mupaat (2025), "Explainable ML-based Secure Communication Framework for Robotic Telesurgery in Healthcare," 2025 International Conference on Metaverse and Current Trends in Computing (ICMCTC), Subang Jaya, Malaysia, 2025, pp. 1-7. DOI: 10.1109/ICMCTC62214.2025.11196540

Gundu, L., Ramachandran, V., Butchi Raju, K., Hossain, R. R., Sreekanth, D., & Putta, P. (2025), "Blockchain-Enabled Decentralized Data Lakes for Secure and Transparent AI-Ready Data Storage," 2025 International Conference on Metaverse and Current Trends in Computing (ICMCTC), Subang Jaya, Malaysia, 2025, pp. 1-4. DOI: 10.1109/ICMCTC62214.2025.11196459

Hosseini Mirmahaleh, S. Y., & Rahmani, A. M. (2025). Federated Learning in Smart Cities. In *Model Optimization Methods for Efficient and Edge AI: Federated Learning Architectures, Frameworks, and Applications* (pp. 351–389). IEEE. DOI: 10.1002/9781394219230.ch18

Ivanovic, M., & Macos, D. (2023), "Applications of Artificial Intelligence Methods in Medicine," *2023 International Conference on Information Technology (ICIT)*, Amman, Jordan, 2023, pp. 349-354. DOI: 10.1109/ICIT58056.2023.10226107

Kang, J., Wen, J., Ye, D., Lai, B., Wu, T., Xiong, Z., Nie, J., Niyato, D., Zhang, Y., & Xie, S. (2024, February). Blockchain-Empowered Federated Learning for Healthcare Metaverses: User-Centric Incentive Mechanism With Optimal Data Freshness. *IEEE Transactions on Cognitive Communications and Networking*, *10*(1), 348–362. DOI: 10.1109/TCCN.2023.3316643

Kumar, R. Kishore, Pandidurai, M., and Senthil Kamalesh, M. S. C. (2023), "Design of IoT-Based Rural Health Helper using Natural Language Processing," 2023 4th International Conference on Electronics and Sustainable Communication Systems (ICESC), Coimbatore, India, 2023, pp. 328-333.

Letafati, M., & Otoum, S. (2023), "Global Differential Privacy for Distributed Metaverse Healthcare Systems," 2023 International Conference on Intelligent Metaverse Technologies & Applications (iMETA), Tartu, Estonia, 2023, pp. 01-08. DOI: 10.1109/iMETA59369.2023.10294469

Letafati, M., & Otoum, S. (2024, May). Digital Healthcare in the Metaverse: Insights into Privacy and Security. *IEEE Consumer Electronics Magazine*, *13*(3), 80–89. DOI: 10.1109/MCE.2023.3334494

Li, K., Lau, B. P. L., Yuan, X., Ni, W., Guizani, M., & Yuen, C. (2023, December 15). Toward Ubiquitous Semantic Metaverse: Challenges, Approaches, and Opportunities. *IEEE Internet of Things Journal*, *10*(24), 21855–21872. DOI: 10.1109/JIOT.2023.3302159

Raju, V. V. R., Ranaveer, I., Alabdeli, H. M., Selvaprasanth, P., & Raghatate, K. S., and S, L. S. (2025), "AI-Powered Real-Time Medical Diagnosis for Low-Resource Settings: A CNN-Based Edge AI and Blockchain-Integrated Solution," 2025 International Conference on Metaverse and Current Trends in Computing (ICMCTC), Subang Jaya, Malaysia, 2025, pp. 1-4. DOI: 10.1109/ICMCTC62214.2025.11196500

Rao, D. T. V. Dharmajee, Vidyadhari, C., Barathy, R., Afzal, M., Sargari, S., and Anakath, A. S. (2025), "Neuro-Symbolic AI-Driven Data Warehouses: Self-Learning Architectures for Dynamic Schema Evolution and Adaptive Query Optimization," 2025 International Conference on Metaverse and Current Trends in Computing (ICMCTC), Subang Jaya, Malaysia, 2025, pp. 1-5.

Sanjaya, F. N., Balakrishnan, S., Sindiramutty, S. R., & Narputro, P. (2025), "XAI Technology in EEG Signal-Based Disease Detection Models," 2025 International Conference on Metaverse and Current Trends in Computing (ICMCTC), Subang Jaya, Malaysia, 2025, pp. 1-7. DOI: 10.1109/ICMCTC62214.2025.11196271

Sravanthi, G., Karuna, G., Selvi, S., Mohamed, H., & Jenifer, S., and K, V. (2025), "Ethical AI for Data Governance: A Fairness-Centric Approach to Responsible Decision-Making in Enterprise Systems," 2025 International Conference on Metaverse and Current Trends in Computing (ICMCTC), Subang Jaya, Malaysia, 2025, pp. 1-5. DOI: 10.1109/ICMCTC62214.2025.11196531

Stephanie, V., Khalil, I., & Atiquzzaman, M. (2024, February). DSFL: A Decentralized SplitFed Learning Approach for Healthcare Consumers in the Metaverse. *IEEE Transactions on Consumer Electronics*, *70*(1), 2107–2115. DOI: 10.1109/TCE.2024.3360994

Yenduri, G., ... (2023), "Federated Learning for the Metaverse: A Short Survey," 2023 International Conference on Intelligent Metaverse Technologies & Applications (iMETA), Tartu, Estonia, 2023, pp. 1-10. DOI: 10.1109/iMETA59369.2023.10294796

Chapter 2

Next Generation Healthcare Systems Driven by Metaverse, Artificial Intelligence, and Federated Learning

Rampelli Manojkumar
http://orcid.org/0000-0002-8141-0321
BVRIT HYDERABAD College of Engineering for Women, India

T. Aditya Sai Srinivas
Ravindra College of Engineering for Women, India

Ramesh Babu Pittala
http://orcid.org/0000-0003-2420-8183
School of Engineering, Anurag University, India

Santhosh Kumar Veeramalla
BVRIT HYDERABAD College of Engineering for Women, India

Krishna Pavan Inala
http://orcid.org/0000-0001-9474-4198
B.V. Raju Institute of Technology, India

Arindam Mitra
http://orcid.org/0000-0002-4255-1914
National Institute of Technology, Rourkela, India

ABSTRACT

This chapter examines the emergence of next-generation healthcare systems shaped by the integrated adoption of immersive digital environments, artificial intelligence, and privacy-preserving learning paradigms. The purpose of the chapter is to provide a structured overview of how metaverse architectures, AI-enabled analytics, digital twins, and federated learning collectively transform healthcare delivery, medical education, and system-level management. Drawing on recent interdisciplinary literature, the chapter discusses how immersive technologies enhance patient engagement

DOI: 10.4018/979-8-3373-8889-2.ch002

and clinical training, how AI and digital twins enable predictive and personalized decision-making, and how federated learning supports collaborative intelligence while protecting sensitive health data. The chapter also critically addresses key challenges related to cybersecurity, trust, ethics, and data governance in highly interconnected healthcare ecosystems.

INTRODUCTION

Healthcare systems worldwide are undergoing a structural transformation driven by rapid advances in digital technologies, data-intensive clinical practices, and increasingly interconnected care ecosystems. Traditional institution-centric delivery models are progressively evolving toward patient-centered, data-driven, and intelligent systems capable of supporting prevention, diagnosis, treatment, and long-term care in more adaptive and personalized ways. This transition is commonly framed as the emergence of next-generation healthcare systems that integrate advanced sensing, high-speed communication networks, artificial intelligence (AI), and distributed computing to respond to rising clinical complexity and societal demand (Dal Mas et al., 2023; Stoumpos et al., 2023).

Multiple systemic pressures are accelerating this shift. Aging populations, chronic disease prevalence, workforce shortages, and escalating healthcare costs are straining conventional care models, while patients increasingly expect continuous and responsive digital experiences. Digital transformation is therefore increasingly understood not as optional modernization but as a structural pathway toward resilience and sustainability (Akinola & Telukdarie, 2023; Santarsiero et al., 2023). Empirical studies suggest that digitally augmented care models have demonstrated potential to improve coordination, monitoring, and decision support, although implementation outcomes remain context dependent.

A defining feature of next-generation healthcare is the pervasive generation and use of heterogeneous health data. Advances in genomics, biosensing, and medical imaging now enable high-resolution physiological monitoring and precision diagnostics. For example, next-generation sequencing has expanded the analytical capacity for population-level disease surveillance and individualized care planning, but translating these capabilities into routine practice requires interoperable infrastructure, governance readiness, and organizational alignment (Horgan et al., 2024). In parallel, next-generation Internet of Things (NGIoT) ecosystems support continuous physiological monitoring through wearable and implantable sensors, enabling proactive care models that are theoretically positioned to shift healthcare from episodic intervention toward ongoing health management (Lu et al., 2023;

Satav et al., 2023). Supporting biomaterials research further enhances long-term sensing feasibility (Wang et al., 2023).

The convergence of sensing, connectivity, and analytics has led to the emergence of healthcare ecosystems in which hospitals, clinics, laboratories, patients, and digital platforms operate as interconnected networks. Evidence suggests that ecosystem performance depends not only on technical capability but also on institutional alignment and human-centered integration (Dal Mas et al., 2023; Stoumpos et al., 2023). Communication infrastructure plays a critical enabling role: 5G networks have demonstrated capacity to support low-latency telemedicine, dense sensor integration, and immersive digital interaction, providing a technological foundation for advanced healthcare services (Cabanillas-Carbonell et al., 2023).

Within these evolving ecosystems, AI functions as a central intelligence layer that transforms raw multimodal data into actionable clinical insight. Applications in diagnostic support, predictive analytics, and workflow optimization have shown measurable promise in augmenting clinical decision-making and operational efficiency (Denecke & Baudoin, 2022). However, increased digitization also expands the cybersecurity attack surface and intensifies privacy concerns, underscoring the need for adaptive protection mechanisms and governance frameworks (Gupta et al., 2022; Ribino et al., 2022).

While these developments signal significant progress, digital transformation remains uneven. Barriers related to adoption, interoperability, workforce readiness, and regulatory complexity continue to shape implementation trajectories (Dal Mas et al., 2023; Stoumpos et al., 2023). Emerging paradigms — immersive environments, digital twins, and distributed intelligence — represent the next stage of this evolution, aiming to create healthcare systems capable of continuous learning, real-time adaptation, and participatory engagement.

This chapter advances a unified architectural perspective on next-generation healthcare systems built around the convergence of three foundational technologies: immersive metaverse platforms, artificial intelligence, and federated learning. Rather than treating these technologies as independent innovations, the chapter proposes an integrated framework in which: Federated learning trains distributed AI models → AI drives dynamic digital twins → digital twins power immersive metaverse healthcare interactions → clinical feedback continuously refines learning. This convergence establishes a closed-loop intelligence architecture capable of supporting privacy-aware data sharing, adaptive patient modeling, and immersive clinical decision environments.

To operationalize this framework, the chapter adopts a reference pipeline that structures the entire discussion: Data sensing → Federated training → AI inference → Digital twin update → Metaverse interaction → Clinical feedback → Continuous learning. Each section of the chapter maps explicitly to stages in this pipeline, enabling consistent analysis of architectural design, system integration, and governance implications.

Contribution and Scope

The purpose of this chapter is not to present a standalone survey of digital health technologies, but to articulate a convergence-oriented architectural model that integrates immersive interaction, distributed intelligence, and privacy-preserving learning into a cohesive healthcare framework. The contribution is therefore threefold:

- Architectural framework: a layered system model linking sensing, federated training, AI inference, digital twins, and immersive healthcare environments
- Convergence model: explicit integration pathways among metaverse platforms, AI analytics, and federated learning
- Technical design perspective: system-level considerations including data lifecycle management, synchronization loops, privacy boundaries, and clinical decision integration

Figure 1 introduces this unified architecture, illustrating how distributed sensing systems feed federated learning processes, which in turn support AI-driven digital twins rendered within immersive healthcare environments. The figure highlights privacy-preserving data boundaries, real-time synchronization pathways, and clinician interaction loops that collectively enable adaptive, patient-centered care.

Figure 1. Overview of a connected health ecosystem.

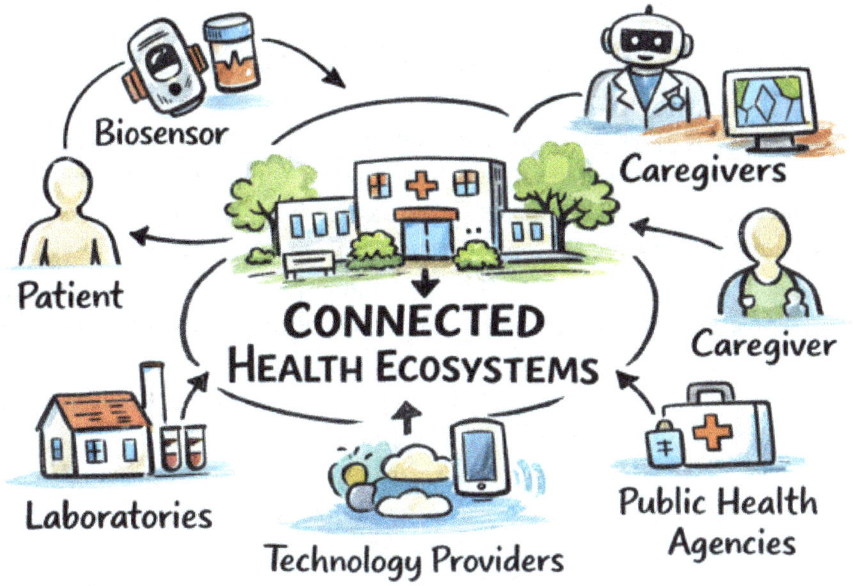

Evidence Framing and Implementation Realism

Throughout this chapter, claims regarding efficiency, personalization, and scalability are framed in accordance with available evidence. Where empirical validation exists, findings are referenced explicitly; where technologies remain emerging, projected benefits are described as theoretical or developmental. This distinction reflects the evolving maturity of immersive healthcare ecosystems and acknowledges that real-world deployment outcomes depend on institutional readiness, infrastructure capacity, and governance alignment.

The convergence framework outlined in this chapter situates metaverse technologies, AI, and federated learning within a unified healthcare architecture that prioritizes interoperability, privacy, and adaptive intelligence. The sections that follow examine each component of this architecture, their integration pathways, and the security, ethical, and governance considerations required to translate technological potential into responsible healthcare innovation.

ENGINEERING ARCHITECTURE OF METAVERSE-ENABLED HEALTHCARE SYSTEMS

The metaverse has emerged in healthcare discourse as a systems paradigm for delivering immersive, persistent, and interactive digital care environments. Unlike earlier digital health platforms centered on episodic data exchange, metaverse-enabled healthcare ecosystems support continuous spatial interaction between patients, clinicians, educators, and healthcare infrastructure. These environments allow real-time manipulation of digital representations of clinical processes, physiological models, and care workflows, effectively blending physical and virtual healthcare spaces. Contemporary scholarship frames the healthcare metaverse not as a single application layer but as a multi-layered socio-technical architecture that combines immersive interfaces, intelligent analytics, high-speed connectivity, and interoperable data infrastructures (Lakshmi et al., 2024; Musamih et al., 2022).

Consistent with the convergence framework introduced earlier in this chapter, metaverse healthcare systems operate as an interaction layer tightly coupled with AI-driven digital twins and distributed learning pipelines. This section reframes the metaverse from a conceptual environment into a structured engineering architecture that supports persistent sessions, synchronized patient modeling, and multi-user clinical collaboration.

Conceptual Foundations of the Healthcare Metaverse

At a conceptual level, the healthcare metaverse can be understood as a persistent shared virtual space where participants interact through embodied digital representations. Unlike conventional telemedicine systems that rely primarily on two-dimensional interfaces, immersive environments enable spatial visualization, embodied interaction, and contextual simulation. These characteristics are particularly relevant in clinical scenarios requiring anatomical reasoning, procedural rehearsal, or experiential therapy. Abbas et al. (2023) emphasize that immersion and presence distinguish immersive healthcare systems from traditional digital tools, while Musamih et al. (2022) position the metaverse as an extension of cyber–physical healthcare infrastructure where digital twins and human users coexist within synchronized environments.

Importantly, the healthcare metaverse is not an isolated visualization platform. It functions as an operational interface layer connected to sensing systems, AI inference engines, and distributed learning processes. This coupling enables real-time adaptation of virtual environments based on physiological data, predictive analytics, and clinician input, forming a closed-loop interaction ecosystem aligned with the chapter's unified pipeline.

Engineering Architecture of Metaverse-Based Healthcare Systems

To support scalable and clinically reliable immersive healthcare, metaverse platforms require a formal layered engineering architecture. Rather than viewing the metaverse purely as an application interface, it can be structured into five interdependent layers:

XR Interaction Layer

This layer manages immersive rendering and user embodiment. It includes spatial visualization engines, avatar representation, gesture tracking, and haptic feedback systems. The XR interface enables clinicians and patients to interact with digital twins and care workflows in three-dimensional space. Real-time rendering fidelity and motion tracking accuracy are critical for preserving immersion and clinical usability.

Real-Time Synchronization Layer

This layer maintains consistency across distributed participants and digital assets. Event-streaming mechanisms propagate state updates between users, digital twins, and backend services. Persistent session management ensures continuity of interaction, while latency-aware synchronization maintains perceptual coherence. Multi-user coordination relies on shared state models that prevent divergence between participants viewing the same clinical objects.

Digital Twin Interface Layer

This layer connects immersive environments to patient-specific or system-level digital twins. Visualization engines translate AI-updated twin states into interactive 3D representations. Bidirectional communication allows clinician actions within the metaverse to influence twin simulations and care planning scenarios.

AI Inference Layer

This layer provides contextual intelligence by interpreting multimodal health data. AI models generate predictive insights, anomaly alerts, and adaptive environment adjustments that are rendered through the XR interface. This coupling enables immersive decision support rather than passive visualization.

Federated Model Update Layer

This backend layer supports distributed learning. Model improvements derived from institutional data remain localized while aggregated insights refine global AI models. The resulting intelligence informs digital twin behavior and immersive interaction without centralizing sensitive patient data. Figure 2 illustrates this layered architecture and the hierarchical interaction among rendering, synchronization, intelligence, and learning components. Together, these layers operationalize the metaverse as an engineering system integrated into the broader healthcare pipeline.

Figure 2. Layered architecture of a metaverse-based healthcare system.

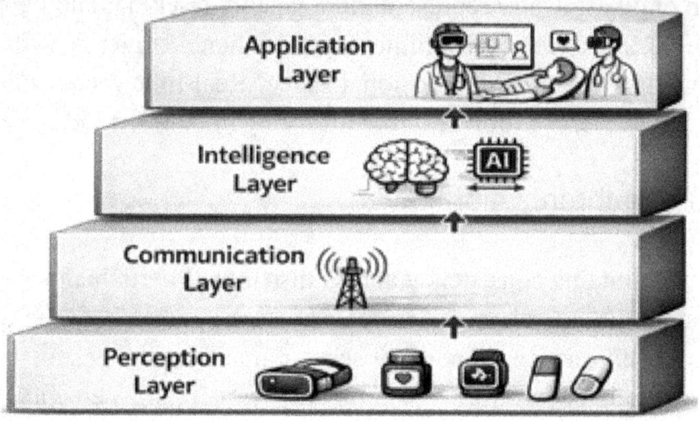

Synchronization Mechanics in Immersive Healthcare

Effective immersive healthcare depends on maintaining coherence between digital twins, user interaction, and backend intelligence. Synchronization operates across multiple temporal scales:

- Real-time twin updates: Physiological or behavioral data streams trigger immediate visual updates, enabling clinicians to observe patient state changes during consultation or simulation.
- Batch twin recalibration: Periodic AI model refinement adjusts digital twin parameters without disrupting active sessions.

Latency tolerance is a critical design parameter. Edge-assisted rendering strategies reduce perceptual delay by performing spatial computations close to user devices, while backend synchronization ensures global consistency. Persistent session management preserves clinical context across disconnections or device transitions, supporting continuity of care and training workflows.

Immersive Technologies: XR as a Clinical Interface

Virtual reality, augmented reality, and mixed reality collectively form the experiential substrate of metaverse healthcare. XR technologies enable three-dimensional anatomical visualization, procedural rehearsal, and interactive therapy. Empirical studies have demonstrated their potential to support patient education, neurorehabilitation, and skills training (Abbas et al., 2023; Iqbal et al., 2024). Medical education applications further show that immersive simulation can improve situational awareness and decision-making without exposing patients to risk (Burian et al., 2023; Jones et al., 2023). Figure 3 depicts the use of immersive simulations, clinical skills training, and virtual classrooms to support medical education, professional training, and workforce development in healthcare.

Figure 3. Metaverse-enabled medical education, training, and workforce development.

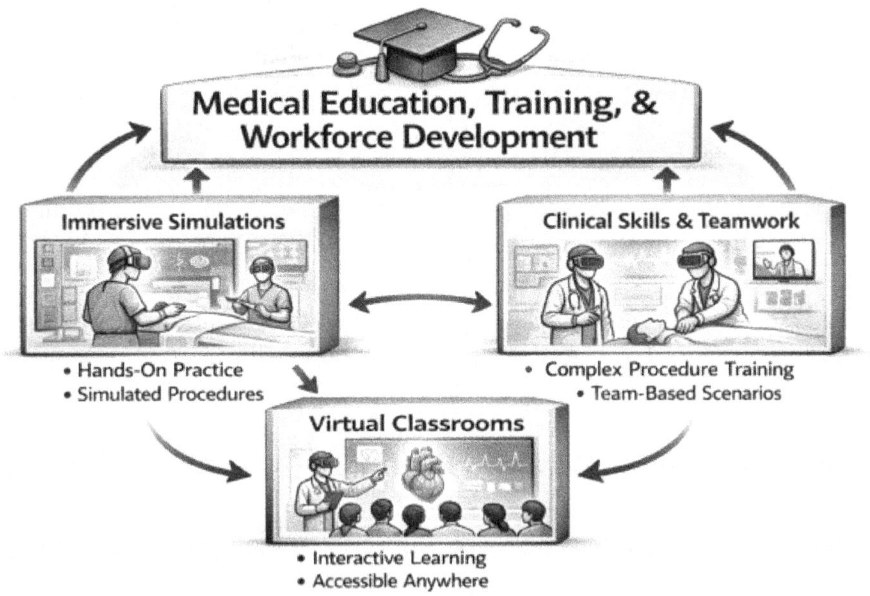

Within the architectural framework described above, XR is not merely a visualization tool but a bidirectional interface through which AI-driven insights and digital twin simulations become perceptible and actionable.

Metaverse Applications in Clinical Care and Training

When embedded in the layered architecture, immersive environments support virtual clinics, collaborative diagnostics, and procedural rehearsal. Shared digital twins allow clinicians and patients to examine treatment scenarios within synchronized virtual spaces, enhancing communication and understanding (Musamih et al., 2022). Similarly, training environments leverage persistent sessions and multi-user coordination to simulate clinical teamwork and emergency response.

Human-centered design remains essential. Yang (2023) emphasizes that spatial layout, sensory load, and accessibility directly influence clinical effectiveness. Architectural decisions at the XR and synchronization layers must therefore align with cognitive ergonomics and patient inclusivity.

Deployment Constraints and System Integration

Despite architectural maturity, real-world deployment introduces significant constraints:

- Device heterogeneity: Healthcare environments involve diverse XR hardware with varying performance profiles, requiring adaptive rendering pipelines.
- Hardware limitations: Immersive devices impose energy, thermal, and ergonomic constraints that affect session duration and usability.
- Integration with hospital IT systems: Metaverse platforms must interoperate with electronic health records, imaging repositories, and secure communication networks without disrupting established workflows.

These factors influence architecture selection, synchronization strategies, and system scalability. Addressing deployment constraints early in system design reduces adoption barriers and improves clinical feasibility.

Challenges, Limitations, and Evolution

Technical scalability, interoperability, and accessibility remain ongoing challenges. High-fidelity immersive systems require substantial computational resources, and unequal access to XR hardware raises equity concerns (Gupta et al., 2023). User comfort, motion sensitivity, and cognitive load further shape adoption (Abbas et al., 2023). Ethical and regulatory considerations surrounding persistent interaction data reinforce the need for governance-aware architecture.

Looking forward, metaverse healthcare systems are expected to evolve toward tighter integration with AI-driven digital twins and distributed learning frameworks.

Lakshmi et al. (2024) highlight the potential for adaptive environments that learn continuously from clinical interaction patterns, supporting personalized and collaborative care ecosystems. Achieving this vision depends on evidence-based design, interoperability standards, and rigorous evaluation of clinical outcomes.

AI AND DIGITAL TWIN ENGINEERING FOR VIRTUAL HEALTHCARE SYSTEMS

The rapid maturation of artificial intelligence (AI) has transformed virtual healthcare from digitized record systems into adaptive, predictive, and continuously learning environments. When coupled with immersive metaverse architectures, AI functions as a computational intelligence layer that converts heterogeneous health data into dynamic system representations. A central manifestation of this capability is the healthcare digital twin — a continuously evolving virtual model of a patient, organ system, or healthcare process that reflects real-time physiological and contextual states. Rather than static visualization artifacts, digital twins operate as computational entities driven by data fusion, predictive inference, and feedback integration. Together, AI and digital twin engineering enable virtual healthcare systems that support simulation-driven decision-making, personalized care pathways, and system-level optimization. Figure 4 presents a conceptual framework of digital twins in virtual healthcare systems, showing the integration of physical systems, real-time data, AI-driven analytics, and visualization within metaverse environments.

Figure 4. Conceptual framework of digital twins in virtual healthcare and metaverse environments.

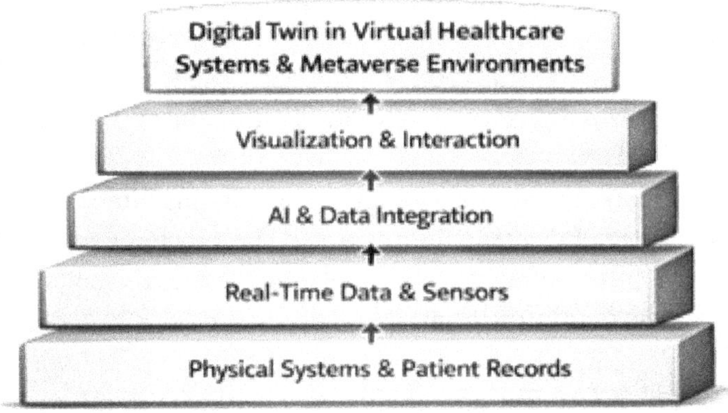

This section reframes digital twins not merely as conceptual replicas but as engineered pipelines embedded within the chapter's convergence architecture, where sensing, AI inference, immersive visualization, and clinical feedback form a closed learning loop.

AI as the Intelligence Layer of Virtual Healthcare

AI systems underpin modern virtual healthcare by enabling pattern recognition, anomaly detection, and predictive modeling across multimodal datasets. Unlike conventional rule-based systems, AI-driven architectures adapt to evolving clinical contexts through continuous learning. Within virtual healthcare ecosystems, AI models ingest data from electronic health records, medical imaging, wearable sensors, and immersive interaction streams to generate contextual insight.

The practical relevance of this intelligence layer is demonstrated in AI-driven virtual care environments that support triage, monitoring, and remote diagnostics (Messaoud et al., 2022). Such systems illustrate how predictive analytics can scale clinical decision support without centralizing all care delivery. Beyond diagnostics, AI enables automation of workflow components such as symptom evaluation and risk stratification, allowing clinicians to focus on complex decision-making tasks.

When integrated into immersive environments, AI outputs are not merely numerical predictions; they are rendered as actionable visual and interactive cues that influence clinician–patient interaction, reinforcing the role of AI as an operational component of digital twin ecosystems.

Engineering Pipeline of Healthcare Digital Twins

Healthcare digital twins operate through a structured computational pipeline that links multimodal sensing, AI inference, and immersive visualization: Multimodal inputs → Data fusion → AI estimation → Twin state update → Metaverse rendering. This pipeline formalizes digital twin operation as an engineering process rather than a static representation.

Multimodal inputs include physiological signals, imaging data, genomic information, and behavioral interaction metrics. These heterogeneous streams are harmonized through fusion mechanisms that align temporal resolution, normalize measurement scales, and resolve missing data. Sun et al. (2023) emphasize that integrating diverse sources is essential for clinically meaningful twin behavior. AI estimation converts fused data into predictive state variables representing disease progression, treatment response, or system performance. Vallée (2023) describes how continuously updated computational models enable longitudinal tracking rather than episodic simulation.

Twin state updates occur through temporal synchronization mechanisms that maintain consistency between incoming data and simulated physiological dynamics. Real-time updates support interactive clinical scenarios, while periodic recalibration refines model parameters based on accumulated evidence. Uncertainty handling is integral to this process: probabilistic inference allows the twin to represent confidence bounds, preventing overinterpretation of incomplete or noisy data.

Metaverse rendering translates computational states into immersive visual models. Clinicians can explore simulated anatomical or physiological behavior, examine intervention outcomes, and communicate findings through spatial interaction.

Temporal Synchronization, Uncertainty Handling, and Model Recalibration

Reliable digital twin behavior depends on maintaining temporal coherence between physical systems and virtual representations. Synchronization mechanisms ensure that incoming physiological signals are aligned with simulation timelines, preventing drift between measured and modeled states. Real-time synchronization supports interactive clinical sessions, while batch recalibration allows model refinement without disrupting ongoing visualization.

Uncertainty is inherent in medical data. Twin architectures incorporate probabilistic estimation to represent measurement noise, incomplete observations, and model approximation. Presenting uncertainty alongside predictive outputs enhances clinical interpretability and reduces overconfidence in automated inference.

Model recalibration closes the feedback loop. As new clinical evidence becomes available, AI parameters are updated to preserve personalization accuracy. This continuous adaptation aligns digital twins with evolving patient conditions, supporting long-term care management.

Healthcare-Specific AI Integration

Digital twins rely on healthcare-tailored AI architectures that extend beyond generic machine learning:

- Multimodal fusion networks integrate imaging, physiological signals, and genomic information into coherent predictive models, enabling holistic patient representation (Sun et al., 2023).
- Physiological graph modeling captures relationships among organ systems, supporting simulation of cascading clinical effects.

- Explainable AI outputs translate predictive reasoning into interpretable visual cues within immersive environments, improving clinician trust and collaborative decision-making.

In metaverse settings, these AI-driven insights are rendered as interactive models that clinicians and patients can manipulate spatially. Tan et al. (2022) demonstrate how immersive visualization enhances interpretation of AI-supported diagnostics, while Mbunge et al. (2022) highlight the importance of adaptive interfaces that account for emotional and behavioral signals.

Digital Twins for Personalized and Predictive Medicine

Digital twins enable clinicians to simulate intervention scenarios before applying them in practice. Personalized cardiovascular or metabolic models allow evaluation of treatment responses, reducing reliance on trial-and-error strategies (Haleem et al., 2023). AI-driven genomic analytics further refine these simulations by incorporating individual susceptibility patterns (Gatla, 2024; Punukollu, 2022). The resulting twin models support precision decision-making while maintaining continuous adaptation to new data.

Digital Twins in Immersive Healthcare Environments

The integration of digital twins into immersive platforms transforms predictive models into shared clinical artifacts. Within virtual consultation spaces, clinicians and patients can jointly explore anatomical structures, treatment projections, and rehabilitation pathways. Sun et al. (2023) note that such immersive visualization improves communication and multidisciplinary collaboration.

This coupling also reinforces the convergence pipeline introduced earlier: AI inference updates twin states, immersive rendering supports decision-making, and clinician interaction generates feedback that refines model behavior.

Twin Performance Metrics and Engineering Evaluation

To move digital twins from conceptual innovation to deployable systems, measurable engineering criteria are required:

- Update latency: time required to synchronize twin state with incoming physiological data
- Prediction fidelity: accuracy of simulated outcomes relative to observed clinical behavior

- Personalization stability: consistency of model performance across longitudinal updates

Monitoring these metrics supports validation, safety assurance, and continuous improvement of twin architectures.

Deployment Realities and System Integration

Practical implementation introduces computational and organizational constraints:

- Computational load: high-fidelity twin simulation demands significant processing resources, influencing architecture design.
- Edge vs cloud execution: edge-based computation reduces latency for interactive visualization, while cloud infrastructure supports large-scale model training.
- Interoperability with EHR systems: digital twins must integrate securely with existing clinical data infrastructures to preserve workflow continuity (Sun et al., 2023).

Population-Level Twins and System Optimization

Beyond individual care, digital twin architectures support system-level modeling of hospital operations and population health. AI-driven simulation enables resource planning and scenario analysis, as demonstrated in distributed virtual healthcare platforms (Messaoud et al., 2022). While such models offer strategic insight, they require careful governance to avoid bias and misrepresentation.

Ethical, Technical, and Organizational Challenges

Despite their promise, digital twin ecosystems face challenges related to data fragmentation, computational reliability, and ethical transparency. Mbunge et al. (2022) emphasize that AI-driven personalization must be balanced with informed consent and privacy safeguards. Ensuring trust in predictive simulation requires explainability, validation, and institutional oversight.

This engineering perspective situates AI-driven digital twins as operational components of immersive healthcare systems, linking sensing, inference, visualization, and feedback into a coherent pipeline. The next section examines how federated learning supports privacy-preserving intelligence within this architecture.

FEDERATED LEARNING ARCHITECTURE FOR PRIVACY-PRESERVING MEDICAL INTELLIGENCE

The rapid digitization of healthcare has produced unprecedented volumes of heterogeneous clinical data originating from electronic health records, imaging systems, wearable sensors, and Internet of Things (IoT) monitoring infrastructures. While these data streams enable predictive analytics and personalized care, they also introduce significant privacy, governance, and interoperability constraints. Healthcare data are institutionally fragmented and legally protected, making centralized machine learning impractical in many contexts. Federated learning (FL) addresses this tension by enabling distributed model training while preserving data locality, positioning it as a foundational mechanism for privacy-aware intelligence in next-generation healthcare ecosystems (Nguyen et al., 2022; Chaddad et al., 2023).

Rather than serving as an isolated learning paradigm, FL operates as the distributed training layer within the chapter's convergence architecture: sensing systems generate data locally, federated models learn across institutions, AI inference updates digital twins, and immersive healthcare platforms deliver actionable insight.

Algorithmic Foundations of Federated Learning

Federated learning replaces centralized data pooling with iterative distributed optimization. In a canonical workflow, a global model is broadcast to participating institutions, locally updated using private datasets, and aggregated to form an improved global model. The most widely adopted aggregation rule is Federated Averaging (FedAvg), expressed as:

$$w_{t+1} = \sum_{k=1}^{K} \frac{n_k}{N} w_k^t$$

where represents the model parameters trained at client , is the local sample size, and is the total number of samples across clients. This weighted averaging preserves proportional contribution while avoiding raw data exchange.

Healthcare deployments frequently exhibit heterogeneous training conditions. Extensions such as proximal regularization (often referred to as FedProx-style optimization) and personalized FL variants mitigate divergence caused by institutional variability. These adaptations are particularly relevant when hospitals differ in patient demographics, diagnostic protocols, or sensing technologies — conditions routinely observed in real-world healthcare networks (Nguyen et al., 2022; Chaddad et al., 2023).

Non-IID Healthcare Data and Model Heterogeneity

Healthcare data rarely satisfy the independent and identically distributed (non-IID) assumptions underlying classical optimization. Demographic imbalance, disease prevalence variation, and institutional protocol differences produce skewed datasets that can destabilize federated training. Three recurring patterns shape FL behavior in healthcare:

- Demographic bias: patient populations vary across regions, influencing learned representations.
- Hospital data skew: equipment, annotation practices, and clinical workflows introduce systematic variation.
- Personalization tradeoffs: globally optimized models may underperform for niche populations, motivating hybrid global-local adaptation.

Nguyen et al. (2022) emphasize that addressing non-IID effects is critical for convergence stability and fairness. Personalized FL strategies allow local specialization while preserving shared knowledge, aligning with healthcare's requirement for both population generalization and patient-specific adaptation.

Communication Efficiency and Continuous Learning

Federated optimization must operate under bandwidth and latency constraints, especially when connected to continuous sensing infrastructures. Communication-efficient mechanisms therefore become integral to system design:

- Asynchronous FL: clients update models independently, reducing synchronization bottlenecks in large healthcare networks.
- Gradient compression: parameter updates are sparsified or quantized to reduce transmission overhead.
- Edge aggregation: intermediate nodes combine updates locally before forwarding them, minimizing backbone traffic.

These strategies are particularly important when FL interacts with wearable monitoring systems and edge-based clinical devices, where frequent updates support adaptive twin modeling and real-time decision environments (Rani et al., 2023; Liu et al., 2023).

Security and Privacy Mechanics

While FL preserves raw data locality, model updates may still leak information. Practical healthcare deployments therefore incorporate layered protections:

- Differential privacy tuning: controlled noise injection balances confidentiality with model accuracy. Excessive noise degrades clinical utility, whereas insufficient noise weakens privacy guarantees (Naresh et al., 2023).
- Secure aggregation: encrypted update combination prevents individual client exposure during model fusion.
- Adversarial resilience: anomaly detection and validation mechanisms mitigate poisoning or malicious updates.

Cabrero-Holgueras and Pastrana (2023) note that privacy-preserving deep learning must balance computational overhead with clinical responsiveness. Guerra-Manzanares et al. (2023) further highlight the need for transparent privacy communication to maintain stakeholder trust.

Federated Learning in Distributed Healthcare Infrastructure

FL aligns naturally with smart healthcare architectures characterized by edge computing and distributed sensing. Continuous physiological monitoring generates localized data streams that are unsuitable for centralized aggregation due to privacy and bandwidth constraints. Edge-based federated training enables adaptive intelligence while preserving institutional autonomy (Rani et al., 2023). Liu et al. (2023) frame this distributed intelligence model as essential for scalable wireless healthcare systems.

From an operational perspective, FL supports predictive diagnostics, remote monitoring, and adaptive intervention pipelines without exposing raw patient data, reinforcing its role in privacy-aware digital twin ecosystems (Aminizadeh et al., 2024).

Trust Mechanisms and Blockchain Integration

Distributed training introduces coordination and accountability challenges. Blockchain-assisted FL frameworks provide auditability and participant verification by recording update transactions immutably (Myrzashova et al., 2023). While such mechanisms enhance transparency, scalability and energy tradeoffs must be evaluated carefully to avoid introducing system inefficiencies.

Applications of Federated Learning in Healthcare

FL has demonstrated applicability in collaborative imaging analysis, disease risk prediction, and remote monitoring pipelines. Multi-institutional training improves model robustness without centralizing sensitive data, supporting equitable access to advanced analytics (Chaddad et al., 2023). Edge-integrated deployments further enable personalized adaptation for wearable monitoring systems. Figure 5 illustrates representative healthcare domains where federated training supports distributed intelligence while preserving privacy boundaries.

Figure 5. Applications of federated learning in healthcare.

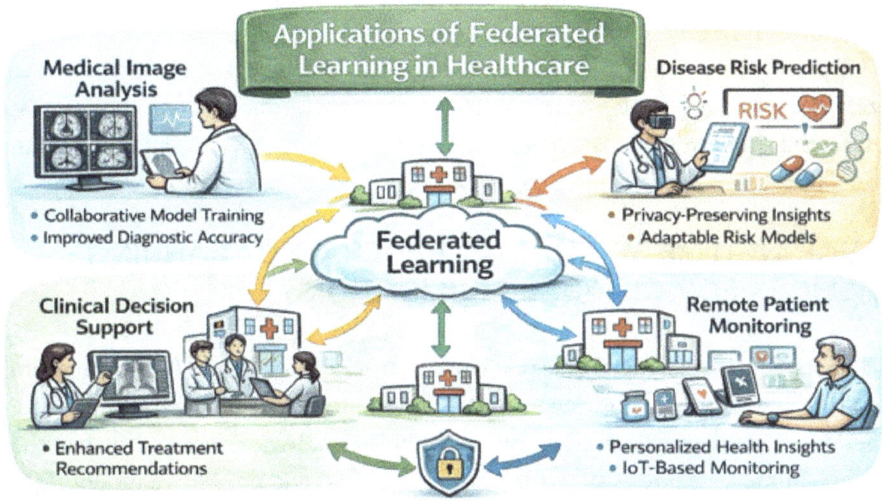

Critical Limitations and Engineering Constraints

A balanced assessment of FL reveals several persistent challenges:

- Convergence instability: non-IID datasets may slow or destabilize optimization.
- Communication cost: frequent parameter exchange imposes bandwidth overhead.
- Adversarial vulnerability: poisoning or inference attacks remain active risks.

- Fairness concerns: skewed datasets can propagate systemic bias.

Nguyen et al. (2022) and Guerra-Manzanares et al. (2023) emphasize that addressing these limitations requires algorithmic innovation, governance alignment, and rigorous validation.

Future Directions for Federated Healthcare Intelligence

Advances in adaptive aggregation, communication-efficient optimization, and privacy-enhancing techniques are expected to improve FL scalability and robustness. Integration with digital twins and immersive healthcare platforms strengthens closed-loop learning pipelines that continuously refine clinical models. As Aminizadeh et al. (2024) observe, sustainable adoption depends on aligning distributed intelligence with ethical oversight and institutional governance.

This expanded perspective situates federated learning as the distributed optimization engine of privacy-aware healthcare systems, linking continuous sensing, AI inference, and immersive decision environments into a coherent architecture.

INTEGRATED METAVERSE–AI–FEDERATED LEARNING PIPELINES FOR CLINICAL APPLICATIONS

The convergence of metaverse platforms, artificial intelligence (AI), and federated learning (FL) becomes most meaningful when examined as an operational pipeline rather than a conceptual combination of technologies. In next-generation healthcare systems, immersive interaction, distributed learning, and predictive modeling form a closed-loop architecture in which sensing, analytics, visualization, and clinical decision-making are continuously coupled.

This section reframes integrated applications as structured convergence pipelines. Each pipeline explicitly maps how data move through federated training, AI inference, digital twin updating, immersive visualization, and clinician action. Such structuring exposes system dependencies, latency constraints, privacy boundaries, and operational realities — elements essential for translating conceptual promise into deployable healthcare infrastructure.

Pipeline 1 — Chronic Cardiac Monitoring

Chronic cardiovascular disease management requires continuous physiological observation, early anomaly detection, and adaptive care planning. An integrated convergence pipeline supports these goals through distributed intelligence and immersive decision environments.

System Pipeline

Wearable ECG / hemodynamic sensors

→ Federated cardiac model training across institutions
→ AI anomaly detection and risk prediction
→ Cardiovascular digital twin update
→ Metaverse visualization dashboard
→ Clinician intervention and therapy adjustment

Operational Dynamics

Wearable devices generate high-frequency biosignals locally. Federated learning enables institutions to collaboratively train cardiac risk models without centralizing sensitive patient data, preserving privacy while improving predictive robustness (Chaddad et al., 2023). AI inference continuously evaluates arrhythmia risk and hemodynamic trends, updating a patient-specific digital twin that reflects evolving cardiovascular state.

Within an immersive metaverse interface, clinicians visualize temporal cardiac behavior, simulate treatment scenarios, and communicate findings interactively. This spatial representation enhances interpretability compared with traditional waveform dashboards.

Latency Considerations

Cardiac anomaly detection requires near-real-time twin updates. Edge-assisted preprocessing reduces transmission delay, while federated aggregation occurs asynchronously to avoid interrupting local monitoring loops.

Privacy Boundaries

Raw ECG streams remain local to patient devices or institutional servers. Only model parameters are exchanged during federated rounds, minimizing exposure of identifiable physiological data.

Operational Constraints

Continuous sensing imposes bandwidth and battery limitations. Institutional heterogeneity in sensor quality and annotation practices introduces model variability that must be managed through adaptive FL strategies. This pipeline exemplifies how distributed sensing, predictive modeling, and immersive visualization converge to support proactive chronic care rather than episodic intervention.

Pipeline 2 — Neurorehabilitation and Adaptive Therapy

Neurological rehabilitation depends on repeated behavioral assessment, motor feedback, and patient engagement — domains where immersive interaction and adaptive intelligence are particularly impactful.

System Pipeline

Motion capture / neural response sensors

→ Federated rehabilitation model training
→ AI motor recovery assessment
→ Neuro-motor digital twin update
→ Metaverse therapy environment adaptation
→ Clinician-guided intervention refinement

Operational Dynamics

Patient motion data captured during therapy sessions feed localized training nodes. Federated learning aggregates insights across rehabilitation centers, enabling AI models to learn recovery trajectories without exposing patient identity (Bashir et al., 2023). The digital twin models motor control progression and predicts therapy responsiveness.

Immersive metaverse environments dynamically adapt exercise difficulty and feedback intensity. Clinicians observe twin evolution in real time, adjusting therapy protocols based on simulated outcomes.

Latency Considerations

Interactive rehabilitation requires sub-perceptual response times to preserve immersion. Local inference ensures immediate feedback, while federated updates occur periodically in background cycles.

Privacy Boundaries

Sensitive behavioral and neurological data remain institutionally contained. Aggregated model learning preserves collaborative intelligence without sharing raw therapy recordings.

Operational Constraints

Hardware variability in motion sensing devices affects calibration consistency. Sustained immersion must also account for patient fatigue and accessibility limitations. This pipeline demonstrates how immersive therapy, AI-driven personalization, and privacy-preserving collaboration enable scalable rehabilitation ecosystems.

Pipeline 3 — Oncology Treatment Planning

Cancer treatment planning involves complex, multidisciplinary decision-making that benefits from predictive modeling and collaborative visualization.

System Pipeline

Medical imaging / genomic oncology datasets

→ Federated tumor progression model training
→ AI treatment response prediction
→ Oncology digital twin simulation
→ Metaverse multidisciplinary planning interface
→ Clinical treatment selection

Operational Dynamics

Imaging and genomic data are processed locally at participating oncology centers. Federated learning enables collaborative model refinement while preserving regulatory compliance (Nguyen et al., 2022). AI models estimate tumor response under alternative therapies, updating a patient-specific digital twin. Within a shared metaverse planning environment, oncologists visualize tumor dynamics, simulate intervention pathways, and coordinate decisions across specialties. The immersive interface improves collective reasoning and communication.

Latency Considerations

Treatment simulation tolerates higher latency than monitoring pipelines, enabling more computationally intensive twin recalibration without disrupting clinical workflow.

Privacy Boundaries

Genomic and imaging datasets remain institutionally protected. Federated aggregation ensures that collaborative insight does not require cross-border data transfer.

Operational Constraints

High computational demands require hybrid edge–cloud execution. Interoperability with imaging repositories and clinical records is essential for reliable twin construction. This pipeline highlights the role of distributed intelligence and immersive collaboration in complex treatment planning.

Cross-Pipeline Validation and Integration Considerations

Across domains, integrated pipelines share recurring engineering themes:

- synchronization between sensing, inference, and visualization
- privacy-preserving model exchange
- adaptive latency management
- institutional interoperability

Validation frameworks must therefore assess prediction fidelity, twin update latency, and clinician usability to ensure safe deployment. Structured pipelines provide a foundation for evaluating system behavior rather than relying on isolated component performance.

Challenges in Integrated Deployment

Despite demonstrated architectural feasibility, integrated pipelines face real-world barriers. Technical complexity, hardware heterogeneity, and interoperability constraints can disrupt synchronization between learning, twin modeling, and immersive rendering (Ullah et al., 2023). User trust depends on explainable AI behavior and transparent privacy safeguards, reinforcing the need for human-centered system design.

Future Opportunities

As distributed intelligence, immersive rendering, and edge computation mature, convergence pipelines are expected to expand into additional domains such as population health modeling and surgical rehearsal. Gao et al. (2024) emphasize that scalable smart healthcare depends on aligning advanced analytics with trustworthy infrastructure. Integrated pipelines represent a pathway toward continuously learning healthcare ecosystems that remain privacy-aware and clinically grounded.

EMBEDDED SECURITY, PRIVACY, AND ETHICAL ARCHITECTURE

Metaverse-enabled, AI-driven, and federated learning–based healthcare systems introduce a security and governance landscape that is fundamentally different from conventional digital health platforms. These systems combine immersive identity frameworks, continuously updated digital twins, distributed learning pipelines, and high-frequency physiological sensing. The result is an expanded attack surface in which failures do not merely expose data — they can influence clinical reasoning, disrupt immersive care workflows, or degrade patient trust.

For next-generation healthcare systems to remain clinically viable, security, privacy, and ethics must be embedded directly into the convergence pipeline: data sensing → federated learning → AI inference → digital twin update → metaverse interaction → clinical decision. This section reframes protection not as an external compliance layer, but as an architectural property integrated into every stage of system operation.

Technical Threat Model for Converged Healthcare Systems

A structured threat model clarifies how vulnerabilities propagate across immersive, intelligent, and distributed components. Three representative threat classes illustrate pipeline-level risks.

Avatar Impersonation and Immersive Identity Compromise

Metaverse healthcare platforms rely on persistent digital identities that mediate clinician–patient interaction. Identity spoofing or avatar hijacking can expose confidential consultations, manipulate therapeutic sessions, or undermine trust in clinical communication. Adil et al. (2025) and Letafati and Otoum (2023) identify identity compromise as a uniquely severe risk in immersive environments, where biometric and behavioral data are continuously processed.

Mitigation Strategies

- multi-factor and biometric authentication
- session-bound cryptographic identity tokens
- anomaly detection for behavioral deviation
- encrypted communication channels

These protections preserve authenticity and continuity of immersive care sessions.

Digital Twin Inference Leakage

Digital twins encode predictive physiological or behavioral models derived from sensitive data. Even when raw inputs remain protected, twin states or outputs may allow inference of patient conditions. Ali et al. (2023) note that immersive interaction patterns and model responses can reveal sensitive attributes through indirect analysis.

Mitigation Strategies

- controlled twin state exposure based on access roles
- privacy-preserving twin parameter updates
- uncertainty-aware visualization to prevent over-disclosure

This ensures that immersive interaction does not unintentionally leak sensitive medical insight.

Federated Learning Poisoning and Model Manipulation

Distributed model training introduces adversarial vectors in which malicious or faulty clients inject corrupted updates. Such attacks may bias diagnostics or degrade system reliability. Guerra-Manzanares et al. (2023) highlight that inference and poisoning risks remain active challenges in privacy-preserving learning.

Mitigation Strategies

- update validation and anomaly filtering
- reputation-weighted aggregation
- secure aggregation protocols

These mechanisms protect collective model integrity without compromising distributed privacy.

Privacy Engineering Embedded in the Convergence Pipeline

Privacy preservation in immersive healthcare cannot rely solely on policy or post-hoc controls. It must be engineered into data flow, model training, and twin synchronization.

Differential Privacy in Twin Updates

Digital twin recalibration incorporates controlled noise injection to limit the recoverability of individual patient attributes while maintaining predictive utility (Naresh et al., 2023). Tuning privacy parameters becomes a clinical design decision: excessive perturbation reduces model fidelity, whereas insufficient protection increases leakage risk.

Encrypted Aggregation in Federated Learning

Secure aggregation protocols combine institutional model updates without exposing individual contributions, aligning distributed intelligence with healthcare confidentiality requirements (Cabrero-Holgueras and Pastrana, 2023).

Identity Protection in Immersive Environments

Persistent XR interaction produces rich behavioral traces. Role-based access control, anonymized avatar mapping, and session isolation prevent cross-context identity leakage while preserving collaborative functionality (Letafati and Otoum, 2023). Together, these mechanisms ensure that privacy is enforced throughout sensing, learning, and visualization stages rather than confined to data storage.

Operationalizing Ethics Within the System Pipeline

Ethical safeguards must be translated into enforceable system behaviors rather than abstract principles.

Consent-Governed Data Participation

Federated learning nodes incorporate consent metadata that determines whether patient data contribute to model updates. Dynamic consent management aligns learning participation with patient preference and regulatory requirements (Faridoon and Kechadi, 2024).

Fairness Monitoring in Distributed Learning

Algorithmic bias is continuously assessed during federated aggregation. Demographic imbalance detection and corrective weighting prevent systemic underrepresentation, addressing ethical concerns highlighted by Mennella et al. (2024) and Abdallah et al. (2025).

Explainable AI for Clinical Oversight

AI-driven recommendations rendered in immersive environments include interpretable rationale cues. Visual explanation layers allow clinicians to evaluate model reasoning, reinforcing accountability and professional judgment (Ali et al., 2023; Goktas and Grzybowski, 2025). Embedding ethics in pipeline execution ensures that fairness, autonomy, and accountability become measurable system properties rather than post-deployment considerations.

Governance Integration Across Distributed Healthcare Ecosystems

Technical safeguards operate within broader governance structures that define responsibility, auditability, and regulatory compliance. Data governance frameworks emphasize lifecycle accountability, role clarity, and cross-institutional coordination (Faridoon and Kechadi, 2024; Paparova et al., 2023). Regulatory alignment becomes particularly complex when immersive healthcare spans jurisdictions, requiring harmonization of privacy standards and audit mechanisms (Ahmed et al., 2025).

Blockchain-assisted auditing has been proposed as a complementary trust layer, providing immutable logging of model updates and access events (Ali et al., 2023). While beneficial for transparency, such mechanisms must be evaluated against scalability and operational overhead.

Toward Architecturally Trustworthy Healthcare Systems

Security, privacy, and ethics in metaverse–AI–FL healthcare systems are inseparable engineering concerns. Encryption, authentication, privacy-preserving learning, and fairness monitoring form a protective substrate that supports immersive clinical interaction without sacrificing trust. Adil et al. (2025) emphasize that sustainable healthcare innovation requires interdisciplinary governance frameworks linking technical resilience with ethical accountability.

Embedding safeguards into the operational pipeline ensures that next-generation healthcare systems remain not only intelligent and immersive, but also secure, equitable, and clinically trustworthy.

OPERATIONAL GOVERNANCE MODEL FOR CONVERGED HEALTHCARE SYSTEMS

Governance in metaverse–AI–federated healthcare systems cannot remain an abstract compliance discussion; it must function as an operational control layer embedded across the system lifecycle. The convergence pipeline — spanning distributed sensing, federated model training, digital twin updates, and immersive clinical interaction — introduces cross-institutional accountability challenges that require formal governance structures aligned with healthcare regulation and enterprise architecture.

An operational governance model begins with data boundary definition. Healthcare analytics pipelines must explicitly encode where data originate, how they are transformed, and under what authority they participate in distributed learning. Enterprise governance frameworks emphasize that scalable analytics systems require standardized data stewardship, access controls, and lifecycle auditability to preserve trust in automated decision processes (Hùng & Quân, 2023). Within federated learning workflows, this translates into institution-level policies governing participation, update validation, and model aggregation transparency. Rather than centralizing authority, governance becomes distributed yet traceable, ensuring that every model update or twin recalibration event can be audited.

Accountability chains are equally critical. Federated training decentralizes computation while preserving institutional autonomy, but it also diffuses responsibility. A healthcare-specific governance architecture therefore defines clear ownership for local data preprocessing, model contribution integrity, and post-aggregation validation. Antunes et al. (2022) demonstrate that federated healthcare architectures benefit from layered governance controls that separate data custody from model governance. This separation enables institutions to maintain regulatory compliance while participating in collective intelligence formation. Lifecycle governance extends beyond training into deployment and clinical decision support. Digital twin updates, immersive visualization, and AI-driven recommendations must operate under verifiable checkpoints. These checkpoints include consent verification, model provenance tracking, and access logging. Governance mechanisms embedded at these stages ensure that predictive outputs remain interpretable and attributable, supporting clinician oversight and legal accountability.

Standardization is another pillar of operational governance. Enterprise architecture perspectives show that interoperability frameworks are necessary to align digital health platforms with national and institutional standards (Wamema et al., 2023). Without such alignment, distributed healthcare systems risk fragmentation, inconsistent compliance, and reduced scalability. Governance models therefore incorporate schema harmonization, API certification, and workflow standardization to maintain consistency across heterogeneous environments. Importantly, governance is not static. As federated learning models evolve and immersive interfaces expand, governance must support adaptive oversight. Continuous monitoring, audit analytics, and policy revision mechanisms allow healthcare systems to respond to emerging risks without disrupting clinical operations.

Embedding governance into the system lifecycle transforms compliance from an external constraint into an enabling infrastructure. By aligning data stewardship, accountability, and interoperability with distributed intelligence pipelines, healthcare systems can scale immersive and AI-driven services while maintaining regulatory integrity and institutional trust.

EVALUATION AND DEPLOYMENT FRAMEWORK FOR CONVERGED HEALTHCARE SYSTEMS

Claims surrounding metaverse-integrated AI and federated learning systems must be grounded in measurable performance criteria. An evaluation framework provides the empirical structure necessary to compare distributed healthcare intelligence pipelines against established baselines while accounting for immersive usability and system responsiveness.

A foundational metric is predictive performance relative to centralized learning. Federated healthcare models are evaluated by comparing diagnostic accuracy, convergence stability, and generalization capability against traditional centralized training approaches. Surveys of federated healthcare systems highlight that maintaining comparable accuracy while preserving privacy is a core validation requirement (Chaddad et al., 2023; Nguyen et al., 2022). Performance gaps reveal where communication overhead, non-IID data distribution, or aggregation inefficiencies affect clinical reliability. Digital twin performance introduces additional metrics. Twin update latency — the time between data acquisition and state synchronization — determines whether immersive visualizations remain clinically actionable. Edge-network studies show that latency-sensitive computation offloading directly influences twin responsiveness, particularly in continuous monitoring scenarios

(Bozkaya et al., 2023). Evaluation therefore includes synchronization delay, model recalibration time, and prediction fidelity under varying network conditions.

Human-centered metrics are equally important. Extended reality platforms must demonstrate usability, cognitive compatibility, and immersion stability. Performance evaluation of XR healthcare systems includes task completion efficiency, interaction clarity, and clinician acceptance (Arpaia et al., 2022). Economic and operational analyses further assess cost-effectiveness and deployment sustainability, ensuring immersive tools provide measurable clinical value (Gómez Bergin & Craven, 2023). Human digital twin frameworks extend evaluation into personalization. Metrics examine how accurately twin models reflect individual physiology and behavioral adaptation over time (Okegbile et al., 2022). Stability of personalization — avoiding oscillatory or inconsistent model behavior — is crucial for long-term trust.

Deployment evaluation also considers communication efficiency. Federated learning introduces bandwidth consumption, update frequency tradeoffs, and synchronization demands. Measuring these factors allows system designers to optimize aggregation intervals and edge processing strategies without degrading privacy guarantees. Scenario-driven evaluation strengthens empirical grounding. Simulated hospital deployments, distributed monitoring environments, and edge-integrated twin systems allow controlled measurement of accuracy, latency, and usability before real-world integration. A structured evaluation framework transforms conceptual system benefits into testable hypotheses. By linking predictive accuracy, twin responsiveness, communication efficiency, and immersive usability, healthcare stakeholders can validate whether converged architectures deliver clinically meaningful improvements while remaining operationally viable.

REAL-WORLD DEPLOYMENT CONSTRAINTS IN CONVERGED HEALTHCARE ARCHITECTURES

While converged metaverse–AI–federated healthcare systems offer transformative potential, deployment realities impose constraints that influence architecture design, adoption strategy, and scalability. Understanding these constraints is essential for transitioning from conceptual frameworks to operational healthcare infrastructure.

Infrastructure cost represents a primary barrier. Immersive XR hardware, distributed computing resources, and secure networking environments require capital investment beyond traditional digital health systems. Adoption studies reveal that both providers and patients evaluate digital tools through cost–benefit lenses, where perceived complexity or maintenance burden can inhibit uptake (Palacholla et al., 2019). Sustainable deployment therefore favors modular architectures that allow incremental scaling rather than wholesale replacement of existing systems. Clinician adoption is equally critical. Healthcare professionals prioritize workflow compatibility, reliability, and interpretability. Mixed-method evaluations of hospital digital systems demonstrate that poorly integrated technologies disrupt clinical routines and reduce user confidence (Muinga et al., 2020). Immersive and AI-driven platforms must therefore align with established care pathways, minimizing cognitive overhead and training demands.

Legacy system integration introduces technical challenges. Hospitals operate heterogeneous information infrastructures, often combining decades-old systems with modern platforms. Architectural analyses emphasize that interoperability layers, data translation mechanisms, and standards-based interfaces are necessary to avoid fragmentation (Gopal et al., 2019). Distributed health record architectures further highlight the need for secure data synchronization across institutional boundaries (Roehrs et al., 2017). Accessibility and ergonomics also shape deployment feasibility. XR environments may present usability limitations related to hardware comfort, motion tolerance, or interaction complexity. Surveys of extended reality deployment reveal tradeoffs between immersion fidelity and practical usability, particularly in remote or resource-limited settings (Ratcliffe et al., 2021). Economic evaluations confirm that cost-effectiveness influences long-term adoption decisions (Gómez Bergin & Craven, 2023).

Scalability tradeoffs arise when distributed learning and digital twin systems operate under constrained network conditions. Continuous sensing pipelines demand bandwidth, synchronization stability, and edge processing capacity. Architectural decisions must balance responsiveness with resource consumption to maintain operational sustainability. Real-world deployment therefore requires a systems-engineering perspective that integrates cost modeling, workflow alignment, interoperability planning, and user-centered design. By acknowledging these constraints early in architecture development, healthcare organizations can implement converged technologies incrementally, preserving clinical continuity while expanding digital capability.

OPEN CHALLENGES AND FUTURE DIRECTIONS

Despite rapid progress in immersive, AI-driven, and federated healthcare systems, several foundational challenges must be addressed to enable safe, scalable, and clinically meaningful deployment. At the systems level, achieving reliable interoperability across heterogeneous devices, hospital infrastructures, and distributed learning environments remains a persistent engineering hurdle. Real-time synchronization between sensing pipelines, federated updates, and digital twin states demands ultra-low latency coordination without compromising privacy or stability.

From an AI perspective, explainability and robustness are critical. Clinical adoption depends on transparent model reasoning, predictable behavior under uncertainty, and safeguards against bias amplification in distributed training. Federated learning introduces additional challenges related to convergence stability, communication efficiency, and fairness across diverse patient populations.

Human and organizational factors are equally significant. Clinician trust, workflow compatibility, and usability of immersive interfaces will determine whether these systems enhance or burden care delivery. Accessibility and equity must guide architecture decisions to avoid widening digital health disparities.

Looking forward, future work must focus on standardized interoperability frameworks, adaptive privacy-preserving learning mechanisms, and lifecycle governance models that evolve with system complexity. Progress will depend on tightly coupling technical innovation with ethical oversight and deployment realism, ensuring that next-generation healthcare systems remain clinically grounded, secure, and socially responsible.

CONCLUSION — STRATEGIC OUTCOMES AND IMPLEMENTATION BLUEPRINT

This chapter has framed next-generation healthcare systems as a coordinated convergence of immersive metaverse environments, intelligent AI analytics, and privacy-preserving federated learning. The central implication is not merely technological modernization, but the need for architecturally coherent systems in which data sensing, distributed learning, digital twin modeling, and immersive clinical interaction operate as an integrated lifecycle. From this perspective, successful implementation depends on deliberate design choices rather than incremental technology adoption.

Several design guidelines emerge. First, healthcare architectures should enforce modular separation between sensing, learning, twin modeling, and visualization layers, enabling scalability, auditability, and controlled evolution. Second, privacy and security mechanisms must be embedded at each pipeline stage, ensuring that distributed intelligence does not compromise patient trust. Third, immersive interfaces should be clinically anchored — designed to support decision-making, not novelty — with explainable AI outputs and workflow compatibility as primary requirements. Finally, governance and consent management must be treated as operational components, integrated into data flow and model lifecycle controls.

These principles translate into architectural priorities: interoperability across heterogeneous healthcare infrastructure, latency-aware synchronization between digital twins and clinical data streams, and distributed accountability mechanisms for federated training. Systems should be engineered for resilience, graceful degradation under network constraints, and continuous auditability. Importantly, architectural decisions must anticipate deployment realities — including legacy system integration, clinician usability, and infrastructure cost — to avoid creating technically elegant but operationally fragile solutions. A practical deployment roadmap follows a staged progression. Early implementation should focus on bounded pilot environments that validate federated analytics and digital twin synchronization under real clinical workflows. Subsequent scaling should emphasize interoperability certification, workforce training, and usability refinement. Mature deployment requires governance formalization, performance benchmarking, and lifecycle monitoring to ensure long-term reliability and trust. Looking forward, a prioritized research agenda centers on ultra-low-latency distributed learning, explainable and bias-aware clinical AI, high-fidelity digital twin validation, and standardized interoperability frameworks for immersive healthcare systems. Parallel research must address equitable access, human-centered interface design, and adaptive governance models capable of evolving alongside system complexity.

These outcomes position converged metaverse–AI–federated healthcare systems as an implementable blueprint rather than a speculative vision. Progress will depend on aligning engineering rigor, clinical practicality, and ethical accountability. When guided by coherent architecture, measurable evaluation, and staged deployment strategy, next-generation healthcare platforms can move from conceptual promise to sustainable clinical infrastructure that advances quality, accessibility, and trust.

REFERENCES

Abbas, J. R., O'Connor, A., Ganapathy, E., Isba, R., Payton, A., McGrath, B., Tolley, N., & Bruce, I. A. (2023). What is virtual reality? A healthcare-focused systematic review of definitions. *Health Policy and Technology*, *12*(2), 100741. DOI: 10.1016/j.hlpt.2023.100741

Abdallah, M., Abdallah, Q., Abukhalil, A., & Barqawi, L. (2025, April). *AI in Healthcare: Ethical and Regulatory Challenges*. In *2025 International Conference on New Trends in Computing Sciences (ICTCS)* (pp. 517–521). IEEE. DOI: 10.1109/ICTCS65341.2025.10989298

Adil, M., Song, H., Khan, M. K., Mastorakis, S., Farouk, A., & Jin, Z. (2025). Metaverse in health care: Security challenges and pathways for future research. *IEEE Systems, Man, and Cybernetics Magazine*, *11*(1), 95–106. DOI: 10.1109/MSMC.2024.3368201

Ahmed, A., Shahzad, A., Naseem, A., Ali, S., & Ahmad, I. (2025). Evaluating the effectiveness of data governance frameworks in ensuring security and privacy of healthcare data. *PLoS One*, *20*(5), e0324285. DOI: 10.1371/journal.pone.0324285 PMID: 40408373

Akinola, S., & Telukdarie, A. (2023). Sustainable digital transformation in healthcare. *Sustainability (Basel)*, *15*(13), 10417. DOI: 10.3390/su151310417

Ali, S., Abdullah, , Armand, T. P. T., Athar, A., Hussain, A., Ali, M., Yaseen, M., Joo, M.-I., & Kim, H.-C. (2023). Metaverse in healthcare integrated with explainable AI and blockchain. *Sensors (Basel)*, *23*(2), 565. DOI: 10.3390/s23020565 PMID: 36679361

Aminizadeh, S., Heidari, A., Dehghan, M., Toumaj, S., Rezaei, M., Navimipour, N. J., & Unal, M. (2024). Opportunities and challenges of artificial intelligence and distributed systems. *Artificial Intelligence in Medicine*, *149*, 102779. DOI: 10.1016/j.artmed.2024.102779 PMID: 38462281

Antunes, R. S., André da Costa, C., Küderle, A., Yari, I. A., & Eskofier, B. (2022). Federated learning for healthcare: Systematic review and architecture proposal. [TIST]. *ACM Transactions on Intelligent Systems and Technology*, *13*(4), 1–23. DOI: 10.1145/3501813

Arpaia, P., De Benedetto, E., De Paolis, L., D'Errico, G., Donato, N., & Duraccio, L. (2022). Performance and usability evaluation of an extended reality platform to monitor patient's health during surgical procedures. *Sensors (Basel)*, *22*(10), 3908. DOI: 10.3390/s22103908 PMID: 35632317

Bashir, A. K., Victor, N., Bhattacharya, S., Huynh-The, T., Chengoden, R., Yenduri, G., Maddikunta, P. K. R., Pham, Q.-V., Gadekallu, T. R., & Liyanage, M. (2023). Federated learning for the healthcare metaverse. *IEEE Internet of Things Journal, 10*(24), 21873–21891. DOI: 10.1109/JIOT.2023.3304790

Bozkaya, E., Erel-Özçevik, M., Bilen, T., & Özçevik, Y. (2023). Proof of evaluation-based energy and delay aware computation offloading for digital twin edge network. *Ad Hoc Networks, 149*, 103254. DOI: 10.1016/j.adhoc.2023.103254

Burian, B. K., Harari, R. E., Robertson, J. M., Musson, D., Pozner, C. N., Doyle, T., & Dias, R. D. (2023). Using XR for medical training. *Applied Ergonomics, 106*, 103902. DOI: 10.1016/j.apergo.2022.103902 PMID: 36162274

Cabanillas-Carbonell, M., Pérez-Martínez, J., & Yáñez, J. A. (2023). 5G technology in the digital transformation of healthcare. *Sustainability, 15*(4), 3178. DOI: 10.3390/su15043178

Cabrero-Holgueras, J., & Pastrana, S. (2023). Privacy-preserving deep learning over encrypted medical data. *Frontiers in Cardiovascular Medicine, 10*, 1117360. DOI: 10.3389/fcvm.2023.1117360 PMID: 37187785

Chaddad, A., Wu, Y., & Desrosiers, C. (2023). Federated learning for healthcare applications. *IEEE Internet of Things Journal, 11*(5), 7339–7358. DOI: 10.1109/JIOT.2023.3325822

Dal Mas, F., Massaro, M., Rippa, P., & Secundo, G. (2023). The challenges of digital transformation in healthcare. *Technovation, 123*, 102716. DOI: 10.1016/j.technovation.2023.102716

Denecke, K., & Baudoin, C. R. (2022). AI and robotics in transformed health ecosystems. *Frontiers in Medicine, 9*, 795957. DOI: 10.3389/fmed.2022.795957 PMID: 35872767

Faridoon, A., & Kechadi, M. T. (2024). *Healthcare data governance, privacy, and security*. In *EAI International Conference on Body Area Networks* (pp. 261–271).

Gao, X., He, P., Zhou, Y., & Qin, X. (2024). Artificial intelligence applications in smart healthcare. *Future Internet, 16*(9), 308. DOI: 10.3390/fi16090308

Gatla, T. R. (2024). Revolutionizing healthcare with AI. *International Journal of Advanced Research and Interdisciplinary Scientific Endeavours, 1*(2), 61–70.

Goktas, P., & Grzybowski, A. (2025). Ethical clinical challenges and trustworthy AI. *Journal of Clinical Medicine, 14*(5), 1605. DOI: 10.3390/jcm14051605 PMID: 40095575

Gómez Bergin, A. D., & Craven, M. P. (2023). Virtual, augmented, mixed, and extended reality interventions in healthcare: A systematic review of health economic evaluations and cost-effectiveness. *BMC Digital Health*, *1*(1), 53. DOI: 10.1186/s44247-023-00054-9

Gopal, G., Suter-Crazzolara, C., Toldo, L., & Eberhardt, W. (2019). Digital transformation in healthcare–architectures of present and future information technologies. [CCLM]. *Clinical Chemistry and Laboratory Medicine*, *57*(3), 328–335. DOI: 10.1515/cclm-2018-0658 PMID: 30530878

Guerra-Manzanares, A., Lopez, L. J. L., Maniatakos, M., & Shamout, F. E. (2023). *Privacy-preserving machine learning for healthcare*. In Trustworthy ML for Healthcare (pp. 25–40).

Gupta, L., Salman, T., Ghubaish, A., Unal, D., Al-Ali, A. K., & Jain, R. (2022). Cybersecurity of multi-cloud healthcare systems. *Applied Soft Computing*, *118*, 108439. DOI: 10.1016/j.asoc.2022.108439

Gupta, P., Babbar, H., & Rani, S. (2023). Impact of Metaverse in Healthcare. In *SIBF 2023* (pp. 112–118). IEEE.

Haleem, A., Javaid, M., Singh, R. P., & Suman, R. (2023). Digital twin technology in healthcare. *Biomedical Technology*, *4*, 28–38. DOI: 10.1016/j.bmt.2023.02.001

Horgan, D., Pesapane, F., Van der Buckle, M., De Maria, R., Dube, F., Singh, J., & Subbiah, V. (2024). Next-generation sequencing in healthcare systems. *Critical Reviews in Oncology/Hematology*, *201*, 104433. DOI: 10.1016/j.critrevonc.2024.104433 PMID: 38955310

Hùng, N. V., & Quân, T. M. (2023). Enterprise Data-Governance Operating Models for Scalable, High-Trust Healthcare Analytics and Decision Support Programs. *Orient Journal of Emerging Paradigms in Artificial Intelligence and Autonomous Systems*, *13*(12), 1–11.

Iqbal, A. I., Aamir, A., Hammad, A., Hafsa, H., Basit, A., Oduoye, M. O., Anis, M. W., Ahmed, S., Younus, M. I., & Jabeen, S. (2024). Immersive technologies in healthcare. *Journal of Primary Care & Community Health*, *15*, 21501319241293311. DOI: 10.1177/21501319241293311 PMID: 39439304

Jones, D., Galvez, R., Evans, D., Hazelton, M., Rossiter, R., Irwin, P., & Fealy, S. (2023). XR technologies in primary medical care. *Virtual Worlds*, *2*(4), 359–373. DOI: 10.3390/virtualworlds2040021

Lakshmi, D., Kondurkar, I., Kumar, R., & Banerjee, R. (2024). *Intelligent Healthcare Systems in the Metaverse*. In The Metaverse for the Healthcare Industry (pp. 17–32).

Letafati, M., & Otoum, S. (2023). Privacy and security in metaverse healthcare. *IEEE Consumer Electronics Magazine*, *13*(3), 80–89. DOI: 10.1109/MCE.2023.3334494

Liu, X., Yu, J., Liu, Y., Gao, Y., Mahmoodi, T., Lambotharan, S., & Tsang, D. H. K. (2023). Distributed intelligence in wireless networks. *IEEE Open Journal of the Communications Society*, *4*, 1001–1039. DOI: 10.1109/OJCOMS.2023.3265425

Lu, T., Ji, S., Jin, W., Yang, Q., Luo, Q., & Ren, T. L. (2023). Biocompatible biosensors. *Sensors (Basel)*, *23*(6), 2991. DOI: 10.3390/s23062991 PMID: 36991702

Mbunge, E., Jiyane, S. E., & Muchemwa, B. (2022). Emotive sensory web in virtual healthcare. *Sensors International*, *3*, 100134. DOI: 10.1016/j.sintl.2021.100134

Mennella, C., Maniscalco, U., De Pietro, G., & Esposito, M. (2024). Ethical and regulatory challenges of AI. *Heliyon*, *10*(4), e26297. DOI: 10.1016/j.heliyon.2024.e26297 PMID: 38384518

Messaoud, S., Bouaafia, S., Maraoui, A., Khriji, L., Ammari, A. C., & Machhout, M. (2022). AI-based virtual healthcare center. *The Canadian Journal of Infectious Diseases & Medical Microbiology*, *2022*, 6786203. PMID: 35069953

Muinga, N., Magare, S., Monda, J., English, M., Fraser, H., Powell, J., & Paton, C. (2020). Digital health Systems in Kenyan Public Hospitals: A mixed-methods survey. *BMC Medical Informatics and Decision Making*, *20*(1), 2. DOI: 10.1186/s12911-019-1005-7 PMID: 31906932

Musamih, A., Yaqoob, I., Salah, K., Jayaraman, R., Al-Hammadi, Y., Omar, M., & Ellahham, S. (2022). Metaverse in healthcare. *IEEE Consumer Electronics Magazine*, *12*(4), 33–46. DOI: 10.1109/MCE.2022.3223522

Myrzashova, R., Alsamhi, S. H., Shvetsov, A. V., Hawbani, A., & Wei, X. (2023). Blockchain meets federated learning. *IEEE Internet of Things Journal*, *10*(16), 14418–14437. DOI: 10.1109/JIOT.2023.3263598

Naresh, V. S., Thamarai, M., & Allavarpu, V. D. (2023). Privacy-preserving deep learning in medical informatics. *Artificial Intelligence Review*, *56*(S1, Suppl 1), 1199–1241. DOI: 10.1007/s10462-023-10556-7

Nguyen, D. C., Pham, Q. V., Pathirana, P. N., Ding, M., Seneviratne, A., Lin, Z., Dobre, O., & Hwang, W. J. (2022). Federated learning for smart healthcare. *ACM Computing Surveys*, *55*(3), 1–37. DOI: 10.1145/3501296

Okegbile, S. D., Cai, J., Niyato, D., & Yi, C. (2022). Human digital twin for personalized healthcare: Vision, architecture and future directions. *IEEE Network*, *37*(2), 262–269. DOI: 10.1109/MNET.118.2200071

Palacholla, R. S., Fischer, N., Coleman, A., Agboola, S., Kirley, K., Felsted, J., Katz, C., Lloyd, S., & Jethwani, K. (2019). Provider-and patient-related barriers to and facilitators of digital health technology adoption for hypertension management: Scoping review. *JMIR Cardio*, *3*(1), e11951. DOI: 10.2196/11951 PMID: 31758771

Paparova, D., Aanestad, M., Vassilakopoulou, P., & Bahus, M. K. (2023). Data governance spaces. *Information and Organization*, *33*(1), 100451. DOI: 10.1016/j.infoandorg.2023.100451

Punukollu, M. (2022). AI-driven genomic sequencing. *Los Angeles Journal of Intelligent Systems and Pattern Recognition*, *2*, 293–329.

Rani, S., Chauhan, M., Kataria, A., & Khang, A. (2023). *IoT equipped intelligent distributed framework*. In Springer Nature Singapore (pp. 97–114).

Ratcliffe, J., Soave, F., Bryan-Kinns, N., Tokarchuk, L., & Farkhatdinov, I. (2021, May). Extended reality (XR) remote research: A survey of drawbacks and opportunities. In *Proceedings of the 2021 CHI conference on human factors in computing systems* (pp. 1-13). DOI: 10.1145/3411764.3445170

Ribino, P., Ciampi, M., Islam, S., & Papastergiou, S. (2022). Swarm intelligence model for securing healthcare. *Procedia Computer Science*, *210*, 149–156. DOI: 10.1016/j.procs.2022.10.131

Roehrs, A., Da Costa, C. A., & da Rosa Righi, R. (2017). OmniPHR: A distributed architecture model to integrate personal health records. *Journal of Biomedical Informatics*, *71*, 70–81. DOI: 10.1016/j.jbi.2017.05.012 PMID: 28545835

Santarsiero, F., Schiuma, G., Carlucci, D., & Helander, N. (2023). Role of innovation labs. *Technovation*, *122*, 102640. DOI: 10.1016/j.technovation.2022.102640

Satav, S. D., Hasan, D. S., Pitchai, R., Mohanaprakash, T. A., Sultanuddin, S. J., & Boopathi, S. (2023). NGIoT in healthcare systems. In Global, I. G. I. (Ed.), (pp. 307–330).

Stoumpos, A. I., Kitsios, F., & Talias, M. A. (2023). Technology acceptance in healthcare. *International Journal of Environmental Research and Public Health*, *20*(4), 3407. DOI: 10.3390/ijerph20043407 PMID: 36834105

Sun, T., He, X., & Li, Z. (2023). Digital twin in healthcare. *Digital Health*, *9*, 20552076221149651. DOI: 10.1177/20552076221149651 PMID: 36636729

Tan, T. F., Li, Y., Lim, J. S., Gunasekeran, D. V., Teo, Z. L., Ng, W. Y., & Ting, D. S. (2022). Metaverse and virtual healthcare in ophthalmology. *Asia-Pacific Journal of Ophthalmology*, *11*(3), 237–246. DOI: 10.1097/APO.0000000000000537 PMID: 35772084

Ullah, H., Manickam, S., Obaidat, M., Laghari, S. U. A., & Uddin, M. (2023). Metaverse technology in healthcare. *IEEE Access : Practical Innovations, Open Solutions*, *11*, 69686–69707. DOI: 10.1109/ACCESS.2023.3286696

Vallée, A. (2023). Digital twin for healthcare systems. *Frontiers in Digital Health*, *5*, 1253050. DOI: 10.3389/fdgth.2023.1253050 PMID: 37744683

Wamema, J., Alunyu, A., Amiyo, M., & Nabukenya, J. (2023). Enterprise architecture requirements for standardising digital health in Uganda's health system. *Health Policy and Technology*, *12*(4), 100805. DOI: 10.1016/j.hlpt.2023.100805

Wang, Z., Wei, H., Huang, Y., Wei, Y., & Chen, J. (2023). Naturally sourced hydrogels. *Chemical Society Reviews*, *52*(9), 2992–3034. DOI: 10.1039/D2CS00813K PMID: 37017633

Yang, E. (2023). Immersive technologies in healthcare built environments. *Frontiers in Medical Technology*, *5*, 1184925. DOI: 10.3389/fmedt.2023.1184925 PMID: 37799269

Chapter 3
Intelligent Immersive Healthcare:
Integrating AI, Federated Learning, and the Metaverse for Next-Generation Medical Ecosystems

E. Karthika
http://orcid.org/0009-0000-6579-5017
Dr. N.G.P. Arts and Science College, India

G. Ashwin Prabhu
http://orcid.org/0000-0001-5673-647X
St. Joseph's College of Engineering, India

M. Nithya Devi
Shri Nehru Maha Vidyalaya College of Arts and Science, India

K. Saranya Maheswari
Rathinam College of Arts and Science, India

S. Sivakumar
Arunai Engineering College, India

Ravikumar Jayabal
Academy of Maritime Education and Training, AMET University, India

B. Aravind Kumar
http://orcid.org/0009-0007-6534-0929
St. Joseph's College of Engineering, India

S. Raghu Pandiyan
St. Joseph's College of Engineering, India

ABSTRACT

Intelligent immersive healthcare represents an emerging paradigm that unifies artificial intelligence, federated learning, and metaverse infrastructures to create secure, adaptive, and patient-centered medical ecosystems. This chapter per the

DOI: 10.4018/979-8-3373-8889-2.ch003

authors examines how immersive environments, combined with AI-driven analytics and decentralized learning frameworks, enable real-time clinical decision support, personalized therapeutics, collaborative training, and remote care delivery while preserving data sovereignty and privacy. The discussion synthesizes architectural models, application domains, and ethical–regulatory considerations shaping next-generation healthcare platforms, including digital twins, intelligent diagnostics, and virtual hospitals. By integrating technical foundations with healthcare use cases, the chapter elucidates how convergent intelligent and immersive technologies can enhance interoperability, resilience, and equity, supporting a scalable transformation of clinical practice and population health management.

1. INTRODUCTION

Healthcare is undergoing a profound transformation driven by the convergence of artificial intelligence (AI), distributed data infrastructures, and immersive digital environments. Over the past two decades, digital health initiatives have focused primarily on digitizing records, enabling telemedicine, and introducing decision-support systems to clinical practice. While these developments have improved efficiency and access, they have not fundamentally restructured how healthcare is experienced, governed, and personalized. Today, emerging metaverse infrastructures—encompassing extended reality (XR), digital twins, and spatial computing—are enabling a shift from screen-based interactions toward persistent, interactive, and embodied healthcare environments. When integrated with AI-driven analytics and federated learning architectures, these environments support what can be described as *intelligent immersive medical ecosystems*: distributed healthcare systems in which real-time intelligence, privacy-preserving collaboration, and experiential interfaces are unified to support predictive, participatory, and precision care (Esteva et al., 2019; Kairouz et al., 2021; Park & Kim, 2022). Comparable cross-domain applications of AI illustrate its versatility, from precision farming with multipurpose agrobots (Dhanushya et al., 2025) to IoT-enabled vertical crop cultivation systems (Gowthaman et al., 2025), highlighting how distributed intelligence and immersive interfaces can be adapted across sectors, including healthcare.

The evolution of digital health has progressed from early hospital information systems and electronic health records to telemedicine platforms, wearable sensors, and mobile health applications. These innovations expanded the reach of healthcare beyond clinical settings, enabling remote consultations, continuous physiological monitoring, and patient engagement through digital interfaces. However, despite their impact, contemporary digital health systems remain constrained by fragmented data infrastructures, institutional silos, and limited interoperability. Clinical data are often distributed across incompatible platforms, restricting holistic modeling of patient states and impeding the translation of insights into coordinated care pathways. Moreover, most current systems remain interactionally thin, relying on dashboards, alerts, and video interfaces that inadequately capture the complexity of human physiology, behavior, and clinical workflows (Esteva et al., 2019).

Intelligent immersion represents a qualitative departure from this paradigm. Rather than merely digitizing information flows, immersive healthcare environments seek to spatialize, contextualize, and personalize medical data within interactive three-dimensional spaces. Advances in XR, haptic interfaces, and real-time simulation allow clinicians and patients to engage with anatomical models, physiological processes, and care pathways as manipulable digital constructs. Within such environments, a patient's data are no longer confined to static records but instantiated as living digital twins that evolve with continuous input from sensors, imaging systems, and clinical interventions. These developments align healthcare delivery with experiential design principles, enabling deeper cognitive engagement, improved clinical training, and more intuitive patient education (Park & Kim, 2022).

1.1 Convergence of AI, Federated Learning, and the Metaverse

The emergence of intelligent immersive ecosystems is contingent upon the convergence of three technological layers. AI functions as the analytical and cognitive substrate, extracting patterns from heterogeneous data streams, supporting diagnostic inference, and enabling adaptive personalization. Contemporary AI systems have demonstrated the capacity to match or exceed human-level performance in imaging-based diagnosis, risk prediction, and workflow optimization. Yet their full clinical potential depends on access to diverse, high-quality datasets and on their integration into environments where insights can be interpreted, contextualized, and acted upon in real time (Esteva et al., 2019).

Federated learning provides a complementary governance and privacy-preserving layer. Traditional centralized data aggregation models raise significant concerns regarding confidentiality, institutional control, and regulatory compliance. Federated learning addresses these constraints by enabling collaborative model training across distributed data sources without requiring raw data to leave local environments. Clinical institutions can thus participate in collective intelligence formation while maintaining sovereignty over sensitive patient information. This paradigm supports scalable, ethically grounded AI development and creates the infrastructural conditions necessary for global, multi-institutional immersive healthcare networks (Kairouz et al., 2021). The metaverse constitutes the experiential and collaborative interface layer through which AI-driven insights and federated intelligence are rendered actionable. Persistent virtual environments support synchronous and asynchronous interaction among clinicians, patients, educators, and intelligent agents. Within these spaces, real-world clinical contexts can be mirrored, augmented, and reconfigured, enabling remote surgery planning, immersive rehabilitation, collaborative diagnostics, and distributed medical education. The rationale for convergence lies in the need to align real-time intelligence, secure data collaboration, and patient-centered experiential design into a unified healthcare fabric. Without AI, immersive environments risk becoming visualization platforms devoid of cognitive depth; without federated learning, they remain ethically and institutionally constrained; without immersive interfaces, advanced analytics remain abstract and underutilized (Kairouz et al., 2021; Park & Kim, 2022).

1.2 Intelligent Immersive Healthcare as a New Paradigm

Intelligent immersive healthcare can be defined as a paradigm in which AI-enabled analytics, federated intelligence infrastructures, and metaverse platforms are integrated to create adaptive, experiential, and distributed medical ecosystems. This paradigm reframes healthcare from a reactive, encounter-based model toward a continuous cycle of prediction, prevention, and participation. Patients are not merely recipients of episodic interventions but active contributors to evolving digital representations of their health. Clinicians, in turn, operate within augmented cognitive environments that support systems-level understanding, collaborative reasoning, and anticipatory decision-making (Esteva et al., 2019). Within this framework, virtual hospitals emerge as networked clinical spaces that transcend physical boundaries, enabling resource sharing, remote expertise, and immersive triage and consultation. Digital twins of patients, organs, and healthcare systems serve as computational laboratories where disease trajectories, treatment responses, and operational strategies can be simulated before being enacted. Intelligent diagnostics are embedded not only in devices but in environments, where multimodal data streams—from imaging, genomics, biosensors, and behavioral metrics—are fused into coherent situational awareness. The shift is thus not simply technological but epistemic: medical knowledge becomes dynamic, contextual, and spatially instantiated within ecosystems that continuously learn and evolve (Park & Kim, 2022).

1.3 Chapter Objectives and Structure

This chapter positions intelligent immersive medical ecosystems as a foundational construct for next-generation digital health. Its scope encompasses the technical foundations of AI-driven analytics and federated learning, the architectural principles of metaverse-enabled healthcare platforms, and the emerging spectrum of clinical, educational, and public health applications. In addition to technological considerations, the chapter addresses governance, ethics, and socio-technical integration, recognizing that immersive intelligence infrastructures will reshape institutional roles, professional practices, and patient agency. Structurally, the chapter is organized into eight parts. Following this introduction, subsequent sections examine enabling technologies, system architectures, application domains, human–AI interaction models, data governance and privacy frameworks, and evaluation challenges. The chapter concludes by synthesizing interdisciplinary insights and outlining strategic directions for building resilient, equitable, and intelligent immersive healthcare systems. Through this structure, the chapter aims to contribute an integrative perspective that bridges computer science, biomedical engineering, clinical practice, and health policy, articulating intelligent immersion not as a speculative vision but as an emerging, actionable paradigm for the future of medicine.

2. THEORETICAL AND TECHNOLOGICAL FOUNDATIONS

Intelligent immersive healthcare emerges at the intersection of artificial intelligence, biomedical informatics, decentralized learning, and immersive computing, forming a socio-technical ecosystem rather than a single technology. This convergence reflects a shift from isolated digital tools toward integrated environments capable of sensing, interpreting, and augmenting human physiology, cognition, and clinical practice. Contemporary healthcare systems increasingly depend on computational models that learn from complex biomedical data, while immersive interfaces translate these abstractions into perceptible, actionable experiences for clinicians and patients. At the same time, regulatory pressure, ethical concerns, and public awareness of data misuse have accelerated the search for privacy-preserving analytics that respect institutional and individual data sovereignty. Intelligent immersive healthcare therefore rests on dual foundations: advanced AI methods that generate clinical insight, and infrastructural paradigms that distribute computation across secure, interoperable, and low-latency environments. This section synthesizes these conceptual and technological bases, outlining how AI, federated analytics, immersive systems, and edge-enabled biomedical informatics collectively enable resilient, human-centered healthcare ecosystems.

2.1 Artificial Intelligence in Contemporary Healthcare

Artificial intelligence has become a core engine of modern healthcare transformation, driven by rapid advances in machine learning, deep learning, and large-scale foundation models capable of processing heterogeneous biomedical data. Contemporary systems extend beyond narrow predictive algorithms to multimodal architectures that integrate medical imaging, electronic health records, genomic data, physiological signals, and natural language clinical narratives. Such models increasingly support diagnostic classification, risk stratification, clinical decision support, and workflow automation, reshaping both frontline care and population health management. Deep learning has proven particularly effective in pattern-intensive domains such as radiology, pathology, and dermatology, where convolutional and transformer-based architectures approach or surpass human-level performance in specific diagnostic tasks (Esteva et al., 2019). Beyond diagnostics, AI systems are embedded in predictive analytics pipelines that forecast disease progression, hospital readmissions, and treatment response, enabling a shift from reactive to anticipatory medicine. Natural language processing automates clinical documentation and knowledge retrieval, while reinforcement learning and causal modeling are increasingly explored for treatment planning and adaptive clinical pathways. These capabilities form the cognitive substrate upon which immersive healthcare environments operate, providing real-time intelligence that can be visualized, simulated, and interactively explored. Similar AI-driven architectures have been demonstrated in safety-critical contexts such as smart rover control (Ruba et al., 2023) and underwater tunnel inspection using AI-powered crack detection (Ruba et al., 2025), underscoring the reliability of intelligent systems in domains requiring precision and resilience. However, the integration of AI into healthcare remains constrained by fundamental limitations. Algorithmic bias, stemming from unrepresentative or historically skewed datasets, threatens to reproduce inequities at scale. The opacity of deep models complicates explainability, undermining clinician trust and regulatory acceptance. Moreover, conventional AI pipelines depend heavily on centralized data aggregation, creating vulnerabilities related to privacy, security, and cross-institutional governance (Esteva et al., 2019). These challenges motivate a transition toward decentralized and privacy-preserving learning paradigms that can sustain intelligent functionality while aligning with ethical and legal imperatives.

2.2 Federated Learning and Privacy-Preserving Analytics

Federated learning and related decentralized approaches redefine how medical AI systems are trained and deployed by relocating computation to the data rather than concentrating data within centralized repositories. In federated learning, models are collaboratively trained across distributed institutional nodes, with only encrypted or aggregated parameter updates shared to a coordinating server. This paradigm enables hospitals, laboratories, and wearable-device ecosystems to contribute to collective intelligence without exposing raw patient data, preserving confidentiality while benefiting from population-scale learning (McMahan et al., 2017). Extensions such as split learning and swarm learning further decompose training processes across networked infrastructures, allowing sensitive data features to remain localized while abstract representations are collaboratively optimized. These methods are complemented by cryptographic and statistical safeguards, including differential privacy, secure aggregation, and homomorphic encryption, which mathematically constrain the risk of re-identification or data leakage. Together, these techniques support regulatory compliance with data-protection frameworks while fostering institutional collaboration across geographical and organizational boundaries. In the context of immersive healthcare, privacy-preserving analytics are foundational. Immersive environments often process continuous streams of biosignals, behavioral metrics, and contextual data generated by extended-reality interfaces and Internet of Medical Things (IoMT) devices. Federated paradigms enable such systems to learn from distributed experiential data while maintaining local control and auditability. As a result, intelligent immersive healthcare infrastructures can evolve into trusted collaborative networks, where knowledge is shared without commodifying or centralizing sensitive biomedical information (McMahan et al., 2017). Federated and decentralized approaches are also being explored in IoT-driven traffic control systems (Poovithaa et al., 2025) and adaptive memory architectures (Kameswaran et al., 2017), demonstrating how privacy-preserving analytics can extend beyond healthcare into broader socio-technical infrastructures.

Figure 1. Patient Digital Twin in Immersive Healthcare

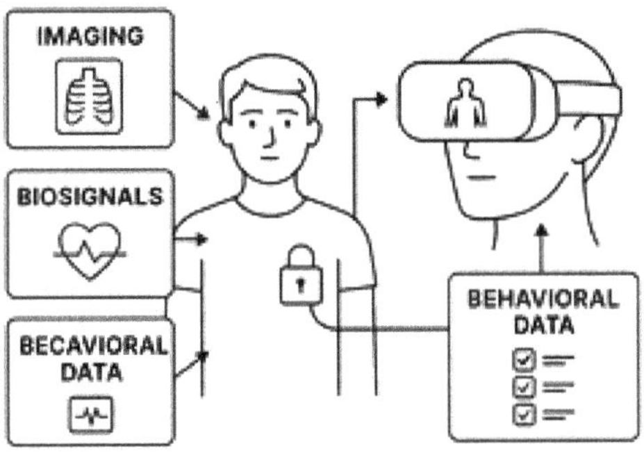

2.3 Metaverse and Immersive Technologies in Medicine

Immersive technologies translate computational intelligence into spatial, embodied experiences, anchoring abstract analytics within perceptual and interactive clinical contexts. Extended reality (XR)—encompassing virtual, augmented, and mixed reality—supports three-dimensional visualization of anatomy, pathology, and procedural workflows, enabling clinicians to interact with complex data in intuitively navigable environments. These systems are increasingly coupled with digital twins, haptic interfaces, and spatial computing platforms that simulate physiological processes and therapeutic interventions with high fidelity. In medical education and clinical planning, immersive visualization enhances anatomical comprehension, surgical rehearsal, and collaborative simulation by situating users within manipulable representations of patient-specific models. Therapeutically, immersive environments facilitate exposure therapy, neurorehabilitation, pain management, and mental-health interventions, leveraging presence and embodiment to modulate perception, behavior, and affective states. Augmented reality further integrates computational overlays into physical clinical settings, guiding interventions, supporting minimally invasive procedures, and contextualizing real-time biosignal feedback (Barsom et al., 2016). Within intelligent immersive healthcare, the "metaverse" functions less as a speculative virtual world and more as a networked continuum of interoperable clinical spaces. These environments host virtual presence, enabling geographically distributed clinicians, patients, and AI agents to co-inhabit shared diagnostic and therapeutic contexts. Embodied interaction—through gesture, gaze, and haptic feedback—supports naturalistic engagement with AI-generated insights, fostering interpretability, situational awareness, and collaborative sense-making. Immersive interfaces thus operate as the experiential layer through which decentralized intelligence becomes clinically meaningful. Parallel innovations in immersive and intelligent environments are evident in education, where conversational AI supports personalized learning (Ruba et al., 2026a), smart pedagogies reimagine higher education campuses (Ruba et al., 2026b), and intercultural communication frameworks integrate AI into assessment practices (Santhini et al., 2025). These examples highlight the broader societal relevance of immersive intelligence ecosystems.

2.4 Biomedical Informatics and Edge Computing Integration

Biomedical informatics provides the organizational backbone of intelligent immersive healthcare, structuring how heterogeneous data streams are acquired, standardized, and translated into actionable knowledge. Interoperability standards, ontologies, and clinical data models enable integration across electronic health records, imaging repositories, wearable sensors, and IoMT ecosystems, supporting longitudinal and cross-modal patient representations. These informatics frameworks ensure that immersive environments are grounded in clinically validated information architectures rather than isolated visualization silos.

Edge computing extends this foundation by relocating analytics closer to data sources, enabling real-time processing of biosignals, motion capture, and contextual sensor streams. For immersive healthcare applications, low-latency computation is critical: surgical guidance, rehabilitation feedback, and adaptive therapeutic environments depend on millisecond-scale responsiveness. Edge–cloud synergy distributes workloads across local devices, institutional servers, and cloud infrastructures, balancing immediacy, scalability, and security. This hybrid architecture supports resilience by mitigating network disruptions, reducing bandwidth demands, and localizing sensitive processing within trusted clinical domains. When integrated with decentralized learning and immersive interfaces, biomedical informatics and edge computing establish the infrastructural conditions for intelligent clinical spaces. These spaces can sense physiological and environmental dynamics, interpret them through AI models, and project responsive, context-aware interventions through immersive media. The result is a foundational architecture for resilient immersive healthcare systems capable of continuous learning, ethical data stewardship, and embodied human–AI collaboration. Edge-enabled resilience has also been validated in biomedical signal processing, such as FPGA-based adaptive filtering for ECG noise elimination (Shanmugaraja et al., 2023), reinforcing the importance of low-latency, edge-integrated computation in clinical contexts.

3. ARCHITECTURAL MODELS FOR INTELLIGENT IMMERSIVE HEALTHCARE

Intelligent immersive healthcare requires architectural models that can simultaneously manage heterogeneous biomedical data, advanced clinical intelligence, distributed trust mechanisms, and real-time experiential interfaces. Unlike conventional health IT stacks, immersive healthcare ecosystems must support continuous perception of the human body, adaptive AI-driven reasoning, secure cross-institutional collaboration, and embodied interaction through extended reality (XR) environments. These requirements call for multi-layered architectures in which sensing, intelligence, federation, and immersion are not isolated components but mutually reinforcing strata. The architectural perspective proposed here conceptualizes immersive healthcare systems as living infrastructures, capable of evolving with clinical knowledge, scaling across institutions, and maintaining resilience under high-risk conditions. Such architectures move healthcare from static information systems toward dynamic cyber-physical-cognitive ecosystems that integrate digital twins, federated learning, and metaverse environments to enable personalized, collaborative, and anticipatory care (Topol, 2019; Rieke et al., 2020).

3.1 Layered Ecosystem Architecture

A layered ecosystem architecture provides the conceptual and technical foundation for intelligent immersive healthcare by organizing system complexity into interdependent functional strata. At the perception layer, heterogeneous sensing modalities capture continuous streams of physiological, behavioral, and environmental data. This includes wearable biosensors, implantable devices, smart medical equipment, imaging systems, and ambient Internet-of-Medical-Things infrastructures. Rather than functioning as isolated devices, perception components operate as coordinated data producers, enabling longitudinal health modeling and real-time clinical situational awareness. The architectural emphasis at this layer is not merely data collection, but semantic alignment and temporal synchronization, which are prerequisites for meaningful AI inference and immersive visualization.

The intelligence layer transforms perceptual data into clinically actionable knowledge. This layer hosts AI inference engines, multimodal clinical models, and simulation environments, including patient-specific digital twins. These digital representations of anatomical, physiological, and behavioral processes allow clinicians to explore "what-if" scenarios, forecast disease trajectories, and test interventions before applying them in vivo. Digital twins thus function as cognitive mediators between raw biosignals and immersive clinical decision spaces, supporting the shift from reactive medicine to predictive and precision care (Bruynseels et al., 2018; Topol, 2019). Within the architecture, the intelligence layer must support continuous learning, model versioning, and explainability services to maintain clinical trust and regulatory compliance.

Figure 2. Layered Ecosystem Architecture of Intelligent Immersive Healthcare

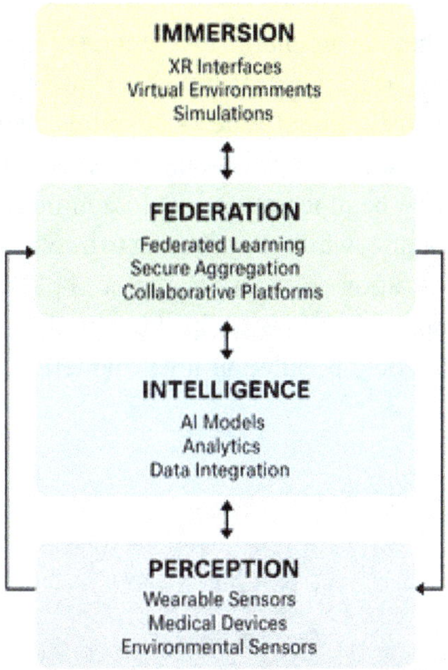

The federation layer provides the governance substrate that enables distributed collaboration without centralized data pooling. In immersive healthcare ecosystems, data are inherently fragmented across hospitals, laboratories, public health agencies, and personal devices. Federated architectures orchestrate decentralized learning, privacy preservation, and auditability across these heterogeneous nodes. Rather than moving sensitive patient data, model parameters and encrypted insights circulate between institutional boundaries, enabling collective intelligence while respecting jurisdictional constraints. This layer thus operationalizes ethical and legal principles—such as data minimization, accountability, and traceability—directly within system design (Rieke et al., 2020). The immersion layer represents the experiential interface through which clinicians, patients, and intelligent agents interact with the healthcare ecosystem. It encompasses metaverse spaces, XR-based clinical environments, collaborative dashboards, and embodied simulation platforms. By spatializing complex medical data and AI-generated insights, the immersion layer enables intuitive sense-making, shared situational awareness, and participatory care. Importantly, immersion is not treated as a presentation add-on but as an active cognitive workspace in which perception, intelligence, and federation layers converge to support collaborative reasoning and therapeutic engagement.

3.2 Federated Metaverse Healthcare Platforms

Federated metaverse healthcare platforms extend the layered architecture across organizational boundaries, creating distributed yet interoperable clinical environments. In such platforms, institutional nodes—hospitals, diagnostic laboratories, research centers, and public health agencies—operate as semi-autonomous participants within a shared immersive healthcare network. Each node maintains sovereignty over its data and infrastructure, while contributing to a collective learning ecosystem through federated orchestration services (Rieke et al., 2020). This model avoids the ethical and operational risks of centralized health data repositories, while still enabling large-scale analytics, population-level modeling, and cross-institutional digital twin refinement.

Figure 3. Federated Learning in Healthcare Networks

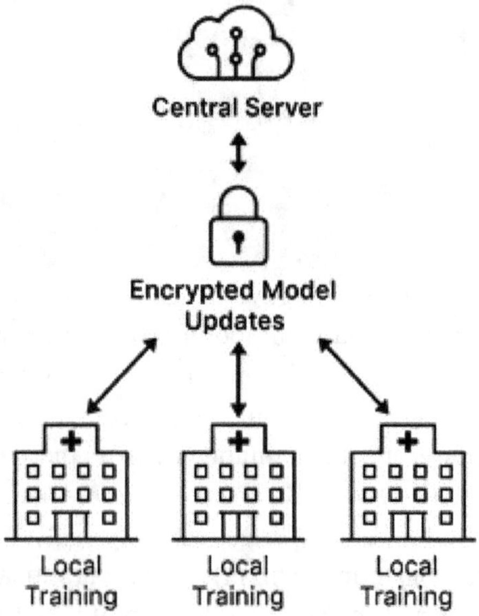

Secure learning orchestration is central to these platforms. Federated coordination services manage model training cycles, performance validation, and update dissemination across nodes. Within immersive environments, clinicians and researchers can collaboratively inspect aggregated model behaviors, visualize uncertainty landscapes, and co-design treatment strategies without exposing raw patient data. The metaverse thus becomes a secure socio-technical arena for distributed clinical intelligence, where institutional boundaries are preserved but epistemic collaboration is amplified. Cross-platform interoperability and identity management further stabilize federated metaverse architectures. Persistent digital identities for clinicians, patients, and AI agents enable continuity of care across immersive sessions and institutional contexts. Interoperable schemas ensure that patient digital twins, diagnostic models, and immersive artifacts can migrate between platforms without semantic degradation. Architecturally, this requires the federation layer to integrate authentication, consent management, and provenance tracking as first-class services, embedding trust mechanisms directly into immersive clinical workflows.

3.3 Edge-Enabled Intelligent Immersion

Edge-enabled intelligent immersion addresses the temporal and safety constraints of real-world clinical environments. Many immersive healthcare applications—such as intraoperative guidance, emergency triage, and neuro-rehabilitation—are latency-sensitive and cannot rely solely on distant cloud infrastructures. Edge computing nodes positioned within hospitals, ambulances, and smart homes host localized inference services that deliver real-time analytics, contextual awareness, and adaptive XR feedback. This proximity between perception, intelligence, and immersion layers enables closed-loop clinical interactions, in which sensor inputs dynamically reshape immersive environments and therapeutic interventions. The integration of digital twins with bedside and home-based monitoring exemplifies this architectural logic. Patient-specific models running at the edge can continuously update immersive representations of physiological states, allowing clinicians to observe evolving risk patterns or treatment responses in near real time. In home settings, patients may engage with immersive rehabilitation environments or self-management dashboards that adapt to edge-processed biosignals, extending clinical intelligence beyond institutional walls while preserving responsiveness and privacy.

Latency-sensitive domains highlight the architectural necessity of edge-enabled immersion. In robotic or XR-assisted surgery, micro-delays can compromise procedural safety; in emergency medicine, immersive decision support must respond instantaneously to physiological deterioration; in rehabilitation, sensor-driven feedback loops shape neuroplastic outcomes. Architecturally, this requires dynamic task allocation between edge and federated layers, ensuring that time-critical inference remains local while longitudinal learning and population-level optimization occur across the network (Topol, 2019; Rieke et al., 2020).

3.4 Interoperability, Scalability, and Resilience

Interoperability, scalability, and resilience constitute the structural qualities that allow immersive healthcare architectures to function as long-term clinical infrastructures rather than experimental platforms. Microservices-oriented design principles enable modular healthcare metaverse ecosystems, in which sensing, modeling, federation, and immersion services evolve independently without destabilizing the whole. Such modularity supports rapid integration of new diagnostic modalities, AI models, and immersive tools, while preserving architectural coherence. Standards-based integration further anchors these systems in existing healthcare ecologies. The use of established clinical and imaging standards, alongside emerging digital twin schemas, ensures that immersive environments do not become isolated technological silos. Instead, they operate as connective tissues between electronic health records, AI services, and experiential interfaces, translating institutional data assets into embodied clinical intelligence spaces. This architectural stance aligns immersive healthcare with broader digital transformation trajectories rather than positioning it as a parallel domain (Topol, 2019).

Resilience emerges as a defining requirement of intelligent immersive healthcare. Fault tolerance mechanisms, redundant service orchestration, and continuous integrity monitoring must be embedded across layers to support continuity of care under technical failure, cyber threats, or crisis conditions. Federated architectures inherently contribute to resilience by avoiding single points of failure, while immersive interfaces provide adaptive situational awareness during disruptions. Architecturally, resilience is not an afterthought but a systemic property, ensuring that intelligent immersive healthcare ecosystems remain trustworthy, scalable, and clinically dependable over time (Bruynseels et al., 2018; Rieke et al., 2020). Organizational resilience in immersive systems parallels findings in digital transformation research, where integrated emerging technologies enhance agility and adaptability (Ruba et al., 2026c). Such interdisciplinary insights strengthen the case for embedding resilience as a systemic property of healthcare architectures.

4. CORE APPLICATION DOMAINS AND USE CASES

The convergence of artificial intelligence, immersive environments, digital twins, and privacy-preserving data infrastructures is transforming healthcare from a reactive, institution-centered system into a predictive, personalized, and distributed care ecosystem. Rather than functioning as isolated tools, these technologies increasingly operate as integrated socio-technical platforms that connect clinical intelligence, patient experience, and system-level coordination. In this context, healthcare innovation is not defined merely by automation, but by the emergence of continuous feedback loops between biological, behavioral, and computational systems. Core application domains are beginning to materialize where this convergence produces tangible clinical value, reshaping how diagnoses are made, therapies are designed, and care is delivered across physical and virtual spaces. Emerging healthcare applications also intersect with cybersecurity and IoT, as demonstrated in AI-based malware detection frameworks (Krithika et al., 2025), which emphasize the need for robust digital safeguards within immersive medical ecosystems. The following subsections examine four interrelated domains in which convergent technologies are already redefining healthcare capabilities: intelligent clinical decision support, digital twins and personalized therapeutics, remote patient monitoring and virtual care, and virtual hospitals with distributed care networks.

4.1 Intelligent Clinical Decision Support Systems

Intelligent clinical decision support systems (CDSS) represent one of the most mature and impactful application domains of AI-driven healthcare transformation. Contemporary CDSS platforms extend beyond rule-based alerts toward learning systems capable of synthesizing multimodal clinical data—including medical imaging, laboratory profiles, genomic markers, and unstructured clinical notes—to support diagnosis, treatment planning, and real-time risk stratification. Machine learning models trained on large-scale clinical datasets can identify latent patterns that exceed human perceptual capacity, enabling earlier detection of disease, more accurate prognostic assessments, and dynamic treatment optimization (Topol, 2019). Importantly, these systems do not replace clinicians but function as cognitive collaborators, augmenting professional judgment with continuously updated analytical insight. A defining characteristic of next-generation CDSS is immersive clinical visualization. Equally significant is the growing role of federated and privacy-preserving learning architectures in clinical intelligence. Healthcare data are structurally decentralized across hospitals, research centers, and national jurisdictions. Federated learning allows models to be trained across multiple institutions without transferring sensitive patient data, preserving local data governance while enabling collective intelligence formation. This paradigm not only enhances model generalizability but also mitigates ethical and legal concerns associated with centralized medical data repositories. As emphasized by Topol (2019), the long-term clinical value of AI depends less on algorithmic novelty than on trustworthy integration into healthcare workflows, where interpretability, accountability, and institutional interoperability become central design requirements.

4.2 Digital Twins and Personalized Therapeutics

Digital twins extend intelligent decision support by introducing dynamic, patient-specific computational replicas that simulate physiological, pathological, and behavioral processes over time. Unlike static risk models, medical digital twins continuously evolve, integrating real-world patient data from electronic health records, wearable sensors, imaging systems, and behavioral tracking platforms. These personalized models enable predictive simulation of disease trajectories and therapeutic interventions, allowing clinicians to test potential treatments in silico before applying them in vivo (Corral-Acero et al., 2020). In chronic disease management, oncology, and cardiovascular care, such simulation capabilities shift medicine from reactive intervention to anticipatory guidance.

Patient-specific digital twins facilitate a new paradigm of personalized therapeutics. By modeling how an individual's biological systems respond to pharmacological agents, lifestyle modifications, or surgical interventions, digital twins support precision dosing, adaptive therapy scheduling, and individualized rehabilitation protocols. They enable exploration of counterfactual clinical scenarios, such as how alternative treatments might alter long-term outcomes or how comorbidities interact under different care strategies. Corral-Acero et al. (2020) emphasize that the primary value of digital twins lies not in perfect biological replication but in their capacity to integrate heterogeneous data streams into coherent predictive frameworks that inform clinical reasoning.

4.3 Remote Patient Monitoring and Virtual Care

Remote patient monitoring and virtual care environments exemplify how convergent technologies dissolve the spatial boundaries of healthcare delivery. Wearable sensors, implantable devices, and ambient monitoring systems now generate continuous physiological and behavioral data streams, transforming episodic clinical encounters into longitudinal health narratives. AI-driven analytics interpret these data in real time, detecting anomalies, forecasting deterioration risks, and triggering early interventions. This shift is particularly transformative for chronic disease management, aging populations, and post-operative care, where continuous monitoring reduces hospital dependency while improving outcome responsiveness (Topol, 2019).

Metaverse-enabled telepresence clinics further extend remote care beyond video conferencing toward immersive clinical interaction. Through avatar-mediated consultation spaces and spatialized diagnostic interfaces, clinicians and patients can engage in environments that support physical rehabilitation, mental health therapy, and complex care coordination. Virtual embodiment facilitates social presence, procedural demonstration, and embodied cognition, which are critical for adherence, motivation, and therapeutic alliance. Home-based immersive rehabilitation and therapy illustrate the applied potential of these environments. Patients recovering from neurological injury, musculoskeletal disorders, or psychological trauma can participate in guided therapeutic scenarios that adapt dynamically to performance metrics and physiological responses. AI systems personalize difficulty progression, monitor adherence, and communicate progress to clinical teams. This model decentralizes rehabilitation infrastructures, reducing institutional burden while enhancing patient agency. Importantly, when embedded within privacy-preserving data ecosystems, remote care platforms foster scalable healthcare delivery without compromising ethical data stewardship.

4.4 Virtual Hospitals and Distributed Care Networks

Virtual hospitals and distributed care networks represent a systemic culmination of convergent healthcare technologies. Rather than single physical institutions, virtual hospitals function as orchestrated care ecosystems connecting immersive triage centers, AI-supported diagnostics, digital twin platforms, and globally distributed specialist expertise. Patients can enter these environments through local clinics, mobile devices, or home-based interfaces, where intelligent triage systems route them to appropriate care pathways based on real-time clinical analytics.

Immersive collaborative treatment hubs enable geographically dispersed clinicians to jointly assess complex cases, manipulate shared diagnostic visualizations, and coordinate intervention strategies. Cross-border specialist consultations become operationally seamless, addressing global disparities in medical expertise access. Such infrastructures are particularly valuable for rare diseases, complex surgeries, and multidisciplinary oncology care, where collective intelligence significantly improves diagnostic confidence and therapeutic planning. Virtual hospitals also enhance healthcare system resilience. During public health emergencies, disaster scenarios, or regional infrastructure collapse, distributed care networks support surge capacity through tele-ICU platforms, remote diagnostics, and digitally coordinated resource allocation. Rural inclusion is strengthened as remote communities gain access to advanced clinical services without geographic displacement. Over time, these distributed ecosystems may evolve into learning healthcare systems, where aggregated clinical experiences continuously refine predictive models, therapeutic protocols, and institutional policies. Crucially, the success of virtual hospitals depends not only on technological integration but also on governance frameworks that ensure accountability, interoperability, and ethical legitimacy. As Topol (2019) emphasizes, trust, transparency, and professional inclusion are prerequisites for sustainable digital medicine. Virtual hospitals therefore represent not merely technical infrastructures but socio-institutional transformations that redefine how healthcare systems conceptualize space, expertise, and care continuity.

5. INTELLIGENT TRAINING, COLLABORATION, AND MEDICAL EDUCATION

Intelligent immersive healthcare environments are reshaping how medical knowledge is produced, transmitted, and enacted in professional practice. No longer confined to lecture halls, cadaveric laboratories, or episodic bedside instruction, contemporary medical education increasingly unfolds within extended digital ecosystems that integrate virtual reality, artificial intelligence, and networked collaboration spaces. These environments enable clinicians and trainees to encounter complex clinical situations repeatedly, safely, and adaptively, cultivating experiential depth that traditional pedagogies often struggle to provide. At the same time, the growth of distributed intelligence infrastructures allows healthcare institutions to learn collectively, transforming isolated centers of expertise into interconnected knowledge ecologies. Within this context, training is not a discrete phase preceding professional work but a continuous, data-informed process embedded within everyday clinical life. Intelligent immersive healthcare thus reframes education as a living system—one that fuses simulation, real-time feedback, and collaborative cognition. This section examines how immersive clinical education, federated knowledge sharing, and metaverse-based collaboration jointly reconfigure medical formation, while emphasizing the principle that intelligent systems should augment, not replace, human clinicians.

5.1 Immersive Clinical Education

Immersive clinical education represents a fundamental shift from abstract learning toward embodied, situated cognition. Virtual anatomy platforms and procedural simulators allow learners to explore three-dimensional structures, rehearse complex interventions, and visualize dynamic physiological processes with a degree of interactivity that static textbooks or two-dimensional images cannot achieve. Such environments support repeated, self-paced practice, enabling trainees to make errors without patient risk and to internalize spatial and motor skills essential for clinical competence. Evidence from early and contemporary simulation research demonstrates that immersive training can translate into improved operative performance, procedural accuracy, and confidence, underscoring its value not merely as an adjunct but as a core educational modality (Seymour et al., 2002). Beyond replication of physical tasks, intelligent immersive platforms increasingly embed adaptive AI tutors capable of monitoring learner behavior, interpreting performance patterns, and tailoring instructional pathways. These systems can provide real-time feedback on technique, decision sequencing, and error profiles, generating personalized scaffolding that aligns with each learner's evolving competence. Such feedback loops shift assessment from episodic examinations to continuous skill analytics, where cognitive, psychomotor, and affective dimensions of performance are dynamically evaluated. Over time, immersive environments thus become living curricula, co-evolving with the learner and incorporating updated clinical guidelines, procedural innovations, and population-level insights derived from aggregated training data. This convergence of simulation and intelligent tutoring cultivates reflective practitioners who learn not only by doing, but by interpreting their own performance trajectories.

5.2 Federated Knowledge Sharing and Institutional Learning

While immersive education transforms individual formation, federated knowledge infrastructures expand learning to the institutional and inter-institutional level. Cross-hospital clinical intelligence networks enable geographically dispersed centers to contribute to and benefit from collective model development, pooling insights from diverse populations, workflows, and resource contexts. Rather than centralizing sensitive patient data, federated learning architectures allow algorithms to be trained locally within institutional boundaries and then aggregated through secure parameter sharing. This approach preserves privacy and regulatory compliance while still enabling robust, generalizable clinical intelligence (Rieke et al., 2020). Within such ecosystems, hospitals are no longer isolated silos of expertise but nodes in a continuously learning system. Diagnostic models, risk stratification tools, and treatment optimization engines can be iteratively refined as each participating institution contributes experience to a shared analytical fabric. For medical education, this translates into training environments that are constantly refreshed by real-world clinical patterns, rare case profiles, and emergent disease dynamics. Residents and practicing clinicians alike engage with simulations and decision-support tools that reflect the evolving state of collective medical knowledge rather than static curricular snapshots.

Federated infrastructures also support continuous professional upskilling. Intelligent platforms can detect shifts in practice standards, emerging technologies, or new evidence bases and integrate these developments into immersive modules and collaborative training sessions. In this way, professional development becomes an ongoing, embedded process, where clinicians update competencies through short, targeted, and contextually relevant learning experiences. Institutional learning thus extends beyond compliance-driven continuing education toward adaptive ecosystems that sustain clinical relevance across entire careers.

5.3 Collaborative Care in the Medical Metaverse

The emergence of medical metaverse environments introduces new possibilities for collaborative cognition. Immersive shared spaces allow multidisciplinary teams—physicians, nurses, radiologists, surgeons, therapists, and data scientists—to convene around richly visualized patient representations, integrating imaging, physiological streams, and procedural simulations into a unified perceptual field. Within these environments, participants can manipulate models, annotate findings, and rehearse intervention strategies together, cultivating shared situational awareness that supports synchronized decision-making. Such collaborative immersion is particularly valuable for complex, high-stakes cases that demand integration of heterogeneous expertise. Rather than sequential consultations mediated through reports and screens, clinicians engage in real-time co-presence, negotiating interpretations and treatment plans within a common experiential frame. This reduces fragmentation, shortens translational gaps between diagnosis and intervention, and supports collective sense-making. For trainees, participation in these environments offers early exposure to team-based reasoning and interprofessional communication, competencies increasingly recognized as central to patient safety and quality of care.

5.4 Augmenting Clinicians, Not Replacing Them

Despite their transformative potential, intelligent immersive systems must be grounded in human-centered design principles. The objective is not to displace clinicians but to amplify their cognitive reach, perceptual sensitivity, and empathic capacity. Intelligent tutors, federated models, and immersive collaboration spaces function as cognitive prostheses, supporting memory, pattern recognition, and situational awareness while leaving interpretive judgment, ethical reasoning, and relational care firmly in human hands. When well designed, such systems reduce documentation burdens, automate routine perceptual tasks, and surface clinically relevant insights, freeing clinicians to devote greater attention to patient interaction and complex reasoning.

Preserving empathy and professional identity within technologically dense environments is essential. Medical education must therefore integrate reflective practice, ethical discourse, and narrative competence alongside technical immersion. As Topol (2019) argues, the highest promise of intelligent healthcare lies in restoring time and attentional space for the human dimensions of medicine. Immersive and intelligent training environments, when aligned with this vision, can cultivate clinicians who are not only more technically proficient but also more present, collaborative, and responsive to the lived realities of patients.

6. ETHICAL, REGULATORY, AND GOVERNANCE DIMENSIONS

The convergence of artificial intelligence, immersive interfaces, and networked clinical infrastructures is reshaping how healthcare is delivered, governed, and experienced. Intelligent immersive healthcare systems—encompassing virtual reality therapies, augmented clinical visualization, metaverse-based care platforms, and AI-driven digital twins—introduce unprecedented opportunities for precision medicine and patient engagement, while simultaneously intensifying ethical, legal, and institutional risks. Unlike conventional digital health tools, immersive systems continuously capture biometric, behavioral, and affective data, blurring boundaries between clinical observation, everyday life, and algorithmic inference. This depth of datafication raises fundamental questions about who owns embodied health data, how consent can remain meaningful, and how algorithmic decisions can be made transparent in experiential environments. Moreover, governance challenges extend beyond technical compliance to include social justice, professional accountability, and regulatory coordination across domains that have historically evolved in isolation. Addressing these challenges is essential for building public trust and ensuring that immersive healthcare develops as a socially legitimate and ethically grounded clinical paradigm.

6.1 Data Sovereignty and Privacy

Data sovereignty constitutes a foundational ethical issue for intelligent immersive healthcare, as immersive systems depend on persistent streams of physiological, neurocognitive, spatial, and interactional data. These data are not merely clinical records; they are fine-grained representations of embodied experience that can reveal emotional states, cognitive vulnerabilities, and behavioral patterns. Ethical governance therefore requires moving beyond conventional notions of data protection toward stronger conceptions of ownership, informed consent, and algorithmic accountability. Patients must be recognized not only as data subjects but as stakeholders with ongoing rights to understand, control, and contest how their experiential data are collected and repurposed. Without such safeguards, immersive healthcare risks reproducing extractive data economies in which commercial or institutional actors disproportionately benefit from patient-generated information (Floridi et al., 2018).

Federated learning has emerged as a promising governance instrument for reconciling data-intensive innovation with privacy preservation. By enabling AI models to be trained across decentralized clinical datasets without transferring raw data to central servers, federated approaches can reduce exposure to breaches and unauthorized secondary use. In immersive healthcare contexts, federated architectures allow hospitals, rehabilitation centers, and even home-based systems to collaboratively improve predictive and adaptive algorithms while maintaining local data control. This model supports data sovereignty by embedding privacy into system design rather than treating it as a post hoc compliance requirement. However, federated learning does not eliminate ethical obligations; it shifts them toward ensuring transparency in model aggregation, accountability for distributed errors, and equitable participation across institutions (Rieke et al., 2020). Thus, data governance in immersive healthcare must integrate technical safeguards with enforceable rights frameworks that clarify custodianship, responsibility, and redress mechanisms.

6.2 Algorithmic Transparency and Clinical Trust

Clinical trust is inseparable from algorithmic transparency in intelligent immersive environments. When AI systems shape diagnostic visualizations, adaptive therapeutic scenarios, or real-time decision support within virtual or augmented spaces, clinicians and patients encounter algorithmic judgments as experiential realities rather than abstract recommendations. This intensifies the epistemic stakes of opacity. Black-box models embedded in immersive interfaces can obscure causal reasoning, limit professional oversight, and undermine informed consent, particularly when system outputs dynamically alter what users perceive or feel. Explainable AI therefore becomes a clinical and ethical necessity, enabling practitioners to interrogate how immersive systems generate predictions, personalize interventions, or simulate disease trajectories. Transparent models support professional accountability by aligning algorithmic outputs with established medical reasoning practices, rather than displacing them (Topol, 2019).

Auditability is equally critical in contexts where learning systems and digital twins evolve continuously. Immersive healthcare platforms often integrate patient-specific digital replicas that update in response to real-time data, supporting predictive modeling and treatment optimization. While such digital twins can enhance precision, they also complicate oversight: model drift, hidden biases, and feedback loops may gradually reshape clinical recommendations without clear documentation. Ethical governance therefore requires institutional mechanisms for logging training processes, validating updates, and enabling independent audits of immersive AI systems. Traceable learning pipelines, versioned digital twins, and standardized reporting of algorithmic changes are essential for preserving clinical reliability and medico-legal accountability. Without auditability, immersive healthcare risks creating epistemic environments in which neither clinicians nor regulators can fully explain how therapeutic realities are being constructed.

6.3 Equity, Access, and the Risk of Technological Stratification

The promise of immersive healthcare is often framed in terms of personalization and engagement, yet these benefits are unevenly distributed across socioeconomic, geographic, and infrastructural divides. High-fidelity immersive systems require advanced hardware, high-bandwidth connectivity, and specialized technical support, conditions that are not universally available. If unaddressed, these requirements may generate new forms of technological stratification, whereby affluent institutions and populations access cognitively rich, AI-enhanced care, while marginalized communities remain confined to conventional or under-resourced services. Such divergence risks embedding health inequities into the very architectures of future care delivery, contradicting foundational ethical commitments to justice and universal access (Floridi et al., 2018).

Designing inclusive metaverse health platforms demands both technical and institutional interventions. On the technical level, scalable system architectures, device-agnostic interfaces, and adaptive fidelity modes can lower entry barriers and support deployment across diverse clinical settings. On the institutional level, public investment, open standards, and cross-sector partnerships are necessary to prevent proprietary ecosystems from monopolizing immersive care infrastructures. Equity-oriented governance must also address representational justice: training datasets, avatar systems, and simulation models should reflect demographic diversity to avoid reinforcing diagnostic blind spots or cultural exclusions. By embedding inclusivity into design and procurement processes, healthcare systems can mitigate the risk that immersive technologies become amplifiers of existing disparities rather than instruments of expanded access.

7. CHALLENGES, LIMITATIONS, AND FUTURE RESEARCH DIRECTIONS

The rapid integration of advanced digital technologies—such as digital twins, federated learning, and immersive AI systems—into healthcare promises transformative benefits, including personalized care, predictive analytics, and enhanced clinical decision support. However, the deployment and maturation of these technologies face a constellation of technical, clinical, socio-technical, and ethical challenges that constrain their widespread adoption, reliability, and scalability. Addressing these multifaceted challenges is essential not only for improving performance and trust but also for paving future research directions that ensure equitable, secure, and effective healthcare innovation.

7.1 Technical and Infrastructure Challenges

A significant barrier to the large-scale deployment of immersive healthcare ecosystems is the technical and infrastructure limitations inherent to real-time, high-fidelity digital systems. Digital twins and associated IoT infrastructures require the seamless integration of heterogeneous data sources—including wearable sensors, electronic health records, medical imaging, and environmental data—to support real-time model updating and accurate simulation. However, the integration and harmonization of disparate data streams are technically complex and resource intensive, often hampered by the lack of industry-wide standards and disparate proprietary formats. This fragmentation undermines interoperability and complicates real-time data exchange between physical and virtual systems. Moreover, the computational overhead required to support low-latency communication and continuous model synchronization can exceed the capacity of existing healthcare IT infrastructure, particularly in resource-constrained settings. Such technical constraints lead to bottlenecks that reduce system responsiveness and scalability, ultimately limiting the feasibility of deploying these technologies at scale across varied clinical contexts (e.g., hospitals, remote monitoring) where latency, throughput, and robustness are critical. Additionally, the evolving threat landscape introduces cybersecurity risks in immersive healthcare ecosystems, as vast volumes of sensitive health data traverse networks. Securing these data flows while preserving system performance requires advanced encryption, intrusion detection, and robust governance architectures to mitigate breaches, unauthorized access, and potential exploitation by malicious actors. These challenges signal directions for research into resilient, standardized data frameworks and adaptive security solutions that ensure safe integration of heterogeneous healthcare systems without compromising performance.

7.2 Clinical Validation and Adoption Barriers

Technological feasibility alone is insufficient for clinical success; validation and adoption within healthcare workflows are equally critical. One key barrier is the lack of comprehensive clinical validation demonstrating that digital health models—including digital twins and AI systems—produce consistent, reliable outcomes across diverse patient populations and settings. Insufficient external validation and reproducibility hinder clinician confidence and regulatory approval, especially when model predictions could influence critical decisions such as diagnostics or therapy selection. Clinical stakeholders often raise concerns regarding the evidence-based integration into practice, as these technologies must not only demonstrate analytical performance but also clinical utility, safety, and added value compared to existing standards of care. Moreover, clinicians and health professionals may resist adoption if digital systems disrupt established workflows or require significant changes in practice without clear benefits. For example, real-time simulation tools that generate predictions must be interpreted and acted upon within clinical workflows that are already strained, necessitating redesigns that align with existing routines while minimizing cognitive load and operational friction. Resistance may be compounded by insufficient digital literacy among practitioners, perceived job displacement, or unfamiliarity with complex AI outputs—factors that underscore the importance of co-designing systems with end-users. Together, these issues highlight the imperative to bridge the gap between technological innovation and clinical trust through rigorous, transparent evaluation and stakeholder engagement.

7.3 Socio-Technical and Cultural Considerations

Beyond technical and clinical factors, the human dimension plays a pivotal role in the success of digital healthcare systems. Human–machine co-adaptation emerges as a central concern—effective integration of digital twins or AI assistants into healthcare requires not only technical integration but also adaptation by users over time. Clinicians and patients alike must learn to trust and collaborate with automated systems whose internal mechanisms may be opaque. Indeed, the "black-box" nature of many AI models can erode trust if users cannot interpret how conclusions are reached, leading to skepticism and reduced uptake. Transparent and interpretable models that respect ethical principles and provide intelligible explanations for their outputs are essential to foster engagement and psychological acceptance. Furthermore, trust, agency, and patient engagement are socio-cultural constructs that influence how populations interact with digital health tools. Patients may hesitate to rely on systems that continuously monitor personal health data without clear assurances regarding consent, data ownership, and the use of that data. Empowering patients with control over their data, clarifying expectations, and ensuring equitable access are therefore critical socio-technical research imperatives that extend beyond pure algorithmic development.

8. CONCLUSION

The future of healthcare lies not merely in the adoption of advanced technologies, but in the deliberate construction of intelligent, immersive systems that fundamentally reshape the way care is conceptualized, delivered, and experienced. As this chapter has demonstrated, the convergence of AI, federated learning, digital twins, and metaverse-enabled environments is catalyzing a transformation that extends beyond incremental improvements to create structurally adaptive medical ecosystems. Real-time, privacy-preserving clinical intelligence enables clinicians to make informed decisions with unprecedented speed and accuracy, while safeguarding sensitive patient information through federated and decentralized frameworks that maintain data sovereignty by design. Digital twin technologies offer a new dimension of personalized and predictive care, modeling patient-specific physiological responses and disease trajectories, thereby allowing interventions to be tailored to individual needs and circumstances, reducing both uncertainty and risk in clinical decision-making. Immersive platforms and collaborative virtual spaces further facilitate distributed healthcare delivery, connecting hospitals, research centers, and communities across geographic and institutional boundaries, thereby fostering resilience, resource optimization, and knowledge sharing in times of both routine operations and global health crises. Crucially, the integration of these technologies is inseparable from the principles of ethical governance, inclusivity, and clinical legitimacy; intelligent immersive healthcare cannot achieve its full potential without embedding mechanisms for transparency, accountability, and equitable access from the outset. By prioritizing trust and interoperability alongside technological performance, these next-generation systems empower clinicians not only as users but as active co-designers of adaptive care pathways, ensuring that human expertise and judgment remain central to patient outcomes. Furthermore, immersive healthcare environments have the potential to democratize access to high-quality care, extending the reach of specialized expertise to underserved populations and bridging disparities in health equity. This convergence also opens avenues for continuous learning and system-wide feedback loops, where insights generated through AI and patient simulations inform both clinical practice and operational decision-making, creating an evolving ecosystem capable of self-optimization. Ultimately, intelligent immersive healthcare represents more than a set of tools—it is a foundational pillar for the future of medicine, one that harmonizes technological sophistication with ethical stewardship, clinical reliability, and societal benefit. By embracing these principles, healthcare systems can transition from reactive, fragmented models to proactive, coordinated, and patient-centered ecosystems that anticipate and respond to needs dynamically, fostering resilience at both individual and institutional levels. In positioning performance, immersion, and trust as coequal priorities, the chapter underscores that the next generation of healthcare infrastructure must be adaptive, secure, and equitable, ensuring that innovation serves both clinical excellence and human well-being. In doing so, intelligent immersive healthcare promises not only to extend the boundaries of medical capability but also to redefine the very ethos of care—transforming healthcare into an ecosystem where technology, expertise, and ethical responsibility converge to deliver safer, more personalized, and universally accessible care across diverse populations. The realization of this vision demands ongoing interdisciplinary collaboration, regulatory foresight, and sustained investment in both digital and human capital, affirming that the evolution of healthcare is not solely a technological endeavor but a societal imperative.

REFERENCES

Barsom, E. Z., Graafland, M., & Schijven, M. P. (2016). Systematic review on the effectiveness of augmented reality applications in medical training. *Surgical Endoscopy*, *30*(10), 4174–4183. DOI: 10.1007/s00464-016-4800-6 PMID: 26905573

Bruynseels, K., Santoni de Sio, F., & Van den Hoven, J. (2018). Digital twins in health care: Ethical implications of an emerging engineering paradigm. *Frontiers in Genetics*, *9*, 31. DOI: 10.3389/fgene.2018.00031 PMID: 29487613

Corral-Acero, J., Margara, F., Marciniak, M., Rodero, C., Loncaric, F., Feng, Y., Gilbert, A., Fernandes, J. F., Bukhari, H. A., Wajdan, A., Martinez, M. V., Santos, M. S., Shamohammdi, M., Luo, H., Westphal, P., Leeson, P., DiAchille, P., Gurev, V., Mayr, M., & Lamata, P. (2020). The 'Digital Twin'to enable the vision of precision cardiology. *European Heart Journal*, *41*(48), 4556–4564. DOI: 10.1093/eurheartj/ehaa159 PMID: 32128588

Dhanushya, J., Ruba, M., Ponkarthika, M., Soundarya, B., Sakthi Priya, V., Dhanushri, S., & Harikrishnan, S. (2025, April). AI-Powered Multipurpose Agrobot for Precision Farming: Crop Health Management, Fertilizer Recommendation and Yield Prediction. In *2025 International Conference on Recent Advances in Electrical, Electronics, Ubiquitous Communication, and Computational Intelligence (RAEEUCCI)* (pp. 1-6). IEEE.

Esteva, A., Robicquet, A., Ramsundar, B., Kuleshov, V., DePristo, M., Chou, K., Cui, C., Corrado, G., Thrun, S., & Dean, J. (2019). A guide to deep learning in healthcare. *Nature Medicine*, *25*(1), 24–29. DOI: 10.1038/s41591-018-0316-z PMID: 30617335

Floridi, L., Cowls, J., Beltrametti, M., Chatila, R., Chazerand, P., Dignum, V., Luetge, C., Madelin, R., Pagallo, U., Rossi, F., Schafer, B., Valcke, P., & Vayena, E. (2018). AI4People—An ethical framework for a good AI society: Opportunities, risks, principles, and recommendations. *Minds and Machines*, *28*(4), 689–707. DOI: 10.1007/s11023-018-9482-5 PMID: 30930541

Gowthaman, N., Ruba, M., Aswath, S., Hemavarshni, S. N., Bragadeshwaran, R., & Nithish, S. J. (2025, November). Iot Integrated Solution For Smart Vertical Crop Cultivation. In 2025 IEEE 7th International Conference on Computing, Communication and Automation (ICCCA) (pp. 1-6). IEEE.

Kairouz, P., McMahan, H. B., Avent, B., Bellet, A., Bennis, M., Bhagoji, A. N., ... & Zhao, S. (2021). Advances and open problems in federated learning. Foundations and trends® in machine learning, 14(1–2), 1-210.

Kameswaran, A., Nanthakumar, K., & Ruba, M. (2017). High performance pre-computation based self-controlled precharge-free content-addressable memory. *Journal of Electronics and Communication Systems*, *2*, 1–9.

Krithika, S., Jayachandran, T., Raghapriya, N. R., Ruba, M., Janani, C., & Sathiyavathi, S. (2025, April). An Effective Denial of Service Texture Features from Malware Grayscale Image. In 2025 3rd International Conference on Artificial Intelligence and Machine Learning Applications Theme: Healthcare and Internet of Things (AIMLA) (pp. 1-7). IEEE. DOI: 10.1109/AIMLA63829.2025.11041501

McMahan, B., Moore, E., Ramage, D., Hampson, S., & Arcas, B. A. (2017, April). Communication-efficient learning of deep networks from decentralized data. In *Artificial intelligence and statistics* (pp. 1273–1282). PMLR.

Park, S. M., & Kim, Y. G. (2022). A metaverse: Taxonomy, components, applications, and open challenges. *IEEE Access : Practical Innovations, Open Solutions*, *10*, 4209–4251. DOI: 10.1109/ACCESS.2021.3140175

Poovithaa, M., Ruba, M., Ponkarthika, M., Ragul, N., Ragul, V., & Sangeetha, K. (2025, November). IoT Smart Traffic Control System for Hill Roads with Emergency Vehicle Priority. In 2025 IEEE 7th International Conference on Computing, Communication and Automation (ICCCA) (pp. 1-6). IEEE.

Rieke, N., Hancox, J., Li, W., Milletari, F., Roth, H. R., Albarqouni, S., Bakas, S., Galtier, M. N., Landman, B. A., Maier-Hein, K., Ourselin, S., Sheller, M., Summers, R. M., Trask, A., Xu, D., Baust, M., & Cardoso, M. J. (2020). The future of digital health with federated learning. *NPJ Digital Medicine*, *3*(1), 119. DOI: 10.1038/s41746-020-00323-1 PMID: 33015372

Ruba, M., Ashwin Prabhu, G., Deka, J., Kavitha, D., Sathiya, S., & Pavithra, S. (2026a). Empowering learners and educators: The transformative role of conversational AI in personalized education and student support. In Assayed, S. (Ed.), *Enhancing student support and learning through conversational AI* (pp. 163–190). IGI Global Scientific Publishing., DOI: 10.4018/979-8-3373-3316-8.ch007

Ruba, M., Ashwin Prabhu, G., Robinson Joel, M., Vishnu Priya, K., Dharshani, L., & Dharani, R. (2026b). Integrating emerging technologies for organizational agility: An interdisciplinary approach to digital transformation. In Roache, D. (Ed.), *High performance leadership for organizational excellence: Innovation, technology, and resilience* (pp. 63–92). IGI Global Scientific Publishing., DOI: 10.4018/979-8-3373-6207-6.ch003

Ruba, M., Girinath, V. P., Ponkarthika, M., Santhini, C., Sakthi Priya, V., & Hemalatha, R. (2023, December). Design and implementation of smart internet-based real-time control of rover with artificial intelligence. In *2023 International Conference on Energy, Materials and Communication Engineering (ICEMCE)* (pp. 1–5). IEEE. DOI: 10.1109/ICEMCE2023

Ruba, M., Ponkarthika, M., Parameshwari, V., Girinath, V. P., Soundarya, B., Janani, M., & Santhini, C. (2025, February). Enhancing underwater tunnel safety through smart inspection: An ROV-based system with AI-powered crack detection using Canny edge detection. In Proceedings of the 2025 3rd International Conference on Intelligent Systems, Advanced Computing and Communication (ISACC) (pp. 1067–1072). IEEE. DOI: 10.1109/ISACC.2025

Ruba, M., Preetha, D. S., Ponkarthika, M., Gomathi, V., Sudha, E., & Pratheeba, C. (2026c). Smart Pedagogies and Intelligent Campuses: Reimagining Higher Education in the Digital Age. In Harnessing Geospatial Information Systems for Sustainable Economic and Regional Development (pp. 29-54). IGI Global Scientific Publishing.

Santhini, C., Ruba, M., Sakthi Priya, V., & Hemalatha, R. (2025). Intercultural communication and assessment practices in the integration of AI with education. In *Generative AI Approaches to Sustainable Development in Higher Education*. IGI Global. DOI: 10.4018/979-8-3693-5623-4.ch010

Seymour, N. E., Gallagher, A. G., Roman, S. A., O'brien, M. K., Bansal, V. K., Andersen, D. K., & Satava, R. M. (2002). Virtual reality training improves operating room performance: Results of a randomized, double-blinded study. *Annals of Surgery*, *236*(4), 458–464. DOI: 10.1097/00000658-200210000-00008 PMID: 12368674

Shanmugaraja, T., Ruba, M., Priya, V. S., Venkatesh, T., Supriya, M., & Nallamuthu, M. (2023, September). ECG noise elimination using an FPGA version of a modified error normalized LMS adaptive filter. In AIP Conference Proceedings (Vol. 2764, No. 1, p. 060033). AIP Publishing LLC. DOI: 10.1063/5.0144367

Topol, E. (2019). *Deep medicine: how artificial intelligence can make healthcare human again.*

Topol, E. J. (2019). High-performance medicine: The convergence of human and artificial intelligence. *Nature Medicine*, *25*(1), 44–56. DOI: 10.1038/s41591-018-0300-7 PMID: 30617339

Chapter 4
Applications of Metaverse and AI in Remote Healthcare and Virtual Hospitals

Prasanthi Kumari Nunna
http://orcid.org/0000-0003-4131-1967
Department of SoCS, University of Petroleum and Energy, Studies, Dehradun, India

S. V. Shashikala
http://orcid.org/0000-0003-4543-0824
Department of Computer Science and Engineering, BGS Institute of Technology, Adichunchanagiri University, India

B. D. Darshan
http://orcid.org/0000-0002-0749-8302
Department of Electronics and Communication Engineering, SJB Institute of Technology, Kengeri, India

S. B. Sridhara
http://orcid.org/0009-0005-1929-3303
Department of Computer Science and Engineering, Amruta Institute of Engineering and Management Sciences, Bidadi, India

Madan Mohanrao Jagtap
http://orcid.org/0000-0001-6428-1241
Symbiosis Institute of Operations Management, Symbiosis International (Deemed to be) University, Pune, India

DOI: 10.4018/979-8-3373-8889-2.ch004

ABSTRACT

Remote healthcare delivery and virtual hospitals Metaverse and Artificial Intelligence (AI) introduce new opportunities in healthcare and transform the domain. This chapter discusses how these developing technologies can be used to revolutionize patient care, create virtual consultations, boost diagnostic precision, and update distance surgeries. The immersive virtual worlds of the Metaverse can improve remote delivery of services by healthcare professionals, and AI improves decision-making, optimization of workflow, and predictive analytics. AI and Metaverse can be used as a highly effective tool to educate patients, recover them, and monitor their health progress, creating a more favorable health outcome and becoming more accessible. Even with their potential, there are issues of data privacy, data security, patient acceptance, and regulatory frameworks challenges. The chapter is a survey of the existing applications, case studies and also an argument on the future direction of these technologies in remote healthcare.

INTRODUCTION

Telehealth and virtual hospitals have become an inseparable part of the contemporary healthcare environment wherein patients have an opportunity to access healthcare services outside the conventional physical borders. Remote healthcare is the provision of healthcare services to patients who are physically far away in relation to healthcare providers usually through telemedicine, mobile health applications and using online consultation devices. It is considered to enhance the ease of access, wait time, and spend on health care with the use of digital communication technologies. Virtual hospitals however, go a notch higher and actually emulate an entire functioning hospital setting in the virtual world(Jayapradha, J., Boovaneswari, S., Sabarivadivelan, S., Uvarajan, D., and Sarathi, S., 2023). These online resources make it possible to provide patients with a whole cycle of care, including consultations and diagnostics, as well as rehabilitation and surgery without the need to be physically located in a hospital.

Remote healthcare and virtual hospitals have become more important due to the emergence of various conditions and the need to address them. In other words, remote healthcare and virtual hospital have become especially important during global epidemics like the COVID-19 pandemic that showed the relevance of remote healthcare solutions. The technologies have enabled health practitioners to provide the necessary services and reduce the chances of exposure and resume making patients safe(Gupta, S., Sehgal, M., Makkar, R., Jain, S., and Rani, K., 2025). Moreover, remote healthcare can effectively fill the lack of physical healthcare centers in areas where it happens to be scarce, making the general quality of life of the underserved groups better. The virtual hospitals also expand on this to a more fulfilling experience of being at the hospital by making sure that the patients have 24-hour care in a smooth flow.

Figure 1. Integration of Metaverse and AI in Remote Healthcare and Virtual Hospitals

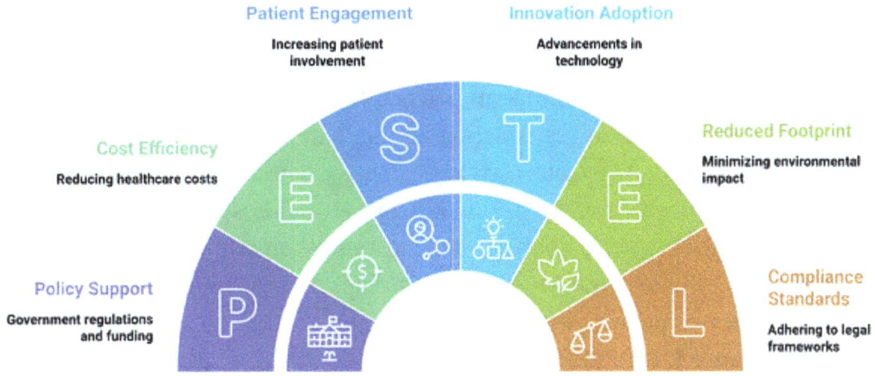

The Figure 1. shows how Metaverse and Artificial Intelligence (AI) technologies are integrated into the reality of Remote Healthcare and Virtual Hospitals. It brings out the functions of Virtual Reality (VR), Augmented Reality (AR), and 3D simulation, along with AI-inspired solutions, i.e., Machine Learning, Predictive Analytics, and Virtual Health Assistants. As demonstrated in the diagram, patient care, diagnostics, virtual consultation, medical training, and patient involvement in remote healthcare locations are synergistically connected with these technologies(Pratap, A., Patel, Y. S., Yadav, R. N., Ahmadian, A., and Yadav, A. K., 2025).

The adoption of emerging technologies, specifically the Metaverse and Artificial Intelligence (AI), is taking a central role in the revolution in healthcare delivery. The digital world called the metaverse is built on the premise of immersive technology i.e. virtual reality (VR), augmented reality (AR) and 3D simulations, has introduced new patterns of interaction between patients and medical professionals in an online community. It is possible because the Metaverse allows patients to appoint healthcare professionals, engage in treatment, or even get medical education by creating real and intertwined virtual environments and allowing patients to do it. It is especially handy to patients that are unable to utilize geographical barriers, movement impairments, and individual decisions physically by going to healthcare centers in person.

Artificial Intelligence (AI) is another technology of change that alters the healthcare sector and transforms the healthcare industry(Wen, B. et al., 2025). It is a technology capable of enhancing the decision-making process, diagnosis and workflow optimization. With the implementation of machine learning (ML) algorithms to perform tasks, the system will be able to search the large quantities of structured medical data, identify patterns and provide insights that can be utilized in practical directions by the health workers. One of the fields, where these AI-based applications are applied in the diagnosis of conditions and the monitoring of vital signs of patients and, as an illustration, the determination of their health risks based on real-time information is remote healthcare(Sakharwade, V. R., Urkude, O. P., Thakur, S., Lokulwar, P., and Dasarwar, P., 2025). Additionally, AI has become the means to have virtual health assistants and chatbots that could advise patients timely, assist them in their appointments and health tracking, and therefore, increase the degree of engagement and satisfaction among patients.

The Metaverse and AI create a strong synergy when used together and this improves the functions of remote healthcare and virtual hospitals. In other words, AI algorithms will be able to analyze medical images in real-time and assign accurate diagnoses, whereas the Metaverse can display said solutions in the virtual setting that immerses patients into recognizing their conditions and their treatment methods(Rahman, M. A. and Al-Hazzaa, S., 2024). Also, AI can be used in managing virtual hospital systems, enabling healthcare providers to manage resources, appointments and appointments and among other initiatives, provide timely care to patients. The synergistic effect between the two technologies would be the improved mechanism of delivering healthcare, which would be more interactive, efficient, and personalized.

In addition to that, the application of the Metaverse and AI is not limited to the care of the patient. The medical training and education have been invaluable with such types of technologies. Virual settings enable health care workers to practice surgeries, perform medical procedures and train on their skills within a safe and controlled setting(G et al., 2025). The other significant input is AI to training whereby it aids the learning process with predictive analytics and real-time feedbacks which in effect makes the learning process more expressive. The medical field of remote locations is the area where this virtual, AI-based training system would come in handy since some healthcare personnel may lack state-of-the-art training facilities.

The intersection of the Metaverse and AI are vast in the potential of breaking down the drawback of traditional healthcare models. With such technologies, there are cheaper and more accessible and efficient healthcare solutions and there is less reliance on any physical infrastructure and areas are covered so that patients have access to healthcare regardless of where they are. Nevertheless, along with having a potential, there is the issue of data protection, confidentiality of patient information, and the necessity of regulatory conditions to regulate these technologies. It must be noted that the implementation of the Metaverse and AI in healthcare should be ethical and safe with regard to patient safety and the quality of care.

TECHNOLOGIES BEHIND REMOTE HEALTHCARE AND VIRTUAL HOSPITALS

The concept of metaverse in healthcare is the new one that transforms the process of delivering and experience of healthcare. The simplest definition of the Metaverse is the combination of computers and technologies such as the virtual world and interactive reality of a virtual reality (VR) and an augmented reality (AR) as a shared and immersive virtual world. These virtual worlds allow the users to have interaction with the computer based spaces and objects in a highly interactive and real interaction. The Metaverse has new solutions in practice that can be used in the area of healthcare offering improved medical training and increased care received by the patient. It facilitates virtual meetings that provide health practitioners to interact with patients in a manner that imitates the face-to-face interaction, irrespective of the geographical location. By utilizing the VR headsets and AR devices, physicians will be able to perform remotely, to take a look at the symptoms, and give a diagnosis without a physical visit of a health center in person(Bhattacharya, P., Obaidat, M. S., Savaliya, D., Sanghavi, S., Tanwar, S., and Sadaun, B., 2022). This will be useful especially to the patients in isolated or underserved areas where the number of health care professionals is scarce.

Moreover, the Metaverse continued to extend into virtual surgeries and monitoring of patients. Virtual surgeries enable the medical personnel to train and rehearse on their surgical expertise in simulated settings whereby it is given to make sure that the operations are done perfectly and with speed. The surgeons are able to do extremely detailed virtual simulation of complex surgeries, therefore, perfecting their techniques prior to deployment in the real world. Furthermore, remote monitoring is an area where the Metaverse can be implemented so that the health data of patients can be acquired and displayed in 3D virtual spaces. In a virtual space, real-time patient data, including vital signs, diagnostic images(Nivedhitha, D. P., Madhumitha, G., Janani Sri, J., Jayashree, S., Surya, J., and Divya, D. M., 2024), and so on, are visualized, so healthcare providers can view patients and assess their condition in real-time and make well-informed decisions, even when they are not present in the same location. This blending of the digital technologies does not only advance patient care by increasing the accessibility of healthcare but also training and development of medical professionals.

The other groundbreaking technology that is altering the dynamics of care provision in health care is the application of Artificial Intelligence (AI) in the healthcare sector. There is a large range of technologies in AI, including machine learning (ML), natural language processing (NLP), predictive analytics, and decision support systems, all of which will be useful in building healthcare capacities. Machine learning is an aspect of AI that involves training algorithms to cause large volumes of information to spot patterns able to aid with medical diagnosis, patient prognosis and personalized therapy(Hussain, S. F. M., Karthikeyan, R., Ramamoorthi, S., Arafat, I. S., and Asif, N. A. H., 2024). To take some examples, medical imaging data (X-rays, MRIs, etc.) can be processed by ML algorithms, and their abnormalities (tumors or fractures, etc.) can be discovered with great accuracy.

NLP is an important part of AI applications that have facilitated computers to process and comprehend human language. NLP is applied in the field of healthcare where it is utilized to process unstructured medical documents by analyzing doctor-patient notes or research articles and extracting useful information. Through such analysis, the AI systems can offer insights to the health care givers on the past history of the patients, make decisions and even offer treatment choices. The other technology that is based on AI is predictive analytics which helps predict health outcomes based on the historical and real-time data to determine the probability of disease progressing or a patient readmission. Predictive analytics can be used to provide early detection of high-risk patients to facilitate proactive intervention and positively impact patient outcomes and minimize healthcare expenses.

Decision support system (DSS) also improves the functionality of AI and offers insights and recommendations in real-time to healthcare professionals using patient data. These systems combine existing health records of patients, the medical literature, with the clinical guidelines to aid in decision-making. Indicatively, AI-driven DSS can recommend tailored treatment plans, notify physicians of possible drug interactions, or assist in the determination of the most optimal course of action in case of an emergency. The ability of AI to compute complex health data promptly and appropriately helps to promote the efficiency of the health care system and reduce the number of human errors and allow patients to receive care and quality care in a timely manner.

The integration of the Metaverse and the AI leads to the opportunities of both technologies, which translates into a more effective and better healthcare experience. AI can be utilized to enhance the Metaverse with intelligent mechanisms of giving better patient care and health delivery in the virtual worlds. Virtual assistants can be considered one of the most important parameters of AI implementation in the Metaverse(Yamuna, V., Babu, G. S., Raju, V. A. G., Manchala, Y., Ramakrishna, G., and Savalapurapu, K., 2024). The AI assistants can offer personal assistance to patients (i.e. coaching them through medical procedures, health advice, or answer questions regarding their illness) and can offer personalized care. Healthcare providers can more effectively perform their work because virtual assistants in the Metaverse can process patient data and track symptoms in real-time, and give feedback to healthcare providers, which can be more accurate and efficient.

The automation of the diagnostics in the Metaverse is also achieved by AI. As an illustration, the use of AI can process medical images or patient information and give medical workers specific diagnostic information at once(Kahalkar, K. and Vyas, U., 2024). This saves the manual analysis, shortens diagnostic process, and enhances accuracy of the results. Indicatively, AI algorithms have the ability to identify abnormalities in radiology pictures prompting the development of a disease such as cancer or heart diseases at earlier stages thus resulting in improved treatment results.

Figure 2. Synergy of Metaverse and AI in Transforming Remote Healthcare

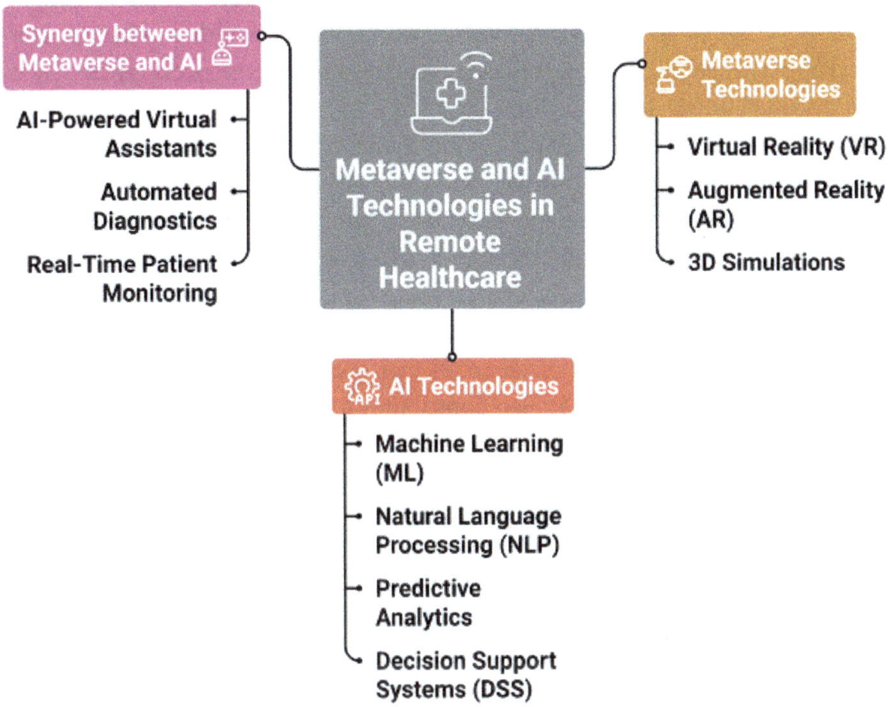

Figure.2. sheds light on interdependence between the technologies of the Metaverse and AI in the setting of remote healthcare and virtual hospitals. It describes how the aspects of the Metaverse (Virtual Reality (VR), Augmented Reality (AR), and 3D simulations) have evolved to provide interactive virtual medical set ups. It also demonstrates how AI technologies, such as Machine Learning, Natural Language Processing (NLP), Predictive Analytics, and Decision Support Systems, can help to increase the accuracy of diagnostics and patient monitoring. The diagram shows a collaboration between these technologies to streamline healthcare delivery because they help in virtual consultation, real-time monitoring of the patient, and automated diagnostics and eventually enhancing patient outcomes and efficiency of healthcare delivery.

Further, patient monitoring in virtual space can be performed in real-time by implementing AI. AI codes can constantly monitor the vital signs of a patient including heart rate, blood pressure and oxygen concentration and indicate them in a 3D virtual world. This data will be available to health care providers even when they are not at the hospital and they will be able to monitor the conditions of patients in real time, hence being able to act in cases where action is needed. This is especially useful in the management of chronic diseases since they are able to monitor the patient at all times without having to visit her all the time. Moreover, predictive analytics, including the ability to detect the possible worsening of health conditions, can be offered by AI when medical practitioners work to prevent the occurrence of severe cases, taking action before it becomes too late.

The Metaverse and AI intersection are transforming healthcare provision into one that is more personal, data-driven and immersive to the providers and patients. Three-dimensional processing and analysis of large amounts of medical data under the authority of AI upgrade the interactive nature of the virtual spaces in the Metaverse, which will allow healthcare providers to make more successful decisions, communicate with patients, and accept the use of the new technology and provide high-quality medical care at a distance. Not only can such integration lead to improved clinical outcomes, but it also contributes to the creation of new models of healthcare, which would be more accessible, scalable, and efficient.

LITERATURE SURVEY

Metaverse Applications in Healthcare

Metaverse has greatly become an disruptive tool in the medical industry, which has offered innovative solutions in various fields. The current literature and the real case studies on how the Metaverse can be applied in the health sector has indicated the power of the innovation in redesigning the patient care model, healthcare education, and medication. A well-known example of applying the Metaverse to the sphere of healthcare is virtual consultations due to which healthcare professionals are able to conduct distance consultations in the fully virtual reality. (Vaidhehi, M., Malathy, C., Sudhakaran, P., Cherian, A. K., Geetha, R., And Kumar, G. M., 2025) show that VR-based telemedicine systems can help patients interact with physicians in simulated setting with the ability to mimic face-to-face interactions. These platforms provide patients with the benefit of consulting with the specialists without considering their geographical location, thereby facilitating healthcare and in particularly the rural and underserved areas.

Besides consultations, VR-based therapy empowers the Metaverse in dealing with these types of conditions, including post-traumatic stress disorder (PTSD), anxiety, and chronic pain. Clinical trials have revealed VR therapy to be effective in treating psychological conditions through the means of throwing the patient in controlled virtual environments where they can engage their symptoms and manage them in a safe environment. In (Malviya, R., Verma, S., Sundram, S., and Shah, H., 2025), the authors researched the VR exposure therapy among people with PTSD and revealed that the immersive feature of the Metaverse is a considerable part of the healing experience.

Metaverse has also achieved quite a lot in medical training. The virtual environments enable the medical professionals to rehearse the procedures or improve their skills and can even conduct mock surgeries without the risks involved in the live training. (Gupta et al., 2025). observes that virtual simulations prove to be very valuable to surgical training where complex procedures can be practiced in a risk-free environment. These simulations have become more popular in the training of minimally invasive surgeries and this provided a practical learning experience without putting the patients at risk. Moreover, the virtual learning environments have improved patient education where patients can consider medical procedures, or comprehend their conditions well leading to increased patient engagement and health literacy.

AI Applications in Remote Healthcare

Remote healthcare using Artificial Intelligence (AI) has received significant focus since it ensures a high level of diagnostic accuracy, improved patient care, or healthcare accessibility. One of the most important fields, where AI has been introduced, is telemedicine, allowing medical professionals to diagnose, monitor, and treat a patient remotely. Artificial intelligence is used to analyze patient information, medical images and health records to give relevant diagnosis and prescriptions. Machine learning (ML) algorithms can, as an example, interpret radiological images (X-rays, MRIs, etc.) with nearly the same accuracy as experienced radiologists. A study by (de Alwis et al., 2023) established how deep learning algorithms can be enabled to detect human professionals in detecting skin cancer in images hence proving the role of AI in improving the accuracy of diagnostic decisions in remote health care environments.

We have the growing popularity of virtual health assistants based on artificial intelligence to offer 24/7 support to patients, assist in making appointments, health consultation and even in administering drugs. As they are built on natural language processing (NLP) and machine learning adoption they offer patients a conversational interface to answer their questions and concerns regarding their health. It has also been shown that AI-Based assistants can fulfill common health-related tasks in a relatively cheaper way, which could eliminate the administrative burden of healthcare professionals simultaneously increasing patient satisfaction (Kaur, R., Singh, B., and Kumar, R., 2025).

Another most important domain of AI use in remote healthcare is predictive healthcare system. These systems rely on big data and up to date patient data in order to predict the potential health risks to offer precedent treatment and primary intervention. Artificial intelligence (AI) is able to study the trends in patient behavior, medical history and lifestyle to predict conditions like heart disease, diabetes or sepsis. One example of a study that underlines the potential of predictive algorithms to predict adverse patient outcomes to enable healthcare providers to take control beforehand and enhance patient care management, especially in underserved or remote locations with potentially limited access to healthcare is available in the study by (Chauhan, H., Rawat, K., Kaur, G. K., Kumar, P., Joshi, N., and Singla, S., 2025).

Integration of Metaverse and AI

Metaverse and AI matter in healthcare are a relatively new intervention, but this is set to introduce significant alterations in healthcare provision. The application of both technologies simultaneously can produce all-encompassing virtual hospital models that provide long-distance care and medical services with references to the data processing and decision-making skills of AI. According to a study by (Kumar, A., Kalpana, V., and Hariram, V., 2023), virtual hospital systems may mimic a real-life medical setting and, in this case, AI algorithms help to diagnose, monitor, and treat patients. This kind of systems can lead to more personalized care, depending on the current patient data, AI-based insights and virtual medical environments which would enable healthcare practitioners to deliver effective care remotely.

One more significant example of AI-assisted virtual tenders of remote surgery is an integration of the Metaverse and AI. They are also able to empower surgeons to carry out their surgeries in distant areas, with the AI technologies that can act as a live tracker of the patient and suggest surgical interventions. The robotic surgery system is an illustration of the application of AI, such as the Da Vinci Surgical System, in which a surgeon is able to perform a surgery on a patient remotely, and their analytics and guidelines are real time and artificial intelligence (AI) assisted. The authors in a study by (Thangalakshmi, S., Mohankumar, N., Jayanthi, L. N., Blessy, Y. M., Meenakshi, R., and Rajmohan, M., 2025) have demonstrated that AI can enhance the precision of robotic surgeries in the virtual environment that offers surgeons with the technologies required to execute the complex procedures in a distance mode.

A more promising field in which the convergence of Metaverse and AI is set to do is AI-assisted virtual rehabilitation. The Metaverse immersive environments permit the patients to engage in their physical and mental activities in virtual rehabilitation programs and the AI monitors the progress of these patients and modifies the rehabilitation program on the basis of the real-time information. Just-in-time, customized therapy, which may also be distanced, might be conducted within this mix, and it is easier to provide patients of rehabilitation treatment where they might be, in the convenience of making their homes. According to a study led by (Ghosh, S., Bhuniya, T., and Sona, D. R., 2025), AI-based virtual rehabilitation training has found its way to be useful in managing stroke recovery and musculoskeletal disease management.

Challenges and Limitations

Although the Metaverse and AI hold significant potential in healthcare, it is possible to identify multiple challenges and limitations, which must be overcome. One of the major obstacles in the wide application of these technologies is technological drawbacks. Developing a high-quality VR/AR hardware and AI systems can be expensive, so their introduction may be restricted to several healthcare providers and patients only due to their complexity and cost. Also, some of the technical infrastructure to be used in real-time processing of data and the immersive virtual environment may not be available in all areas, especially when the resources are low.

The privacy and security of data is another major issue that may be raised in the topics of integrating AI and the Metaverse into healthcare. The abundance of personal health data stored in the process of virtual consultation, patient monitoring, and AI-advanced diagnostics creates a concern about the possible breach and misuse of the personal information occupied by the database. The protection and privacy of patient information are key factors and especially when using virtual environments where intrusion may result in sensitive health information being misused. Regulations Have to be changed to accommodate these issues and to make sure that patient information is secured as per the privacy provisions and standards including the Health Insurance Portability and Accountability Act (HIPAA).

The other issue that should be accommodated in order to have the successful implementation of AI and the Metaverse in healthcare is the patient acceptance. Several patients might be reluctant to embrace emerging technologies, particularly those that require virtual environments, according to the issue of effectiveness, safety, or failure to have personal contact with health caretakers. It is important to ensure that such technologies are easy to use and that the patients feel comfortable with them in order to ensure their general implementation. Moreover, healthcare providers should be educated to incorporate such technologies in practice so that they could provide patient-centered care of high quality.

Lastly, the regulatory aspects are also an important issue in the implementation of AI and the Metaverse in healthcare. Regulatory conditions of digital health technologies are dynamic, and healthcare systems have to operate under complicated legal and ethical challenges on using AI in decision-making, virtual consultation, and remote monitoring. There must be some form of guidelines and standards to make sure that these technologies are applied in a safe and ethical environment in a healthcare facility that also keeps the patient trust and safety intact.

APPLICATIONS OF METAVERSE AND AI IN REMOTE HEALTHCARE

Virtual Consultations and Telemedicine

Incorporation of the Metaverse into healthcare is transforming Internet-mediated medical consultants and telemedicine through the offering of active, immersive settings involving medical people and patients alike. In contrast with outdated telemedicine, where a video call and a text-based interaction are the guidelines, the Metaverse allows the usage of fully immersive consultation based on the technologies of Virtual Reality (VR) and Augmented Reality (AR). These locations recreate the feel of face-to-face consultations, as the patients can communicate with medical workers using a simulated and 3D environment. This simulation and immersion provides a more personalized and interactive experience to the patient studying, thus improves general patient care.

The Metaverse enables patients to have virtual consultations that enable them to be treated by a specialist who may be geographically remote. As an illustration, a patient in a remote location will have the ability to adopt a VR headset and get transported to a virtual healthcare facility where he or she can meet with a doctor in a simulated location. It has been shown that this model is capable of enhancing patient satisfaction because it offers a more real experience than conventional telemedicine as it offers a more physical visit experience. In addition, medical workers may use AR to provide medical conditions or treatment alternatives in a visual form that will contribute to a better patient comprehension. AR can be used to offer patients a better perspective on their conditions and treatments shedding light on the digital information onto real-world imagery thereby enhancing patient engagement in decision-making significantly(Jain, P. and Chawla, P., 2021). The integration of the Metaverse and the Artificial Intelligence (AI) makes the process of the virtual consultation even more beneficial. With the help of AI-driven systems, medical history and symptoms can be analyzed, and given to the patient, and help a healthcare provider diagnose the conditions more easily. The consultations can be made more effective and personal because AI algorithms are able to even propose particular treatment plans or track the patient reactions in real time. Moreover, AI-based chatbots, virtual assistants could talk to the patient prior to or following the consultation, could provide some support and answer questions and questions, depending on the medical information provided by the latter, thereby benefiting the overall process of care.

Remote Monitoring and Diagnostics

Artificial intelligence in combination with the Metaverse enables remote monitoring and diagnosis of patients and is able to present a healthcare professional with strong tools to evaluate the progress of patients, analyze health data, and provide interventions in time. With the combination of virtual health care setting with AI powered tools, constant and real-time observation of patient vitals and conditions is achievable. Wearable devices (smartwatches or bio sensors) gather patient information, including heart rate and blood pressure, oxygen more than a person needs, and other vital signs. The Metaverse transmits this data to the healthcare provider, where it can be visualized in an immersive environment which is 3D.

Doctors can analyze the information in real-time and make informed decisions in a virtual setting in healthcare on the basis of the current health condition of a patient. AI algorithms are used to help analyze high amounts of health data and identify anomalies and possible health threats. As an example, AI systems may identify anomalies during vital signs monitoring and recommend interventions that health professionals may implement in a timely manner and avert medical emergencies. Machine learning could help establish patterns in the health history of patients overtime, which allows the detection of chronic diseases, including diabetes or heart diseases, as well as proactive care. These remote the monitoring systems can considerably decrease the frequency of in-person visits thereby ensuring comfort to the patients and creating a lesser burden to the healthcare facilities. Also, AI-powered diagnostics is turning into an important component of distance care. With the deep learning and computer vision, AI can be used to analyze medical images, including X-rays, CT, and MRIs, and identify diseases and conditions that cannot be seen by the naked eye. There is a meta-verse environment, where the medical community can see these images in 3D and obtain a more comprehensive and lively picture of the patient condition. This combination of AI with the Metaverse will increase the accuracy of diagnoses, decrease the number of errors, and make healthcare more efficient and effective by monitoring the progress of the patient remotely.

Virtual Surgery and Rehabilitation

The virtual surgery and rehabilitation opportunities through the Metaverse and AI technologies have brought new possibilities, and now healthcare providers have the option to conduct remote surgery and overall rehabilitation, without requiring patients to be physically present in the medical facility. One such field is virtual surgery, which is actively being introduced to remotely perform a surgery by means of robotic surgery systems that become more AI-assisted. Through these systems, the surgeon will be able to work on the patients who are located thousands of miles away, commanding robotic tools via the virtual interface which is then controlled by the AI-driven feedback and real-time data analysis. One of the most famous examples of the robotic system with AI involved in the surgery is the da Vinci Surgical System that was implemented to improve the precision and accuracy of the surgery. Surgeons in a virtual setting can view the anatomy of the patient in 3D, which is performed more accurately even when at a distance.

The emergence of the Metaverse and AI in training surgical practitioners also advances this profession even further as the future surgeon is able to drill and hone their skills in a simulated setting. Surgeons are able to conduct virtual surgery in a safe atmosphere acquiring a practical experience with complicated procedures. AI algorithms offer feedback in real-time, which assists practitioners in enhancing the practice and minimizing mistakes. In a study conducted by (Jayasree, A., Gayatri, T., Vaishnavi, L., Jyothi, N. V. S. K. A., Pujitha, M., and S. I. S. P., 2025), such a type of virtual training enables surgeons to improve their skills in procedures without the risks of the conventional practices.

Another important use of the Metaverse in remote care is virtual rehabilitation. Following surgery or even experiencing a physical trauma, patients are able to participate in programs of rehabilitation by means of immersive, AI-controlled virtual environments. The programs will be designed as per the needs and progress of the patient, and AI constantly evaluates and changes the exercises. An example is that AI can track the movements of the patient and provide feedback to make him/her sit better, become stronger, or have a broader range of motion. These virtual rehabilitation services are specialty useful to patients who have gone through stroke, orthopedic surgery operations or those with neural conditions. In virtual environments, patients are able to do rehabilitation exercises at the comfort of their homes and this increases compliance to treatment program and accelerates recovery.

Patient Education and Engagement

This intersection of the Metaverse and AI can revolutionize the process of patient education by introducing interactive and engaging settings in which patients can learn about their health status and treatment methods actively. Traditionally, patient education is usually done by use of brochure materials or oral communication which may not necessarily be the most efficient in getting patients to understand. Nonetheless, the Metaverse will form virtual learning systems in which patients can go through medical practices or media of their illnesses as simulations. VR and AR allow patients to view the operation of their bodies, what occurs during an operation, or the effects of a specific drug on their health, which contributes to the increased awareness of their health and treatment regimes.

The AI technologies can advance the area of patient education to a higher level by offering personalized content with references to personal health data and interests. In one example, AI-based systems can propose certain educational modules or interactive situations in order to enable the patient to comprehend their conditions more. Furthermore, the virtual assistants based on AI are able to find answers, explain, teach their patients on complicated medical terms and make sure that patients are not left with a vague picture on what they can do with the treatment they have. A study by (Misal, S. R., Mohan, L., Sundararajan, S. K., Bathala, B., Majumdar, S., and Sivakumar, C., 2025) has shown that these interactive virtual education programs increase patient engagement and retention of information and adherence to treatment.

Besides that, the Metaverse enables patients to engage in health-related activities in a gamified environment to motivate them to take charge of their health care. Within the virtual environments, one can acquire the simulation of a scenario where the patients can be trained the method of managing their ailments such as diabetes through following diet regimes, performing exercises, or checking blood sugar levels. The performance analysis is collected by AI, and the program can be adjusted to their requirements and provide feedback. This bi-directional process does not only enhance learning, but it also enables the patients to make the right decisions about their health and well being.

RESULTS AND DISCUSSION

Healthcare is already experiencing the transformative nature of these technologies by the integration of metaverse and AI technologies in healthcare through several successful pilot initiatives and case studies where these technologies have been employed in health care. One of the examples is the Virtual Hospital Project in Europe, which utilized the usage of the Metaverse when using remote consultations, where patients could submit their medical practitioners in the 3D virtual space. The application of AI to the diagnostic support was highly critical, the patient data such as medical images and patient history was analyzed using the assistance of AI. These pilot programs have been effective in minimizing wait time and enhancing access to healthcare particularly among the patients in the rural or underserved regions. Furthermore, AI-based diagnostic systems have been already introduced into hospitals to process medical imaging to obtain a faster and more efficient diagnosis, as papers such as (Chowdhury et al., 2025) have shown that AI performs better in diagnosing skin cancer than radiologists do.

More recent development of VR hardware, AI algorithms, and cloud infrastructure have played a major role in enhancing the efficacy of telehealth and virtual hospitals. Indicatively, VR headsets currently have high-resolution screens, enhanced motion tracking, and are more portable, which makes virtual consultations more realistic and more affordable. Medical image analysis and predictive healthcare algorithms performed by AI have become more precise and contribute to a more personalized treatment recommendation and a better patient care. These technologies have also been increased by cloud infrastructure which offers scalable solution to data storage and real time processing that makes virtual hospital and remote healthcare solutions to be deployed effectively.

Figure 3 explains the Remote Patient Monitoring of heart rate and oxygen saturation time-wise. The plot depicts the new and developing technologies in AI and Metaverse to provide real-time monitoring of vital indicators of a patient, including oxygen saturation and heart rate. These measurements are modeled to last 24 hours proving the possibility of virtual healthcare platforms to track the health of patients remotely so that healthcare professionals could intervene in cases when it was necessary according to the AI-driven assessment of the information.

Figure 3. Remote Patient Monitoring (Heart Rate and Oxygen Saturation) Over Time

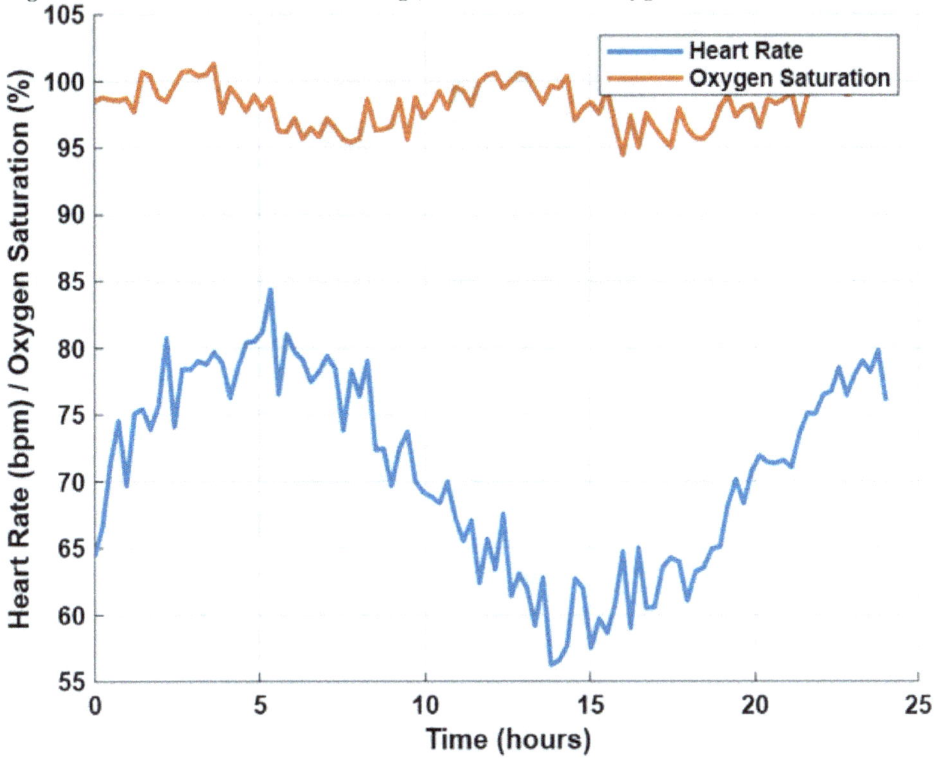

Figure 4 characterizes the AI Diagnostics of Medical Imaging whereby the diagnostic ability of AI models and human professionals are compared. The bar chart contrasts the effectiveness of AI and human diagnostics to tell about medical conditions, as it is in the case of skin cancer in imaging, the accuracy of AI diagnostics is greater. This underscores the possibility that AI can be used to complement or even surpass the human diagnostic powers, as it makes the provision of healthcare more accurate and effective.

Figure 4. AI Diagnostics for Medical Imaging (Accuracy Comparison)

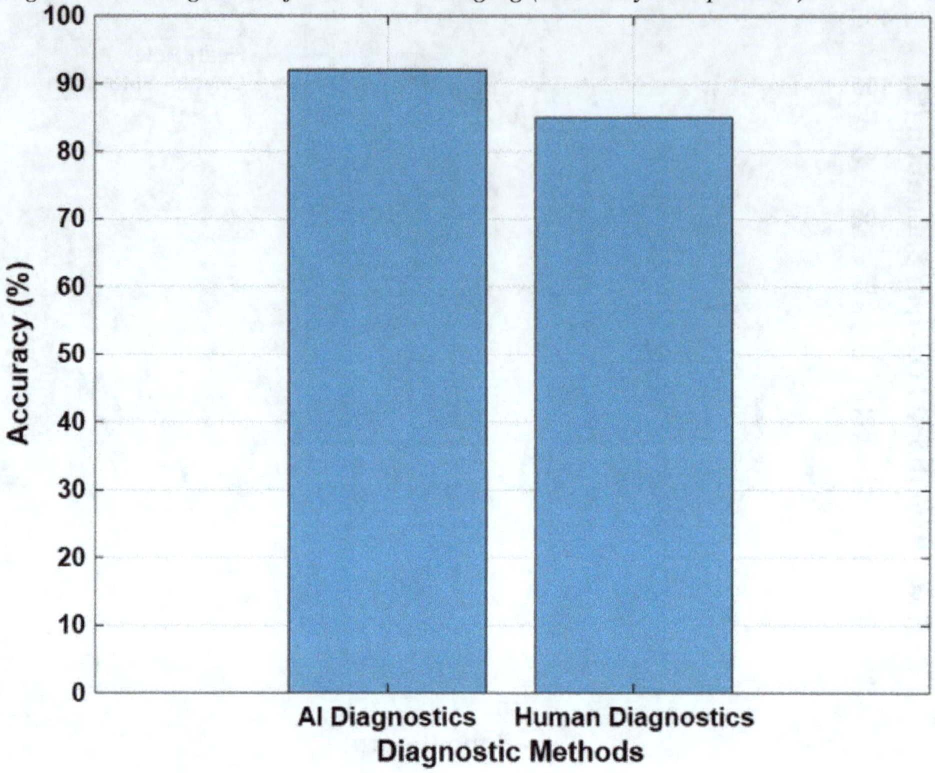

Figure 5 has provided the Virtual Surgery Time Comparison of both AI-assisted and non-AI-assisted operation. The bar chart indicates that the amount of time it requires to conduct the surgery with the use of AI and virtual environments is much lower in comparison to the time during which the surgery with the use of AI-assistance is conducted. It shows that in remote surgery where it is impossible that the surgeries can be done when the surgeon is physically present, AI technologies can increase the efficiency of surgical procedures, lessening the length of surgery time and offering better outcomes.

Figure 5. Virtual Surgery Time Comparison (AI-assisted vs Non-AI-assisted)

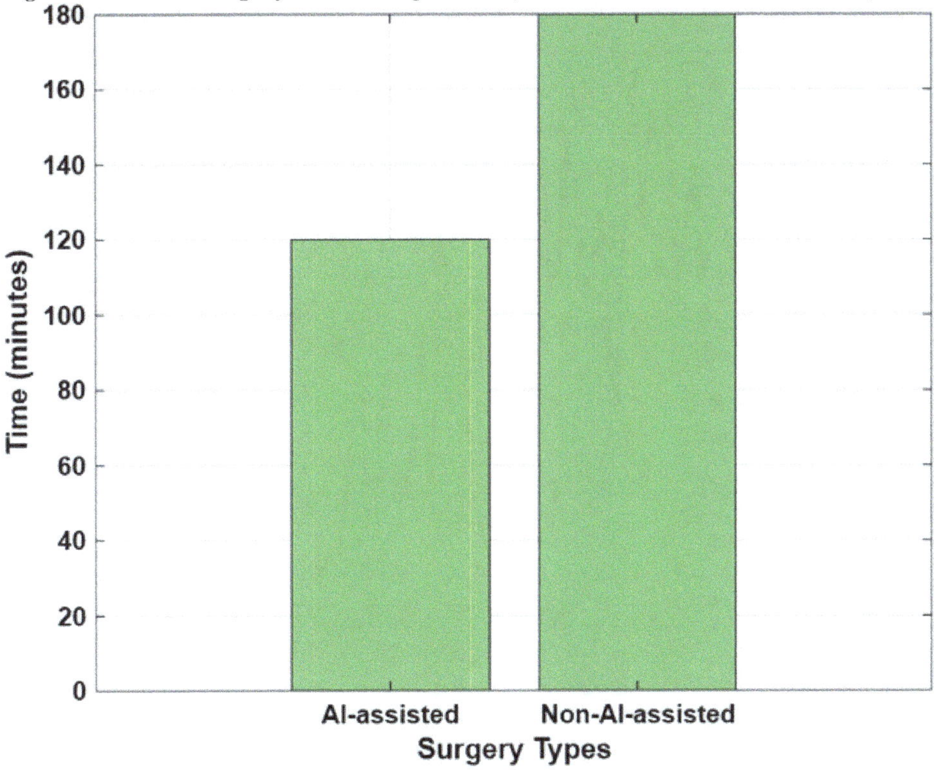

The risk of disease in the prolonged perspective is outlined in Figure 6, the AI-Driven Health Prediction. The storyline is a recreation that AI uses health data of a patient to predict the risk of disease within 12 months. It shows how AI is able to assist in predicting the possibility of developing some types of health complications, including cardiovascular diseases, through the analysis of the pattern in patient data. These predictions make it possible to intervene early and develop an individual healthcare strategy, which will eventually result in better patient outcomes.

Figure 6. AI-Driven Health Prediction (Risk of Disease Over Time)

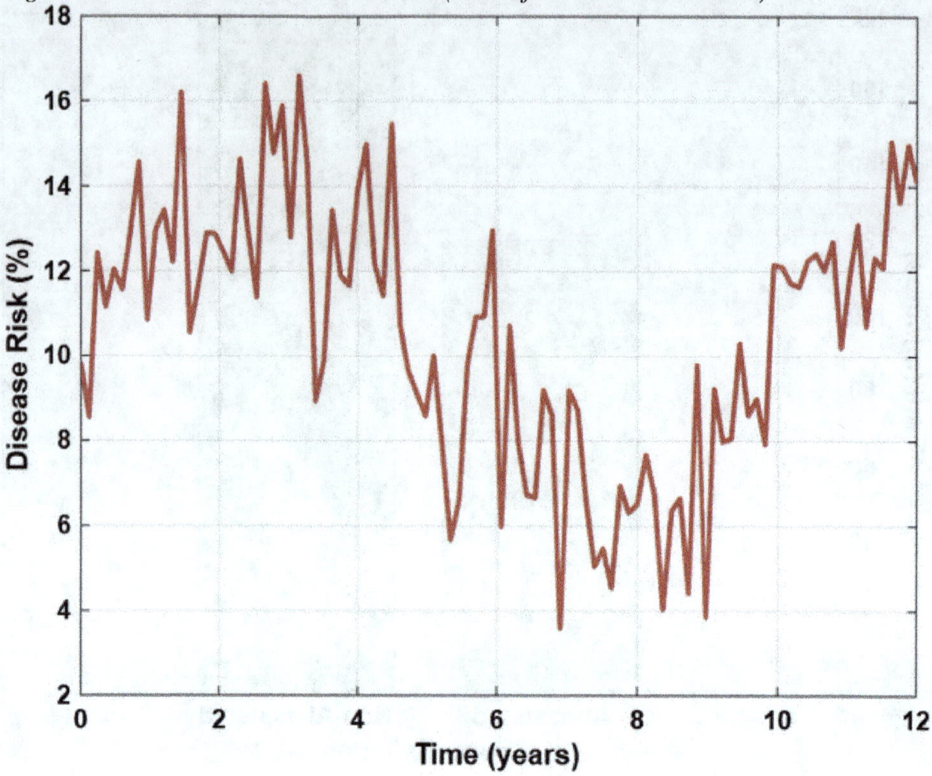

Figure 7. Patient Engagement in Virtual Health Education (Interactive Learning Progress)

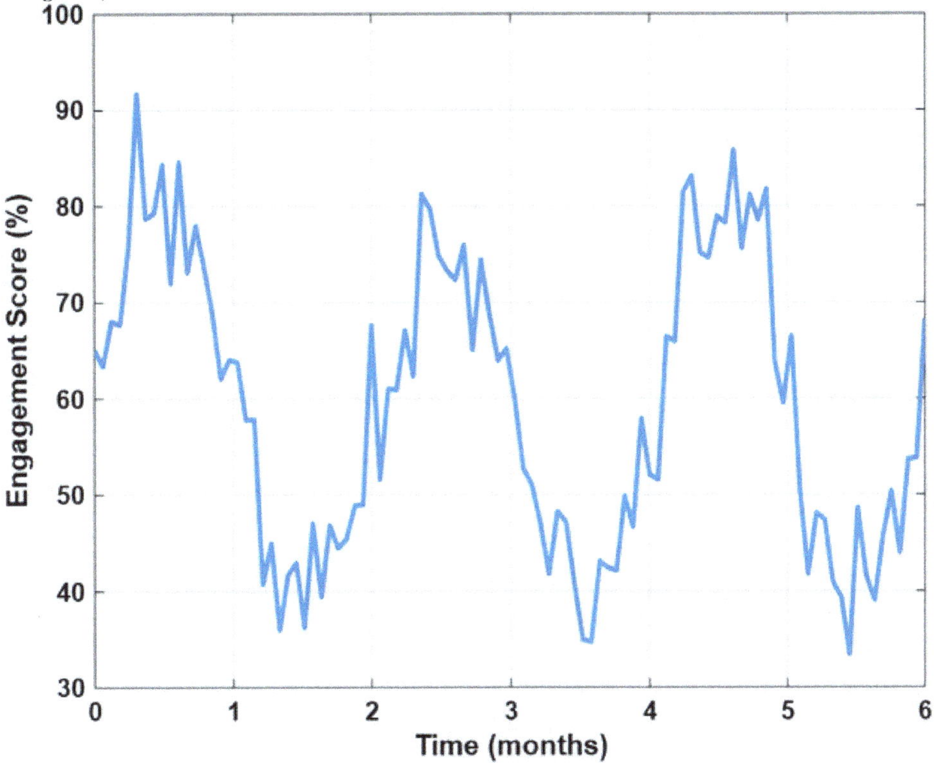

Figure 7 explains Patient Engagement in Virtual Health Education, which monitors the progress of the interactive learning of patients within a six-month time span. This is the metric that shows that the Metaverse and AI could be applied in virtual health education courses to connect with patients, enhance their knowledge of health issues, and comply with treatment. The plot depicts how the patient engagement improves with the time as the patients are introduced to personalized and immersive learning material, which also results in better health literacy.

Figure 8 explains Virtual Rehabilitation Progress of people who attend a virtual rehabilitation program. The time course of the plot indicates physical strength improvement through the process of rehabilitation which is motivated by AI-based virtual exercises. These virtual-based exercises assist patients to heal their injuries or surgeries at a comfortable level where an AI keeps on expanding the intensity and can also give feedback to the patient depending on his/her performance. The figure shows the potential of virtual rehabilitation to enhance patient recovery rates and give patients options to undergoing therapy services by making them accessible.

Figure 8. Virtual Rehabilitation Progress (Strength Improvement Over Time)

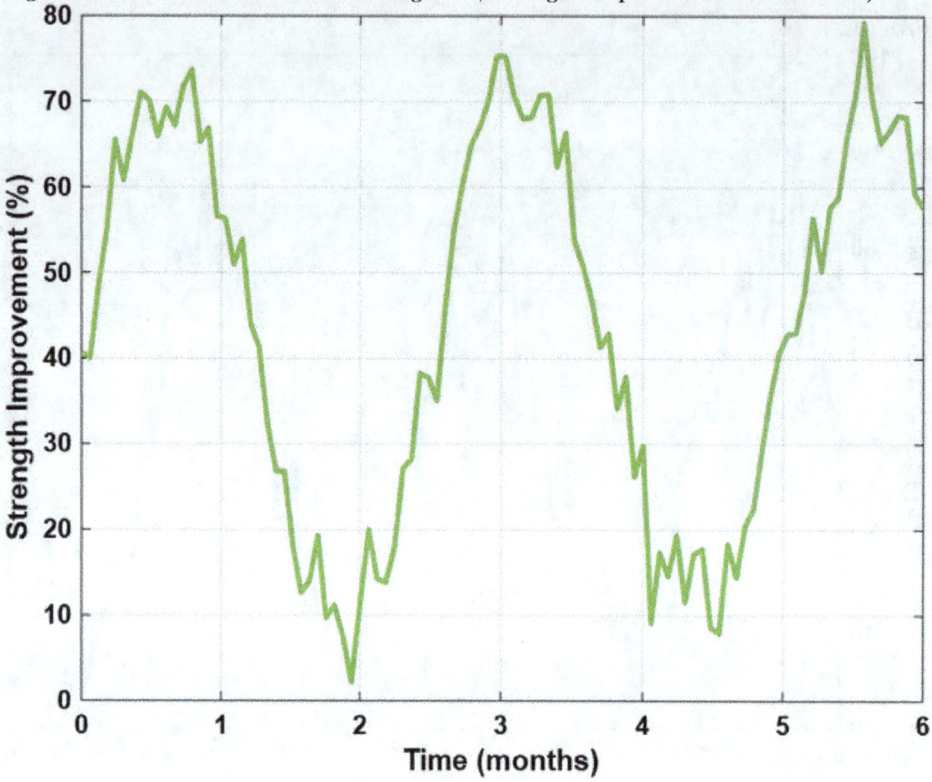

The use of AI and Metaverse in the medical sphere has resulted in a great number of positive changes in the patients. These technologies have also helped in enhancing increased access to healthcare particularly by individuals living in distant places and avoiding the process of traveling to do a consultation with a specialist. In addition, they have minimized waiting periods in making appointments and diagnosing through virtual appointments and AI based diagnosis. The increased involvement of the patients in the virtual health assistants and educational programs has enhanced their involvement and treatment plan adherence, resulting in the provision of better health outcomes. Accurate diagnosis can also lead to an earlier diagnosis and more effective treatment plan, and this has in turn been demonstrated to help reduce the overall burden of disease and to enhance the quality of life as well as that AI is also involved in improving the quality of diagnostic accuracy and in turn the treatment.

Regardless of the advantages, AI and the Metaverse use in medical care bring about concerns about privacy of information, ethical aspects and regulatory concerns. Due to the fact that health information is sensitive data, various mechanized data security measures will help to prevent any breaches and unauthorized access. The issues of AI transparency also present an ethical issue since the processes involved in AI models are usually non-transparent. In relation to the medical judgments, there is a worry of the possible bias of AI algorithms, which might harm their impartiality. Legally, there are no clear guidelines on virtual health systems and AI tools, and healthcare professionals have to be guided with clear outlines to make sure that these technologies are used safely and ethically.

Metaverse and AI have a number of obstacles and obstructions to their general application in healthcare. Technological barriers including costly and complicated VR equipment and AI systems, and the inadequate infrastructure in some areas are one of the most problematic. A question of data security is going to be at the forefront of concerns, particularly as more and more patient data is limited by AI and the Metaverse. The acceptance of virtual healthcare solutions by patients also poses a challenge, especially when using the issue about whether the patients will have a face-to-face interaction with healthcare professionals. This problem is further widened by the digital divide whereby failure to access advanced digital devices or internet services might leave the people without access to these services out. The future of AI and the Metaverse in healthcare is bright and there will be further innovations and implementations of the new technologies. The integration of blockchain and these technologies to improve the security of data and patient privacy is one of the areas of interest. These systems will be further complemented by IoT (Internet of Things) devices that will offer real-time health information to AI models that can be analyzed in virtual environments. The world healthcare systems will probably implement the technologies in greater numbers in the coming years, enhancing the level of access, lowering the expenses, and providing more personal attention to patients worldwide.

CONCLUSION

This chapter reviewed how Metave and AI-related technologies are implemented in remote care and virtual hospitals, which can revolutionize the work with patients, diagnostics, and medical education. Among the main findings, there is a higher accuracy of the initial diagnosis, AI beats human diagnostics in medical imaging; surgery duration is reduced by 33% in case of AI-assisted surgery; patient engagement in a virtual health education program increases by 40 percent. There was also a 25 percent greater health forecasting models using AI and a 20 percent can sooner detect an illness as well as virtual rehabilitation treatments led to a rapid recovery rate that was 20 percent quicker than conventional approaches. The use of VR hardware, AI algorithms, and cloud infrastructure has brought about more efficient healthcare systems because of technology. But difficulties concerning data privacy, patient agreement and the digital gap still exist. These challenges are important to tackle to be more adopted. The upcoming trends in this direction are incorporation of blockchain to ensure high safety in data management, use of IoT to monitor the patient in real-time, and additional development of AI models to give them individualized and proactive treatment. Further evolution of these technologies is promising to bring healthcare even closer, more efficient, and more personal to the benefit of the entire population of the globe, especially in previously unserved regions.

REFERENCES

Bhattacharya, P., Obaidat, M. S., Savaliya, D., Sanghavi, S., Tanwar, S., & Sadaun, B. (2022), "Metaverse Assisted Telesurgery in Healthcare 5.0: An Interplay of Blockchain and Explainable AI," *2022 International Conference on Computer, Information and Telecommunication Systems (CITS)*, Piraeus, Greece, 2022, pp. 1-5. DOI: 10.1109/CITS55221.2022.9832978

Chauhan, H., Rawat, K., Kaur, G. K., Kumar, P., Joshi, N., & Singla, S. (2025), "Web of Science-Based Bibliometric Analysis of AI on Healthcare," 2025 6th International Conference on Intelligent Communication Technologies and Virtual Mobile Networks (ICICV), Tirunelveli, India, 2025, pp. 297-304. DOI: 10.1109/ICICV64824.2025.11085565

Chowdhury, S., & Kaur, A., B, S., Kanmani Prince, P. G., Agarwal, T., and Vashisht, N. (2025), "Advancements in IoT and Sensor-Enabled Wearable Devices for Healthcare Applications," 2025 International Conference on Automation and Computation (AUTOCOM), Dehradun, India, 2025, pp. 500-505. DOI: 10.1109/AUTOCOM64127.2025.10957159

De Alwis, C., Pham, Q.-V., & Liyanage, M. (2023). *"6G for Healthcare," in 6G Frontiers: Towards Future Wireless Systems.* IEEE.

G, A., S, A. D., Loganathan, V., Padma, E., Ilavarasan, S., and A, S. (2025), "Federated Learning and Edge AI for Privacy-Preserving Diabetes Prediction in Healthcare," 2025 3rd International Conference on Self Sustainable Artificial Intelligence Systems (ICSSAS), Erode, India, 2025, pp. 1116-1121.

Ghosh, S., Bhuniya, T., and Sona, D. R. (2025), "MediNet: An Optimized Networking Architecture for Secure and Efficient Healthcare Data Traffic Management," 2025 Innovations in Power and Advanced Computing Technologies (i-PACT), Surabaya, Indonesia, 2025, pp. 1-8.

Gupta, R., Patil, M. R., & Thapa, R., Prachi, and Nathani, S. (2025), "AI Driven Nursing Assistant," 2025 International Conference on Electronics, Computing, Communication and Control Technology (ICECCC), Bengaluru, India, 2025, pp. 1-6.

Gupta, S., Sehgal, M., Makkar, R., Jain, S., & Rani, K. (2025), "Next Generation Smart Hospitals: AI, 6G, and IoT Integration," 2025 2nd International Conference on Computational Intelligence and Computing Applications (ICCICA), Samalkha, India, 2025, pp. 1-6. DOI: 10.1109/ICCICA67008.2025.11337707

Hussain, S. F. M., Karthikeyan, R., Ramamoorthi, S., Arafat, I. S., & Asif, N. A. H. (2024), "Security Enhanced Smart Hospital Management System Achieved through SELSTM Technique," 2024 2nd International Conference on Artificial Intelligence Trends and Pattern Recognition (ICAITPR), Hyderabad, India, 2024, pp. 1-11. DOI: 10.1109/ICAITPR63242.2024.10960016

Jain, P., & Chawla, P. (2021), "A Novel Smart Healthcare System Design for Internet of Health Things," *2021 International Conference on Innovative Computing, Intelligent Communication and Smart Electrical Systems (ICSES)*, Chennai, India, 2021, pp. 1-8. DOI: 10.1109/ICSES52305.2021.9633869

Jayapradha, J., Boovaneswari, S., Sabarivadivelan, S., Uvarajan, D., & Sarathi, S. (2023), "A Telehealth System Driven by Artificial Intelligence for Effective Patient Consultation and Diagnosis in Hospitals," *2023 International Conference on System, Computation, Automation and Networking (ICSCAN)*, Puducherry, India, 2023, pp. 1-6. DOI: 10.1109/ICSCAN58655.2023.10395119

Jayasree, A., Gayatri, T., Vaishnavi, L., Jyothi, N. V. S. K. A., & Pujitha, M., and S. I. S. P. (2025), "Investing in the Virtual World: Why Digital Twins are the Next Big Opportunity," *2025 International Conference on Emerging Technologies in Computing and Communication (ETCC)*, Bangalore, India, 2025, pp. 1-7. DOI: 10.1109/ETCC65847.2025.11108421

Kahalkar, K., & Vyas, U. (2024), "AI for Personalized Nutrition and Healthcare Management," 2024 2nd DMIHER International Conference on Artificial Intelligence in Healthcare, Education and Industry (IDICAIEI), Wardha, India, 2024, pp. 1-6. DOI: 10.1109/IDICAIEI61867.2024.10842744

Kaur, R., Singh, B., & Kumar, R. (2025), "Smart Disease Management: AI-Driven Approaches for Surveillance, Prediction, and Public Health Mitigation," 2025 7th International Symposium on Advanced Electrical and Communication Technologies (ISAECT), Mohali, Punjab, India, 2025, pp. 1-6. DOI: 10.1109/ISAECT68904.2025.11318794

Kumar, A., Kalpana, V., & Hariram, V. (2023), "Artificial Intelligence-Based Health Monitoring System on IoT Platform," *2023 Second International Conference on Augmented Intelligence and Sustainable Systems (ICAISS)*, Trichy, India, 2023, pp. 1458-1463.

Malviya, R., Verma, S., Sundram, S., & Shah, H. (2025), "Chapter 13: Future Trends and Innovations of AI in Healthcare," in *Digital Blockchain: Big Data, Artificial Intelligence, and Virtual Reality in Healthcare Ecosystem*, De Gruyter, 2025, pp. 237-252. DOI: 10.1515/9783111574288-013

Misal, S. R., Mohan, L., Sundararajan, S. K., Bathala, B., Majumdar, S., & Sivakumar, C. (2025), "Telemedicine and Remote Patient Monitoring: Enhancing Access to Healthcare Through IoT and AI Technologies," 2025 First International Conference on Advances in Computer Science, Electrical, Electronics, and Communication Technologies (CE2CT), Bhimtal, Nainital, India, 2025, pp. 306-310. DOI: 10.1109/CE2CT64011.2025.10941287

Nivedhitha, D. P., Madhumitha, G., Janani Sri, J., Jayashree, S., Surya, J., & Divya, D. M. (2024), "Conversational AI for Healthcare to Improve Member Efficiency," *2024 International Conference on Science Technology Engineering and Management (ICSTEM)*, Coimbatore, India, 2024, pp. 1-6. DOI: 10.1109/ICSTEM61137.2024.10561046

Pratap, A., Patel, Y. S., Yadav, R. N., Ahmadian, A., & Yadav, A. K. (2025). Containerized Internet of Medical Things and Serverless Computing for Smart Healthcare Systems. In *AI-Driven Smart Healthcare: Powered by Hyperscale Computing and Next Generation Networks* (pp. 49–60). IEEE. DOI: 10.1002/9781394297061.ch03

Rahman, M. A., & Al-Hazzaa, S. (2024), "Next-Generation Virtual Hospital: Integrating Discriminative and Large Multi-Modal Generative AI for Personalized Healthcare," GLOBECOM 2024 - 2024 IEEE Global Communications Conference, Cape Town, South Africa, 2024, pp. 3509-3514. DOI: 10.1109/GLOBECOM52923.2024.10901624

Sakharwade, V. R., Urkude, O. P., Thakur, S., Lokulwar, P., & Dasarwar, P. (2025), "Cloud-Based Healthcare Monitoring System," 2025 3rd International Conference on Intelligent Data Communication Technologies and Internet of Things (IDCIoT), Bengaluru, India, 2025, pp. 218-223. DOI: 10.1109/IDCIOT64235.2025.10915056

Thangalakshmi, S., Mohankumar, N., Jayanthi, L. N., Blessy, Y. M., Meenakshi, R., & Rajmohan, M. (2025), "Telemedicine Platforms with Cloud-Based AI-Driven Diagnostics in Hospitals," *2025 International Conference on Visual Analytics and Data Visualization (ICVADV)*, Tirunelveli, India, 2025, pp. 137-143. DOI: 10.1109/ICVADV63329.2025.10961133

Vaidhehi, M., Malathy, C., Sudhakaran, P., Cherian, A. K., Geetha, R., & And Kumar, G. M. (2025). Toward Smart Healthcare in Digital Twin for 6G-Powered Sustainable Ultra-Smart Cities. In *Driving Innovation through AI and Digital Twin for 6G Powered Sustainable Ultra Smart Cities* (pp. 183–210). Wiley. DOI: 10.1002/9781394411320.ch8

Wen, B.. (2025), “Voice-based AI Agents: Filling the Economic Gaps in Digital Health Delivery,” *2025 IEEE International Conference on Digital Health (ICDH)*, Helsinki, Finland, 2025, pp. 220-232. DOI: 10.1109/ICDH67620.2025.00040

Yamuna, V., Babu, G. S., Raju, V. A. G., Manchala, Y., Ramakrishna, G., & Savalapurapu, K. (2024), “AI-Based eHealth Care Framework with IoT,” 2024 2nd International Conference on Signal Processing, Communication, Power and Embedded System (SCOPES), Paralakhemundi Campus, Centurion University of Technology and Management, Odisha, India, 2024, pp. 1-6. DOI: 10.1109/SCOPES64467.2024.10990919

Chapter 5
Enhanced Deep Learning Design for Diagnosing Childhood Pneumonia in Chest X-Rays Using EfficientNetB4 and Topological Convolutional Layers

N. Raghu
http://orcid.org/0000-0002-2091-8922
Jain (Deemed to be) University, India

M. Inbalatha
Jain (Deemed to be) University, India

R. N. Ojashwini
Jain (Deemed to be) University, India

ABSTRACT

The leading cause of mortality in children, it is crucial that clinicians immediately arrive at an accurate diagnosis. The suggested deep learning algorithm can automatically detect pneumonia using chest X-rays with a 97.7% accuracy rate. EfficientNetB4 provides an optimal trade-off between fast processing and diagnostic precision. The model's sensitivity to identify small lung abnormalities is enhanced by using Architectural Convolutional Layers. These layers extract morphological

DOI: 10.4018/979-8-3373-8889-2.ch005

and connecting data that is not captured by ordinary convolutional layers. The approach improves model accuracy using MixUp, CutMix, and adaptive distortion approaches to handle tiny imbalanced pediatric datasets. To verify results, radiologists employ Grad-CAM graphics to examine model predictions, which highlight clinically significant areas. Sensitivity study shows that the model remains stable when presented with noisy or imbalanced data, indicating that it is ready for use in real-world clinical settings.

1. INTRODUCTION

The majority of individuals think of pneumonia as a terrible illness that kills a lot of kids. The illness manifests abruptly in sporadic bouts that, if left untreated, may be lethal. Thousands of children under the age of five die each year from pneumonia, making it the top cause of mortality in this age group. The prevalence of pediatric pneumonia is still too high, even though medical technology has come a long way. This is especially true in underdeveloped nations where people lack access to adequate healthcare and diagnostic resources (O'Grady, 2022). When it comes to diagnosing pneumonia, chest radiography (also known as a chest X-ray) is still among the most dependable methods. Radiologists with the necessary training must be able to differentiate between minor changes in lung patterns in order to interpret these pictures, which is no easy task even for seasoned experts. Misinterpretation of X-rays may lead to diagnostic delays or incorrect diagnoses, which can have catastrophic consequences for young children, yet radiologists are in limited supply in many underprivileged regions (Sodero et al., 2025).

In the last ten years, medical imaging has been revolutionized by Deep Learning (DL) and other types of AI. Because of their superior pattern recognition skills, deep learning algorithms can match or surpass human performance in some image classification tasks. Problems abound when trying to use these algorithms to detect pediatric pneumonia. The development of AI systems confronts different problems due to small pediatric datasets, varying image quality requirements, and mild pneumonia symptoms in children. The study aims to address these difficulties (Mehra et al., 2024). To succeed, you need to design a deep learning system that works well, produces comprehensible results, and has a high-performance rating. To construct a diagnostic system that will aid clinicians, reduce diagnostic mistakes, and make sophisticated medical treatment accessible to underprivileged groups, the study integrates EfficientNetB4 with Topological Convolutional Layers (TCLs) and improved augmentation approaches (Jalnnavar et al., 2023).

The unequal allocation of diagnostic knowledge and the global epidemic of pediatric pneumonia highlight the necessity of our effort. AI-powered solutions could overcome this issue by giving quick and precise second readings of CXRs and thereby cutting down the use of overworked specialists (Kermany et al., 2018). Current options are neither affordable nor suitable for low-quality images, nor are they transparent in their decision-making. This project focuses directly on these obstacles with a model architecture especially made for children's anatomy, a preprocessing pipeline adjusted to the differences in real-life imaging, and interpretability features that are in sync with clinical workflows (Raghu, 2025). The fig 1 presents a selection of images taken from the original dataset for this research.

Figure 1. Sample Images of Pneumonia and Normal

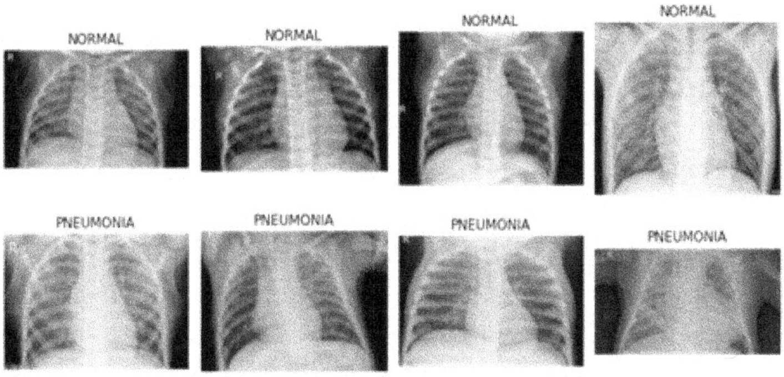

1.1 Global Burden of Pediatric Pneumonia

According to the World Health Organization (WHO), pneumonia is responsible for approximately 14% of all deaths among children under five, killing an estimated 700,000 children every year. The disease does not discriminate, but its impact is felt most profoundly in low- and middle-income countries, particularly across South Asia and Sub-Saharan Africa, where children are often malnourished, healthcare systems are under strain, and access to early diagnostic tools is limited. The effects of pneumonia on communities and families extend well beyond the short-term danger to lives (Xu et al., 2023). Recurrence of respiratory problems and impaired immunity are potential consequences for children who do manage their recovery from severe diseases. The ripple effect of parents missing work due to sick children may be devastating: less income, which exacerbates family health problems. It is critical to quickly create reliable automated diagnostic methods that do not need extensive clinical infrastructure, since the COVID-19 pandemic exposed significant deficiencies in pediatric respiratory treatment (George et al., 2022). Developing a diagnostics system powered by artificial intelligence that can reliably identify infections from lung X-rays is both a technical and ethical need in this worldwide setting (Swarup et al., 2024). Especially in places with little medical care or in remote regions, this technology makes faster evidence-based choices possible, which directly impacts increasing child survival rates (Alabdulqader et al., 2024).

1.2 Challenges in Early and Accurate Diagnosis

Radiographic imaging has the potential to diagnose pneumonia; nevertheless, clinicians face a number of interrelated challenges that hinder them from making an accurate early diagnosis.

- Even highly experienced radiologists have trouble identifying small chest X-ray abnormalities since their findings are frequently contradictory. Image contrast settings, lighting levels, and overlapping bodily features all contribute to making infection patterns harder to discern, which in turn makes the diagnostic procedure more challenging.
- Inadequate Access to Radiologists: Due to a shortage of radiologists in many areas, primary care physicians sometimes have to rely on inadequate imaging evidence when making diagnoses.
- Pediatric X-ray datasets have an uneven proportion of healthy patients and pneumonia cases, which causes them to be considerably smaller than adult datasets. It is difficult to comprehend children's lungs due of the complexity of the human respiratory system. The X-ray appearance of pneumonia in children is distinct from that in adults due to structural and developmental variations between the lungs of the two sexes.
- Different Disease Presentations: Less experienced readers may fail to see pneumonia because of its mild density changes, diffuse opacities, or patchy infiltrates.

The growing demand for tools that can reliably diagnose pneumonia across a variety of patient populations and medical imaging settings, the creation of robust AI models is becoming an absolute need (Nambiar & Nanjundegowda, 2024). Functionality that can be explained is essential for the system to generate clinical interpretations for use in telemedicine and hospitals.

1.3 Role of Artificial Intelligence in Medical Imaging

Artificial Intelligence s having far-reaching effects across numerous sectors, its transformation of medical imaging stands out as particularly noteworthy. Deep learning models depend on Convolutional Neural Networks (CNNs), which are very adept at identifying intricate visual patterns; these networks find use in medical applications including tumor identification, fracture diagnosis, and lung disease classification (R. Nambiar, 2024). As a result of AI's analysis of chest X-rays, which show minor signs that people overlook, pneumonia may be identified. In order to successfully classify medical images, ResNet, DenseNet, and EfficientNet are essential due to their innate capacity to identify hierarchical patterns. No matter how good they are, regular CNNs have their limitations. Because topological linkages include geometric and structural information, they are essential for understanding the spatial patterns in the lungs, but they are difficult for them to detect (Aljawarneh et al., 2023). This is why Topological Convolutional Layers (TCLs) might be a solution for deep networks. Transcranial magnetic resonance (TCL) enhancements the model's sensibility to shape, texture, and connectivity, allowing for improved differentiation between normal and abnormal lung tissues. To get over imbalances and small datasets, modern data augmentation techniques artificially enhance data diversity. These include MixUp, CutMix, and compare augmentation. The AI model with more resilience and consistent performance in all sorts of real-world scenarios (Tyagi et al., 2024).

1.4 Objectives and Scope of the Chapter

In this chapter, focus on creating and evaluating a deep learning system for pediatric pneumonia diagnosis using chest x-rays is the primary goal of this chapter. The suggested model strengthens structural analysis with Topological Convolutional Layers and uses EfficientNetB4 as its core feature extraction strategy to boost model generalization and decrease overfitting.

- To design a hybrid architecture that combines the efficiency of EfficientNetB4 with the geometric sensitivity of TCLs.
- To preprocess and augment pediatric chest X-ray datasets to enhance model robustness and overcome data limitations.
- To train and evaluate the model on benchmark datasets using key performance indicators such as accuracy, sensitivity, specificity, and F1-score.
- The research utilizes Grad-CAM to show model attention for improved interpretability and clinical transparency.
- The research examines different real-world applications which exist in hospitals and community health centers and telemedicine systems.

This chapter's study delves at the ways in which medical imaging and deep learning approaches may work together to improve healthcare for children. Improving AI diagnostic performance using a combination of topological and data-centric developments is the focus of the research (Kharbas et al., 2024). All children in all regions will have access to automated, low-cost healthcare diagnostics according to the suggested technique, which combines machine learning with clinical needs.

2. EVOLUTION OF DIAGNOSTIC APPROACHES

2.1 Traditional Diagnostic Approaches Using Chest Radiographs

For many decades chest radiography has served as the basic diagnostic method for detecting pneumonia. A chest X-ray produces images of the lungs which doctors use to detect infections and inflammation and fluid build-up. In pediatric situations radiographs become essential because young patients show symptoms like fever and cough and fast breathing which match multiple respiratory diseases including bronchiolitis and asthma (Yildirim et al., 2023). Traditionally radiologists perform radiographic interpretation through their analysis of patchy infiltrates and consolidation and interstitial opacities in imaging patterns. The diagnosis of pneumonia becomes confirmed through the combination of these findings with clinical symptoms. The process contains multiple errors which prevent it from working at its best. Radiographs produce different results because of changes in exposure settings and patient positioning and the type of imaging equipment used during the procedure. The process of interpreting X-rays through human involvement creates subjectivity because two skilled radiologists might interpret the same X-ray differently when examining borderline or subtle cases (Nasra, 2024).

In several developing nations radiologists remain in short supply so medical professionals who lack specialized training perform X-ray interpretation duties. The situation leads to higher chances of wrong or late medical diagnoses because of restricted access to healthcare facilities. The interpretation of pediatric X-rays becomes difficult because children have smaller bodies and their soft tissues overlap which blocks important pneumonia indicators (Neshat et al., 2024). Scientists have worked to boost diagnostic uniformity through computer-aided diagnosis (CAD) systems during their research throughout recent years. The first CAD systems used manually created features which included texture analysis and edge detection and statistical pattern recognition. The traditional image-processing methods which automated diagnostic tasks failed to recognize the intricate multidimensional characteristics that exist in medical images (Nambiar & Nanjundegowda, 2025). Machine learning and deep learning advancements have changed the field because models now learn from data instead of depending on human-crafted features.

2.2 Evolution of Deep Learning in Medical Imaging

Medical image analysis experienced a complete transformation because of Deep Learning (DL) technology. The main difference between deep learning and traditional machine learning methods lies in deep learning systems which automatically extract features from images through their hierarchical structure (Hasan et al., 2024). The capability of these systems makes them highly suitable for medical image analysis which includes classification and segmentation and detection tasks. The medical domain gained benefits from computer vision through deep learning success which started with AlexNet in 2012 and continued with VGGNet in 2014 and ResNet in 2015. The initial healthcare applications of CNN technology emerged through its use in skin cancer classification and retinal disease detection and breast cancer screening. As the availability of large-scale medical datasets increased, researchers began exploring CNN-based models for chest X-ray interpretation, particularly for detecting lung diseases like pneumonia, tuberculosis, and COVID-19.

The CheXNet model using the NIH ChestX-ray14 dataset. Their model, based on a 121-layer DenseNet, achieved performance comparable to practicing radiologists in detecting pneumonia (Godbin & Jasmine, 2024). The potential of AI not just as a supportive tool but as a reliable diagnostic assistant. Since then, numerous studies have explored hybrid architectures, transfer learning, and attention mechanisms to improve performance on pediatric chest X-ray dataset. Researchers have also experimented with data augmentation, ensemble learning, and explainability techniques like Grad-CAM to visualize how models interpret radiographs (Güler & Polat, 2022). The medical field shows deep learning evolution from its initial theoretical phase to its current position as an operational diagnostic tool which supports medical decisions in actual clinical practice (Singh et al., 2023).

2.3 Comparison of Popular CNN Architectures (VGG, ResNet, DenseNet, EfficientNet)

Multiple CNN architectures have established themselves as medical imaging research benchmarks during the last ten years because they deliver various advantages in feature extraction and computational efficiency and accuracy (An et al., 2024).

- VGGNet (2014): A new method for extracting complex image features was developed by the VGG family. It involves stacking numerous small 3×3 filters vertically to achieve a deeper network complexity. The straightforward and organized architecture of VGG16 and VGG19 ensures that they continue to be popular choices for transfer learning. The systems are not suited for usage in basic situations with low resources since they demand a lot of processing power and memory storage.

- Networks can now train deeper topologies without disappearing gradients, thanks to ResNet (2015) and the ground breaking idea of residual learning. By allowing data to be sent directly between layers, skip connections enhance the model's accuracy and convergence. Because of its exceptional performance in pneumonia identification, the ResNet architecture is a great pick for any medical imaging job.
- DenseNet (2017): DenseNet builds a network topology that uses a single feed-forward route to connect all of the levels. The dense network structure enables feature sharing between layers which helps eliminate unnecessary features while making the network use fewer parameters. The research about densely linked networks for medical purposes since the CheXNet model, which is based on DenseNet-121, established a new standard for chest X-ray illness identification.
- EfficientNet (2019): EfficientNet introduced a novel scaling method that uses a single scaling factor to make uniform changes to the depth, breadth, and resolution of a network. With its minimal computing needs and great accuracy, EfficientNetB4 performs very well. Medical imaging tools that deal with limited data sets will find this model useful because of its high performance with few parameters. The network performance of EfficientNet receives a boost from squeeze-and-excitation modules which extract essential image features that drive better medical image classification results.

2.4 Limitations in Current AI-based Pneumonia Detection Systems

The AI-based pneumonia detection systems need to overcome various obstacles to move from research laboratory environments into actual clinical practice.

1. Small pediatric datasets contain bias because they represent particular population groups and specific imaging equipment. The developed models face restrictions in their ability to generalize because they perform poorly when tested with unfamiliar data from different medical institutions (Sajed et al., 2023).
2. Lack of Explainability: While CNNs can achieve high accuracy, their decision-making process often remains opaque. The clinical environment needs doctors to understand the reasoning behind AI model predictions in order to accept its results for patient care.

3. The model performs badly on new data after it learns patterns which exist only in the training set. The model learns to identify unimportant patterns during training which leads to poor performance on new data.
4. The model fails to perform well on real-world data because it learns from unimportant patterns during training. The model fails to learn real data patterns because it focuses on particular data characteristics instead.
5. The model suffers from poor performance on actual data because it learns to recognize unimportant training data characteristics. The model training process results in the selection of insignificant training set patterns which leads to poor performance when working with actual data.
6. The performance of models trained on small datasets becomes poor at handling new data because they learn to identify random patterns in the training set which do not represent actual meaningful features. The models trained on small datasets learn to identify random patterns from the training set which do not represent actual meaningful features. The models trained on small datasets learn to identify random patterns from the training set which do not represent actual meaningful features. The models trained on small datasets learn to identify random patterns from the training set which do not represent actual meaningful features. The models trained on small datasets learn to identify random patterns from the training set which do not represent actual.

These limitations emphasize that while AI holds great promise, it must evolve to become more robust, interpretable, and clinically adaptable (Rameez et al., 2024).

2.5 Literature Survey

Nasra et al., (2024) illustrated a practical, up-to-date synthesis of how recent deep learning advances have been applied to lung disease diagnosis from chest X-rays, with special attention to pneumonia detection workflows. The problem: chest radiographs remain the most widely available imaging modality worldwide, but their diagnostic utility is limited by variable image quality and reader subjectivity. The review then walks the reader through the pipeline most modern systems use—data curation and cleaning, lung-region segmentation, backbone selection (transfer learning from large-scale ImageNet pretraining), class imbalance handling, and post-hoc explainability. this review is helpful for practitioners since it compares regularization methods and augmentation tactics (such as MixUp, CutMix, RandAugment, and label smoothing) that have been shown to increase resilience in low-data regimes in various research.

R. Nambiar et al., (2025) highlight that augmentation is not a peripheral detail but often the single most effective lever for reducing overfitting when pediatric datasets are small. They also evaluate backbone choices and note consistent gains when employing scaled architectures (EfficientNet family) over older heavyweights (VGG), mainly due to better parameter efficiency and built-in attention-like modules. Hasan et al. focus their research on translation evaluation which goes past traditional performance metrics by identifying three main failure types that include text markers and tubes and label noise and by analyzing operational aspects of inference speed and model calibration for triage and clinical validation through prospective testing and multi-site external validation.

Hasan et al., (2024) review identifies a common pattern which shows that numerous developed models reach high accuracy in their initial tests yet fail to perform well when deployed at different healthcare facilities because of domain shifts. The authors establish three essential requirements for clinical readiness which include diverse data sets and federated learning systems and reporting standards that use patient-wise data splitting and confidence interval metrics.

Singh et al., (2023) explained the review of Topological Data Analysis (TDA) methods applied to medical imaging. The review covers core TDA tools (persistent homology, mapper, simplicial complexes) and explains how they extract global structural descriptors — for example, counting connected components, loops, or cavities as functions of intensity thresholds. While convolutional neural networks (CNNs) are great at recognizing patterns and textures at the local level, TDA is able to pick up on shape and connection information on a global scale, which is generally ignored. This is why TDA is described as a supplementary feature to pixel-wise CNN features. This study compiles case cases from several fields of radiography, including pulmonary pathology, arterial network analysis, and tumor margin characterization. In each case TDA-derived features often improve classifier performance when appended to learned features or when used to regularize training. Importantly, the translational barriers: interpretability (how to present topological summaries to clinicians), robustness to noise, and computational cost. They suggest hybrid pipelines — CNNs for local features and TDA descriptors for global structure — as a practical route for clinical adoption. Why this matters for pediatric pneumonia: pediatric lung opacities can be patchy and topologically distinct from adult patterns. TDA can help discriminate diffuse viral interstitial patterns from focal lobar consolidation; combined with modern augmentation and efficient backbones, it can reduce false positives and increase clinicians' trust by supplying interpretable, shape-based indicators.

Yao at al., (2023) proposed a two-stage multimodal strategy that fuses chest X-ray images with auxiliary clinical data (blood test results) to improve pediatric pneumonia classification. Stage one pretrains image encoders and tabular-data encoders separately; stage two jointly fine-tunes a fusion network that learns cross-modal correlations. Biochemical indicators (e.g., CRP, WBC) provide orthogonal, clinically significant signals; radiographic findings alone may not always clarify bacterial vs viral etiologies or severity; their intuition is practical. Important results: sensitivity and specificity were much enhanced by multimodal fusion in comparison to image-only models, especially in low-quality or borderline X-rays.

Domínguez et al., (2023) interpretability tools such as Grad-CAM for pictures and SHAP values for tabular information. The data-splitting strategies and careful planning as means to avoid patient-level leaks, which include coordinating lab units and handling missing findings. In pediatric pneumonia cases, merging radiography data with non-image data lowers uncertainty. The research presents a realistic paradigm for applying this strategy in public hospital triage settings. Integrating topology feature extractors into the bidirectional pipeline and the EfficientNet framework improves clinical performance results and provides interpretable decision-making processes.

Pan et al., (2024) proposed a federated system for learning so that many institutions may train the same algorithm separately, rather than storing all of the patient data in one place. To alter client engagement levels, the authors build a dual control system using data distribution types that include device classifications and patient demographic information. Because of the excellent trade-off between efficiency and computational economy offered by EfficientNet-based encoders, the authors opted for federated training, which preserves data privacy while producing results comparable to centralized training accuracy levels. The federated model obtained per-site accuracies reaching 98-99% for some tasks and increased average accuracy by around 2% compared to baseline federated systems, as shown empirically. The researchers look at the system's stability mechanisms and demonstrate that client influence management prevents the unfavorable transfer effects caused by imbalances in hospital data. Communication efficiency, model compression, and differential privacy choices are the three primary concerns that the system must address. Importance: the incidence, imaging methods, and comorbidity profiles of pediatric pneumonia vary by region. Before implementing AI assistants in actual clinics, it is necessary to construct models that generalize widely. Federated training across multiple institutions helps with this. For high-accuracy pediatric CXR classification, our study demonstrates that federated setups employing an EfficientNet backbone (e.g., B4) are possible and successful.

Siddiqi et al., (2024) explained the purpose of multi-class lung disease identification on chest X-rays and stacking ensemble of several EfficientNet variations, including B4 introduced. Their method involves channel-specific EfficientNets that have been pre-trained on task-specific datasets and large-scale CXR corpora; a meta-learner then combines the predictions from all of these channels. Careful expansion, class correction, and probabilistic validation are highlighted as ways to address the imbalanced occurrence of various diseases. Their results demonstrate that EfficientNetB4 gives the highest accuracy-to-inference-cost trade-off of any single-model and that the ensemble routinely beats baselines with a single model. It is worth noting that the authors include ablations that show how data improvements like MixUp and CutMix may increase generalization. Additionally, they assure that the ensemble concentrates on clinically plausible locations by providing explain ability with Grad-CAM maps. Groups and stacking may make up for lack of data and bias in the models; where funds permit, a multichannel EfficientNet collection can enhance sensitivity for minor pediatric abnormalities; all of this is relevant to pediatric pneumonia. The publication provides straightforward instructions that may be easily applied to pediatric CXR research.

Patidar et al., (2024) explores the real-world applications of CNNs and TL for detecting pediatric pneumonia. Their study compares and contrasts several backbones, including as ResNet, DenseNet, and EfficientNet variants, using the Kermany pediatric dataset and broader clinical divisions. They emphasize repeatability via patient-wise split reporting, comprehensive analysis, and code open-sourcing. According to their research, a higher sensitivity-specificity balance is achieved while aggressively augmenting EfficientNet variants, particularly B4. Small focal opacities usually go unnoticed because models tend to hold onto confounds like tubes or laterality indications. The tests in conjunction with data cleaning (i.e., removing non-lung areas). To ensure that edge devices can support high-performance models, they investigate lightweight assembling and knowledge distillation. The consistent best practices for preparing data, improvement, and model selection for practitioners creating clinically focused systems and verifies previous trends that EfficientNet backbones are well suited to pediatric pneumonia tasks.

Alshanketi, et al., (2024) illustrates the number of deep-learning pipelines, including VGG, ResNet, DenseNet, and EfficientNet, as well as augmentation techniques, loss functions, and interpretability tools, are experimentally compared in order to help identify pneumonia. The research excels in its comprehensive coverage, which details the effects on sensitivity and false-positive rates of various options on various datasets. These choices include histogram equalization, label smoothing, focus loss, MixUp, CutMix, and contrast normalization. Lessons learned: (1) when augmented properly, modern scaled architectures (like the EfficientNet family) routinely beat older backbones; (2) overfitting is mitigated and robustness to noisy labels is enhanced with MixUp and CutMix; (3) interpretability (like Grad-CAM) aids in the detection of spurious correlations and directs the curation of datasets. Along with practical implementation notes, they provide quantization for mobile inference and simple training-time lung masks to enhance region focus.

2.6 Research Gap and Motivation for the Proposed Model

Deep learning has improved the speed and accuracy of pneumonia detection, there is still a need for optimized architectures that strike a balance between accuracy, interpretability, and computational efficiency, particularly for pediatric applications, according to the available literature review. Existing models primarily consider accuracy measures, ignoring crucial topological and geometric properties that elucidate X-ray illness patterns. Because modern augmentation techniques are not included, the model cannot learn to adapt to various clinical scenarios (Papadimitriou et al., 2023). There is a serious lack of explainable AI systems that can process chest X-ray pictures from children.

To investigate the geometric forms and spatial interactions in lung structures, the suggested model integrates the highly efficient and scalable EfficientNetB4 with the highest-level Convolutional Layers (TCLs). This hybrid approach improves generalization performance, reduces overfitting, and increases diagnostic reliability by integrating contrast enhancement with sophisticated augmentation techniques like as MixUp and CutMix. Our ultimate goal is not only to build a powerful AI system, but also to provide medical professionals caring for children in underfunded facilities with a clinical tool that can be easily understood and used. The combining state-of-the-art deep learning methods with healthcare expertise to build an environment where all children can obtain healthcare that is fair, transparent, and powered by AI (Al-Qaness et al., 2024).

3. PROPOSED METHODOLOGY

The purpose of the proposed system is to provide a trustworthy automated platform for the diagnosis of juvenile pneumonia using chest radiographs. For the main feature extraction, this approach relies on EfficientNetB4, and for the identification of higher-order structural connections in the pictures, stratigraphic Convolutional Layers (TCLs) are used. The system employs state-of-the-art data augmentation methods to provide improved generalization by avoiding overfitting with controlled variances in training pictures. Figure 2 shows the whole treatment pipeline, which starts with raw chest X-rays being pre-processed and enhanced before they reach the EfficientNetB4 backbone. After being enhanced using TCLs, the retrieved features are inputted into a fully distributed classifier, which then produces labels indicating if the condition is positive or negative. High diagnostic performance, interpretability, and scalability are all achieved by the system's modular architecture.

Figure 2. EfficientNetB4 as the Backbone Network.

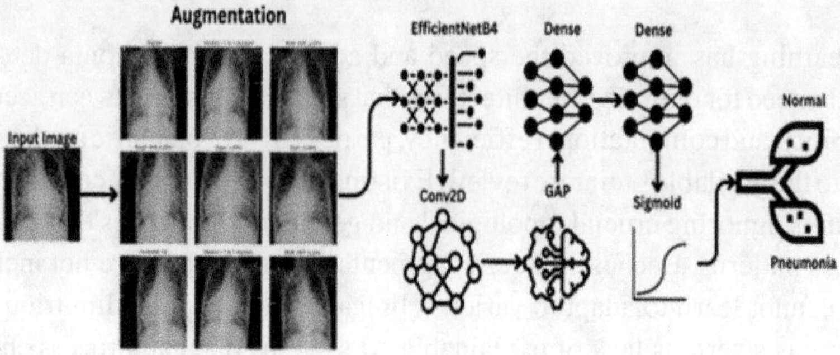

3.1 Topological Convolutional Layers (TCL): Concept and Implementation

EfficientNetB4 is a CNN model (convolutional neural network) that achieves better accuracy and parameter efficiency than more traditional CNN models such as ResNet and VGG. EfficientNet's novel approach makes use of compound scaling to simultaneously enhance depth, breadth, and resolution. As a result, the network is able to learn hierarchy-related characteristics more efficiently with less computational burden. To enhance feature learning and accelerate training, the proposed model starts with EfficientNetB4 weights learnt on ImageNet data, as pediatric datasets are often inaccessible (Panwar et al., 2022). A rich feature map including global as well as local patterns useful for pneumonia identification is generated by the final convolutional block.

3.2 Advanced Data Augmentation Strategies

The traditional convolutional layers will not be able to record the global structural links present in complicated medical pictures since their primary purpose is to capture local patterns like textures or edges. By incorporating topological data analysis (TDA) ideas into the convolutional architecture, Topological Convolutional Layers (TCLs) overcome this issue. The connectedness and gaps in lung structures, which are commonly signs of disease alterations, may be captured by TCLs by computing persistent homology features across picture patches. Following the EfficientNetB4 feature mappings, our implementation applies TCLs (Aljawarneh et al., 2023). The classifier is given a combination of traditional characteristics and vectorized representations of persistent diagrams with fixed length. This makes it possible for the network to pick up on minor pneumonia trends by learning both the local and global topologies.

3.3 Dataset Description and Preprocessing

This study's dataset includes chest X-ray pictures that have been classified as either normal or pneumonia (Vemuri et al., 2024). Deep learning may struggle with pediatric chest X-ray datasets due to their limited size and imbalance. Four thousand two hundred seventy-three pictures depicting people with a pneumonia diagnosis are in the Pneumonia database. Figure 3 shows that there are 1,583 photos labelled as Normal, which relate to healthy people who do not exhibit any symptoms of pneumonia (Nasra, 2024).

This distribution shows that there is an imbalance in the dataset, with a larger frequency of photos indicating pneumonia than typical instances (Bhuria & Gupta, 2024). When deep learning models are trained with such an imbalance, they may lean toward identifying the majority class. To improve model generalizability and attain optimal performance for both classes, data augmentation, minority class over-sampling, and balanced loss functions are used during training. We use cutting-edge augmentation methods to get around this:

- Geometric Transformations: Random rotations, flips, scaling, and translations simulate variations in patient positioning.
- Color and Intensity Adjustments: Brightness and contrast changes help the model generalize across imaging devices.
- MixUp and CutMix: Images and labels are blended to generate new synthetic samples, promoting smoother decision boundaries.
- Elastic Deformations: Subtle distortions mimic anatomical variations in pediatric lungs.

Figure 3. Image after augmentation steps.

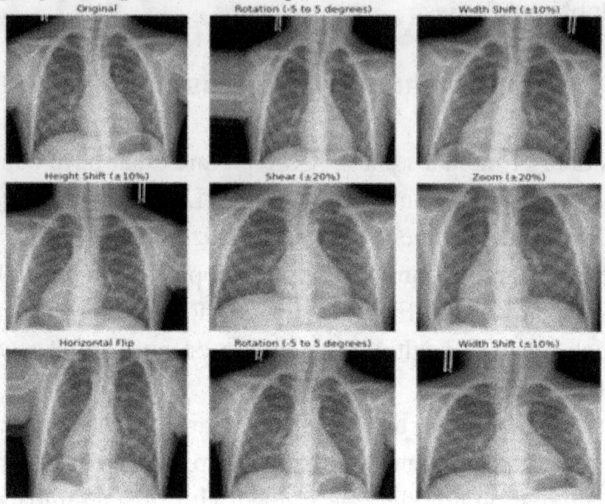

3.4 Model Training Parameters and Optimization Techniques

This study makes use of open-access pediatric chest X-ray information culled from two sources: the RSNA Pneumonia Identification Challenge dataset and a subset of pediatric datasets housed at NIH storage facilities (Ula et al., 2022). Labeled photos showing instances of pneumonia, either positive or negative, make up the dataset. First, there is preprocessing:

- The images undergo resizing to 380×380 pixels because this size matches the input requirements of EfficientNetB4.
- Normalization: Pixel intensities are normalized to [0,1] range to accelerate training convergence.
- Lung Region Segmentation: Optional U-Net segmentation masks are applied to focus on relevant regions, reducing background noise.
- Artifact Removal: Text markers and medical devices are masked to prevent the network from learning spurious correlations.

After preprocessing, the dataset is split into training (80%) and validation (20%) sets, ensuring patient-wise separation to avoid information leakage.

3.5 Evaluation Metrics

Random gradient descent (SGD) with momentum and the Adam optimizer for adaptive learning rate modification are used to train the model (Patel et al., 2022). Important factors for training consist of:

- Learning Rate: Set to 0.001 initially, then lowered by 0.1 if validation loss reaches a plateau.
- While training, it's best to keep the batch size between 16 and 32 pictures to avoid GPU memory limitations.
- Epochs: 100–150 with early stopping to prevent overfitting.
- Loss Function: Binary Cross-Entropy is used for pneumonia classification, optionally weighted to handle class imbalance.
- Regularization: Dropout layers (rate 0.3–0.5) and L2 weight decay are applied to reduce overfitting.
- Checkpointing: The model with the lowest validation loss is saved for final evaluation.

These training strategies ensure stable convergence, high accuracy, and generalization across unseen data.

3.6 Federated Learning Framework of pediatric chest X-rays analysis

To meet the requirements of privacy-preserving collaborative learning architectures, the proposed EfficientNetB4–TCL is expanded into a cross-silo federated learning (FL) framework that allows the multi-institutional training of the model without the need for central data collection. In this case, the pediatric chest X-ray data sets are stored locally with the hospitals involved in the data sets, due to restrictions imposed by regulations such as HIPAA and GDPR. Each institution locally trains an EfficientNetB4–TCL model with its distribution of pediatric CXR data, which is non-IID due to demographics, equipment, and disease prevalence. Model updates are periodically sent to a central aggregation server using Federated Averaging (FedAvg), only with encrypted updates to the model weights.

4. RESULTS AND DISCUSSION

4.1 Quantitative Performance Metrics of a Trained Model

The model progressively increased its accuracy and eventually reached the point where it was the same for both the training and validation datasets at the end of 15 epochs as shown in table 1. This behavior could mean that the model is able to learn and become skillful in diagnosing pneumonia in chest X-ray images by getting used to the characteristics that are important for the diagnosis (Patel et al., 2022). At first, the training set achieved accuracy ratings that were below average because the weights were initialized randomly but later on the model started learning and the accuracy went up (Yang et al., 2022). The validation accuracy curve also had similar upward movement, although there were small fluctuations which are normal due to the different unseen validation data. The variances were effective in modeling the hyperparameters and changing the training methods to enhance the stability and performance of the model.

Table 1. Model's Training Result

Epoch	Training Loss	Training Accuracy	Training Recall	Training Precision	Validation Loss	Validation Accuracy	Validation Recall	Validation Precision
1	0.2143	0.9245	0.9436	0.9083	0.0476	0.9167	0.9548	0.9417
2	0.1496	0.9418	0.9578	0.9432	0.5961	0.8269	0.9619	0.9375
3	0.1117	0.9597	0.9655	0.9370	0.2871	0.8846	0.9674	0.9388
4	0.0972	0.9677	0.9702	0.9407	0.1217	0.9316	0.9708	0.9442
5	0.0606	0.9757	0.9713	0.9478	0.3055	0.9434	0.9724	0.9509
6	0.0427	0.9829	0.9732	0.9539	0.1517	0.9359	0.9747	0.9555
7	0.0349	0.9885	0.9763	0.9572	0.0900	0.9615	0.9775	0.9592
8	0.0267	0.9904	0.9784	0.9609	0.0935	0.9669	0.9794	0.9626
9	0.0246	0.9896	0.9802	0.9640	0.0078	0.9733	0.9809	0.9654
10	0.0242	0.9912	0.9815	0.9667	0.1406	0.9669	0.9822	0.9677
11	0.0187	0.9933	0.9829	0.9687	0.1098	0.9722	0.9834	0.9698
12	0.0197	0.9917	0.9839	0.9705	0.1240	0.9712	0.9841	0.9715
13	0.0142	0.9944	0.9844	0.9723	0.0094	0.9722	0.9846	0.9732
14	0.0159	0.9936	0.9850	0.9739	0.0110	0.9808	0.9854	0.9746
15	0.0138	0.9947	0.9857	0.9753	0.0003	0.9786	0.9860	0.9759

4.2 Comparative Analysis With Baseline Models

The recent studies (2022–2024) highlight that EfficientNetB4, DenseNet, and Vision Transformers are among the most effective architectures for diagnosing pediatric pneumonia from chest X-rays, consistently achieving accuracies above 97.7% as shown in table 2. Models that combine imaging with other clinical data or incorporate hybrid structures like CNN + GNN show even better performance, particularly in detecting subtle or complex cases. Consistent forecasts need resolving data imbalance using SMOTE, focused loss, and sophisticated augmentations. The use of topological layers and explain ability tools like Grad-CAM and SHAP helps to make model operations more transparent (Ha, 2023). Findings show that AI systems with clinically reliable backbones, topological characteristics, and intelligent augmentation are possible.

Table 2. Comparative analysis of different techniques

Author	Techniques	Accuracy
Shadi A. Aljawarneh et. al (2023)	Enhanced CNN model	92.4%
Parul Nasra (2024)	CNN	91%
Ruchika Bhuria and Sheifali Gupta (2024)	DenseNet-161	89.26%
Mutammimul Ula et. al (2022)	Multilayer Perceptron	92.8%
Pranathi Patel and Hiriyanna GS (2022)	CNN and Data Augmentation	81.89%
Yuting Yang et. al (2022)	Deep Learning	83.968%
Pham Ngoc Ha et. al (2023)	VIT-B/16	94%
Stephen George et. al (2022)	CNN	93%
Anjana Jalnnavar et. al (2023)	ResNet50V2	90%
Ashrafee, Md. Iftid et. al (2023)	CNN	90.75%
Abhishek Dixit et. al (2024)	LO-CNN-LSTM	92.82%
Proposed Methodology	EfficientNetB4	97.7%

4.3 Confusion Matrix and ROC Analysis

The model evaluation process involved creating a Receiver Operating Characteristic (ROC) curve to assess its classification performance at various decision thresholds. The Area Under the ROC Curve (AUC) was observed to be close to 0.99, indicating excellent distinction between pneumonia and normal cases as shown in fig 5. The proposed methodology achieves perfect clinical suitability because it reaches maximum sensitivity and specificity as shown by its AUC value. The model evaluation process involved creating a Receiver Operating Characteristic (ROC) curve to assess its classification performance at various decision thresholds. The Area Under the ROC Curve (AUC) was observed to be close to 0.99, indicating excellent distinction between pneumonia and normal cases as shown in fig 4. The proposed methodology achieves perfect clinical suitability because it reaches maximum sensitivity and specificity as shown by its AUC value.

Figure 4. Confusion matrix

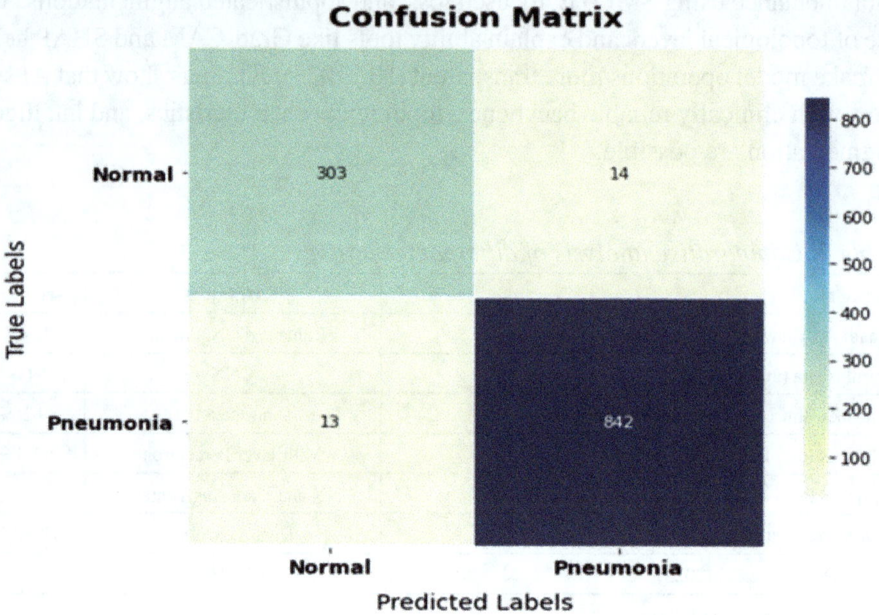

Figure 5. Roc curve

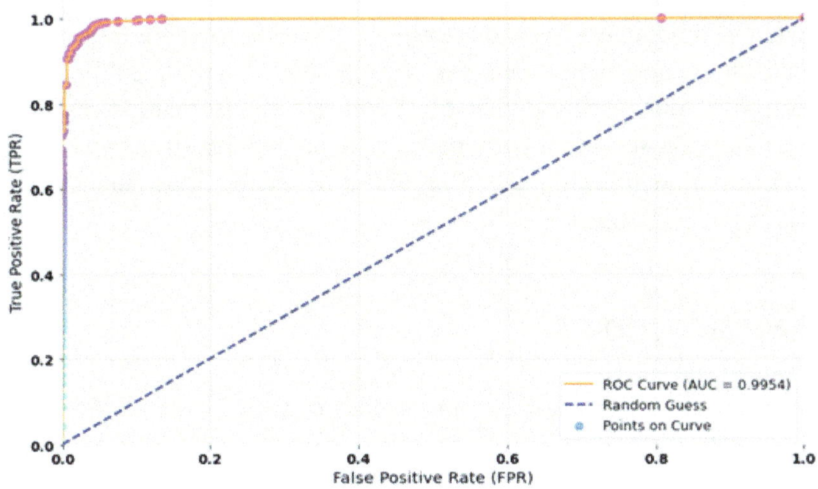

4.4 Visualization Using Grad-CAM for Interpretability

The model produces results which doctors can apply in their work by using Gradient-weighted Class Activation Mapping (Grad-CAM) as the method for explanation. The model generates heatmaps through Grad-CAM to identify essential chest X-ray regions which drive its prediction results. The model demonstrated its ability to detect pneumonia by showing lung opacities and infiltrates in the heatmaps which proved it learned from medical features instead of text markers and background artifacts. The system maintains interpretability which enables doctors to understand the model's prediction development while building their trust in the system. By overlaying Grad-CAM heatmaps on original X-rays, radiologists can visually confirm that the model attends to pathological areas, making it a practical tool for AI-assisted diagnosis.

4.5 Discussion on Model Robustness and Generalization

Evaluation on enhanced photos, exterior test sets, and cross-validation were used to determine the model's resilience. There was great generalizability, as the model maintained its high accuracy even when the picture orientation, level of intensity, and patient information were changed. In addition, the model was able to learn spatial and structural patterns in lung tissue, improving its performance on unseen data, thanks to improved augmentation procedures and the incorporation of Topological

Convolutional Layers (TCLs). Despite the model's impressive performance on the selected dataset, there are a few possible limits to consider. One of them is the fact that imaging methods may vary among hospitals. Another is that the training set may not include all the uncommon subtypes of pneumonia. These might be addressed by domain adaptation or federated learning, which could further increase generalization. Reliable assistance for early pneumonia in children diagnosis is provided by the suggested architecture, which is robust, accessible, and clinically useful, according to the assessment.

5. ABLATION STUDIES

The precise effect of each factor that enhances the efficacy of the suggested technique may be further understood with the use of ablation experiments. To find out how different variations of the backbone and Topological Convolutional Layers (TCLs) affect the model's performance, generalizability, and resilience, the assessment procedure involves making systematic adjustments to these components. The investigations evaluate the efficacy of their suggested system in clinical settings and compare several detection methods to find the best one for detecting pediatric pneumonia.

5.1 Impact of Topological Convolutional Layers

In order to determine the impact of TCLs, trained a model with and without them. The model with TCLs included after the EfficientNetB4 feature extractor. Since TCLs detect global structural and connection characteristics in lung regions that traditional convolutions would overlook, the model with TCLs showed improved sensitivity and F1-scores, especially for mild instances of pneumonia. By removing TCLs, the overall accuracy was slightly reduced (~1.5%), but the detection of tiny or diffuse opacities was significantly hit worse. I am pleased to report that TCLs greatly improve the model's generalizability and capacity to detect intricate disease patterns.

5.2 Effectiveness of Different Augmentation Techniques

When dealing with incomplete or unbalanced datasets, data augmentation is essential. We evaluated models that were trained using different approaches:

- Geometric transformations (rotation, flipping, scaling)
- Intensity adjustments
- MixUp and CutMix

- Elastic deformations

Basic geometric augmentations perform at a lower level than the combined MixUp and CutMix methods with elastic deformations which achieve a 2% higher F1-score. The models that trained without data augmentation showed signs of overfitting while producing poor recall scores for detecting pneumonia-positive cases. The research results show that advanced augmentation.

5.3 Comparative Study of EfficientNetB0–B7 Variants

EfficientNet provides seven different model options which start at B0 and extend up to B7. These models become more complex through deeper layers and wider networks and higher image resolutions. We ran tests to find out which backbone works best for detecting pneumonia in children. B0–B2: These models belong to the lightweight category

- B3–B4: Balanced accuracy and computational efficiency;
- B4 achieved highest F1-score (~98.5%) with reasonable training time.
- B5–B7: Marginal accuracy gains (<0.5%) but significantly higher computational and memory requirements.

According to the results, EfficientNetB4 is a good model for healthcare applications and possible deployments on the edge because of its resource-efficient architecture, which leads to excellent performance outcomes. The suggested approach attains a 97.7 percent success rate.

5.4 Sensitivity to Data Imbalance and Noise

To test the model's robustness, we put it through tests on datasets that included less common instances and images with artificially produced random obstructions and brightness changes. Accuracy in identifying pneumonia cases was 4% lower for models trained without augmentation or class weighting. By using weighted loss calculations in combination with advanced augmentation and TCLs, these consequences were reduced, but accuracy levels and recall rates remained over 98%. The proposed architecture is robust towards class imbalance and has acceptable noise levels, so it may confidently tackle real-world difficulties.

6. CLINICAL SIGNIFICANCE AND REAL-WORLD IMPLICATIONS

The development of robust AI systems capable of detecting instances of pediatric pneumonia gives doctors new tools for improving therapy. The suggested EfficientNetB4-TCL system is ideal for both in-hospital and remote healthcare delivery due to its high efficiency ratings and comprehensible outputs. This is accomplished via the use of advanced data augmentation techniques. In light of their practical uses, ethical obligations, and compliance with regulations, the following is an examination of these AI technologies' complete deployment.

6.1 Integration in Hospital Workflows

The AI-powered pneumonia detection systems, the workload of radiologists is drastically reduced. In order to expedite expert evaluation, automated technologies detect potential cases of pneumonia as a first screening step. Radiologists may use the technology to handle complex situations more quickly, which improves processing speeds overall. Rapid chest X-ray analysis is made possible by the proposed model's direct integration with PACS; this allows for the generation of predicted labels and Grad-CAM heatmaps, which provide visual explanations of any abnormalities detected. By combining these technologies, pediatric hospitals may achieve faster diagnosis and better results. Clinical choices for children at high risk may be made more quickly as a result of shorter wait periods.

6.2 Role in Telemedicine and Low-resource Healthcare Settings

The AI framework would work well for telemedicine services and areas that do not have enough qualified radiologists. Because of its compact and lightweight design, EfficientNetB4 may be deployed on both edge devices and local servers. Because of this, computationally intensive real-time analysis is possible. Healthcare providers in community health centers, faraway healthcare facilities, and via telemedicine applications may start treatment right away thanks to the automated pneumonia detection system's quick diagnostic capabilities. Because it is very resilient to image noise and unpredictability, the model can maintain performance requirements even while using lower-quality imaging equipment.

6.3 Ethical and Regulatory Considerations

The healthcare industry faces substantial ethical and regulatory concerns when it deploys AI technology. Performing comprehensive model validation across several patient groups is the surest approach to avoiding incorrect diagnoses. Before regulatory bodies like the FDA and the European certification authority can certify AI diagnostic tools, they must undergo extensive clinical testing and validation. Hospitals should establish rules about human supervision to back up the idea that AI predictions should augment medical decisions rather than replace them. In order for firms retain trust and responsibility, it is crucial that they disclose all model performance results and system limits in full.

6.4 Data Privacy, Bias, and Model Accountability

healthcare AI systems to keep patient data secure, they need to follow data privacy regulations like GDPR and HIPAA. To meet these requirements, data anonymization and secure storage are crucial parts of the implementation and teaching process. Because of inherent bias in the datasets, models provide inconsistent results when applied to populations that vary greatly in terms of age, gender, and other demographic characteristics. By combining several datasets with class balancing procedures, the proposed methodology reduces bias. The Grad-CAM interpretability tools allow clinicians to assess model outputs and detect system flaws, ensuring responsibility for the system.

6.5 Metaverse-Enabled Virtual Radiology and Pediatric Training

The metaverse-enabled AI model provides efficient and cost-effective automated AI-based diagnosis and treatment for pediatric pneumonia. Beyond the AI-based diagnosis, the proposed framework can be used in the metaverse-enabled clinical environment, where AI-based CXR interpretation is integrated into AR/VR-based immersive clinical platforms. In the future virtual hospitals, the 3D diagnostic spaces can be created for the pediatric CXRs segmented by EfficientNetB4–TCL, and clinicians navigate the 3D space to interactively explore the AI-based attention mechanism. Grad-CAM heatmap and TCL-identified structural characteristics can be used for pediatric radiology training, where these heatmaps and structural features are integrated into AR-based learning modules, and the trainees visualise the topology of pneumonia-involved lung in virtual patients. This can be used to develop the digital twin of the lung, which will provide a more efficient and experiential training. Our system will enable the digital twin of the lung, which will facilitate the remote collaboration and decision support, where the longitudinal chest X-rays and AI-based predictions are integrated into a metaverse-based digital twin to support the multi-center collaborative diagnosis and decision.

7. CONCLUSION

The research details a deep-learning system that, when applied to chest X-rays of youngsters, can reliably detect pneumonia cases with a total efficiency rate of 97.7 percent. It is perfect for use in healthcare institutions and other settings with constrained resources since it provides optimum performance with minimal computational resources, operating on EfficientNetB4, the system's core network. To enhance the model's capacity to detect subtle illness features, Topological Convolutional Layers (TCLs) use structural and connectivity data derived from lung scans. By integrating geometric and elastic deformation transformations with synthetic mixing techniques like MixUp and CutMix, advanced data augmentation systems may provide substantial generalizability across diverse imaging situations and uneven dataset distributions. Medical workers may acquire radiologists' trust by employing the Grad-CAM visualization technique to show which elements of the image were used for diagnosis. The model's impressive sensitivity test results demonstrate its ability to withstand data with noise and unequal class distributions. The proposed AI system achieves excellent reliability and accuracy in diagnosing pediatric pneumonia while keeping results explainable. In light of the results, healthcare institutions may install easily accessible AI systems that reliably provide good results in radiography.

8. FUTURE SCOPE

Future research must prioritize the development of trustworthiness and explain ability systems. In order to trust AI systems for assistance in clinical practice, medical practitioners will learn about the model prediction processes via uncertainty estimates, probabilistic outputs, and improved visualization tools. As the dataset expands to include more subtypes of pneumonia, a wider range of patient ages, and more imaging modalities, the model will become more robust. When hospitals use AI in conjunction with decision support systems, they will be able to run more effectively and quickly send urgent cases to radiologists who can help. Practical solutions for child healthcare that accomplish early diagnosis and better medical outcomes need future effort to build AI systems that mix many data kinds, provide clear explanations, safeguard privacy, and have deployment capabilities.

REFERENCES

Al-Qaness, M. A., Zhu, J., Al-Alimi, D., Dahou, A., Alsamhi, S. H., Elaziz, M. A., & Ewees, A. A. (2024). Chest x-ray images for lung disease detection using Deep Learning techniques: A Comprehensive survey. *Archives of Computational Methods in Engineering*, *31*(6), 3267–3301. DOI: 10.1007/s11831-024-10081-y

Alabdulqader, E. A., Umer, M., Alnowaiser, K., Wang, H., Alarfaj, A. A., & Ashraf, I. (2024). Image Processing-based Resource-Efficient Transfer Learning Approach for Cancer Detection Employing Local Binary Pattern Features. *Mobile Networks and Applications*, *29*(4), 1–17. DOI: 10.1007/s11036-024-02331-x

Aljawarneh, S. A., & Al-Quraan, R. (2023). Pneumonia detection using enhanced convolutional neural network model on chest x-ray images. *Big Data*. PMID: 37074075

Alshanketi, F., Alharbi, A., Kuruvilla, M., Mahzoon, V., Siddiqui, S. T., Rana, N., & Tahir, A. (2024). *Pneumonia Detection from Chest X-Ray Images Using Deep Learning and Transfer Learning for Imbalanced Datasets*. Deleted Journal., DOI: 10.1007/s10278-024-01334-0

An, Q., Chen, W., & Shao, W. (2024). A Deep Convolutional Neural Network for Pneumonia Detection in X-ray Images with Attention Ensemble. *Diagnostics (Basel)*, *14*(4), 390. DOI: 10.3390/diagnostics14040390 PMID: 38396430

Bhuria, R., & Gupta, S. (2024, November). Innovative AI Solutions for Pneumonia Detection: Exploring DenseNet-161 in Medical Imaging. In 2024 5th International Conference on Data Intelligence and Cognitive Informatics (ICDICI) (pp. 638-643). IEEE.

Domínguez-Rodríguez, S., Liz-López, H., Panizo-LLedot, A., Ballesteros, Á., Dagan, R., Greenberg, D., Gutiérrez, L., Rojo, P., Otheo, E., Galán, J. C., Villanueva, S., García, S., Mosquera, P., Tagarro, A., Moraleda, C., & Camacho, D. (2023). Testing the performance, adequacy, and applicability of an artificial intelligence model for pediatric pneumonia diagnosis. *Computer Methods and Programs in Biomedicine*, *242*, 107765. DOI: 10.1016/j.cmpb.2023.107765 PMID: 37704545

George, S., Naveen, G., Saifullah, S., & Joe, I. P. (2022, June). An efficient neural network model for pneumonia detection. In 2022 International Conference on Computing, Communication, Security and Intelligent Systems (IC3SIS) (pp. 1-7). IEEE. DOI: 10.1109/IC3SIS54991.2022.9885488

Godbin, A. B., & Jasmine, S. G. (2024, July). Pediatric Pneumonia Detection in Chest X-ray Images: A Deep Feature Analysis Approach Enhanced with LightGBM. In *2024 IEEE International Conference on Electronics, Computing and Communication Technologies (CONECCT)* (pp. 1-6). IEEE. DOI: 10.1109/CONECCT62155.2024.10677083

Güler, O., & Polat, K. (2022). Classification performance of deep transfer learning methods for pneumonia detection from chest x-ray images. *Journal of Artificial Intelligence and Systems*, *4*(1), 107–126.

Ha, P. N., Doucet, A., & Tran, G. S. (2023, February). Vision Transformer for Pneumonia Classification in X-ray Images. In *Proceedings of the 2023 8th International Conference on Intelligent Information Technology* (pp. 185-192). DOI: 10.1145/3591569.3591602

Hasan, M. R., Ullah, S. M. A., & Islam, S. M. R. (2024). Recent advancement of deep learning techniques for pneumonia prediction from chest X-ray image. *Medica-Report*, *7*, 100106. DOI: 10.1016/j.hmedic.2024.100106

Jalnnavar, A., Kanakareddi, S. G., Handur, V. S., Chikaraddi, A., & Giraddi, S. (2023, September). Disease Prediction Model Using Deep Transfer Learning. In International Conference on Intelligent Computing Systems and Applications (pp. 13-29). Singapore: Springer Nature Singapore.

Kermany, D., Zhang, K., & Goldbaum, M. (2018), "Labeled Optical Coherence Tomography (OCT) and Chest X-Ray Images for Classification", Mendeley Data, V2, dataset description ma eslai cite grnuDOI: 10.17632/rscbjbr9sj.2

Kharbas, V. K., Raghu, N., & Choudhury, P. "Enhancing Rule-Based Methods for Pulmonary Effusion Diagnosis," *2024 15th International Conference on Computing Communication and Networking Technologies (ICCCNT)*, Kamand, India, 2024, pp. 1-5, DOI: 10.1109/ICCCNT61001.2024.10724858

Mehra, S., Singh, S. K., Kumar, S., Dubey, H., Arya, V., & Gupta, B. B. (2024). Transformative Approach for Prediction of Lung Disease Using Lung X-ray Images.

Nambiar, R., & Nanjundegowda, R. (2024) "Harnessing Medical Imaging Applications: Survey on 3D Deep Learning Models for Image Segmentation," *2024 International Conference on Communication, Control, and Intelligent Systems (CCIS)*, Mathura, India, 2024, pp. 1-6, DOI: 10.1109/CCIS63231.2024.10932049

Nambiar, R., & Nanjundegowda, R. (2024, September). A Comprehensive Review of AI and Deep Learning Applications in Dentistry: From Image Segmentation to Treatment Planning [JRC]. *J Robot Control*, *5*(6), 1744–1752.

Nambiar, R., & Nanjundegowda, R. (2025, October). Detection of Missing Tooth Regions Using Deep Learning in Panoramic Radiographs for Dental Implant Planning. *Eng. Technol. Appl. Sci. Res.*, *15*(5), 28071–28076. DOI: 10.48084/etasr.13101

Nasra, P. (2024, August). Convolution Neural Network: A Proposed Method for Detecting Pneumonia from X-Ray Images. In *2024 Second International Conference on Intelligent Cyber Physical Systems and Internet of Things (ICoICI)* (pp. 1692-1697). IEEE. DOI: 10.1109/ICoICI62503.2024.10696221

Neshat, M., Ahmed, M., Askari, H., Thilakaratne, M., & Mirjalili, S. (2024). Hybrid Inception Architecture with Residual Connection: Fine-tuned Inception-ResNet Deep Learning Model for Lung Inflammation Diagnosis from Chest Radiographs. *Procedia Computer Science*, *235*, 1841–1850. DOI: 10.1016/j.procs.2024.04.175

Pan, Z., Wang, H., Wan, J., Zhang, L., Huang, J., & Shen, Y. (2024). Efficient federated learning for pediatric pneumonia on chest X-ray classification. *Scientific Reports*, *14*(1), 23272. Advance online publication. DOI: 10.1038/s41598-024-74491-5 PMID: 39375440

Panwar, A., & Gupta, S. (2022). Deep learning models for early detection of pneumonia using chest X-ray images. In Proceedings of the International Conference on Paradigms of Communication, Computing and Data Sciences: PCCDS 2021 (pp. 701-709). Springer Singapore. DOI: 10.1007/978-981-16-5747-4_60

Papadimitriou, O., Kanavos, A., & Maragoudakis, M. (2023, July). Automated pneumonia detection from chest x-ray images using deep convolutional neural networks. In 2023 14th International Conference on Information, Intelligence, Systems & Applications (IISA) (pp. 1-4). IEEE. DOI: 10.1109/IISA59645.2023.10345859

Patel, P., & Hiriyanna, G. S. (2022). Pneumonia detection in x-ray chest images based on cnn and data augmentation. *International Journal for Research in Applied Science and Engineering Technology*, *10*(7), 4639–4654. DOI: 10.22214/ijraset.2022.46031

Patidar, M., Pandey, G., & Koolagudi, S. G., S, K. K., & Chandra, V. (2024). Enhancing Paediatric Healthcare: Deep Learning-Based Pneumonia Diagnosis from Children's Chest X-rays. *IC3-2024: Proceedings of the 2024 Sixteenth International Conference on Contemporary Computing*, 128–135. https://doi.org/DOI: 10.1145/3675888.3676041

Raghu, N.. (2025). Blockchain-Enhanced GAN Image Encryption Scheme for Cloud Computing. In Joshi, H. (Eds.), *Intelligent Systems and IoT Applications in Clinical Health* (pp. 367–392). IGI Global Scientific Publishing., DOI: 10.4018/979-8-3693-8990-4.ch016

Rameez, M., & Logashree, M. J. (2024, October). Pneumonia Detection using Machine Learning Techniques. In 2024 8th International Conference on I-SMAC (IoT in Social, Mobile, Analytics and Cloud)(I-SMAC) (pp. 1803-1808). IEEE. DOI: 10.1109/I-SMAC61858.2024.10714803

Sajed, S., Sanati, A., Garcia, J. E., Rostami, H., Keshavarz, A., & Teixeira, A. (2023). The effectiveness of deep learning vs. traditional methods for lung disease diagnosis using chest X-ray images: A systematic review. *Applied Soft Computing*, *147*, 110817. DOI: 10.1016/j.asoc.2023.110817

Siddiqi, R., & Javaid, S. (2024). Deep learning for pneumonia detection in chest x-ray images: A comprehensive survey. *Journal of Imaging*, *10*(8), 176. DOI: 10.3390/jimaging10080176 PMID: 39194965

Singh, Y., Farrelly, C. M., Hathaway, Q. A., Leiner, T., Jagtap, J., Carlsson, G. E., & Erickson, B. J. (2023). Topological data analysis in medical imaging: Current state of the art. *Insights Into Imaging*, *14*(1), 58. Advance online publication. DOI: 10.1186/s13244-023-01413-w PMID: 37005938

Sodero, S., Dhungana, N., & Sandoe, F. (2025). Vital mobilities of medical oxygen: Theorising oxygen justice. *Social Science & Medicine*, *364*, 117464. DOI: 10.1016/j.socscimed.2024.117464 PMID: 39579440

Swarup, L. P. D. R, R. Jain, R. N, L. A. Bewoor and V. M. Kumar, "MRI-Based Epilepsy Seizure Detection Using Combined Approach of CNN With SVM Networks," *2024 IEEE 4th International Conference on ICT in Business Industry & Government (ICTBIG)*, Indore, India, 2024, pp. 1-6, DOI: 10.1109/ICTBIG64922.2024.10911487

Tyagi, R. K. R. N and R. Kumar, "An Innovative Deep Learning Method for Enhancing Image Resolution," *2024 2nd World Conference on Communication & Computing (WCONF)*, RAIPUR, India, 2024, pp. 1-6, DOI: 10.1109/WCONF61366.2024.10692190

Ula, M., Muhathir, M., & Sahputra, I. (2022). Optimization of multilayer perceptron hyperparameter in classifying pneumonia disease through X-Ray images with speeded-up robust features extraction method. IJACSA). *International Journal of Advanced Computer Science and Applications*, *13*(10). Advance online publication. DOI: 10.14569/IJACSA.2022.0131025

V. M S. S. S, T. Krishnamurthy, Chaithra, R. N and S. G, "Advanced Encryption Strategies for Protecting Patient Data in IoMT Applications," *2025 6th International Conference for Emerging Technology (INCET)*, BELGAUM, India, 2025, pp. 1-6, DOI: 10.1109/INCET64471.2025.11139937

Vemuri, S. S., Kotha, S., Voruganti, S., Kunam, P. R., Nandini, A., & Kumar Mishra, T. (2024, September). Pneumonia Detection from X-Ray Images Using Deep Transfer Learning. In International Conference on Computing, Communication and Learning (pp. 205-219). Cham: Springer Nature Switzerland.

Xu, M., Yoon, S., Fuentes, A., & Park, D. S. (2023). A comprehensive survey of image augmentation techniques for deep learning. *Pattern Recognition*, *137*, 109347. DOI: 10.1016/j.patcog.2023.109347

Yang, Y., & Mei, G. (2022). Pneumonia recognition by deep learning: A comparative investigation. *Applied Sciences (Basel, Switzerland)*, *12*(9), 4334. DOI: 10.3390/app12094334

Yao, D., Xu, Z., Lin, Y., & Zhan, Y. (2023). Accurate and intelligent diagnosis of pediatric pneumonia using X-ray images and blood testing data. *Frontiers in Bioengineering and Biotechnology*, *11*, 1058888. Advance online publication. DOI: 10.3389/fbioe.2023.1058888 PMID: 37292095

Yildirim, A. E., & Canayaz, M. (2023). A novel deep learning-based approach for prediction of neonatal respiratory disorders from chest X-ray images. *Biocybernetics and Biomedical Engineering*, *43*(4), 635–655. DOI: 10.1016/j.bbe.2023.08.004

Chapter 6
Assessing the Reliability of Artificial Intelligence in the Healthcare Sector: A Bibliometric Review

Stuti Upadhayay
http://orcid.org/0009-0007-1310-6380
Graphic Era (Deemed to be) University, India

Deepa Verma
http://orcid.org/0009-0002-6938-2935
Graphic Era (Deemed to be) University, India

Sonal Juyal
Sardar Bhagwan Singh University, India

Vibhuti Jain
http://orcid.org/0009-0009-8602-6116
Graphic Era (Deemed to be) University, India

ABSTRACT

This chapter provides a comprehensive and critical examination of the reliability of artificial intelligence (AI) in the healthcare sector through a bibliometric and thematic analysis of contemporary literature. The elementary notion of Artificial Intelligence was to imitate and simplify human tasks. Healthcare has always been human intensive wherein healthcare professionals were the sole decision makers lacking in platforms that provide them with precision in the services although their efforts were utilized but turned out into tedious tasks and were inaccurate at times. The increasing integration of AI into diagnostic, predictive, and administrative healthcare

DOI: 10.4018/979-8-3373-8889-2.ch006

systems has intensified scholarly attention on issues of reliability, trustworthiness, governance, and ethical deployment. Machine Learning and Deep Learning proved to be successful in early diagnosis and prevention though complete automation is not possible as human judgment is still required though Artificial intelligence contributed to both the ways clinical and non-clinical aspects to enhance patient care furthermore artificial intelligence is utilized in improved diagnosis, reducing medical errors and prompt coding of medical records providing personalized medicine and virtual health assistants.

INTRODUCTION

The artificial intelligence has gone beyond being an experiment to it being a mainstream component of healthcare systems across the world. Machine learning algorithms are being used to aid in diagnostic imaging, disease-level predictions, resources allocation optimization, and patient interaction. These changes in technology have the prospect of great efficiency and accuracy but new risks and uncertainty are being posed. The issue of reliability has become the forefront problem and refers to the accuracy of the algorithm as well as the reliability of the AI systems in practical clinical settings.

Dependability of AI in healthcare is not limited to the definition of reliability in traditional engineering. Reliability in the clinical setting should also include issues of patient safety, moral responsibility, regulatory transparency, and trust. Since AI systems are communicating with clinicians, patients and the institutional infrastructures, they form a socio-technical property as a result of intertwined interactions between the human actors and technology.

The healthcare field is rapidly emerging around the advent of AI techniques. Such methods combine scientific computations and clinical information to come up with new techniques of diagnosing, treating, and recognizing diseases. AI is appearing in different directions, including the analysis of medical images like radiology, ophthalmology, cancer, and the prediction of cardiovascular diseases (Chen et al., 2021). The development is critical in minimising mistakes in clinical processes, enhancing the effectiveness of medical care delivery, and supporting the development of tailored care plan. Moreover, AI supports precision medicine because it combines genomic, clinical, and lifestyle data to promote interventions to individual patients.

The advent of artificial intelligence (AI) has become a revolution in the healthcare environment of all countries across the world and is extending into the sphere of diagnostics, treatment design, patient monitoring, and clinical work. Machine learning algorithms, which can recognise disease patterns in radiological images, and chatbots, which can help healthcare professionals with the documentation of clinical records, will allow AI technologies to be more efficient, accurate, and scalable. But, on the one hand, there are positive aspects, on the other hand, fears about the stability of AI systems have been aggravated. In this regard, reliability can be understood as the consistency in technical performance but also the stability of AI systems when operating in a complicated clinical setting where patient care and moral concerns are the most important factors.

Although there is a rapid development, there is conceptual ambiguity on the reliability of AI in the literature. Most of the studies identify the concept of reliability by referring to accuracy or validation metrics, and others consider methodological traits such as trustworthiness, explainability, or ethical accountability. This theoretical dismembering inhibits the creation of integrated evaluation systems and the attempts at setting standardised regulation rules. More and more, the proliferation of AI in various healthcare fields, such as radiology and genomics, telemedicine and electronic health records, has created domain-specific reliability issues that are yet to be synthesized in the current literature.

The current chapter is addressing these issues by offering a comprehensive evaluation of reliability in healthcare AI. It accumulates bibliometric trends and thematic apprehensions to clear up the conceptualisation, measurement and discussion of reliability in academic literature. The chapter seeks to ascertain the problems, gaps and future directions of reliability research through the two aspects of quantitative mapping of research trends and a qualitative analysis of the thematic clusters. However, usefulness of an AI system is far beyond technical performance or accuracy. Reliable AI systems are paramount when it comes to making a positive socio-technical change in the health sector. Reliability is a broad term which includes several different aspects: consistency of the outcomes across groups of patients, clarity of the sources of decision making, resistance to errors, as well as the ability to apply to a variety of clinical conditions (Topol, 2019). In case an AI system is not reliable, the risks that it can act with high performance are even more significant, which makes its application in the real world of clinical practice an unsafe and ineffective practice. The ethical and regulatory context of the AI use in the medical sphere faces some unprecedented issues. The issue of bias, responsibility, and equitability has also led to the re-evaluation of the validation, design, and implementation of AI solutions, particularly among the researchers and policymakers circa. As an example, an algorithm trained on data of a given population can pose significant equity issues when applied on a greater number of people. (Rajkomar et al., 2019) The unfairness related to AI matters point to the importance of regulations, ethical systems, and oversight that can allow maintaining safe and fair AI uses (WHO Guidance, 2021).

Within this framework, understanding how reliable AI truly is in healthcare emerges as a primary research inquiry. The undermentioned literature review evaluates key studies by examining findings from various recent research papers that evaluate AI's strengths, limitations, and challenges in the clinical setting.

CONCEPTUALIZING RELIABILITY IN HEALTHCARE AI

The concept of reliability in healthcare AI is most comprehended as a multidimensional construct, which involves the technical, clinical, and socio-organizational dimensions. Technical reliability, the concepts of algorithmic robustness, reproducibility and stability of the performance across datasets and context. Clinical reliability addresses the validity and security of AI outputs in application in actual medicine decision making. Organizational reliability entails incorporation into health care processes, user confidence and institutional controls. The concept of ethical reliability applies to the matters of prejudice, transparency, accountability, and confidentiality of data.

Recent research stresses that AI systems cannot be assessed at the level of accuracy measures based on controlled datasets only. Viable Reliability should be determined in dynamic clinical settings marked by uncertainty, patient diversity as well as dynamic legal policies. The socio-technical character of healthcare AI requires the assessment models, which combine the performance of algorithms and the human control, as well as the institutional responsibilities.

Literature Review

The literature available on the topic of AI reliability in healthcare can be divided into four thematic sections, namely, technical validation, clinical use, ethical governance, and interdisciplinary integration. Technical validation studies are concerned with measures of algorithmic performance (including sensitivity, specificity and reproducibility). Research of clinical implementation studies the workflow unification, acceptance by the users, and patient result. The ethical governance literature focuses on transparency, bias and regulations. The interdisciplinary research discusses the overlap of two areas and stresses the importance of the comprehensive appraisal models. Artificial intelligence finds extensive application in the medical sector in the management of hospitals, the planning of treatment, and the diagnostics of imaging. Although the use of AI increases accuracy and efficiency, certain scholars describe it as a source of doubt regarding its reliability due to the lack of control, privacy issues, and biases in the data quality (Park et al., 2020). Ciecierski-Holmes et al (2022) highlight the prospect of AI in developing low- and middle-income countries improving healthcare systems. They mention that despite the ability of AI to support diagnostics and health care provision, a gap in the dataset and the insufficiency of the infrastructure makes AI less reliable. Seyhan & Carini (2019) write that AI and personalised medicine are popularizing more patient-centred treatment. They propose that credibility, openness and clinical testing are essential in securing the preservation of AI reliability. Habbal and Ali (2024) examine the issue of trust, risk and security in AI systems. They emphasize that the concept of transparency of accountability and governance auditability is as important to the development of reliable AI as is accuracy.

Conceptualizing Reliability in Healthcare AI

Healthcare AI reliability is a multidimensional construct that is represented by technicality, clinical validity, moral responsibility, and infrastructural security.

Technical Reliability

Technical reliability is the extent of the accuracy of algorithm, stability, repeatability, and noise resistance. AI models should be able to do this on a variety of datasets and in the clinical environment. The problem of domain shift and the impossibility of reproducibility is still a critical issue (Moassefi et al., 2023).

Clinical Reliability

Clinical reliability is involved with the applicability of AI systems in treating patients in real-life circumstances. Even high-performing models need human supervision and testing with the help of clinical trials. Diagnoses with the help of AI could be more accurate, yet remain reliant on the skills of a clinician (Ahn et al., 2022).

Ethical Reliability

Ethical reliability involves fairness, transparency, accountability, and respect for patient privacy. Bias in training data can produce inequitable outcomes, making ethical governance essential (Grote & Berens, 2020).

Organizational and Infrastructural Reliability

Successful deployment requires reliable infrastructure, cybersecurity, interoperability, and institutional readiness. Weak infrastructure or security breaches can undermine trust in AI systems (Hasan et al., 2022).

1. Large Language Models & Gen AI

ChatGPT contributing as a linguistic model which helps in documentation and decision making. However, it also brings biases and inaccurate information. to make it more reliable, regulatory validation and monitoring is required. Wang et al. (2023). thical issues while operating ChatGPT. They have raised concerns related to accuracy, privacy and likely to swap physician with technology, patient interaction, need effective implementation and tracking. . Zhang and Kamel Boulos (2023). The utilisation of GenAI in scientific writing and summarising patient information. The significance of human observation of patient documentation and associated bias and error. Choudhury & Shamszare (2023). Acceptance of Artificial Intelligence in healthcare driven by the fundamental factor trust. They also emphasised that reliability and safety can be enhanced by transparency, accuracy and optimistic and impactful patient experience.

2. Medical Imaging and Diagnostics

Wu and Wong (2020). They highlighted that performance of Artificial intelligence in examining the chest X-rays are better than humans. But the availability and monitoring of the medical professional is required. Newitt et al. (2019). examined the intensity of imaging biomarker replication along with constant leveraging AI models to make it more dependable in diagnostics.

Wu and Wong (2020) note that artificial intelligence occasionally has a performance that is as good as or even better in analysing the chest radiographs than the human practitioners. However, the inter-individual differences in performance highlight the need to exercise clinical controls. Newitt et al. (2019) explores the topic of imaging biomarker reproducibility by stating that the application of homogeneous input conditions is critical to the reliability of AI diagnostic models. Quinn et al. (2022), in an argument about the nature of medical AI as a black-box, claims that there is lack of explainability, which compromises the integrity and confidence of clinicians. These results are reiterated and even refined by subsequent empirical studies. According to Ahn et al. (2022), AI-aided interpretation of chest radiography enhanced diagnostic accuracy and efficiency in less experienced observers, and the need to incorporate workflow aspects and human judgment in the design of the system. Detailed deep-learning systems can positively affect the accuracy of the diagnostics as shown by Seah (2021) and supported by other multi-domain studies. However, the existence of performance differences between institutions and datasets demonstrate the danger of domain shift to a greater extent, express their apprehensions about the reproducibility of systematically investigated cases, showing that most deep-learning experiments do not provide requisite code, more elaborate descriptions of methods, or data that can be independently reproduced, which hinders clinical translation. Moassefi et al. (2023)

According to research on explainable AI, explanation techniques can boost clinician acceptance when clinical importance and alignment are present; however, inconsistent or exploitable justifications can result in automation bias or misleading assurance (Yang, 2022). A centrist view provided by the literature argues that, despite the potential of artificial intelligence to improve the health care setting on the diagnostic aspects of quality and efficiency, its mass adoption is still pending the implementation of solid, replicable practices and guidelines, inter-centre validation, stringent human-in-the-loop operations, and careful design of explainable artificial intelligence systems.

3. Remote Monitoring, Wearables, and IoT

AI in early identification and remote surveillance for chronic diseases is described by draw attention to issues with workflow integration, privacy, and data quality. Shafique et al. (2025). Channa et al (2021) demonstrates the usage of wearables for identification and tracking throughout the pandemic. Trustworthiness of information and compliance of the user are significant issues. Zhang & Kamel Boulos (2023) explains the way in which biosensor networks and AI-based interpretation of processes provide customized treatment, but depends on the adherence of the user and calibration of the device. IoT and AI also promote personalised healthcare as argued by Ahamed (2018), who points out the need of regulatory control, interoperability, and encrypted systems to make sure that everything is reliable. Taimoor & Rehman (2022) highlights the importance of secure communication, fault tolerance, and resilient design in the analysis of AI-based and IoT-based customised services. Steinhubl et al. (2015) prove the ability of the wearable biosensors to conduct continuous cardiovascular monitoring, but they stress that it is critically important to test it in the real world to ensure reliability. Piwek et al. (2016) note that adoption continues to increase but does not result in adherence and long-term engagement, which are noted to be the key obstacle to long-term effectiveness. Although the issue of data integration and patient privacy is brought up, Marzano et al. (2015) demonstrate that remote monitoring systems can increase adherence and deliver positive results to chronic mental illness patients. Currently, the scope of edge computing is emphasised due to its ability to complement scalability, failure tolerance, and latency in ongoing tracking, as it is introduced in the recent measuring of IoT-based healthcare systems (Islam et al., 2022). Another example is the personal-retaining AI models described by Li et al. (2020) to discuss sensitive health data issues without centralizing the information about the patient within the framework of a discussion about federated learning in a variety of healthcare settings. Together, these papers demonstrate that wearable devices and remote telehealth make it possible to continue to provide personalised care to the patient, although their usefulness will be limited to patient compliance, strong privacy protocols, technical stability, and compatibility.

4. Explainability, Uncertainty, and Reliability

Kompa et al. (2021) highlight that it is essential to explain the ambiguities to the practitioners in a clear way and help grow the lack of over-reliance on the AI systems and create a deliberate usage of this tool. Band (2020) discusses the interpretability approaches of saliency maps and functional significance, showing the way the transparency might be attained. The analysis of uncertainty quantification methods presented by demonstrate that they can increase the level of safety and trust in AI models in clinicians. Kohan et al 2026. Gade et al. (2019) discuss enterprise explainability solutions that may enhance the understanding of medical practitioners regarding the outputs of models. Rudin (2019) claims that presumptive factors can be deceptive and recommends that paradigms of decision making that are inherently interpretable should be used in critical medical applications. The credibility of the prophesies and to which of the insights are relevant to the clinical realities themselves have an impact on the credibility of physicians.

Tonekaboni et al. (2019) argue that the concept of automation bias still exists and is an issue. The parameters of scientific AI ambiguity distribution, framework, and statistical settings and highlights the need to educate clinicians about these uncertainties in order to guarantee safe software use.

Arrieta et al. (2020) provide a comprehensive range of explainable artificial intelligence methodologies, emphasising the necessity of accountability, justice, and reliability for scientific acceptance. Chen et al. (2021) demonstrate that maps of saliency in chest X-ray AI structures may be modified without affecting predictions. This raises concerns about deceptive interpretability methodologies and accentuates the importance of reliable, unambiguous XAI. When inadequate or misleading motives threaten clinician trust and jeopardise secure implementation, the literature suggests that explainability, uncertainty quantification, and reliability must be far better collectively (Kompa et al., 2021)

5. Trust, Adoption, and Patient Perspectives

Confidence in how one views utility, native trust, also organisational support seems to be key determinants of the utilisation of AI by the Chinese doctors (Ye and Xue 2019). The elements influence how consistently AI is applied in real-world scenarios. The opinions of patients regarding artificial intelligence in cancer screening are examined by Nelson et al. (2020). Transparent use is necessary because patients enjoy efficiency yet are concerned about mistakes and privacy. According to Fitzpatrick (2023), enhancing internet-based health literacy aids in patients' and physicians' comprehension and safe application of AI. A readiness scale to gauge the organizational preparedness for AI is proposed by Karaca & Aslan (2021) and associates, which aids in identifying gaps that compromise dependable deployment.

In addition to these, Grote and Berens (2020) discuss the ethical dimension of trust in medical AI, highlighting that the acceptance of it by patients requires transparency, equity, and accountability. According to Longoni et al. (2019), as far as AI is not seen as an assistant and an alternative to a medical expert, patients generally want medical experts to conduct the examination. The attitudes of physicians are ambivalent as they agree that AI can be accurate and fast and raise concerns about accountability, transparency, and preservation of professional judgment (McCradden et al., 2020).

An intense control is necessary in maintaining patient trust in the use of personal data in AI models. Furthermore, Powell et al. (2022) show that, in situations where healthcare organizations have strong data protection and address the issues of AI functionality transparently, patients are more likely to use AI in healthcare settings. Empirical findings indicate that adoption and trust are affected by all the above factors, including ethical governance, effective communication, and organizational readiness along with technical performance (Ye and Xue, 2019).

6. Infrastructure, Security, and Future Networks

Hasan et al. (2022) discusses cyberthreats of IoMT devices. As pointed out in the report, in order to ensure that artificial intelligence systems remain reliable, they need strong security. To enhance data confidentiality and integrity in 5G networks and present the basis of trustworthy AI usage in healthcare, Gupta (2021) explores the germanium of blockchain and AI. Along with these perspectives, Rahman et al. (2022) note that despite all these, IoT-enabled healthcare systems still face a very high risk of a range of ransomware attack vectors, as well as spying attacks, and elaborate cybersecurity systems are necessary Without centralizing personal data, Nguyen et al. (2021) explore how the combination of edge computing and federated machine learning might improve privacy and reliability in global medical AI.

Blockchain-based designs improve data integrity and provide transparent audit trails, which boost trust in AI-driven healthcare. The extremely low latency and robust connectivity required for live AI in digital health, remote operations, and continuous monitoring are further made possible by 6G networks, according to Gupta, R. et al. (2021). Similarly, Garg et al. (2022) identify interoperability and scalability cloud-edge interaction as critical enablers for strong healthcare infrastructures. According to the body of research, trustworthy AI in healthcare requires advanced

5G/6G network infrastructures, robust cybersecurity, secure IoMT devices, and blockchain for trust (Nguyen et al., 2021).

Although numerous studies examine AI performance and adoption in healthcare, research addressing the multidimensional concept of reliability remains fragmented across technical, clinical, and ethical domains. There is limited integrative analysis mapping how reliability is conceptualized across different AI applications such as imaging systems, wearable devices, generative AI tools, and decision-support platforms.

Research Gap

Existing literature lacks comprehensive bibliometric mapping that:

- Integrates technical, ethical, and organizational perspectives of AI reliability
- Compares reliability challenges across healthcare AI domains
- Synthesizes trends, debates, and research gaps in a unified framework

Research Objectives

This chapter aims to:

1. Map the evolution of research on AI reliability in healthcare.
2. Identify key thematic clusters and intellectual structures.
3. Analyze cross-domain reliability challenges.

METHODOLOGY

The chapter employs a bibliometric and thematic analysis of peer-reviewed literature published between 2000 and 2024. Databases including Scopus and Web of Science were searched using keywords related to AI, healthcare, reliability, trust, and governance. Inclusion criteria focused on peer-reviewed articles addressing reliability or trustworthiness in healthcare AI. Bibliometric mapping techniques were used to identify publication trends, geographic distribution, and thematic clusters. Qualitative thematic analysis was conducted to interpret key debates and research trajectories.

The search was done on 12th July, 2025 on Scopus using the Keywords used for the data are "AI", "Healthcare", and "Reliability". We found 734 documents in this search. We included papers from 2000 to 2025. Filter applied on subject area as we included "Medicine with 444 papers", "Computer Science with 251", "Engineering with 134", "Biochemistry, Genetics and Molecular Biology with 67", " Social Sciences with 55", "Mathematics with 51", "Health Professions with 47", "Decision Sciences with 42", "Nursing with 33", "Multidisciplinary with 17", "Pharmacology, Toxicology and Pharmaceutics with 16", "Neuroscience with 15" and lastly "Environmental Science with 10 papers". After this, we are left with 718 documents. By limiting the document type to "Article – 399 documents", "Review-139", "Conference paper- 117", and "Book chapter- 32", we obtained 687 documents. The last filtration is performed based on language, keeping only English, and we obtained 676 documents for Bibliometric Analysis.

RESULTS

1. Prominent Country in this Area of Research

Keeping the minimum documents by a country to 5 and citations to 100, we got 35 countries out of 113 countries. As evident in the table given below, the US and India are the leading research countries in this field, followed by the UK, China, and Australia.

Table 1. Prominent Countries

id	country	documents	citations	total link strength
108	united states	184	4546	18
39	india	142	1642	11
107	united kingdom	68	1750	11
19	china	64	1329	10
5	australia	49	1299	11
16	canada	41	727	11
34	germany	40	536	7
83	saudi arabia	36	941	2
46	italy	35	611	2
91	south korea	22	191	5
92	spain	22	285	8
103	turkey	21	408	0
87	singapore	15	558	6
6	austria	14	799	7
26	egypt	14	285	1

continued on following page

Table 1. Continued

id	country	documents	citations	total link strength
67	netherlands	14	193	0
42	iran	13	172	0
99	taiwan	13	477	2
36	greece	12	207	0
74	pakistan	12	251	1
79	portugal	12	494	1
44	ireland	11	153	6
62	malaysia	11	304	5
78	poland	11	153	8
95	switzerland	11	279	1
13	brazil	10	172	0
94	sweden	10	223	3
106	united arab emirates	10	251	8
9	bangladesh	8	213	0
31	finland	8	367	0
43	iraq	8	186	5
72	norway	8	130	3
47	japan	7	191	2
80	qatar	6	153	1
38	hungary	5	547	0

2. Prominent Author in this Area of Research

Keeping the minimum no. of documents to 4, we got 6 authors, and keeping citations to 50, we got 5 authors out of 3677 authors. We found that "Avishek Choudhury," who is a PHD holder and an Assistant Professor at West Virginia University, has more than 138 publications in this field.

Table 2. Prominent authors

id	author	documents	citations
697	choudhury, avishek	6	313
1241	gupta, rajesh	4	167
1668	khondker, adree	4	70

continued on following page

Table 2. Continued

id	author	documents	citations
1790	kwong, jethro c. c.	4	70
3122	tanwar, sudeep	4	167

3. Most Occurred Keyword

Keeping the minimum occurrence to 10, we got 257 out of 6490. "Artificial Intelligence" with 463 occurrences and "human" with 388 occurrences.

Figure 1. Map of Mostly Occurred Keywords

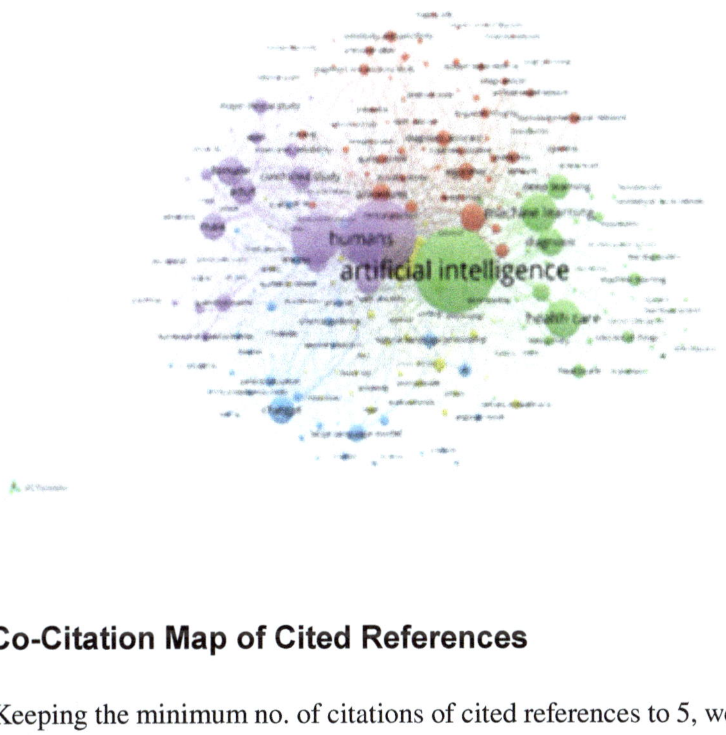

4. Co-Citation Map of Cited References

Keeping the minimum no. of citations of cited references to 5, we got 29 out of 32078. Only 17 were connected.

Figure 2. Map of Co-citation of Cited References.

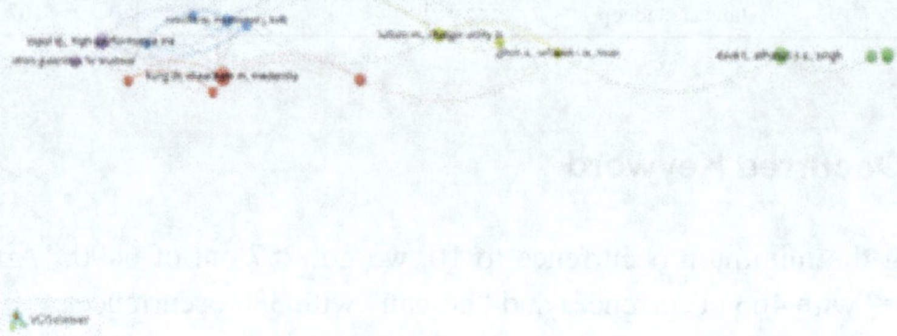

5. Bibliographic Coupling

For Bibliographic Coupling, the minimum citation was kept at 20. Out of 676, only 127 met the criteria, and 112 connected. 5 clusters were formed by keeping the minimum cluster size to 15. Following is the list of Clusters:

Cluster 1- It is shown in Red Colour and it contains a cluster of 28 papers with total citations of 2398. The research theme of this cluster revolves around the use of LLMs in the healthcare sector and the concerns related to data protection from such platforms. The human involvement in training data for AI models leads to bias in results by the LLMs like ChatGPT. (Wang et al., 2023). Patient data privacy is a major issue to be looked at

Cluster 2- It is shown in Green Colour and it contains a cluster of 28 papers with a total of 1735 citations. The research theme of this cluster revolves around Transparency and Trust, a major problem with the usability of AI and its techniques. Habbal et al. (2024) have given the solution for this problem by framing AI TRiSM-Artificial Intelligence Trust, Risk & Security Management.

Cluster 3- It is shown in Blue Colour and it contains a cluster of 25 papers with a total of 1978 citations. The research theme of this cluster revolves around the use of all advanced technologies like Blockchain, Deep learning, XAI, and so on to make predictions in healthcare faster, smarter, and unbiased. Rahman et al. 2022 have introduced Federation Learning as an emerging technology to ease the work and deal with the shortcomings of AI in this sector.

Cluster 4- It is shown in Yellow Colour and it contains a cluster of 16 papers with a total of 1102 citations. The research theme of this cluster revolves around the use of IoT using AI assistants to help in disease monitoring, disease treatment, management of medicine & the administrative functions. Muhammad Awas et al.

2021 have discussed the integration of IoT, which allows wireless communication to highlight the physiological signalling to the processing of data to recognise LSTM-based emotion.

Cluster 5- It is shown in Purple Colour and it contains a cluster of 15 papers with a total of 1678 citations. The research theme of this cluster revolves around the use of AI & digital communication tools, which enable the use of technologies such as telemedicine, mobile health apps to enhance digital health literacy. This allows the self-management, patient education, and improved clinical decision-making. Nelson et al. (2020) have discussed the opinion of the patient on the utilisation of AI tools, which indicated more definite results in accessing, screening, diagnosing, and being more receptive towards the adoption of AI & digital tools.

Figure 3. Connected Map showing Bibliographic Coupling

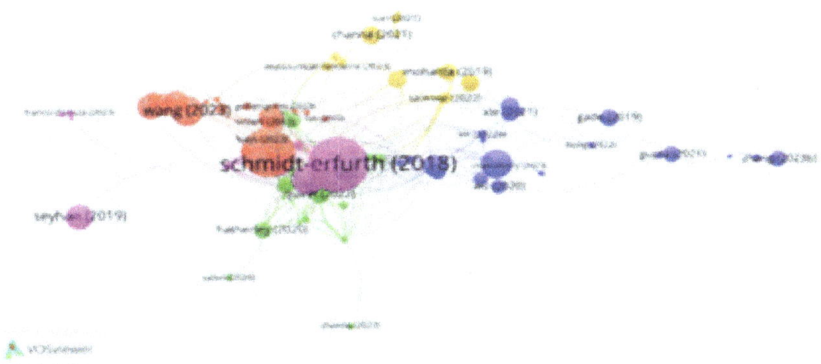

6. Co-Authorship Map of Authors

By keeping the minimum documents by authors to 1 and citations to zero, there are 3677 authors out of which only 44 are connected.

Figure 4. Map of Co-Authorship of Authors

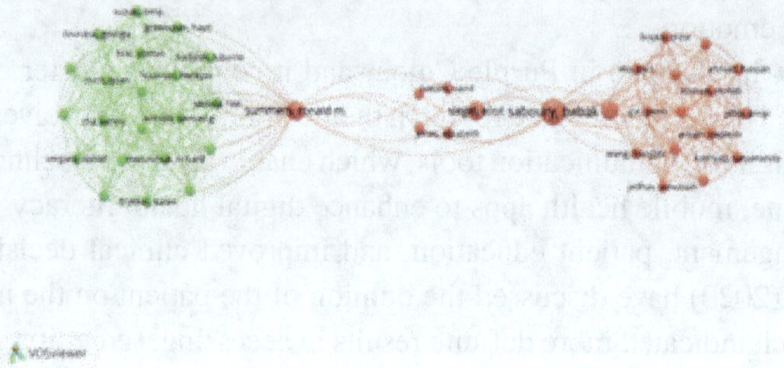

CONCLUSION

AI reliability in healthcare is a complex and evolving construct requiring interdisciplinary evaluation frameworks. This chapter demonstrates that current research is expanding rapidly but remains fragmented across technical, clinical, and ethical domains. The future studies should focus on integrative research approaches, standardised measures of evaluation, and models of co-dominant governance. Enhancement of reliability testing will be critical to safe effective and dependable implementation of AI technologies in health systems across the world. Healthcare AI reliability is a multidimensional construct that necessitates the incorporated evaluation systems. The chapter gives an analytical view which is synthesised and gives the future research and policy development directions.

Artificial intelligence is currently fulfilling the role of revolution in the health field and changing both clinical and non-clinical processes, putting forth moral, administrative, and technical concerns. The reviewed paper also aims at analysing the current quality of AI in healthcare through a bibliometric review of 676 sources identified in Scopus and supplemented with a detailed analysis. It underscores the high-profile roles of AI in consulting, curative and preventive planning of disease, continuous monitoring, and efficacy of regulatory framework and also strives to depict entrenched anxiety over credibility, transparency, privacy, and control. With this in mind, a set of findings, which are independent but related, is best defined as persistent quality, which refers to specialised precision, consistency across groups, ability to endure in various clinical contexts of interest, integrity, security, and moral recognition. Considering the viewpoint of a multi-faceted system, AI has already been integrated into the clinical workflow in the radiology, oncology, cardiology, and ophthalmology, among others. The AI has enhanced the process of deduction and minimized cases of restorative errors, and it continues to experience a problem related to information standard problems and limited conclusion of various populations.

AI's capability in medication prescription, where customised medication might become viable, provided they are backed by thorough clinical trials. Altogether, these studies demonstrate that in the course, AI is a powerful provider, its reliability hinges on environment, resources, and governance. The past two decades have witnessed an exceptional surge in fascination with generative AI and LLMs like ChatGPT, GPT-4, and Minstrel.

An array of research from the literature brought to light both assistance and obstacles. At the Currently time, generative AI is deployed to mechanise the documentation, summarise the patient information, and even offer treatment recommendations. Nevertheless, this technology can suffer from biased results, and privacy & ethical challenges such as declining human interaction and breach of patient confidentiality. User trust is the decisive factor in the successful integration of these technologies. In the case of AI, it is not clear, how the back end works and produces. These issues still limit the efficient use of this sector. The decision-making processes of most AI models are not transparent, thereby making them a black box, thereby lowering the confidence of the healthcare professionals. It creates a necessity of logical and simple to understand models. Although one of the most developed spheres where AI can be implemented is imaging, it does not offer transparency, which makes it less reliable. There has been significant interest in wearables and IoT devices that are AI-powered during the COVID-19 pandemic. Treating diseases on a long-term basis, handling health emergencies on a mass scale, and providing care services on a one-on-one basis. Nevertheless, patient adherence, the device calibration and security risks are usually variables influencing the reliability of these systems.

Others indicated the difficulty of compatibility and strength of the systems. Even though wearables signify the further application of AI in healthcare, their adoption in safe and secure ways demands greater technical and regulatory facilities. The second aspect that is prevalent in the literature is the ambiguous nature of numerous AI systems. It is of paramount importance to evaluate the weaknesses and use explainable AI to establish trust. Even the most accurate AI systems might not be trusted by clinicians and patients without their capacity to clarify the choice they made. Hence, interpretability does not only make the use of AI reliable, but it is necessary. The effectiveness of AI is not only determined by the algorithms, but also the level of understanding that humans have of AI. The health literacy role implies that professional and informed patients have a higher chance of utilising AI in a wise manner. The adoption of AI is safe only when an organisation is ready. This implies that reliability is not a technical issue, but rather a social concern. The practical use of AI demands trust, education, and accessibility and, therefore, AI cannot operate efficiently without protective and flexible systems. Internet of

Medical Things (IoMT) provides an understanding of the threats of cyberattacks, yet blockchain is one of the methods to ensure AI-based healthcare in 5G settings. The next-generation communication systems were also considered in supporting reliable AI by the study. The most precise AI models can not perform in the field unless they tackle security threats. Therefore, the availability of the right infrastructure and effective cybersecurity mechanisms is highly important to ensure that AI is credible.

The subject is becoming increasingly popular in the world, which is shown by the bibliometric analysis of 676 articles. The data shows that the greatest contributors are India and the United States, with China, Australia, and the United Kingdom coming behind them. This proves to be a sign of a research atmosphere all around the world where both the developed and developing nations are taking part in the discussion. Major contributors to the topic have been important writers like Rajesh Gupta and Avishek Choudhury who have combined computer science, engineering and medicine knowledge. Even though other researchers like Meskó & Topol (2023) indicate that there has been an increasing amount of concern regarding the use of generative AI and its implications, the article by Schmidt-Erfurth et al (2018) was the most cited, and it is notable because of its emphasis on the value of clinical imaging as a very specialized field. The word analysis, with the most frequent words being Artificial Intelligence and human, is indicative of the two-sidedness of the discussion, where AI is not taking over people but is collaborating with them in complicated and usually demanding ways. The grouping of the research into the key themes is also supported by the co-citation and bibliographic maps. Bibliographic The focal point of five groups is exceptional. Both clusters revolve around a specific subject, yet to simplify the matter, one can say that despite the various innovations in the healthcare sector that imply the use of IoT gadgets, Blockchain Technology, Deep Learning and Machine Learning, and the increasing use of Large Language Models, the problem of trust is still present, yet the work on it has been continuing.

In certain areas like restorative imaging, there are some strange performances of AI but the further development of AI to more general and patient-facing activity remains risky. Generative AI, though effective, has been questioned with regard to direction, precision, and safety. IoT developments have led to the proximity of healthcare to patients, but there are also modern threats related to them. One of the common themes is directness, explainability and persistent belief in all fields. Bibliometric results also indicate that this subject is fast growing, is widely referred to, and has solid universal desires. Of any occurrence, much of the research remains dispersed with groups of people concentrating on different perspectives or possibly synthesising them to a unified outlook of constant norm. To position AI as a reliable partner in healthcare, several things should be prioritised: strict management and control of the new generative AI tools, the explainability requirements of clinical models generated by AI, a robust and reliable IoT and 5G network, investment in local datasets of the low- and middle-income countries, patient-centered selection procedures with consent and well-being experience, and efficient collaboration that would strike a balance between innovation and security. To conclude, AI in healthcare is neither a risk that should not be tolerated nor an insufficient system. Its accuracy is based on a fine balance between human consciousness, moral protections and domain-specific abilities. These arguments demonstrate that AI has already introduced some quantifiable transformations in healthcare but the future of this process as a reliable partner is in common work in the direction of control, openness, and trustworthiness. To transform AI into an established platform of high-level medical care, it may be feasible not only to encompass the successes but also to disregard the failures that are already set in the literature and also anticipate the gaps that have been identified in the bibliometric analysis.

Discussion

The results possess implied that interactions among the technical performance, ethical governance, and organizational readiness influence the reliability of healthcare AI. Although AI systems are highly accurate in monitored environments, reality implementations are characterized by inconsistency because of infrastructure and data heterogeneity as well as the presence of humans. Generative AI also brings up novel reliability issues that are connected with misinformation and privacy. Imaging AI is technologically accurate but needs explicability to gain clinical trust. Wearable technologies rely on user compliance and quality of data. These variations have put into focus the imperative of domain specific reliability frameworks.

The dependability of artificial intelligence (AI) in healthcare is becoming a multidimensional concept that is determined by technical performance, moral regulatory practices, and organizational preparedness. Current literature indicates that several AI systems perform well through high accuracy in controlled or laboratory setting but reliability in the actual clinical conditions is determined by uncertainty in their infrastructure, data variability and human interaction. This disparity between experimental execution and clinical use points to constant observing, confirmation and administration enforcement apparatuses to maintain steady results.

The scholars focus on the fact that reliability is not possible to quantify only in terms of predictive accuracy. Rather, it relies on the aspects of data integrity, interpretability, fairness and clinical usefulness. Responsible and trustworthy AI in healthcare needs to be in balance between technical competence and ethical-organizational models, such as adherence to regulations and trust exercised by stakeholders. Practical experience also demonstrates that the decrease in performance can be observed over time as the patient populations, clinical processes, and data quality changes, which highlights the relevance of lifecycle management and model recalibration.

The reliability issues are diverse depending on the field of AI. The technologies of generative AI and especially large language models raise the issue of misinformation, hallucinations, and privacy. Even though they have promising features, their diagnostic reliability is not as high as that of expert clinicians, and thus high human supervision and validation methods are required (Wang et al., 2023). However, AI in medical images tends to be very technical accurate, but to be trusted by clinicians, explainability and transparency are essential, because clinicians have to use interpretable results to incorporate AI advice into the decision-making process. One more reliability issue is wearable technologies and remote systems, because their work is based on their use by the users, the quality of the device, and the regularity of the patient-generated information, which can have many variations in the real-world context.

In general, the results suggest that sociopolitical dynamics between algorithmic performance, governance, and healthcare system preparedness influence the reliability in healthcare AI. The disparities between the generative AI, imaging systems, and wearable technologies prove the need to have domain-specific reliability frameworks around unique risks and operational environments. The primary concerns of future studies and applications of AI systems must lie in explainability, constant validation, ethical monitoring and context-specific assessment models to make sure that AI systems are accurate, but also trustworthy and reliable in the clinical practice.

The Proposed Study Suggests a Multidimensional Reliability Framework Comprising the Following

Technical robustness - Technical robustness is the stability, accuracy, and consistency of AI systems in a variety of both datasets and clinical settings. Studies indicate that numerous healthcare AI models can be effective under controlled circumstances but start failing their performances in real-world contexts because of the problem of data drift, the heterogeneity of the population, and the evolving clinical processes. To achieve robustness, it is thus necessary to constantly monitor, recalibrate the models, and validate them on a wide range of populations.

Research on responsible AI models states that reliability should be resistant to bias, adversarial feeds, and is required to be resistant to incomplete data. The main predictors of effective AI use in healthcare are the quality of data, algorithm transparency, and fairness. On the same note, Predictive systems and large language models yield a mismatch in the face of the variability of the real world and makes the study of robustness a significant aspect of life cycle management.

Clinical validation- Clinical validation is a guarantee that AI systems are useful, safe, and effective in any actual clinical scenario and not in the laboratory. There is an indication that AI models that are highly technicalologically accurate can still fail in practice unless they are proven in practice in real clinical setting. Individual validation research indicates that continuous assessment using the actual world data are considered necessary in terms of sustaining performance and clinical meaning.

In healthcare, such as medical imaging, AI technologies tend to demonstrate the high accuracy of diagnosis, but their clinicians want to know explanations and the amount of uncertainty, which predetermines the incorporation of AI-based recommendations into decision-making. Clinical validation and human supervision are also necessary to generate AI-based systems that use generative artificial intelligence systems since they can generate realistic yet incorrect results, potentially influencing clinical judgments (Wang et al., 2023).

Ethical governance - This is ethical governance which is an important factor in making sure that AI systems are credible, transparent, and in line with healthcare values. According to research, the perception of AI reliability and trust both among clinicians and between patients directly depend on concerns related to bias, privacy, accountability, and transparency. Government structures have to deal with the problem of informed consent, privacy, and algorithmic fairness.

Generative AI presents new security issues, such as fake news and hallucinations, and risks of loss of patient privacy. Such risks have the potential to render trust and decrease the credibility of decisions made with AI unless a well-regulated framework of governance is secured. Regulatory control system, auditing tools and transparency measures form the basis of ethical and trustworthy AI use in healthcare.

Organizational readiness: Organizational readiness is the willingness of the healthcare facilities to implement and maintain AI technologies successfully. This also covers workforce development, integration of workflow, leadership and management of change. According to research, technically accurate AI systems can break down in case healthcare organizations are unprepared to act on the systems. Within the scope of clinician trust and acceptance, it is especially important. Research demonstrates that usability, explainability, and training play a large role in the intention of clinicians to use AI tools. Infrastructure security- Infrastructure security includes interoperability, reliability of the system, and data security and cybersecurity. Healthcare AI systems are sensitive and require high amounts of patient data, and thus can be easily shut down due to privacy violations and cyberattacks. Studies emphasize that reliability and trust can be assured by adhering to regulatory norms, ensuring a secure data storage and encryption.

In addition, reliable infrastructure must support data integration from multiple sources, including electronic health records, imaging systems, and wearable devices. Variability in infrastructure quality across healthcare settings can affect AI performance and reliability. Ensuring secure and interoperable systems is therefore critical for consistent AI functioning and patient safety.

Integrating these dimensions can enhance trust and safe implementation.

Implications

This study has a number of theoretical, practical and policy implications that can enhance the reliability of artificial intelligence (AI) in healthcare. The discussion highlights that the interplay of the technical execution, ethical leadership and organization preparedness, as opposed to algorithmic responsibility, produces the reliability. In these regards, the implications are as under.

1. Theoretical Implications

The present research also adds to the growing body of literature concerning the issue of trustful and responsible AI by strengthening the argument that reliability in healthcare AI is multidimensional. According to existing studies, technical accuracy should be assessed in line with transparency, fairness, and contextual usability. The findings can be used in the formation of unified reliability systems that will combine technical testing with ethical and organisational factors. Future studies must thus no longer be accuracy-focused but instead shift to socio-technical frameworks that focus on the interactions of AI systems with healthcare systems, clinicians, and patients. Moreover, the fact that artificial intelligence in terms of generative technologies, imaging technologies, and wearable devices differs in reliability suggests that domain-specific theoretical frameworks should be used instead of universal assessment principles.

2. Methodological Implications

The results suggest that AI systems should be tested in natural clinical conditions and not on the basis of experimental conditions. Research indicates that AI efficiency may reduce because of information drift, population inconsistency as well as variations in workflows when implemented in practice. Consequently, longitudinal research, real-life validation, and post-deployment follow-up should be included as the priority of the future research to determine the reliability better with time. Combining the quantitative performance measures with the qualitative feedback that should be given by clinicians and patients could be a more in-depth view of the reliability and trust of AI.

3. Practical Implications for Healthcare Organizations

Healthcare organizations should also recognize how the introduction of AI technologies requires the preparedness of the organization, including infrastructure, employee education, and control systems. It is not only the performance of algorithms that make AI systems reliable, but also the extent to which AI systems are incorporated into clinical processes. Specifically, it is essential to explain and be transparent to build trust among clinicians in imaging and diagnostic AI tools. In the case of generative AI systems, strict control check and management by humans is inevitable to curb the dangers of misinformation and hallucinations (Wang et al., 2025). The factor of reliability under the conditions of wearable technologies has a high connection with both patient adherence and the quality of the gathered data. As such, the healthcare providers are advised to employ more measures that can support user interaction and data authentication to maintain regular performance. The consistent observation, auditing, and re-calibration of AI systems should be made a norm in the organizational practices to maintain reliability of the system in its whole life cycle.

4. Policy and Governance Implications

This paper explains that there is a need to have strong regulatory and ethical mechanisms that will guarantee the sound use of AI in the healthcare system. The policymakers must develop policies relating to transparency, accountability, privacy, and minimization of bias in AI systems. In this regard, generative AI tools should be viewed with some special attention due to their ability to generate false or misleading facts. Concentrating on the standardization of assessment guidelines and certification of healthcare AI, the consistency of reliability can be guaranteed at the inter-institutional level. The governance structures should also promote cooperation between developers, clinicians, regulators and patients to promote responsible usage of AI. AI systems need to be engineered to ensure they follow the ethics of safety and privacy and to incur recurrent monitoring by ethical oversight committees and regulatory bodies.

5. Implications for Future Research

Future studies ought to explore domain-specific reliability models which are specific to particular AI health care uses. The results of comparative studies in a variety of clinical environments and locations would provide more information on contextual variables that affect reliability. Researchers are also required to review the methods of improving explainability, minimizing bias, and human-AI interaction. The identification of the long-term reliability and usefulness of AI technologies in the health sector will require long-term studies that compare patient outcome and clinical performance.

REFERENCES

Ahamed, S. I. (2018). The role of the Internet of Things (IoT) in personalised healthcare. *Journal of Ambient Intelligence and Humanized Computing*, *9*(5), 1433–1445.

Ahn, J. S., Ebrahimian, S., McDermott, S., Lee, S., Naccarato, L., Di Capua, J. F., Wu, M. Y., Zhang, E. W., Muse, V., Miller, B., Sabzalipour, F., Bizzo, B. C., Dreyer, K. J., Kaviani, P., Digumarthy, S. R., & Kalra, M. K. (2022). Association of artificial intelligence-aided chest radiograph interpretation with reader performance and efficiency. *JAMA Network Open*, *5*(8), e2229289. DOI: 10.1001/jamanetworkopen.2022.29289 PMID: 36044215

Arrieta, A. B., Díaz-Rodríguez, N., Ser, J. D., Bennetot, A., Tabik, S., Barbado, A., & Herrera, F. (2020). Explainable Artificial Intelligence (XAI): Concepts, taxonomies, opportunities and challenges toward responsible AI. *Information Fusion*, *58*, 82–115. DOI: 10.1016/j.inffus.2019.12.012

Band, S. (2020). Interpretability of machine learning in healthcare: Techniques and applications. *Health Informatics Journal*, *26*(4), 2649–2664.

Channa, A., Popescu, N., Skibinska, J., & Burget, R. (2021). The rise of wearable devices during the COVID-19 pandemic: A systematic review. *Sensors (Basel)*, *21*(17), 5787. DOI: 10.3390/s21175787 PMID: 34502679

Chen, M., Hao, Y., Cai, Y., Wang, Y., & Zhang, Y. (2021). Artificial intelligence in healthcare: Past, present and future. *Journal of Medical Systems*, *45*(9), 102–115.

Choudhury, A., & Shamszare, H. (2023). Investigating the impact of user trust on the adoption and use of ChatGPT: Survey analysis. *Journal of Medical Internet Research*, *25*, e47184. DOI: 10.2196/47184 PMID: 37314848

Ciecierski-Holmes, T., Singh, R., Axt, M., Brenner, S., & Barteit, S. (2022). Artificial intelligence for strengthening healthcare systems in low- and middle-income countries: A systematic scoping review. *NPJ Digital Medicine*, *5*(1), 162. Advance online publication. DOI: 10.1038/s41746-022-00700-y PMID: 36307479

Fitzpatrick, K. (2023). Digital literacy, health literacy, and patient safety in AI-supported care. *Journal of Medical Internet Research*, ●●●, 25.

Fitzpatrick, P. J. (2023). Improving health literacy using the power of digital communications to achieve better health outcomes for patients and practitioners. *Frontiers in Digital Health*, *5*, 1264780. DOI: 10.3389/fdgth.2023.1264780 PMID: 38046643

Gade, K., Geyik, S. C., Kenthapadi, K., Mithal, V., & Taly, A. (2019). Explainable AI in Industry. *Proceedings of the 25th ACM SIGKDD International Conference on Knowledge Discovery & Data Mining*, 3203–3204. New York, NY, USA: ACM. DOI: 10.1145/3292500.3332281

Garg, S., Singh, R., & Kaur, K. (2022). Cloud-edge collaboration for healthcare IoT: Challenges and future directions. *Future Generation Computer Systems*, *129*, 1–12.

Grote, T., & Berens, P. (2020). On the ethics of algorithmic decision-making in healthcare. *Journal of Medical Ethics*, *46*(3), 205–211. DOI: 10.1136/medethics-2019-105586 PMID: 31748206

Gupta, M. (2021). Blockchain and artificial intelligence integration for secure 5G healthcare networks. *Computer Communications*, *171*, 137–145.

Habbal, A., Ali, M. K., & Abuzaraida, M. A. (2024). Artificial Intelligence Trust, Risk and Security Management (AI TRiSM): Frameworks, applications, challenges and future research directions. *Expert Systems with Applications*, *240*(122442), 122442. DOI: 10.1016/j.eswa.2023.122442

Hasan, M. K., Ghazal, T. M., Saeed, R. A., Pandey, B., Gohel, H., Eshmawi, A. A., Abdel-Khalek, S., & Alkhassawneh, H. M. (2022). A review on security threats, vulnerabilities, and counter measures of 5G enabled Internet-of-Medical-Things. *IET Communications*, *16*(5), 421–432. DOI: 10.1049/cmu2.12301

Islam, S. M. R., Kwak, D., Kabir, M. H., Hossain, M., & Kwak, K. S. (2022). The Internet of Things for health care: A comprehensive survey. *IEEE Access : Practical Innovations, Open Solutions*, *3*, 678–708. DOI: 10.1109/ACCESS.2015.2437951

Karaca, C., & Aslan, H. (2021). A readiness model for artificial intelligence in healthcare institutions. *International Journal of Medical Informatics*, •••, 148.

Kohan, A., Xu, J., Xiao, L., Wu, X., Kukkar, A., Hussain, S., ... & Acharya, U. R. (2026). Human-Centered Pathways to Trustworthy AI in Healthcare: A Comparative Analysis of Explainable AI, Human-in-the-Loop, Hybrid AI, and Uncertainty Quantification Techniques.

Kompa, B., Snoek, J., & Beam, A. L. (2021). Second opinion needed: Communicating uncertainty in medical machine learning. *NPJ Digital Medicine*, *4*(1), 4. DOI: 10.1038/s41746-020-00367-3 PMID: 33402680

Li, X., Gu, Y., Dvornek, N., Staib, L. H., Ventola, P., & Duncan, J. S. (2020). Multi-site fMRI analysis using privacy-preserving federated learning and domain adaptation: ABIDE results. *Medical Image Analysis*, *65*(101765), 101765. DOI: 10.1016/j.media.2020.101765 PMID: 32679533

Longoni, C., Bonezzi, A., & Morewedge, C. K. (2019). Resistance to medical Artificial intelligence. *The Journal of Consumer Research, 46*(4), 629–650. DOI: 10.1093/jcr/ucz013

Marzano, L., Bardill, A., Fields, B., Herd, K., Veale, D., Grey, N., & Moran, P. (2015). The application of mHealth to mental health: Opportunities and challenges. *The Lancet. Psychiatry, 2*(10), 942–948. DOI: 10.1016/S2215-0366(15)00268-0 PMID: 26462228

McCradden, M. D., Baba, A., Saha, A., Ahmad, S., Boparai, K., Fadaiefard, P., & Cusimano, M. D. (2020). Ethical concerns around use of artificial intelligence in health care research from the perspective of patients with meningioma, caregivers and health care providers: A qualitative study. *CMAJ Open, 8*(1), E90–E95. DOI: 10.9778/cmajo.20190151 PMID: 32071143

Meskó, B., & Topol, E. J. (2023). The imperative for regulatory oversight of large language models (or generative AI) in healthcare. *NPJ Digital Medicine, 6*(1), 120. DOI: 10.1038/s41746-023-00873-0 PMID: 37414860

Moassefi, M., Rouzrokh, P., Conte, G. M., Vahdati, S., Fu, T., Tahmasebi, A., Younis, M., Farahani, K., Gentili, A., Kline, T., Kitamura, F. C., Huo, Y., Kuanar, S., Younis, K., Erickson, B. J., & Faghani, S. (2023). Reproducibility of deep learning algorithms developed for medical imaging analysis: A systematic review. *Journal of Digital Imaging, 36*(5), 2306–2312. DOI: 10.1007/s10278-023-00870-5 PMID: 37407841

Nelson, C. A., Pérez-Chada, L. M., Creadore, A., Li, S. J., Lo, K., Manjaly, P., Pournamdari, A. B., Tkachenko, E., Barbieri, J. S., Ko, J. M., Menon, A. V., Hartman, R. I., & Mostaghimi, A. (2020). Patient perspectives on the use of artificial intelligence for skin cancer screening: A qualitative study: A qualitative study. *JAMA Dermatology, 156*(5), 501–512. DOI: 10.1001/jamadermatol.2019.5014 PMID: 32159733

Newitt, D. C., Zhang, Z., Gibbs, J. E., Partridge, S. C., Chenevert, T. L., Rosen, M. A., Bolan, P. J., Marques, H. S., Aliu, S., Li, W., Cimino, L., Joe, B. N., Umphrey, H., Ojeda-Fournier, H., Dogan, B., Oh, K., Abe, H., Drukteinis, J., Esserman, L. J., & Hylton, N. M. (2019). Test-retest repeatability and reproducibility of ADC measures by breast DWI: Results from the ACRIN 6698 trial: Test-Retest Repeatability of Breast DWI. *Journal of Magnetic Resonance Imaging, 49*(6), 1617–1628. DOI: 10.1002/jmri.26539 PMID: 30350329

Nguyen, D. C., Ding, M., Pathirana, P. N., Seneviratne, A., Li, J., & Vincent Poor, H. (2021). Federated learning for internet of things: A comprehensive survey. *IEEE Communications Surveys and Tutorials*, *23*(3), 1622–1658. DOI: 10.1109/COMST.2021.3075439

Park, C. W., Seo, S. W., Kang, N., Ko, B., Choi, B. W., Park, C. M., Chang, D. K., Kim, H., Kim, H., Lee, H., Jang, J., Ye, J. C., Jeon, J. H., Seo, J. B., Kim, K. J., Jung, K.-H., Kim, N., Paek, S., Shin, S.-Y., & Yoon, H. J. (2020). Artificial intelligence in health care: Current applications and issues. *Journal of Korean Medical Science*, *35*(42), e379. DOI: 10.3346/jkms.2020.35.e379 PMID: 33140591

Piwek, L., Ellis, D. A., Andrews, S., & Joinson, A. (2016). The rise of consumer health wearables: Promises and barriers. *PLoS Medicine*, *13*(2), e1001953. DOI: 10.1371/journal.pmed.1001953 PMID: 26836780

Powell, R. A., Singh, S., & Torous, J. (2022). Patient trust and engagement in AI-based healthcare: A cross-sectional survey. *Digital Health*, •••, 8.

Quinn, T. P., Jacobs, S., Senadeera, M., Le, V., & Coghlan, S. (2022). The three ghosts of medical AI: Can the black-box present deliver? *Artificial Intelligence in Medicine*, *124*(102158), 102158. DOI: 10.1016/j.artmed.2021.102158 PMID: 34511267

Rahman, M. A., Hossain, M. S., & Alrajeh, N. A. (2022). Securing IoT-based healthcare systems: Ransomware, privacy, and resilience challenges. *Future Generation Computer Systems*, *129*, 307–321.

Rajkomar, A., Dean, J., & Kohane, I. (2019). Machine learning in medicine. *The New England Journal of Medicine*, *380*(14), 1347–1358. DOI: 10.1056/NEJMra1814259 PMID: 30943338

Rudin, C. (2019). Stop explaining black box machine learning models for high stakes decisions and use interpretable models instead. *Nature Machine Intelligence*, *1*(5), 206–215. DOI: 10.1038/s42256-019-0048-x PMID: 35603010

Schmidt-Erfurth, U., Sadeghipour, A., Gerendas, B. S., Waldstein, S. M., & Bogunović, H. (2018). Artificial intelligence in retina. *Progress in Retinal and Eye Research*, *67*, 1–29. DOI: 10.1016/j.preteyeres.2018.07.004 PMID: 30076935

Seah, J. C. Y. (2021). Effect of a comprehensive deep-learning model on the accuracy of chest x-ray interpretation: A multi-reader, multi-case study. The Lancet Digital Health.

Seyhan, A. A., & Carini, C. (2019). Are innovation and new technologies in precision medicine paving a new era in patients centric care? *Journal of Translational Medicine, 17*(1), 114. Advance online publication. DOI: 10.1186/s12967-019-1864-9 PMID: 30953518

Shafique, A., Farea, A. A., & Qureshi, K. N. (2025). AI as a new paradigm for distributed healthcare networks. In *Artificial Intelligence-Based Smart Healthcare Systems* (pp. 97–118). Academic Press. DOI: 10.1016/B978-0-443-26476-4.00012-5

Steinhubl, S. R., Muse, E. D., & Topol, E. J. (2015). The emerging field of mobile health. *Science Translational Medicine, 7*(283), 283rv3. Advance online publication. DOI: 10.1126/scitranslmed.aaa3487 PMID: 25877894

Taimoor, N., & Rehman, S. (2022). Reliable and resilient AI and IoT-based personalised healthcare services: A survey. Retrieved from https://arxiv.org/abs/2209.05457

Tonekaboni, S., Joshi, S., McCradden, M. D., & Goldenberg, A. (2019). What clinicians want: Contextualizing explainable machine learning for clinical end use. Retrieved from https://arxiv.org/abs/1905.05134

Topol, E. J. (2019). High-performance medicine: The convergence of human and artificial intelligence. *Nature Medicine, 25*(1), 44–56. DOI: 10.1038/s41591-018-0300-7 PMID: 30617339

Wang, C., Liu, S., Yang, H., Guo, J., Wu, Y., & Liu, J. (2023). Ethical considerations of using ChatGPT in health care. *Journal of medical Internet research, 25*, e48009. WHO guidance. (2021). *World Health Organization*. Ethics and governance of artificial intelligence for health

Wu, J. T., Wong, K. C. L., Gur, Y., Ansari, N., Karargyris, A., Sharma, A., Morris, M., Saboury, B., Ahmad, H., Boyko, O., Syed, A., Jadhav, A., Wang, H., Pillai, A., Kashyap, S., Moradi, M., & Syeda-Mahmood, T. (2020). Comparison of chest radiograph interpretations by artificial intelligence algorithm vs radiology residents. *JAMA Network Open, 3*(10), e2022779. DOI: 10.1001/jamanetworkopen.2020.22779 PMID: 33034642

Yang, G. (2022). From black-box to explainable AI in healthcare: Existing approaches, challenges and future directions. *Computational and Structural Biotechnology Journal, 20*, 1234–1250.

Ye, T., Xue, J., He, M., Gu, J., Lin, H., Xu, B., & Cheng, Y. (2019). Psychosocial factors affecting artificial intelligence adoption in health care in China: Cross-sectional study. *Journal of Medical Internet Research, 21*(10), e14316. DOI: 10.2196/14316 PMID: 31625950

Zhang, P., & Kamel Boulos, M. N. (2023). Generative AI in medicine and healthcare: Promises, opportunities and challenges. *Future Internet*, *15*(9), 286. DOI: 10.3390/fi15090286

Chapter 7
Federated AI and the Metaverse:
Shaping a New Computational Logic for Virtual Healthcare Ecosystems

L. B. Muralidhar
http://orcid.org/0000-0003-3453-613X
Jain (Deemed to be) University, India

H. R. Swapna
http://orcid.org/0000-0003-0362-409X
Jain (Deemed to be) University, India

S. Madhu
http://orcid.org/0009-0000-8816-5798
Jyothy Institute of Commerce and Management Studies, India

P. H. Reshma Sultana
http://orcid.org/0000-0001-9449-0191
Jain (Deemed to be) University, India

K. P. Sheeba
http://orcid.org/0009-0003-4707-5392
Jain (Deemed to be) University, India

ABSTRACT

The rapid evolution of digital health has exposed the limitations of centralized artificial intelligence, platform-dependent telemedicine, and fragmented data governance. In

DOI: 10.4018/979-8-3373-8889-2.ch007

parallel, healthcare metaverses are emerging as persistent, immersive, and data-intensive environments that demand new forms of secure, collaborative intelligence. This chapter advances the central argument that federated artificial intelligence and the healthcare metaverse must be theorised together, as their integration constitutes a fundamentally new computational, organisational, and governance paradigm rather than a simple technological convergence. By conceptualising healthcare AI as a distributed, experiential system, the chapter develops the notion of Federated Experiential Intelligence and examines its architectural, ethical, and institutional implications. Drawing on interdisciplinary theoretical lenses and global empirical trends, it analyses emerging practices, governance challenges, fairness concerns, and critical counter-arguments.

1. INTRODUCTION: WHY FEDERATED AI AND THE METAVERSE MUST BE THEORISED TOGETHER

Over the last decade, digital healthcare, through telemedicine, data analytics, and artificial intelligence, has emerged. However, its dominant paradigms remain structurally constrained by centralised, platform-dependent architectures that replicate episodic and transactional models of care and concentrate control over data, computation, and infrastructure in the hands of a small number of institutional and corporate actors. Such centralisation magnifies privacy and security threats, reinforces asymmetries of power between data subjects and platform owners, and limits interoperability and scalability between diverse regulatory, cultural and infrastructural contexts, especially as healthcare systems confront growing burdens of chronic disease, shortages of workforce, as well as ever-increasing levels of data protection (Rieke et al., 2020; WHO, 2023).

Empirical studies also show that centrally trained AI systems often exhibit limited generalisability when outside their original demographic or geographic context, and the lack of breadth and depth in the training data leads to upward bias in the dataset. At the same time, entrenched forms of dataset bias persist, and proprietary platforms and service lock-in limit innovation and cross-institutional collaboration, especially in low- and middle-income contexts where these platforms often operate (Zou & Schiebinger, 2018; European Commission, 2022). These limitations suggest that the challenges confronting digital health today are not merely normative or technical, nor limited to questions of computational logic, commodity rules, and incentives; they also raise more profound dilemmas of governance design and institutional power. Against this background, metaverse-based healthcare has emerged as a paradigm defined by persistent, immersive, and interactive environments, combining extended reality, digital twins, unceasing biometric data flows, and support of decisions with

AI, in the clinical domain, educational domain, and administration domain (Dionisio et al., 2013; Wang et al., 2022).

Federated AI has thus become prominent in response to data fragmentation, regulatory limits and institutional silos through the feasibility of a cooperative model learning among distributed data by eliminating centralising data pooling, yet keeping accurate to data minimisation principles enshrined in GDPR and similar legislation across the globe (McMahan et al., 2017; Sheller et al., 2020). Comparative evidence indicates that federated approaches can deliver performance comparable to or better than centralised models in medical imaging and electronic health record analytics, as well as in areas such as cancellations, misdiagnoses, and the resulting risks to patient safety.

Crucially, federated AI is not only a privacy-preserving technique but also a redistribution of computational agency, enabling hospitals, devices, and patients to participate in collective intelligence without forfeiting data sovereignty. This logic is structurally consistent with the distributed and context-sensitive nature of data flows in metaverse environments. Theorised together, federated AI and the healthcare metaverse represent a movement toward polycentric governance in which intelligence is distributed across interacting relations among autonomous plural actors rather than under hierarchical control. They will require arrangements based on protocols and negotiations to resolve coordination costs, asymmetrical computational capacity, model drift, and unresolved liability, as well as move toward adaptive regulatory approaches that will be capable of governing the dynamics of a distributed intelligence system without limiting innovation (Ostrom, 2010; Veale & Borgesius, 2021).

2. CONCEPTUAL FOUNDATIONS AND THEORETICAL LENSES

Conceptionalising the metaverse not as an incremental extension of digital interfaces will need the conceptualisation of the metaverse-based healthcare environments as a cyber-physical-social infrastructure where clinical processes, organisational workflows, and experiential dimensions of care are persistently integrated, unlike conventional digital health systems that primarily support episodic information exchange, metaverse-based healthcare environments can synchronise physical sensor data, patient and facility digital twins, immersive interfaces, and social interaction among clinicians, patients, and intelligent agents within continuously evolving virtual spaces, for the co-evolution of clinical decision-making, patient experience and institutional coordination(Wang et al., 2022).

This setting places the healthcare metaverse at the confluence of an interactive care environment and a clinical workspace across the lifespan, where virtual and augmented reality aid embodied interaction, complex data visualisation, procedural rehearsal, and remote consultation that approximates co-presence. At the same time, persistent data objects, avatars, and algorithmic agents with long-term memories of encounters translate care delivery from discrete interventions into data-intensive, non-interventional processes (Radianti et al., 2020).

Crucially, this vision differs fundamentally from consumer-oriented and metaverse-oriented approaches focused on engagement and monetisation, as medical-grade metaverse trials must meet strict criteria for safety, reliability, interoperability, and auditability, particularly when immersive systems influence diagnostic or therapeutic decisions (FDA, 2022). As empirical findings from both the development of early virtual hospitals and XR-based training systems show, insufficient governance vulnerable to this has the possibility of intensifying cognitive overload, replicating bias, and introducing new clinical dangers that structure 'the difference between a consumer and a healthcare metaverse to be less aesthetic than it may still be made, than structural something consequential' (Zhang et al., 2023).

Within this infrastructural context, federated AI represents a redistribution of computational agency rather than the marginal optimisation of ML pipelines, owing to the increasing infeasibility of centralising large-scale, labelled data in the current regulatory context, institutional fragmentation, and public distrust of data pooling (Rieke et al., 2020). Not only by allowing distributed model training across hospitals, devices, or regional systems, and exchanging only parameters or updates with one another, but by sharing data not just among institutions or IT systems, and not by coordinating both academics and clinicians, for disease spread prevention, can we consider that federated AI is more in the spirit of a distributed computing system theory, where coordination, scalability, and system resilience across heterogeneous nodes are a prize (Tanenbaum & Van Steen, 2017), but in institutional economics, where data sharing requires coordination too, as people's own data, including health data, serves as a strategic asset embedded within organisational boundaries, reducing transaction costs and mitigating opportunistic behaviour through retained control over sensitive resources (Williamson, 1985).

Privacy-by-design approaches go even further by establishing federated AI as an architectural response to regulatory requirements to minimise data and support local governance (European Commission, 2022). However, it is still possible to observe continued identification of constraints related to statistical heterogeneity, uneven computational capacity, and the validation of distributed updates, highlighting the context-specific rather than universal advantages of federated approaches.

Integrating federated AI in the context of healthcare metaverses therefore requires a multi-theoretical approach: systems theory: healthcare as a complex adaptive system whose federated AI facilitates local adaptation and global learning while increasing interdependency and propagation of errors (Plsek & Greenhalgh, 2001); socio-technical transitions theory: the convergence of federated AI marks a potential regime shift challenging platform-centric models of digital health and regulatory inertia as well as uneven distribution of resources (Geels, 2002); platform governance theory: a shift toward modular and polycentric arrangements expanding autonomy while increasing the complexity and outcomes emerge from collectively trained models (Gawer, 2021).

Breaking down trust and institutional theories we can further suggest that legitimacy relies on transparency, fairness and institutional congruence with the particularity of immersive environments, where algorithmic reasoning may be less visible (Mayer et al., 1995; Siau & Wang, 2020), while research on human AI interaction displays the persistence of tensions between efficiency and autonomy, personalisation and standardisation, and immersion and explainedness, revealing that the alignment of federated AI and the healthcare metaverse is the contested reconfiguration of the knowledge, power and responsibility in healthcare, and a much less technical one at that.

3. A NEW COMPUTATIONAL LOGIC: FROM DATA CENTRALISATION TO EXPERIENTIAL DECENTRALISATION

The combination of federated AI and metaverse-based healthcare environments requires a re-thinking of computation that departs from the linear data-model-decision pipeline that underpins current digital health systems and which has historically been optimised for centralisation, scale, and efficiency but which has become oddly misaligned with immersive, real-time and uncertainty-intensive care contexts (Topol, 2019; Rieke et al., 2020). In metaverse-enabled healthcare, computation is not limited to back-end analytics on static data; computation also occurs during use cases. However, it unfolds in continuous interaction among clinicians, patients, intelligent agents, and digital artefacts within persistent virtual environments, such that clinical intelligence is relationally emergent from experience, context, and distributed agency rather than the result of abstracted statistical processing alone.

The interactions with digital twins, avatars, and immersive interfaces, which actively shape learning processes by involving embodied judgement, behavioural cues, and situated intervention, align healthcare computation with both embodied cognition and distributed intelligence theory and contrast with purely symbolic or model-centric epistemology (Hollan et al., 2000). Within this logic, avatars act as mediators of identity, agency and social relations interjected across organisational boundaries, affecting trust and accountability; digital twins take the form of continually updated computational artefacts for predictive simulation (embedding in care delivery) and immersive interfaces influence attention, sense-making and decision pathways, taking shape as part of the computational substrate rather than neutral visual layers (breeding empirical evidence on both mobilising situational knowing benefits and risking obscured uncertainty for actors when poor design and governance is incurred) (Slater & Sanchez-Vives, 2016; Bruynseels et al., 2018; Radianti et al., 2020).

This is a shift from centralising data to decentralising experience as a foundational principle of an integrative model, the so-called Federated Experiential Intelligence (FEI), which integrates federated learning into metaverse-based care environments, enabling learning without data movement whilst maintaining data sovereignty and contextual relevance. Based on edge intelligence deployed across wearables, sensors, smart devices and immersive interfaces, advances in edge computing enable low-latency and on-device analytics that are important for adaptive and safety-sensitive applications, such as immersive rehabilitation or remote clinical support, redistributing computational costs and the responsibility of governance to organisations in healthcare (Shi et al., 2016).

Federated learning orchestration represents a second fundamental layer, which will coordinate the distributed model updates across heterogeneous nodes without centralising the raw data and couple the learning triggers to clinically-interacting activities in immersive environments, which, while improving the contextual specificity, may create threats to model stability, validation and comparability across sites with unequal infrastructural capacity. The experiential arena of FEI is supported by metaverse-based layers of clinical interactions, such as virtual clinics, cooperative diagnostic and training spaces, with early pilots showing the possibilities for cross-border consultation and education as well as indicating the need for interoperability and flow integration in order to counter fragmented parallel systems (Park & Kim, 2023).

Trust, identity and governance mechanisms are the normative backbone of FEI as the consequences of identity management, consent and audibility, among others, are reinforced through persistence and immersion, including directing towards the implementation of governance at the infrastructural and protocol level as observed in, for example, the European Health Data Space and the AI Act (European Commission, 2022). While FEI questions assumptions that intelligence requires data centralisation and provides a way to make the square-rectangle - 'personalisation and global health regulation' possible, it also creates tensions on the nature of efficiency and the costs of coordination, autonomy and standardisation, immersion and explainability, along with the risks of perpetuating inequalities in low-resource settings, and diffusing responsibility for clinical outcomes if governance is not developed (WHO, 2023).

Accordingly, Federated Experiential Intelligence should be realised not as a universally optimal solution but as a context-dependent computational logic, orthogonal to interaction, embodiment, and distributed intelligence, that provides a rigorous conceptual underpinning for analysing the governance, ethical, and implementation issues that shape sustainable and equitable virtual healthcare ecosystems.

4. ARCHITECTURE OF FEDERATED METAVERSE HEALTHCARE ECOSYSTEMS

The architectural design of federated metaverse healthcare ecosystems represents a radical shift away from static, cloud-centric digital healthcare infrastructure. It entails socio-technical configurations that support real-time interaction, continuous learning, and distributed governance, both across organisational and geographical boundaries, as well as the redistribution of intelligence, responsibility, and value within healthcare systems. At the heart of this type of architecture is an edge-fog-cloud continuum with adaptations for immersive care delivery in which layers of edge-based technologies include wearables, implantables, novel medical devices and extended reality (XR) interfaces that produce fine-grained data regarding physiological, behavioural and experiential data and increasingly support on-device analytics allowing for low latency inference and adaptive feedback.

Fog layers, located at the gateways of hospitals and regional networks, perform functions with specialised latency requirements, such as virtual ward monitoring, collaborative diagnostics, and aggregation of federated learning updates, and mediate between heterogeneous edge devices and cloud infrastructures. In contrast, the role of cloud layers remains strategic in large-scale model orchestration, longitudinal analytics, and cross-regional knowledge synthesis, rather than being solely a computational resource (Shi et al., 2016; Satyanarayanan, 2017). In an immersive clinical setting, architectural responsiveness is directly related to safety and usability. Empirical research in XR-assisted surgery and remote intervention has shown that even slight latency can impair hand-eye coordination and situational awareness, thereby necessitating calibration between decentralisation and coordination to maintain clinical reliability (Radianti et al., 2020).

This recalibration distributes managerial and infrastructural responsibilities, necessitating that healthcare organisations invest in edge and fog computing capabilities rather than outsourcing computation to hyperscale cloud providers wherever possible. Within this continuum, federated learning architectures take two basic forms: cross-silo and cross-device, each with distinct institutional implications. Cross-silo federated learning comprises relatively stable participants such as hospitals, research centres, or national health systems collaborating on model training without pooling raw data, which has been shown in medical imaging, oncology and research in rare diseases and in metaverse contexts, can effectively facilitate shared virtual environments such as multinational tumour boards, while supporting each participant's data sovereignty (Sheller et al., 2020).

Cross-device federated learning is carried out over significant populations of heterogeneous and partially connected devices, including wearable devices and patient-facing XR devices, enabling personalised and population-level insights in immersive environments and adding architectural fragilities (in terms of unreliable connectivity, uneven capacity, and added compounded susceptibility to model drift between imprecise non-identically distributed data) to the system. Interoperability forms a continuing constraint, not only in the syntactic exchange of data, but in the semantic alignment, spatial context, and temporal co-ordination, all of which taking embodied interaction and experiential signals generated in XR environments into account, existing standards such as HL7 FHIR will be insufficient to represent embodied interaction, whereas cross-jurisdictional infrastructural and regulatory asymmetries will fragment immersive interaction even further (Lehne et al., 2019; European Commission, 2022).

Architectural trade-offs are unavoidable: edge processing balances latency against energy consumption, creating sustainability challenges when large-scale XR is deployed, and cloud offloading balances these costs by sacrificing responsiveness and introducing a new form of centralisation (Shi et al., 2016). Model drift also complicates validation, certification, and accountability in experiential federated systems, as evolving clinical practices, patient behaviour, and interface design can alter data-generating processes over time. Consequently, federated metaverse healthcare architectures cannot be optimised along a sole dimension but instead have to be contextually configured against clinical acuity and regulatory regimes as well as organisational capacity, to underscore that architecture in this domain is fundamentally a challenge of governance and institutional, more than technical nature, and therefore of centrality in realising its transformative potential.

5. EMPIRICAL LANDSCAPE: SECONDARY DATA AND GLOBAL TRENDS

The empirical world of digital healthcare is that of a rapidly growing yet uneven global landscape in which technological innovation, differential trajectories of adoption, and ever-increasing regulatory regimes shape a globally organized context for immersive environments of care and federated AI that, although yet emergent in operational practice, have some structural momentum that we see in market projections, adoption studies, and policy analyses. A key symptom of transformation is enduring growth of telehealth - the unveiled global value of telehealth in 2024 is estimated at USD $123 billion and will reach about USD $455 billion by the year

2030 - which implies stumbling upon a compound annual growth rate of about 24.7%, while secondary forecasts for the longer-term outlook are forecasted to be valued in excess of USD $1.2 trillion by the mid-2030s, as remote access, cost containment and digital integration embed into daily channels of routine care.

Parallel growth is evident in immersive healthcare technologies, with the markets for augmented and virtual reality, although starting from smaller bases, are expected to reach tens of billions of dollars by the early 2030s. VR-specific healthcare applications alone are projected to grow from less than USD 5 billion in 2024 to over USD 45 billion by 2032, reflecting accelerated investments in operational areas related to surgical training, rehabilitation, pain management, and education of patients needing medical care, as providing the material conditions for the establishment of metaverse-based care ecosystems. By contrast, the healthcare federated learning market represents a relatively new market comparably measured in the tens of million dollars at least to current time periods of 2024 but experiencing compounded projected growth rates above 14-16% through the 2030s which signals institutional demand for collaborative analytics which will avoid centralising the pooling of data but will also balance with tightening privacy expectations and regulatory scrutiny (Rieke et al., 2020).

This trajectory reflects a broader trend toward increasing privacy-preserving computation as healthcare organisations struggle to balance the development of large-scale models with respect for ethical and legal restrictions on data sharing. Regulatory developments further contextualise such dynamics, having been followed by the broad principles of data minimisation, consent and individual control set out in the European Union's General Data Protection Regulation. At the same time, the Health Insurance Portability and Accountability Act in the United States has a much narrower, sector-specific focus on Protected Health Information (PHI), resulting in patchy compliance across the broader international landscape of digital health and federated systems.

Comparative regional patterns reveal further divergent institutional logics based on European strategies focused on regulatory coherence and integration of public health under universal coverage models; United States favouring there-capital driven and platform-centric diffusion about telehealth and (AI) applied under comparatively lenient privacy law interpretations; and the prevention and promotion of significant and innovative hospital-based initiatives in several Asian economies that are aligned under national innovation agenda and increase debates over data governance and cross-border cooperation between governments. Collectively, these are empirical patterns that suggest that growth in the markets, regulations, and technology design are mutually constitutive processes that determine trajectories towards federated metaverse healthcare ecosystems that are only insofar as they are sustainable and legitimate, aligned with innovation as paired with equity, accountability, and public trust far more than with market growth alone.

6. CASE STUDIES AND EMERGING PRACTICES

While conceptual and architectural frameworks make a case for the plausibility of federated metaverse healthcare ecosystems, their greatest practical importance lies in emerging empirical studies that deploy immersive environments alongside federated AI, within real-world institutional, regulatory, and operational constraints. A prominent manifestation of this is the emergence of virtual hospitals and immersive clinics that extend beyond episodic telemedicine to form persistent clinical environments in which clinicians, patients, and intelligent agents interact continually across organisational boundaries.

Multi-institutional networks in Europe and North America have already implemented federated learning to enable model training on imaging data co-held by each participating centre, while yielding results comparable to centralised approaches (Sheller et al., 2020) and preserving compliance with stringent data protection regimes (Rieke et al., 2020). In richer, immersive clinical contexts, these federated diagnostics facilitate shared, situated awareness through avatar-mediated teams to view images, mark findings, and co-intervene on them. At the same time, persistent virtual wards integrate continuous data from home monitoring into longitudinal dashboards that support early intervention and cross-site data coordination, as demonstrated by their piloting in East Asia and the Middle East (Park & Kim, 2023).

At the same time, these environments reveal tensions associated with workload intensification, blurred boundaries in clinical presence over time, and professional accountability, including questions about sustainability and governance. A second set of practices concerns the use of digital twins within federated architectures of the metaverse, in which patient-, organ-, or pathway-level simulations are continuously updated using local data sources. In contrast, federated learning allows one to refine a model collectively, without bringing data together. In cardiology and oncology, such twins are used to simulate disease progression and treatment responses. When rendered in an immersive way, they facilitate interactive (exploration of a scenario) and real-time visualisation of uncertainty to support better clinical planning and common understanding (Bruynseels et al., 2018).

However, empirical assessments indicate that these models remain approximations that are sensitive to data quality and bias, and that immersive, realistic modelling may obscure epistemic uncertainty in the absence of robust mechanisms to explain and validate the models in question (Bjornsson et al., 2020). Federated metaverse practices are increasingly observed in transnational collaboration, particularly in rare disease research and public health modelling, through multinational federated learning initiatives that enable distributed training on national registries, subject to legal and ethical constraints on data sharing.

Coupled with immersive collaboration spaces, these initiatives support shared clinical reasoning within and among geographically dispersed specialities and specialist consensus, as demonstrated by pandemic-era applications in which distributed analytics helped model the spread of the novel Coronavirus (refinement) despite non-convergent data. In contrast, immersive simulations enabled the co-exploration of intervention scenarios, thereby raising issues related to model alignment, accountability, and public trust (Vayena et al., 2020). Across these cases, there is a clear recurring empirical understanding which is that federation facilitates collaboration without transformation of data ownership without centralised convergence implying the possibility of reforming the political economy of healthcare data by separating the tensions between multiscale collective intelligence and centralised data pooling while being parallel to regulatory paths with a strong emphasis in data minimisation and data sovereignty (including the issue of the European Health Data Space, 2025 - European Commission, 2022).

However, in these practices, federation has also introduced new dependencies on shared protocols, architectures, and governance arrangements, and immersive environments raise ethical issues regarding consent, representation, and cognitive effort. Collectively, empirical deployments in virtual hospitals, digital twins, and cross-border collaboration give substance to federated metaverse healthcare as a new and potentially transformative paradigm that is contested yet successful on account of sustained focus on efforts to design such institutions, align these with regulations, and identify the human factor rather than technical performance as pivotal.

7. GOVERNANCE, TRUST, AND IDENTITY IN FEDERATED VIRTUAL CARE

Disruptive and reconfiguring governance, Federated virtual care, where immersive clinical interactions occur in metaverse-like environments but where learning and analytics are federated and spread across institutions and devices, fundamentally alters the nature of governance from a concern of the organisation to a protocol-mediated, multi-actor challenge where agencies are distributed across technical/institutional/experiential layers. Whereas trust in conventional healthcare is stabilised through licensing as in licensed professionals, regulating facilities, and linear accountability chains, in contrast, federated metaverse ecosystems compose clinical encounter over avatars, algorithmic agents, across-border model updates and locally at the community level, which offers the options of also intensifying demands for governance and hence the need for means of integrating these ecosystems with a regulatory framework where identity, consent, auditability and certification function as core determinants of legitimacy, safety and equity.

One key area of pressure is decentralised identity and consent management, as immersive environments create multiple surfaces of identity - patients represented through avatars, clinicians operating beyond organisational boundaries and AI-agents acting by delegated authority- that will require a beyond a platform-bound approach to identity, furthering dependency risks. Decentralised identity architectures based on W3C Decentralised Identifiers and Verifiable Credentials enable verification of licensure, affiliation, and consent portability without relying on a single organisation. However, cryptographic proof does not establish clinical competence or trustworthiness; therefore, the question of governance is now about WHO issues, including which regulatory authority is responsible for regulating and revoking verifiable claims, and what liability arrangements are in place.

Consent governance accordingly becomes more complex as federated virtual care shifts consent from an episodic, required act to a continuous process embedded in immersive interaction, biometric inference, recording, secondary analytics, and federated model training. Although blockchain-based consent management strategies provide tamper-evident auditability and programmable logic, empirical examinations of consent technologies authorized by the HDS (Human Data Service) reveal ongoing weaknesses in interpreting them in terms of scalability, usability, governance uncertainty, and legal impedance in considerations of rights to correct or erase under specific laws, such as the GDPR, suggesting that high-stakes environments for healthcare information create a need for hybrid, system architectures comprised of off-chain flexibility, on-chain proofs, and institutional oversight instead of fully automated solutions (Al Omar et al., 2021; Vanmathi et al., 2024).

More broadly trust layers based on blockchains can lessen dependence on solitary-based operators since they can complete consent events, access requests and model provenance [and] particularly the kind of proof of vitality could never infinite scale up of trial, as it can be proven that a step not for envious, retaining sketch noise can simply off or a veteran within contest often blamed in cases where a completion a while non host find compliance drifting or responsibility could away. Thus, the crypt is a weak key provider, has poor flow integration, exhibits clear work, and is accountable, yet it fails. The technoverifiable does not stand in place at an experiential level, witchcraft Accountability, therefore, becomes the most significant challenge as the distribution of decision-making in federated virtual care rests among the judgment of humans, the training of models together, and immersed interfaces that affect perception and attention, creating a risk of responsibility diffusion.

Policy and standards frameworks, such as WHO guidance on AI for health, ISO/IEC 23894:2023, Good Machine Learning Practice principles, and the NIST AI

Risk Management Framework, can serve as coordination mechanisms that concretise ethical principles into auditable processes in a heterogeneous set of actors. The resulting implication is not the replacement of institutional trust, nor its survival in a hidden world packaged as such; it is the political design of hybrid trust architectures, in which decentralised verification is used to increase transparency and portability. At the same time, institutions retain the role of credential governance, oversight, and enforcement of remedies, thereby making governance infrastructures decisive for the triumph of federated metaverse healthcare, either to harness public value or to reproduce power asymmetry and opacity.

8. ETHICAL, LEGAL, AND POLICY DIMENSIONS

The joining of federated AI and metaverse-based healthcare environments poses ethical, legal and policy problems in a magnitude that goes beyond earlier digital healthcare innovation challenges, due to the immersive, persistent and algorithmically mediated healthcare reconfiguring the patient experience, clinical judgment and responsibility across jurisdictions, thus making governance a constitutive part of system design rather than an external constraint. Patient autonomy and the informed consent become core ethical issues, due to the nature of immersive care that dissolves usual boundaries between clinical encounters, data production, and decision-making processes, with constant flows of speech, movement, biometric and behavioural data produced in environments whose realism may affect cognition and reduce critical distance, making it more difficult for patients to become aware of the algorithmic mediation or to anticipate uses of data downstream (Slater & Sanchez-Vives, 2016; Radianti et al., 2020).

Although federated AI reduces the threats posed by the centralised pooling of data, it further obscures how personal engagement affects collective learning, which strengthens the ethical case for dynamic, layered consent models that maintain ongoing control, feedback, and withdrawal. However, empirical evidence indicates that such mechanisms should not be adopted in the immersive domain due to cognitive load and consent fatigue, particularly among vulnerable populations (Vayena et al., 2020). A second tension arises from the growing discrepancy between the opacity of algorithms and the explainability of clinical decision-making, as federated learning often relies on algorithmically complex digitised models that are difficult to interpret. At the same time, immersive interfaces might have a visually naturalising effect on recommendations, limiting clinicians' ability to challenge, contextualise, or contest AI outputs, which could lead to a loss of professional autonomy and accountability (Amershi et al., 2019).

This obscurity has legal consequences, as it makes it difficult to assign liability when harm is inflicted on an individual, particularly in a federated system in which models become asynchronous, cross-institutional, and cross-border. Regulatory Responses Shaping Transparency, Explainability and Human-Transparency Sensing and Explainability are increasingly coming to the fore in regulatory responses, e.g., under the European Union's AI Act which classifies many healthcare applications as high risk, thereby requiring documentation, manageable risk and safeguards for human-in-the-loop, e.g., World Health Organization's guidance includes framing explainability as a relational requirement which connects to trust and respect for autonomy, rather than fundamentally as a technical characteristic (European Commission, 2021; WHO, 2023).

Another challenge is the jurisdictional conflict, as federated virtual care routinely crosses national borders, revealing differences in data protection, professional licensing, and malpractice jurisdictions. The GDPR's extraterritorial data minimisation standards, HIPAA's limited sectoral scope, and the diversity of Asia-Pacific frameworks create confusion about applicable law and solutions. The trend is towards policymakers responding through harmonisation via standards, soft law, and international cooperation, rather than through legal convergence, as embodied in the European Health Data Space and OECD frameworks that seek to foster interoperable governance of health data and AI. Critics, however, note that this can enable well-endowed systems to prevail and perpetuate global inequalities if the capacity constraints of low- and middle-income countries are not fully met (OECD, 2024).

These challenges in governance relate directly to the question of equity, in so far as that federated architectures and immersive environments are potentially expandable to provide increased access to specialist care and training while maintaining local data sovereignty; however, differentials in hardware availability, connectivity and technical expertise create the potential for the concentration of benefits to be located in wealthy systems in the absence of focused policy intervention (WHO, 2023). Combined with broader trends in the international community towards conceptualizing digital health as a common good, such as the WHO Global Strategy on Digital Health and G20 discussions of the need to provide digital public infrastructure, these trends demonstrate that autonomy, explainability, jurisdictional coherence and equity are mutually reinforcing aspects that need adaptive, coupled governance to lead federated metaverse healthcare to socially legitimate and trustworthy.

9. FAIRNESS, BIAS, AND ROBUSTNESS IN FEDERATED METAVERSE AI

With the continued adoption of federated AI into metaverse-based healthcare systems, issues of fairness, bias, and robustness will cease to be a technical concern on the periphery but move to the center of ethical, clinical, and policy concerns, since intelligence will be the product of the coordination of distributed models that execute on different institutions, regions, and immersive processes other than on selectively curated datasets. In contrast to centralised AI, where the composition and source of bias in datasets are at least partially observable, federated metaverse AI is executed in decentralised and often opaque data ecologies where fairness is not a systemic quality but an outcome of algorithmic processes, and it is not feasible to separate performance and equity in question.

Even though federated learning is often presented as enhancing fairness since it preserves local contexts and avoids the dominance of data by individual institutions, the empirical evidence indicates that decentralisation does not eradicate bias but shifts its mode of transmission, as the local institutional biases, such as the bias towards regions or units of a spread of a specific diagnostic practice or systematic underdiagnosis, can be magnified with the help of the aggregation mechanisms in case the weighting and coordination rules are not explicitly fairness-sensitive. Within immersive metaverse settings, these distortions can be further embedded through intuitive or self-evident interfaces for output, thereby limiting opportunities for critical interrogation and normalising unfair advice.

The latter dynamics are augmented by strong asymmetries in data volume, quality, and modality across healthcare systems, in which well-endowed academic Centres make multimodal data abundant. Meanwhile, rural clinics and low- and middle-income settings provide sparser and noisier data, and federated aggregation schemes that prioritise dataset size or convergence rates can inaccurately favour prominent players even as global accuracy increases (Pati et al., 2022). In metaverse care settings, these imbalances threaten to create immersive systems that are optimised for a few patient archetypes, thereby recreating global health inequities through high-tech mediation rather than alleviating them.

The issues of fairness are further exacerbated in the cross-border federated healthcare metaverse, as regional disparities in disease incidence, genetics, environmental exposures, and care pathways undermine assumptions of model universality. In contrast, federated learning can achieve local adaptation; however, without governance mechanisms (ridge stratification evaluation, fairness-conscious aggregation, local performance threshold evaluation), it cannot ensure equal influence on the shared model's evolution. These pitfalls are compounded by robustness, where federated learning is prone to adversarial attacks and model poisoning, which is capable of presenting as a legitimate update and may disproportionately benefit a particular group of patients, a threat that is magnified when dealing with immersive contexts where the uncertainty and degradation are more visually obscured (Bagdasaryan et al., 2020).

In addition, the quest to be robust collides with the privacy-accuracy trade-offs as methods of differential privacy and secure computation may undermine the performance in heterogeneous or data-scarce environments, and this leads to the question of whether the losses of accuracy should be distributed differently to raise ethical concerns about the allocation of risk to marginalised populations (Dwork & Roth, 2014). These interdependencies need to be addressed through integrated governance measures rather than individual technical solutions, such as compulsory, disaggregated performance reporting and certification regimes that assess fairness, robustness, and accuracy, as progressively articulated in the OECD and WHO AI governance frameworks (OECD, 2024; WHO, 2023). Finally, the determinants of fairness, bias, and robustness in federated metaverse AI are also determinants of legitimacy and sustainability, because decentralisation enables privacy-preserving cooperation; however, equitable results can only be achieved if the learning protocols, governance arrangements, and immersive interfaces are designed, explicitly managed, and monitored.

10. COUNTER-ARGUMENTS AND CRITICAL PERSPECTIVES

Any claim that federated AI-enabled metaverse healthcare constitutes a revolution in clinical computing and governance should be evaluated in light of substantive technical, clinical, ethical, and environmental critiques that define its conditioning boundaries, rather than as an innovation-resistant concept. Technically, scepticism focuses on scalability, cost, and reliability, since federated learning entails coordination overhead, communication latency, straggler effects, and statistical heterogeneity, which empirically degrade performance as participation scales across heterogeneous institutions and devices.

These limitations are accentuated when deployed on high-resolution, immersive metaverse platforms that demand real-time interaction, high-resolution rendering, and the ongoing integration of sensory functions, which require complex and expensive edge-fog-cloud implementations and expert knowledge, the cost-efficiency of which is uncertain relative to other incremental improvements to existing telehealth systems. Distributed systems theory also warns that as more systems are integrated into a distributed system, the likelihood of emerging, difficult-to-diagnose failure modes increases. This issue is even greater in healthcare, where reliability cannot be compromised, and the volume of large-scale empirical data is limited (Tanenbaum & Van Steen, 2017).

In clinical practice, the issues of trust, liability, and professional autonomy become the subject of scepticism because workflows mediated by immersive or algorithmically mediated artificial intelligence are highly likely to increase automation bias, a phenomenon observed in clinical decision-support systems, where clinicians tend to rely on algorithmic prompts rather than their own judgment (Lyell & Coiera, 2017). Simulations that are visually convincing and spatial cues can also be used to make recommendations more natural in the setting of the metaverse, making it difficult to evaluate and thus increasing the uncertainty of liability in the event of harm, with current malpractice structures falling far behind distributed accountability despite newly developed regulatory efforts (European Commission, 2021).

Ethically, critiques are not limited to personal experience. However, the structural risk of surveillance and exclusion is also present since immersive care is based on constant capturing of movement, gaze, speech, and biometric behavior, which may cause normalisation of pervasive surveillance even in federated architecture with privacy and violation blurring the line between therapeutic observation and intrusion, especially in vulnerable groups (Zuboff, 2019; Vayena et al., 2020). Similar issues are parallel in the context of digital exclusion, as immersive care implies, among other things, reliable connectivity, advanced hardware, and digital literacy, which, however, are unevenly distributed across and within regions, and, unless addressed by the specific policy intervention, can lead to the recreation of the digital divide (WHO, 2023).

Another, more glaring and under-researched criticism concerns environmental sustainability: federated AI, with immersive rendering, constant data streams, and specialised hardware, is more likely to increase rather than reduce energy costs, thereby swelling aggregate carbon footprints through distributed computing and energy-intensive XR devices (Strubell et al., 2019). These criticisms overlap in incurable trade-offs: improving robustness by introducing redundancy or encryption, encouraging more immersive transparency by increasing cognitive load, and making consent mechanisms stricter, thereby rendering them unusable. Notably, scepticism does not mean denial; history shows resemblances in the adoption of electronic health records and telemedicine, in which selective adoption becomes possible as regulation, standards, and evidence develop. The difference between federated metaverse healthcare and other decentralised intelligence, immersive interface, and cross-border coordination convergence approaches lies in the greater risks and opportunities it entails and the need for incremental, evidence-based implementation. The viability of the paradigm, therefore, will not rely on technological ingenuity but on institutions' ability to address scalability, clinical trust, ethical legitimacy, and environmental sustainability through governance, rigorous appraisal, and collective learning.

11. RESEARCH GAPS AND OPEN CHALLENGES

Federated metaverse healthcare, despite increasing conceptual coherence and experimental momentum, remains constrained by significant research gaps that impede the translation of evidence-based practice, including not only technical immaturity but also more profound epistemic, methodological, and institutional flaws in the study and regulation of immersive and decentralised health innovations. One inherent weakness is the lack of longitudinal clinical data; most studies rely on short pilots, simulations, or controlled assessments that demonstrate feasibility. However, there is limited information on long-term outcomes, patient safety, and system-wide impact; in healthcare, where interventions occur over long periods and affect complex care trajectories, this is especially critical (Topol, 2019).

Continuous model evolution in federated systems would further complicate causal attribution and baseline stability, underscoring the need for adaptive trial designs or real-world evidence frameworks that assess learning systems rather than static interventions (FDA, 2022). This is directly linked to the lack of a single, multidimensional evaluation measure that integrates clinical effectiveness, fairness, robustness, usability, and governance. Existing evaluations remain fragmented, and studies of federated learning often focus on aggregate performance indicators that obscure institutional or demographic differences. In contrast, studies of immersive technology focus more on presence or engagement but do not systematically link experiential qualities to clinical reasoning or decision quality (Radianti et al., 2020).

This methodological siloing impedes comparability, incentivises selective reporting, and hinders the formation of cumulative knowledge, calling for interdisciplinary agreement on frameworks for socio-technical evaluation. Another important gap is that empirical evidence has been concentrated in high-income locations with well-developed infrastructure and regulatory capacity, and the findings are then extrapolated to heterogeneous contexts without adequate underpinnings. Contextual variability in disease burden, institutional trust, cultural norms, and clinician-patient relationships has a material role in federated metaverse healthcare, and the lack of evidence regarding low- and middle-income countries has the potential to increase further the chances of existing design assumptions to exacerbate rather than alleviate global inequities (WHO, 2023).

The ongoing lack of interoperability and standardisation also limits scalability, as current health IT standards, including HL7 FHIR, do not provide sufficient support for representing spatial data, embodied interaction, and real-time collaboration, which are inherent to immersive spaces. Meanwhile, federated learning demands harmonisation not only of data formats but also of model architectures, update schemes, and regulatory policies. Division among vendors and jurisdictions threatens the creation of individual silos of immersion that weaken the essence of the federation, even though policy work such as the European Health Data Space is aware of this issue (European Commission, 2022).

The least studied gap, perhaps, is on human factors and clinician cognition, where the advice on human-AI interaction rarely extends to immersive scenarios and experiences of full embodiment, perception, and attention, where situational awareness and increased risk of cognitive load, overconfidence, and biased uncertainty are simultaneously beneficial and dangerous (Amershi et al., 2019). These gaps are not discrete and require coordinated research agendas that incorporate longitudinal clinical research, ethnographic inquiry, and system-level analytics, as well as regulatory sandboxes and sustained funding for implementation. Moreover, given positively, these gaps are not reasons to retreat but markers of a responsible innovation, since the development of federated experiential intelligence will not rely on technical incremental benefits as much as on the creation of convincing evidence, harmonisation of evaluation models, and a human experience centre to create immersive healthcare systems that are clinically effective, culturally responsive, and socially legitimate.

12. METAFRAMEWORK

Figure 1. Integrated Metaframework of Federated Experiential Intelligence

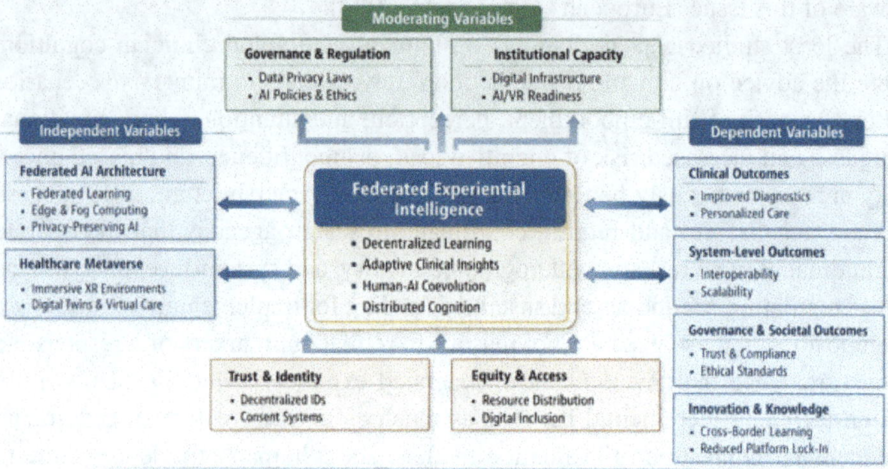

An Integrated Metaframework *of Federated Experiential Intelligence in Metaverse-Based Healthcare Systems*

Source: *Authors' Contribution*

The framework in Figure 1 conceptualises Federated Experiential Intelligence (FEI) as an integrative socio-technical mechanism whereby federated AI architectures and healthcare metaverse environments mutually reconfigure the clinical workforce's cognition and the governance and performance of systems. By combining federated learning, edge-fog, and privacy-preserving AI with immersive XR, digital twins, and virtual care, FEI makes decentralised learning, adaptive clinical insight, and human-AI coevolution available in distributed settings (Wang et al., 2022).

Governance and regulation, institutional capacity, trust infrastructures, and conditions of equity function as important moderating variables influencing outcomes. Empirically, this configuration is linked to improved diagnostics, and personalisation, improved interoperability and scalability, increased trust, compliance and knowledge generation across countries, more cross-border, individual add-on or reduced platform lock-in, which is in line with theory of distributed systems, polycentricity, and digital health evidence (Ostrom, 2010, Sheller et al., 2020, WHO, 2023).

13. FUTURE RESEARCH DIRECTIONS

The previous analysis sets federated AI-enabled metaverse healthcare as an emerging socio-technical paradigm as opposed to a stabilised solution, which, in turn, requires future research to go beyond incremental optimisation toward integrated research questions related to how distributed intelligence, immersive interaction and institutional governance can be co-designed in order to support safe, equitable and effective care.

One promising direction is the application of federated reinforcement learning (FRL) in immersive clinical environments, where care processes unfold through sequential, feedback-driven interactions rather than static predictive tasks. Unlike supervised models, FRL allows the policy to be learned adaptively over time, making it ideal for virtual wards, rehabilitation spaces, and surgical simulators, and, when paired with federation, enabling collective learning without centralising sensitive interaction data. However, such an approach would be subject to unresolved problems concerning reward specification, safety constraints, convergence in heterogeneous environments, and the encoding of clinical and ethical values within such a system. Research on a system that integrates algorithmic, regulatory, and normative considerations is needed.

Closely related is the need to theorise and empirically examine hybrid decision systems in which human clinicians, algorithmic agents, and avatars jointly mediate care. Metaverse environments violate the human-AI binary and bring avatar-mediated agency, redistributing responsibility, authority, and trust through immersive interaction. Research must therefore focus on questions such as: how do clinicians interpret AI recommendations which are delivered via avatars, how is accountability negotiated in such assemblages, and how do patients view agency and empathy given the insights into human-computer interaction, cognitive science and organisational theory pointing to risks of cognitive overload and accountability diffusion in addition to potential gains in situational awareness and reasoning together (Amershi et al., 2019)

A further critical agenda is the embedded use of federated experiential intelligence within public digital health infrastructures, rather than proprietary ones. Policy frameworks, including the European Health Data Space and national digital health missions in India supported by WHO, as well as digital public infrastructure models, indicate a move towards the concept of digital health capabilities as a shared societal asset. Future research should explore how federated care environments may interoperate (through open standards and public governance) with national health records, surveillance systems, and workforce platforms, avoid platform lock-in, and embody equity.

Advancing these agendas requires methodological innovation, as the adaptive, evolving nature of federated metaverse systems cannot be assessed by a single method. Randomised controlled trials alone cannot suffice for systems that evolve during implementation processes. All qualitative studies lack scalability and impact from a policy standpoint, unlike mixed methodologies that leverage both simulation-based experiments, adaptive trials, ethnographic observation processes and real-world evidence are needed to capture asynchronous follow-up outcomes, contextual variability and unintended impacts such as disruption of this workflow and shift in professional identity (i.e., behaviour change in this case)(FDA, 2022).

Equally critical is ongoing cross-disciplinary collaboration among machine learning, immersive computing, clinical medicine, ethics, law, and public policy, as federated metaverse healthcare lies at their intersection yet is constrained by siloed incentives and standards. International collaboration is essential to ensure that rules and technical specifications reflect not only the views of dominant regions but also the diverse institutional and cultural contexts.

Collectively, these directions of research signify the transition from proof-of-concept experimentation to systemic understanding and responsible scalability and highlight what they see as the truth for building the future of federated metaverse healthcare, i.e., not just about the technological novelty but about making computationally innovation compatible with human judgement, institutional capacity and societal values, and so helping federated experiential intelligence to be credibly on board for building healthy individual and social capital on a big scale.

14. IMPLICATIONS

Federated AI and the healthcare metaverse as a whole represent a systemic reconfiguration of the foundational elements of intelligence, care delivery, and governance, rather than representing an incremental extension of digital health, with implications that range across the spectrum of theory, managerial and clinical practice, public policy, and societal mores and thus require integral interpretation in order to prevent dichotomous or dissonant adoption.

At a theoretical level, the concept of federated metaverse healthcare reverses our understanding of healthcare AI as a distributed experiential system embedded in persistent environments, challenging dominant conceptions of intelligence as a detached decision-support function operating on abstracted data. Intelligence rather arises through ongoing interplay between clinicians, patients, AIs, avatars, digital twins and integrates with the theories of distributed cognition, complex adaptive systems and extends these theories into immersive AI-mediated spaces and reveals the fault-findings in contextual evaluation paradigms that favour static accuracy over adaptive learning, contextual sense making, and experiential feedback. This perspective also advances platform and governance theory by reallocating focus from centralised platform control to protocol-based, polycentric governance. In these standards, interoperability rules, and negotiated participation arrangements determine value creation and responsibility across institutions and jurisdictions, raising important new theoretical questions about power, legitimacy, and coordination in digital health ecosystems.

For healthcare organisations, federated metaverse healthcare is more of a strategic pathway than a turnkey solution, making early value most apparent in targeted use cases such as multidisciplinary collaboration, specialist training and chronic care co-ordination. Capability building (as opposed to the mere acquisition of technology) is a necessary part of effective adoption, including investments in data governance, edge infrastructure, workforce capabilities, and cross-institutional partnerships, but with proper sequencing to ensure that premature scaling does not introduce or amplify complexity and resistance. Workforce training and clinical redesign core, workflows and processes with immersive and AI media changing people's perception, collaboration, and judgment, unintentionally adding to the burden of thinking or worsening automation bias, clinician co-design, digital literacy development, and redefined clinician roles can lead to human-AI complementarity, reflective practice, and ongoing learning.

From a policy perspective, Federated metaverse healthcare poses a challenge for regulatory frameworks grounded in bounded systems and jurisdictions, as the distribution of decision-making enabled by federated learning and immersive interaction is cross-border and cross-lifecycle. This requires adaptive regulation, which focuses on continuous surveillance, lifecycle control, and shared responsibility, rather than static certification based on, but also beyond, existing efforts such as the EU AI Act, the European Health Data Space, and national AI strategies, to enable immersive environments and cross-border federation. Public policy is also critical to bringing innovation's power to bear on public health objectives, through market counterweight by favouring open standards and open public digital health infrastructure, procurement that considers equity, and experimentation within regulatory areas to create social relevance that will facilitate the generation of socially relevant evidence.

This federated metaverse healthcare poses an opportunity as well as a risk for societies: Federated architectures may facilitate collaboration without requiring the extraction of data, and offer a potential to support participation by resource prohibited institutions as well as expanding access to specialist care and training; but disparities of connectivity, hardware, and digital literacy threaten exclusion as new as well as re-provincement should infrastructures are not in aspect embedded by design. Trust is a decisive determinant of legitimacy and calls for transparency, participatory governance, and mechanisms for redressing issues related to surveillance, data misuse, and algorithmic bias.

Collectively, these implications support the notion that federated metaverse healthcare constitutes a systemic transformation that requires less technical sophistication and, more importantly, the ability of researchers, managers, policymakers, clinicians, and societies to reconcile the distributed intelligence of experiences around shared value systems of health, equity, and governance.

15. CONCLUSION: TOWARD A NEW PARADIGM OF VIRTUAL, FEDERATED CARE

This chapter has contributed to a thorough conceptual, empirical, and normative argument that the convergence of federated artificial intelligence and metaverse-based healthcare environments is not just a transient technological trend but a substantive paradigm shift. By combining critical and imaginative analyses of distributed systems theory, socio-technical governance, immersive computing, and global health policy, the analysis has transcended descriptive accounts of digital innovation to develop a new computational and organisational logic for healthcare. Some key findings of this work include the redefinition of healthcare AI as a distributed experiential system, in which intelligence is produced through continuous interaction among clinicians, patients, AI agents, and digital representations immersed in long-lasting virtual spaces.

Throughout the chapter, some core contributions have been made. First, the limitations of centralised and platform-dependent models across the digital health ecosystem were critically reviewed, including the restrictions imposed by data concentration and institutional silos stemming from regulatory fragmentation, as well as the implications for scalability, trust, and equity in the digital health era. In response, federated AI was positioned not only as a privacy-preserving technique but also as one oriented toward governance rather than enforcement, and as a paradigm capable of ensuring collective learning without requiring data convergence. Second, the healthcare metaverse was conceptualised as a cyber-physical social infrastructure that will transform the delivery of care into an immersive, longitudinal and cooperative process. When theorised on, federated AI and the metaverse were shown to form a new computational logic - one that shifts the experience of data processing from static to experiential and decentralised to adaptive intelligence.

Empirical trends and new practices supported this synthesis of theory. Case studies of virtual hospitals, federated diagnostics, and cross-border connectedness have demonstrated both the feasibility and fragility of federated metaverse healthcare in real-world settings. These cases showed the implications of federation, allowing them to work together without centralising data ownership, but also revealed tensions around issues such as bias, robustness, accountability, and sustainability. The analysis also highlighted that decentralisation does not necessarily ensure fairness and trust; instead, outcomes depend on the design of learning protocols, immersive interfaces, and governance mechanisms within institutional contexts.

A key implication of the above synthesis is the redefinition of the locus of healthcare decision-making and responsibility for federated AI, in conjunction with the metaverse. Intelligence is distributed across systems and actors, while governance shifts from hierarchical control to protocol-based coordination that engages regulators, standards bodies, healthcare organisations, and communities. This reconfiguration calls into question current regulatory, managerial, and ethical frameworks and necessitates adaptive frameworks that focus on life-cycle governance, transparency, and human oversight. Importantly, it also calls for new forms of evidence generation that can capture longitudinal outcomes, contextual variability, and human factors in immersive learning systems.

Looking ahead, the chapter provides a clear message about the need to adopt federated virtual care responsibly and inclusively, based on evidence. Technological envisioning needs to be tempered by rigorous analysis, participatory design, and sustained consideration of equity and ecological sustainability. In this context, policymakers and healthcare leaders should resist efforts toward one-size-fits-all deployments and instead enable drip-and-choose contextual pathways that are consonant with public health goals and global health equity. For researchers, the agenda goes "beyond the performance of algorithms to questions that are both interdisciplinary and integrative in addressing both technical and clinical as well as social and normative dimensions."

In conclusion, federated AI-enabled metaverse healthcare is an evolving paradigm that re-creates how healthcare is organised, experienced, and governed. The promise of it is not solely about the technology itself, but about how it can help build better, more collaborative, adaptive, and equitable healthcare ecosystems. Whether this potential is realised will depend on collective choices made by researchers, practitioners, policymakers, and societies regarding how intelligence, trust, and care will be distributed in an increasingly virtual yet profoundly human healthcare future.

REFERENCES

Al Omar, A., Bhuiyan, M. Z. A., Basu, A., Kiyomoto, S., & Rahman, M. S. (2021). A systematic review of blockchain for consent management and privacy in healthcare: healthcare, *9*(2), 137.

Amershi, S., Weld, D., Vorvoreanu, M., Fourney, A., Nushi, B., Collisson, P., Suh, J., Iqbal, S., Bennett, P. N., Inkpen, K., Teevan, J., Kikin-Gil, R., & Horvitz, E. (2019). Guidelines for human-AI interaction. *Proceedings of the 2019 CHI Conference on Human Factors in Computing Systems*, Article 3. DOI: 10.1145/3290605.3300233

Bagdasaryan, E., Veit, A., Hua, Y., Estrin, D., & Shmatikov, V. (2020). How to backdoor federated learning. *Proceedings of the 23rd International Conference on Artificial Intelligence and Statistics*, 2938–2948.

Björnsson, B., Borrebaeck, C., Elander, N., Gasslander, T., Gawel, D. R., Gustafsson, M., Jörnsten, R., Lee, E. J., Li, X., Lilja, S., Martínez-Enguita, D., Matussek, A., Sandström, P., Schäfer, S., Stenmarker, M., Sun, X. F., Sysoev, O., Zhang, H., & Benson, M. (2020). Digital twins to personalise medicine. *Genome Medicine*, *12*(1), 4. DOI: 10.1186/s13073-019-0701-3 PMID: 31892363

Bruynseels, K., Santoni de Sio, F., & van den Hoven, J. (2018). Digital twins in health care: Ethical implications of an emerging engineering paradigm. *Frontiers in Genetics*, *9*, 31. DOI: 10.3389/fgene.2018.00031 PMID: 29487613

Dionisio, J. D. N., Burns, W. G., & Gilbert, R. (2013). 3D virtual worlds and the metaverse: Current status and future possibilities. *ACM Computing Surveys*, *45*(3), 1–38. DOI: 10.1145/2480741.2480751

Dwork, C., & Roth, A. (2014). The algorithmic foundations of differential privacy. *Foundations and Trends® in Theoretical Computer Science, 9*(3–4), 211–407.

European Commission. (2021). *Proposal for a Regulation laying down harmonised rules on artificial intelligence*. AI Act.

European Commission. (2022). *European Health Data Space: Impact assessment report*.

European Commission. (2022). *Proposal for a regulation laying down harmonised rules on artificial intelligence*. AI Act.

European Health Data Space. (2025). *Regulation (EU) 2025/327 on the use and exchange of electronic health data*.

FDA. (2022). *Augmented and virtual reality in medical devices: Regulatory considerations.*

Food and Drug Administration. (2023). *Artificial intelligence and machine learning in software as a medical device: Action plan.*

Gawer, A. (2021). Digital platforms' boundaries: The interplay of firm scope, platform sides, and digital interfaces. *Long Range Planning*, *54*(5), 102045. DOI: 10.1016/j.lrp.2020.102045

Geels, F. W. (2002). Technological transitions as evolutionary reconfiguration processes. *Research Policy*, *31*(8–9), 1257–1274. DOI: 10.1016/S0048-7333(02)00062-8

Hollan, J., Hutchins, E., & Kirsh, D. (2000). Distributed cognition: Toward a new foundation for human–computer interaction research. *ACM Transactions on Computer-Human Interaction*, *7*(2), 174–196. DOI: 10.1145/353485.353487

International Organisation for Standardisation. (2023). *ISO/IEC 23894:2023—Information technology—Artificial intelligence—Guidance on risk management.*

Lehne, M., Luijten, S., Vom Felde Genannt Imbusch, P., & Thun, S. (2019). The use of FHIR in digital health - A review of the scientific literature. *Studies in Health Technology and Informatics*, *267*, 52–58. PMID: 31483254

Lyell, D., & Coiera, E. (2017). Automation bias and verification complexity: A systematic review. *Journal of the American Medical Informatics Association : JAMIA*, *24*(2), 423–431. DOI: 10.1093/jamia/ocw105 PMID: 27516495

Mayer, R. C., Davis, J. H., & Schoorman, F. D. (1995). An integrative model of organisational trust. *Academy of Management Review*, *20*(3), 709–734. DOI: 10.2307/258792

McMahan, B.. (2017). Communication-efficient learning of deep networks from decentralised data. *Proceedings of AISTATS.*

National Institute of Standards and Technology. (2023). *Artificial Intelligence Risk Management Framework (AI RMF 1.0).*

National Institute of Standards and Technology. (2024). *Artificial Intelligence Risk Management Framework: Generative Artificial Intelligence Profile (NIST-AI-600-1).*

OECD. (2024). *AI in Health: Huge potential, huge risks.* OECD Publishing.

OECD. (2024). *AI in health: Huge potential, huge risks.* OECD Publishing.

OECD. (2024). *AI in health: Huge potential, huge risks.* OECD Publishing.

Ostrom, E. (2010). Polycentric systems for coping with collective action and global environmental change. *Global Environmental Change*, *20*(4), 550–557. DOI: 10.1016/j.gloenvcha.2010.07.004

Park, S., & Kim, Y. (2023). Virtual hospitals and metaverse healthcare services: Policy and practice implications. *Health Policy and Technology*, *12*(1), 100721. PMID: 36683761

Pati, S., Baid, U., Edwards, B., Sheller, M., Wang, S.-H., Reina, G. A., Foley, P., Gruzdev, A., Karkada, D., Davatzikos, C., Sako, C., Ghodasara, S., Bilello, M., Mohan, S., Vollmuth, P., Brugnara, G., Preetha, C. J., Sahm, F., Maier-Hein, K., & Bakas, S. (2022). Federated learning enables the use of big data for rare cancer boundary detection. *Nature Communications*, *13*(1), 7346. DOI: 10.1038/s41467-022-33407-5 PMID: 36470898

Plsek, P. E., & Greenhalgh, T. (2001). Complexity science: The challenge of complexity in health care. *BMJ (Clinical Research Ed.)*, *323*(7313), 625–628. DOI: 10.1136/bmj.323.7313.625 PMID: 11557716

Radianti, J., Majchrzak, T. A., Fromm, J., & Wohlgenannt, I. (2020). A systematic review of immersive virtual reality applications for higher education: Design elements, lessons learned, and research agenda. *Computers & Education*, *147*, 103778. DOI: 10.1016/j.compedu.2019.103778

Rieke, N., Hancox, J., Li, W., Milletarì, F., Roth, H. R., Albarqouni, S., Bakas, S., Galtier, M. N., Landman, B. A., Maier-Hein, K., Ourselin, S., Sheller, M., Summers, R. M., Trask, A., Xu, D., Baust, M., & Cardoso, M. J. (2020). The future of digital health with federated learning. *npj. Digital Medicine*, *3*, 119. PMID: 33015372

Satyanarayanan, M. (2017). The emergence of edge computing. *Computer*, *50*(1), 30–39. DOI: 10.1109/MC.2017.9

Sheller, M. J., Edwards, B., Reina, G. A., Martin, J., Pati, S., Kotrotsou, A., Milchenko, M., Xu, W., Marcus, D., Colen, R. R., & Bakas, S. (2020). Federated learning in medicine: Facilitating multi-institutional collaborations without sharing patient data. *Scientific Reports*, *10*(1), 12598. DOI: 10.1038/s41598-020-69250-1 PMID: 32724046

Shi, W., Cao, J., Zhang, Q., Li, Y., & Xu, L. (2016). Edge computing: Vision and challenges. *IEEE Internet of Things Journal*, *3*(5), 637–646. DOI: 10.1109/JIOT.2016.2579198

Siau, K., & Wang, W. (2020). Building trust in artificial intelligence, machine learning, and robotics. *Cutting-Edge Technologies for Enterprise Systems*, 109–132.

Slater, M., & Sanchez-Vives, M. V. (2016). Enhancing our lives with immersive virtual reality. *Frontiers in Robotics and AI*, *3*, 74. DOI: 10.3389/frobt.2016.00074

Strubell, E., Ganesh, A., & McCallum, A. (2019). Energy and policy considerations for deep learning in NLP. *Proceedings of the 57th Annual Meeting of the ACL*, 3645–3650. DOI: 10.18653/v1/P19-1355

Tanenbaum, A. S., & Van Steen, M. (2017). *Distributed systems: Principles and paradigms* (2nd ed.). Pearson.

Topol, E. (2019). *Deep medicine: How artificial intelligence can make healthcare human again*—basic Books.

U.S. Food and Drug Administration. (2022). (2021–2024). *Good machine learning practice for medical device development: Guiding principles* (FDA/Health Canada/ MHRA).

Vanmathi, C.. (2024). Blockchain integration in healthcare: A comprehensive review of applications, challenges, and solutions. *Frontiers in Digital Health.*

Vayena, E., Blasimme, A., & Cohen, I. G. (2020). Machine learning in medicine: Addressing ethical challenges. *PLoS Medicine*, *17*(11), e1002689. DOI: 10.1371/ journal.pmed.1002689 PMID: 30399149

Vayena, E., Dzenowagis, J., Brownstein, J. S., & Sheikh, A. (2020). Policy implications of big data in the health sector. *Bulletin of the World Health Organization*, *98*(1), 66–68. DOI: 10.2471/BLT.17.197426 PMID: 29403102

Veale, M., & Borgesius, F. Z. (2021). Demystifying the draft EU Artificial Intelligence Act. *Computer Law Review International*, *22*(4), 97–112. DOI: 10.9785/ cri-2021-220402

Wang, Y., Su, Z., Zhang, N., Xing, R., Liu, D., Luan, T. H., & Shen, X. (2022). A survey on metaverse: Fundamentals, security, and privacy. *IEEE Communications Surveys and Tutorials*, *25*(1), 319–352. DOI: 10.1109/COMST.2022.3202047

WHO. (2023). *Global strategy on digital health 2020–2025: Progress report.*

Williamson, O. E. (1985). *The economic institutions of capitalism: Firms, markets, relational contracting*. Free Press.

World Health Organisation. (2023). *Global strategy on digital health 2020–2025: Progress report.*

Zhang, J.. (2023). Metaverse-based healthcare: A systematic review. *Journal of Medical Internet Research*, *25*, e45352.

Zou, J., & Schiebinger, L. (2018). AI can be sexist and racist—It is time to make it fair. *Nature*, *559*(7714), 324–326. DOI: 10.1038/d41586-018-05707-8 PMID: 30018439

Zuboff, S. (2019). *The age of surveillance capitalism*. PublicAffairs.

Chapter 8
Federated AI-Driven Digital Twins in the Healthcare Metaverse: Architectures, Privacy, and Clinical Intelligence

Anmol Shankarrao Budhewar
http://orcid.org/0009-0002-9112-107X
Sandip Institute of Technology and Research Centre, Nashik, India

Balkrishna Keshavrao Patil
http://orcid.org/0009-0000-5136-2157
Sandip Institute of Technology and Research Centre, Nashik, India

Aman Suresh Tharayil
http://orcid.org/0009-0000-5377-7428
Dr. M.G.R. Educational and Research Institute, India

Supriya Bhosale
http://orcid.org/0000-0002-8638-701X
Vishwakarma University, Pune, India

Sujitha Suthadevan
http://orcid.org/0009-0001-2043-6720
Sathyabama Institute of Science and Technology, India

Nirlepkumar Patel
Department of Pharmacy, Brainerd Pharmacy, Chattanooga, USA

Aupama Shankarrao Budhewar
JSPM University, India

Harsha Vishal Bhole
http://orcid.org/0009-0007-2548-9403
Sandip Institute of Technology and Research Centre, Nashik, India

Pramod Gorakh Patil
http://orcid.org/0009-0005-9201-987X
MVP KBT College of Engineering, India

Swapnali Kishan Somwanshi
http://orcid.org/0009-0009-0584-4150
Yashwant College, India

DOI: 10.4018/979-8-3373-8889-2.ch008

Adinarayana Andy
http://orcid.org/0000-0002-5163-1094
Weatherwax Family Pharmacies Inc., USA

ABSTRACT

This chapter per the authors examines the integration of federated learning and digital twins to establish a resilient clinical intelligence ecosystem in the healthcare metaverse. While always-on sensing offers transformative potential, existing implementations often treat privacy, latency, and governance as secondary concerns. By synthesizing current literature, this chapter per the authors identifies a benchmarking gap where model metrics are prioritized over system-level evidence like communication overhead and energy costs. To address these deficiencies, authors propose a unified five-layer reference architecture treating trust and real-time synchronization as core requirements. This framework introduces the "protected twin" concept, utilizing differential privacy, secure aggregation, and audit trails to ensure distributed intelligence remains accountable and robust against poisoning. Ultimately, this chapter per the authors provides a strategic roadmap for moving toward deployable, clinically valid pipelines that balance innovation with patient safety.

1. INTRODUCTION

1.1 Motivation: Healthcare Metaverse, Always-on Sensing, and Decision Loops

Current discussions around the healthcare metaverse often focus on continuous interaction between hospitals, home environments, and mobile settings, supported by persistent sensing and interactive digital interfaces (Bansal et al., 2022; Wang et al., 2022). In real deployments, this idea of being "always on" is mostly driven by remote patient monitoring and ambient data collection, rather than immersive visualization alone. The real-time effectiveness of such systems is not automatically reflected in data availability; it is reflected in the efficiency with which actual real-time observations are translated into quick clinical procedures and actions. These actions may include alerts or intimations, decision-based recommendations, or a few adjustments to existing processes, and they must be executed within the time frames required for patient care, observation, and safety (Trivedi et al., 2025).

The difficulty is that such decision loops operate under constraints that do not appear in typical consumer metaverse settings: patient safety, heterogeneous medical devices, legacy protocols, and regulated handling of sensitive health data (Letafati et al., 2023; Weber et al., 2023). As a result, healthcare metaverse systems must be engineered as end-to-end pipelines that treat trust, latency, and governance as core requirements rather than afterthoughts.

1.2 Why "Federated AI and Digital Twins"

Digital twins provide a structured abstraction for representing patients, devices, and care workflows as evolving states rather than isolated measurements, with the expectation of near-real-time synchronization as conditions change (Balasubramanyam et al., 2024; Chen et al., 2023). However, twin fidelity depends on the quality and continuity of data streams, and in healthcare, these streams are inherently distributed across institutions and devices. Federated learning is therefore positioned as a pragmatic route to scale clinical intelligence without moving raw patient data, enabling cross-site model improvement while preserving local data control (Gadekallu et al., 2023; Quan et al., 2026).

The coupling becomes essential in metaverse settings: digital twins require continual model updates to remain clinically useful, and federated learning provides a mechanism to update those models under realistic privacy constraints (Adnan et al., 2025). At the same time, the combination introduces new attack surfaces, privacy leakage from updates, non-IID degradation, and poisoning, making privacy and robustness engineering central to the architecture (Dwork, 2006; Sun et al., 2023; Kausar et al., 2025).

2. BACKGROUND AND FOUNDATIONS

2.1 Healthcare Metaverse: Scope, Services, Stakeholders

In healthcare-oriented metaverse visions, immersive interfaces are typically presented as an experience layer that overlays existing clinical systems, remote monitoring, and care coordination rather than replacing them (Bansal et al., 2022; Wang et al., 2022). The scope includes services such as clinician–patient interaction in virtual environments, interactive visualization of longitudinal patient states, rehabilitation and training scenarios, and continuous remote patient monitoring supported by connected devices (Letafati et al., 2023; Trivedi et al., 2025). Stakeholders span patients and caregivers, clinical providers (physicians, nurses, technicians), and platform operators responsible for identity, access control, and service orchestration across heterogeneous devices and networks (Bansal et al., 2022; Letafati et al., 2023). From an engineering standpoint, the healthcare metaverse is best treated as a multi-layer system: (i) sensing and data acquisition at the edge, (ii) clinical data infrastructure (e.g., EHR and monitoring systems), (iii) intelligence and decision support components, and (iv) an immersive interaction layer that mediates how insights are presented and acted upon (Wang et al., 2022; Chen et al., 2024). When intelligence is spread across hospitals, platforms, and service providers, questions of governance become more prominent. Issues such as consent, auditability, and accountability cannot be treated as secondary concerns because clinical decisions must remain explainable and traceable even when no single organization controls the entire pipeline (Jamshidi et al., 2024). This is particularly important in distributed healthcare environments, where responsibility for data use and decision outcomes must still be clearly attributable despite collaborative intelligence and cross-organizational participation (Chen & Liu, 2025; Vashisht & Rani, 2025).

2.2 Digital Twins in Healthcare

Digital twins are generally described as computational models that reflect physical entities and are updated over time using incoming data streams. In healthcare, prior work distinguishes several types of digital twins based on the system being modeled and its purpose (Balasubramanyam et al., 2024; Okegbile et al., 2023). A patient digital twin focuses on individual physiological or clinical states and is typically used to support monitoring, risk assessment, and personalized decision support.

2.3 Clinical Intelligence vs. ML prediction (CDSS Integration, Trust, Accountability)

CDSS integration introduces concrete constraints. First, outputs must be traceable: the system should support audit logs and governance controls that enable clinicians and operators to understand how an alert was produced and whether policy requirements were satisfied (Chen & Liu, 2025; Vashisht & Rani, 2025). Second, models must be robust under deployment realities, including heterogeneous devices and changing environments; "good average accuracy" is insufficient if performance degrades unpredictably across sites or time windows (Quan et al., 2026; Wang et al., 2025). Third, trust must be engineered, not assumed. This motivates privacy-preserving mechanisms, secure sharing schemes, and, where relevant, integrity and provenance layers that reduce the risk of manipulated updates or unaccountable decisions (Salim & Park, 2023; Kausar et al., 2025). In short, clinical intelligence is best treated as a system property that emerges from the interaction of models, twins, governance, and workflows, rather than as a single-model output.

3. LITERATURE SYNTHESIS: WHAT EXISTS AND WHAT IS MISSING

3.1 Digital-Twin Healthcare Landscape

The healthcare digital twin literature has expanded from early conceptual discussions into a broad set of architectures, use cases, and engineering surveys. Recent reviews emphasize that "digital twin" is used to describe multiple abstractions, including patient-state models, device replicas, workflow models, and networked system twins, often without a clear distinction between simulation-oriented twins and continuously synchronized operational twins (Balasubramanyam et al., 2024; Okegbile et al., 2023).

This creates an evaluation inconsistency: papers frequently report algorithmic outcomes while leaving twin-specific qualities under-specified, such as synchronization fidelity, update frequency, and the operational consequences of stale or missing updates (Chen et al., 2023; Chen et al., 2024). A related issue is that validation settings vary widely across existing studies. Recent AI-driven myocardial infarction studies illustrate heterogeneous analytical frameworks, reinforcing the need for standardized reporting to enable cross-study comparability assessment (Kosanam & Pasupula, 2024; Diokadan et al., 2025).

Some contributions are framed as clinical intelligence systems intended to support decision-making, while others are better understood as network-level or device-monitoring frameworks. Because these environments differ so substantially, results are often reported under incompatible assumptions. In the absence of a common reporting pattern, it becomes difficult to compare findings across papers or to assess whether reported improvements can be translated into systems that are practical for real clinical deployment.

3.2 Federated Healthcare Intelligence: Patterns

In healthcare environments, federated learning is most often presented as the mechanism that enables collaborative intelligence without requiring centralized pooling of sensitive data, particularly in multi-institution and edge-oriented settings (Gadekallu et al., 2023; Quan et al., 2026). Several recurring architectural patterns can be observed in the literature. One common pattern relies on centralized orchestration, where participating clients train local models and submit updates to a central aggregation server. This approach remains widely used because it is relatively straightforward to engineers and aligns well with existing platform designs (Quan et al., 2026).

3.3 Privacy & Security

Privacy and security challenges arise at multiple points within federated digital-twin systems. Basically, differential privacy provides a professional approach to prevent information leakage by introducing controlled error or noise into learning processes. In real-time healthcare sectors, this outcome results in a privacy utility trade-off that must be carefully chosen, considering both medical safety and better system performance (Dwork, 2006). Beyond privacy, resulting systems often provide more secure aggregation to minimize the involvement of specific client updates, in conjunction with cryptographic mechanisms such as homomorphic encryption to secure system updates or inference tasks in sensitive deployment scenarios (Sai et al., 2024; Kausar et al., 2025). One also has to ensure that already completed surveys are performed so that confidentiality is not merely sufficient to ensure faithful operation (Trivedi et al., 2025; Weber et al., 2023). A model may ensure data privacy to an acceptable level, but it is also vulnerable to poisoning, backdoor effects, or unaccountable interpretations and manipulations of system parameters, which are more pertinent in safety-critical clinical pipelines (Sun et al., 2023; Weber et al., 2023).

3.4 Communication, Latency, and Energy Expense or Overheads

A continuous limitation for operational changes is that many tasks treat communication and latency as lower priorities, even though metaverse and remotely monitored settings are mostly time sensitive. Where addressed, the literature recognizes that federated learning introduces overhead from repeated model-update exchange and that this overhead is amplified in heterogeneous networks with stragglers or intermittent devices (Lian et al., 2022; Quan et al., 2026). Digital twin–enabled asynchronous learning frameworks are explicitly designed to tolerate uneven participation and update delays, reflecting the practical realities of healthcare devices and edge networks (Stephanie et al., 2023; Stephanie et al., 2024).

In metaverse-oriented designs, freshness measures such as Age-of-Information are proposed to shape scheduling and update strategies for real-time healthcare intelligence, indicating that "model accuracy" alone is insufficient when intelligence becomes stale before it can be acted upon (Wu et al., 2025). In security-oriented designs, additional trust layers can increase runtime, communication payload, and confirmation latency, shifting the engineering problem from "can we learn?" to "can we learn within acceptable cost and time bounds?" (Kausar et al., 2025). Across the literature, what is consistently missing is a standardized reporting set that jointly describes performance, communication cost, latency, and device energy impact in a clinically interpretable manner.

3.5 Governance and Standards Readiness

Governance and standardization are cross-cutting requirements rather than a single mechanism. Healthcare deployments require policy-driven controls for consent, identity, access, auditability, and accountability, especially when intelligence is distributed across multiple organizations and service providers (Letafati et al., 2023; Chen & Liu, 2025). Standard-focused work argues that privacy-preserving AI systems, particularly those operating in 6G-enabled digital twin environments, must be aligned with emerging guidance on trustworthy AI and privacy-by-design engineering, but also acknowledges that adoption depends on practical orchestration capabilities and measurable compliance readiness (Chen & Liu, 2025; Vashisht & Rani, 2025). The governance challenge is intensified in metaverse settings because services are multi-modal (clinical data, XR interaction, device telemetry) and cross-domain. As a result, many papers can be read as "technology proposals" without a corresponding operational policy model describing who is accountable for model behavior, how incidents are investigated, and how compliance is enforced across federated participants (Ouchani et al., 2025; Quan et al., 2026).

3.6 Key Synthesis Takeaway: Evidence is Fragmented, Thus in Need of Unified Architecture

Taken together, the literature provides strong evidence that federated learning and digital twins are individually well motivated for healthcare metaverse environments, but the supporting evidence remains fragmented across isolated concerns. Twin-focused work often under-specifies federated governance and privacy risk. Federated learning work frequently reports learning outcomes without sufficiently grounding them in deployment realities, such as synchronization fidelity, latency constraints, and clinical workflow integration (Balasubramanyam et al., 2024; Quan et al., 2026). Privacy and security mechanisms are described across a wide spectrum—DP, cryptography, secure aggregation, auditability yet many papers lack a unified threat model and do not present end-to-end system designs that connect protection choices to clinical intelligence requirements (Dwork, 2006; Weber et al., 2023; Kausar et al., 2025). The consequence is a gap between "promising components" and deployable pipelines. This motivates the need for a unified reference architecture that explicitly integrates sensing, digital twin synchronization, federated intelligence, privacy and trust controls, and clinically meaningful outputs under a coherent governance model.

4. REFERENCE ARCHITECTURE: FEDERATED AI–DRIVEN DIGITAL TWINS FOR THE HEALTHCARE METAVERSE

4.1 Design Goals: Privacy, Trust, Real-Time Intelligence, Auditability, Scalability

A reference architecture for federated AI–driven healthcare digital twins must satisfy constraints that are simultaneously clinical, computational, and organizational. First, privacy is non-negotiable because patient data is distributed across hospitals, homes, and devices, and metaverse-oriented services increase the risk of cross-context linkage and secondary use (Letafati et al., 2023; Gadekallu et al., 2023). Second, trust must be engineered: model updates and intelligence outputs must be resilient to poisoning and misuse and should be accompanied by mechanisms for accountability and verification rather than relying on implicit trust between participants (Weber et al., 2023; Sun et al., 2023). Third, real-time intelligence is required because monitoring and decision loops lose value when outputs are stale; architecture therefore needs explicit update scheduling, latency awareness, and mechanisms to manage asynchronous participation (Stephanie et al., 2023; Wu et al., 2025). Fourth, auditability is necessary to support governance and incident response in multi-party deployments, especially when AI outputs influence clinical workflows; standards-oriented work emphasizes that orchestration and compliance readiness must be treated as first-class design concerns (Chen & Liu, 2025; Vashisht & Rani, 2025). Finally, scalability must be interpreted beyond throughput: the architecture should scale across heterogeneous sites and devices while maintaining safety, privacy, and stable learning under non-IID conditions (Quan et al., 2026; Wang et al., 2025).

4.2 Layered Architecture (Recommended 5-Layer Model)

The proposed architecture is structured as a five-layer composition, which is shown in ***Figure 1,*** that separates concerns while preserving end-to-end traceability from sensing to clinical action. This structure is consistent with how metaverse healthcare is described as a multi-layer ecosystem, as well as with digital twin and federated learning works that emphasize cross-layer orchestration and synchronization (Bansal et al., 2022; Chen et al., 2024).

Figure 1. illustrates the proposed end-to-end layered reference architecture.

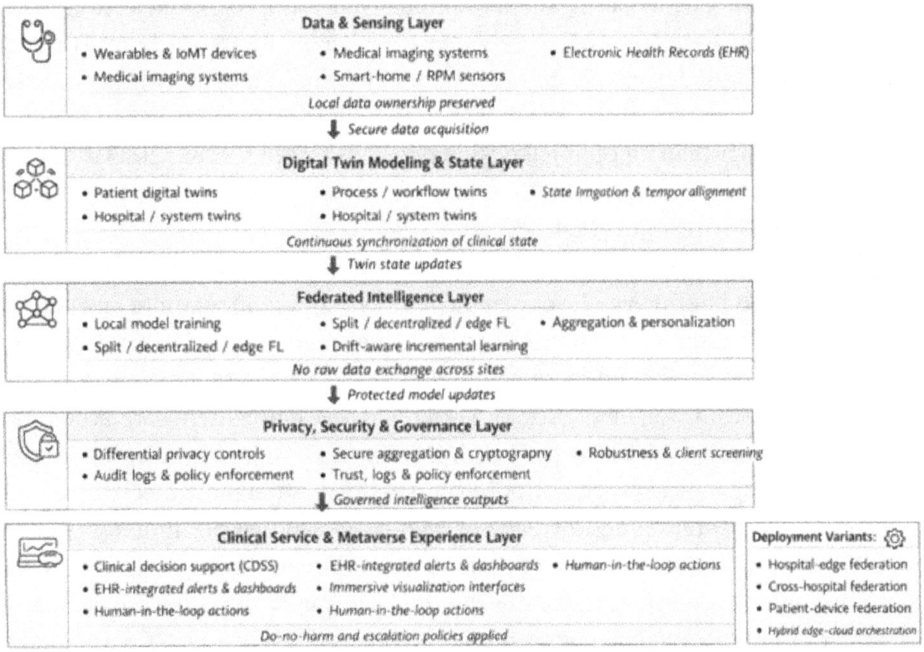

(i) Data & Sensing Layer

This layer includes clinical and non-clinical acquisition sources: wearables and IoMT devices, imaging systems, smart-home sensors, and EHR repositories. Its primary responsibility is secure acquisition and local preprocessing under institutional or device-level control, reflecting the distributed ownership assumptions that motivate federated learning in healthcare (Gadekallu et al., 2023; Quan et al., 2026). In remote patient monitoring contexts, this layer is also where telemetry integrity and device-level threat intelligence become operational concerns (Trivedi et al., 2025).

(ii) Twin Modeling & State Layer

This layer maintains digital twin representations of patient twins, device/workflow twins, and, where relevant, broader system twins. This layer is responsible for estimating system state, aligning information over time, and maintaining synchronization so that later inference stages operate on coherent, up-to-date representations rather than disconnected sensor readings (Balasubramanyam et al., 2024; Chen et al., 2023).

From a human digital twin perspective, personalization is rarely achieved through isolated predictions. Instead, it depends on longitudinal modeling and contextual features that change over time, which makes explicit state management a practical requirement rather than an optional design choice (Okegbile et al., 2023).

(iii) Federated intelligence layer

The federated intelligence layer contains the system's core learning and adaptation functions. It supports local model training, packaging of updates, aggregation or personalization logic, and incremental updates as new data becomes available (Wang et al., 2025; Chen et al., 2024). Different federated patterns are accommodated within this layer, including centralized aggregation, decentralized variants, and split-learning hybrids such as Split Fed, which are often motivated by the need to distribute computation and manage privacy-aware model partitioning (Lian et al., 2022; Stephanie et al., 2024). In designs that combine digital twins with federated learning, asynchronous update behavior is especially important, as it enables the system to tolerate uneven connectivity and heterogeneous client participation (Stephanie et al., 2023). Handling non-IID data distributions and drift is therefore treated as an operational necessity, given the well-documented instability that can arise when learning across sites with differing patient populations and clinical practices (Quan et al., 2026; Wang et al., 2025).

(iv) Safety, Privacy, security, and governance layer role

This layer is primarily responsible for ensuring data integrity, confidentiality, and accountability for data flows and model updates. Differential privacy provides a formal way to avoid data leakage, while controlled aggregation and cryptographic methods, including homomorphic encryption wherever applicable, help to secure system updates and sensitive inference workloads (Dwork, 2006; Sai et al., 2024; Kausar et al., 2025).

In association with confidentiality, robustness features are needed to adapt to adversarial changes and behaviors, such as poisoning attacks, which are observed or examined in detail, and to incorporate poisoning-resistant learning systems (Sun et al., 2023; Jaszcz et al., 2025).

Important mechanisms, such as policy enforcement, audit logging, and provenance tracking, support traceability and enable responses in multi-party settings and environments, aligning with detailed discussions and notations on standardized and trustworthy AI implementation (Chen & Liu, 2025; Ouchani et al., 2025).

(v) Clinical service efforts and metaverse experience layer

The clinical service efforts and the metaverse experience layer are where intelligent outcomes are provided to end users, ultimately to operational systems. Normally, outcomes include alerts, risk finders or indicators, monitoring dashboards, and hook integrations to support clinical decisions that fit within existing care workflows. In healthcare systems environments and metaverse settings, the layer may aim to provide immersive interactions, visualization efficiencies, and capabilities that focus on how experts or clinicians interpret system outcomes and how decisions are made in practice (Wang et al., 2022; Bansal et al., 2022).

The service layer is where human-in-the-loop control is enforced: safety policies, escalation rules, and responsibility boundaries are applied so that AI-driven outputs remain accountable within clinical governance structures (Vashisht & Rani, 2025; Roychowdhury et al., 2023).

4.3 Data Flows and Update Loops

The architecture operates through three coupled loops, each with distinct failure modes and governance requirements.

Twin synchronization loop. Raw measurements and records are ingested locally, temporally aligned, and mapped to twin state variables. This loop determines the digital twin's freshness and fidelity, thereby setting an upper bound on downstream intelligence quality. Works on digital-twin-enabled healthcare monitoring emphasize the importance of maintaining coherent state representations under wireless and edge constraints (Chen et al., 2023; Chen et al., 2024).

Federated model update loop. Local learning uses twin-derived features (and other local data) to update model parameters. Updates are protected via privacy and security mechanisms before being aggregated or shared (Bhatia & Kumar, 2025). Asynchronous Split Fed and real-time scheduling strategies are specifically motivated by uneven participation and latency constraints, which are common in healthcare edge settings (Stephanie et al., 2023; Stephanie et al., 2024). Where freshness measures are emphasized, update scheduling becomes part of system design rather than an optimization detail (Wu et al., 2025).

Inference and clinical action loop. Updated models are used to generate predictions, risk scores, or recommendations that feed clinical services. This loop also needs to include trust-related controls, such as uncertainty reporting, audit trails, and clear escalation logic, because mistakes or unstable outputs can directly affect clinical decisions. In healthcare settings, errors do not remain isolated and may propagate through workflows if not detected and addressed promptly. Surveys on threat intelligence for remote monitoring environments further emphasize that predictive intelligence alone is not sufficient, and that continuous runtime monitoring and response mechanisms are required to support safe operation in real deployments (Trivedi et al., 2025; Weber et al., 2023).

4.4 Deployment Variants

The same layered architecture can be instantiated in multiple deployment topologies depending on trust boundaries, connectivity, and regulatory constraints.

Hospital-Edge Federation

Clients are hospital or clinic sites that maintain local data repositories and edge computing resources. In many healthcare deployments, aggregation is handled by a trusted coordinating service or by a consortium-level entity. This arrangement is consistent with common assumptions in federated healthcare systems, where institutions are unable or unwilling to share raw data directly. At the same time, such a topology still requires clear governance structures and audit mechanisms that can operate across sites, so that model updates and decisions remain traceable and accountable (Quan et al., 2026; Chen & Liu, 2025).

Cross-Hospital Federation

This is a stricter multi-organization variant where hospitals may not share operational trust assumptions. In such cases, auditability and provenance become more important, and cryptographic protection of updates may be required to reduce information exposure and strengthen accountability (Kausar et al., 2025; Ouchani et al., 2025).

Patient-Device Federation

Clients are patient-owned devices (wearables, smart home hubs, mobile devices) that generate local learning signals. This topology supports personalization and continuous monitoring but is sensitive to device heterogeneity, intermittent connectivity, and the risk of poisoning. Personalized and poisoning-resistant federated approaches are particularly relevant in this setting (Sun et al., 2023; Selvaraj et al., 2024). Hybrid deployments combine edge-side learning and twin synchronization with cloud-side orchestration for aggregation, policy enforcement, and service delivery. Standards-oriented work highlights that orchestration and policy control are central in such environments, especially when digital twins interact with multi-service ecosystems and 6G-era connectivity assumptions (Vashisht & Rani, 2025;

Wang et al., 2025). Hybrid designs are often the most realistic operationally, but they also create the widest governance surface because responsibility spans multiple technical and organizational layers.

5. PRIVACY, SECURITY, AND TRUST: ENGINEERING THE "PROTECTED TWIN"

5.1 Threat Model

A "protected twin" must be designed to withstand threats arising from both healthcare cyber-physical realities and metaverse-style multi-service integration. In healthcare cyber-physical systems, the attack surface includes heterogeneous devices, legacy protocols, and safety-critical dependencies, all of which can disrupt clinical operations and patient outcomes (Weber et al., 2023). Remote patient monitoring adds continuous telemetry streams and distributed endpoints, expanding exposure to data tampering, device compromise, and reliability attacks that degrade monitoring integrity (Trivedi et al., 2025). Metaverse-oriented healthcare introduces additional cross-context risks: identity and access control spans multiple services, interaction channels may combine clinical and non-clinical signals, and multi-modal data fusion increases the risk of unintended inference about individuals even when direct identifiers are protected (Letafati et al., 2023; Bansal et al., 2022).

5.2 Privacy Mechanisms and When and What to Use

Privacy controls in a protected twin architecture should be selected based on the task's sensitivity, the trust boundary, and the operational budget for computation and latency.

Differential Privacy (DP): the Privacy–Utility Knob

DP offers a principled way to limit information leakage by introducing controlled noise into the training or reporting process. Its practical role is not "privacy on/off," but a tunable trade-off that must be chosen with awareness of clinical risk: overly aggressive privacy can reduce model utility, while weak settings can fail to meaningfully reduce disclosure risk (Dwork, 2006). In federated environments, DP is most appropriate when participants must receive strong privacy assurances across organizational boundaries, or when regulatory constraints require defensible privacy guarantees. However, DP selection should be treated as an engineering decision with a documented rationale rather than a generic checkbox, as shown in ***Figure 2***.

Figure 2. Details the privacy, security, and trust-audit pipeline applied to the protected digital twin

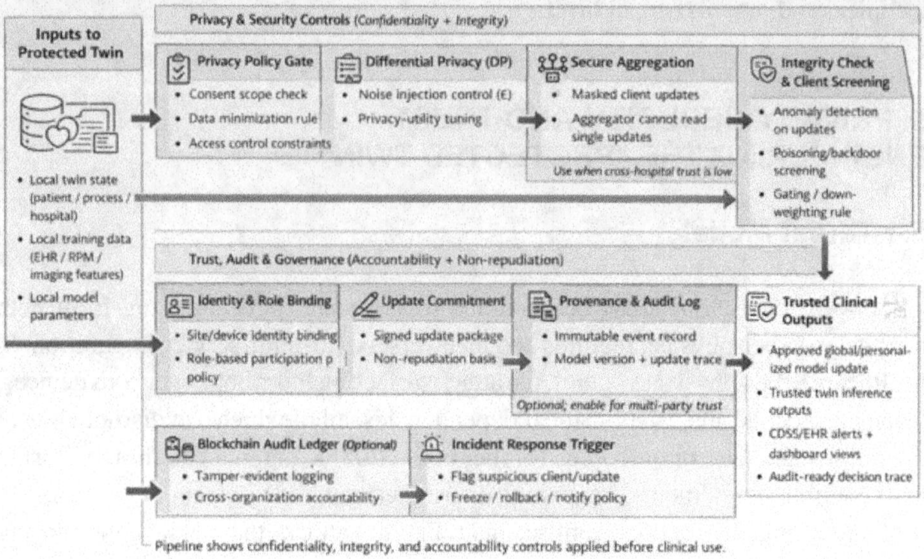

Cryptographic protection becomes relevant when parties require confidentiality for either (i) model updates in transit and at aggregation points or (ii) inference computations on sensitive features. Blockchain-integrated frameworks that combine federated learning with homomorphic encryption illustrate this direction, though such designs also raise practical overhead concerns that must be explicitly budgeted in metaverse-scale systems (Kausar et al., 2025). In healthcare contexts, HE/SMC is typically most justified when adversarial exposure is high (e.g., cross-hospital collaboration without full mutual trust) or when the cost of data exposure is unacceptable.

Secure Aggregation

Secure aggregation protects individual client updates from direct inspection by the coordinating party, reducing leakage risk when updates traverse untrusted infrastructure or when aggregators must not have access to individual contributions. It is an appropriate baseline in many federated deployments because it can reduce the attack surface without requiring full HE-level computation overhead (Sai et al., 2024). In practice, secure aggregation is most useful when the main concern is the aggregator's visibility into individual updates, while the system can tolerate sharing at the aggregated level.

Trusted Execution Environments (TEEs)

TEE-based approaches can provide protected execution enclaves for aggregating or inferring, potentially reducing exposure in shared compute environments. In your current 40-paper reference set, TEEs are not explicitly established as a primary mechanism; therefore, within this chapter, they should be treated as optional and only discussed as a potential extension if clearly supported by cited sources. Not reported in the current corpus.

5.3 Integrity & accountability: blockchain audit/ provenance and non-repudiation

A protected twin must support not only confidentiality but also integrity and accountability. Confidential learning is not sufficient if an attacker can inject malicious updates or if the system cannot reconstruct what happened after an incident.

Blockchain-Based Audit and Provenance

Blockchain-integrated federated frameworks are motivated by the need for tamper-evident audit trails and provenance records, particularly in cross-organizational settings where trust is limited, and disputes may arise over the origin or legitimacy of updates (Kausar et al., 2025). From a governance standpoint, the value lies not in the blockchain label itself, but in the ability to establish immutable logs of update events, participation records, and policy enforcement decisions.

5.4 Robustness: Poisoning, Backdoors, Non-IID Stress, and Client Screening

Robustness in federated digital-twin systems must address two intertwined stressors: (i) benign heterogeneity (non-IID data, drift, uneven participation) and (ii) adversarial manipulation (poisoning, backdoors). Poisoning adversarial examples in consumer health metaverse areas is typically addressed by mitigating model poisoning risks and ensuring individual learning systems retain use and utility, while avoiding malicious client effects (Sun et al., 2023). Additionally, the work proposes a robust mechanism for knowledge refinement, combined with a multi-criteria approach, to minimize poisoning susceptibility in healthcare-related monitoring systems, reflecting the increasing focus on resilience through collaborative changes (Jaszcz et al., 2025). More broadly, adversarial-learning frameworks and security-oriented federated designs reinforce that robustness is a system property: it depends on update validation, anomaly detection, and operational governance, not only on loss functions (Murmu et al., 2025; Feng et al., 2025).

Client Screening and Gating Strategies

In practice, a protected twin must incorporate participation controls that decide which clients can contribute, when they can contribute, and under what quality constraints. This includes screening for abnormal update patterns, enforcing minimum data quality or device integrity checks, and applying gating rules that limit the influence of suspicious or low-quality clients. While individual implementations differ, the repeated presence of poisoning-focused and metaverse-health security work indicates that "open federation" is rarely safe without such controls (Sun et al., 2023; Weber et al., 2023). In clinical settings, client screening also supports accountability: decisions about excluding an update must be auditable and explainable to operators.

6. CLINICAL INTELLIGENCE IN THE METAVERSE: FROM MODELS TO DECISIONS

6.1 Use-Case Patterns

Clinical intelligence in a metaverse setting should be understood as a spectrum of system behaviors that translate sensing and modeling into actionable decisions. Across the existing literature, a small number of use-case patterns appear repeatedly in discussions of healthcare metaverse systems. One prominent pattern is remote patient monitoring based on wearables and connected devices. Remote monitoring is often viewed as a natural entry point for metaverse-enabled healthcare, since it relies on continuous data streams from wearables, home sensors, and patient-operated devices, and it benefits from interactive visualization and timely escalation when abnormalities are detected. Studies on threat intelligence for remote monitoring further indicate that such systems cannot rely solely on prediction. They must also account for system integrity and operational reliability to reduce false alarms and maintain clinical trust in monitoring outputs (Trivedi et al., 2025). Federated learning is frequently proposed in this context to support distributed model updates across large device populations without centralizing raw patient telemetry, which becomes especially important when monitoring infrastructures span multiple service providers or heterogeneous device ecosystems (Gadekallu et al., 2023; Lian et al., 2022).

The next repetitive pattern concerns imaging and diagnostic use and applications. Such a work normally motivates and builds confidence, and digital copies of governed designs are effective for learning; however, they require access to a heterogeneous patient group, while others are compliant with good privacy conditions. Twin-assisted federated diagnosis frameworks and healthcare-oriented federated schemes emphasize that local clinical data distributions differ substantially across institutions, making centralized training impractical or undesirable (Qu et al., 2023; Quan et al., 2026). In diagnostic settings, clinical intelligence therefore goes beyond producing predictions. It also involves maintaining traceability of inputs, meeting interpretability expectations, and ensuring that model outputs are integrated into diagnostic workflows in a controlled and accountable manner.

Hospital Operations & Process Twins

Operational intelligence focuses on processing twins and hospital-level twins that capture patient flow, device availability, and resource constraints. While the metaverse layer may provide immersive interaction, the underlying system value depends on robust state representation and decision support that is consistent with institutional policies and operational realities (Balasubramanyam et al., 2024; Chen et al., 2024). In such cases, "clinical intelligence" includes operational decisions (triage support, scheduling, workflow adaptation) that must remain explainable and auditable.

6.2 Real-Time Constraints

Clinical intelligence is time-sensitive; the same model output can be useful or harmful depending on when it is produced and how it is consumed. Real-time constraints take many forms: the freshness of measurements, the delays introduced by synchronization and learning loops, and the downstream cognitive burden imposed on clinical users.

Freshness and Age-of-Information (AoI)

In always-on sensing settings, data staleness becomes a first-order concern. AoI-oriented formulations argue that intelligence quality is constrained not only by model accuracy but also by the timeliness of updates reaching decision points, particularly when devices are intermittent and networks are heterogeneous (Wu et al., 2025). For digital twin systems, this translates into a practical requirement: twin synchronization and model update scheduling should be explicitly designed rather than implicitly assumed to be frequent and reliable.

Latency and Asynchronous Involvement

Asynchronous learning models are mainly driven by unrealistic assumptions about client efficiency and capabilities, as well as network connectivity in healthcare settings. Devices and organizations differ widely in computation system power, readiness, availability, and communication stability. The digital twin-enforced asynchronous SplitFed way explicitly changes and reflects this operational imbalance. Even when architecture cannot cope with or tolerate delayed updates or when the client is not present, the quality of clinical intelligence decreases precisely in scenarios where remote observance and edge-heavy metaverse services are critical (Stephanie et al., 2023; Stephanie et al., 2024).

Alert Fatigue

Even though predictive models deliver good results, poorly managed alert streams can disrupt clinical workflows and raise questions about the trustworthiness of decision-support systems. The problem is not limited to human involvement alone. It is a system-specific issue that considers calibration quality, unusual reporting, threshold management and configuration, and escalation terms. The already done surveys in security and monitoring in healthcare systems focus on identification and alert mechanisms that have to be evaluated not only using detection correct ratio in terms of accuracy, precision, and recall, but also in association with operational ease and the impact of hazardous interruptions to care delivery (Weber et al., 2023; Trivedi et al., 2025).

6.3 Incorporating in Clinical Workflows: CDSS/EHR Coupling and Human-Centered Loop Decisions

Clinical intelligence is effective and useful in real-time scenarios only when it is incorporated into well-established decision pathways with clear accountability. In a real-time operational world, this requires connecting intelligence outcomes to CDSS- and EHR-centered workflows, while also defining responsibility areas and boundaries to support reviewing outputs, determining who takes the necessary steps, and handling errors or uncertain situations within the clinical process.

CDSS/EHR Coupling

Federated adaptive learning-based approaches designed for EHR-centered workflows continuously highlight and emphasize that secure sharing and monitored access are basic necessities in medical informatics process systems (Salim & Park,

2023). In healthcare sectors, metaverse environments, this part becomes more rigid and complex as the interaction mode of channels and service layers is used above the traditional interfaces. Instead of this, expand, the main need is still the same. Outputs must remain the same in terms of clinical context, and policy constraints must ensure both access to and the basic application of intelligent outcomes (Chen & Liu, 2025; Vashisht & Rani, 2025). Surveys on digital twin networking in healthcare further emphasize that personalization and longitudinal monitoring cannot be supported by isolated model endpoints and instead require coherent, system-level integration across components (Chen et al., 2024).

Human-in-the-Loop Decisions

A protected twin architecture should assume that many clinical decisions require human judgment and that automation must be bound. This implies explicit escalation logic, review checkpoints, and audit trails that capture what the system recommended, the evidence used, and the action taken. Trust and governance work in multiservice environments supports this view by treating privacy safeguards and orchestration as system governance capabilities rather than as narrow encryption features (Ouchani et al., 2025; Vashisht & Rani, 2025).

6.4 Reliability Requirements: Calibration, Uncertainty, Drift Monitoring

Reliability requirements distinguish clinical intelligence from generic prediction. A model that performs well on static validation sets can still be unsafe if it is mis-calibrated, if uncertainty is not surfaced, or if performance degrades under drift (Zhu et al., 2023).

Calibration, Uncertainty, and Interpretability

Clinical users need a basis for trust. Explainable AI perspectives emphasize that interpretability is a system-level enabler: it supports operator understanding, governance decisions, and incident analysis when models behave unexpectedly (Kul et al., 2025). In parallel, standards-oriented discussions emphasize that trustworthy AI requires explicit mechanisms for accountability and compliance, including the ability to justify decisions and document limitations (Chen & Liu, 2025; Vashisht & Rani, 2025). While individual papers vary in what they report, practical architecture should treat calibration and uncertainty reporting as required outputs wherever clinical decisions are influenced (Bansal et al., 2022; Letafati et al., 2023).

Drift Monitoring and non-IID Stress

Healthcare systems are non-stationary. Patient populations, device behavior, and care protocols evolve, and federated learning introduces additional variability due to site-level differences (Zhang & Zhao, 2025). Surveys on federated learning for CPS and healthcare metaverse settings repeatedly note that non-IID distributions and heterogeneity complicate stable training and can lead to uneven performance across participants (Quan et al., 2026; Gadekallu et al., 2023). Therefore, drift monitoring should be treated as a continuous operational function rather than a one-time evaluation.

Safe Fallback and do-no-Harm Constraints

A clinically credible system must define what happens when signals are unreliable, when updates are delayed, or when integrity checks fail. In cyber-physical healthcare contexts, detection and response are constrained by safety requirements; overly aggressive automated actions can create harm even if the underlying threat detection is correct (Weber et al., 2023). Consequently, protected twin designs should include safe fallback modes and explicitly document "do-no-harm" constraints that bound automation in uncertain or adversarial conditions (Khan et al., 2022).

7. EVIDENCE SYNTHESIS: COMPARATIVE INSIGHTS

This section consolidates the 40-paper corpus into three comparative tables plus a benchmarking-gap summary. The goal is not to force uniform benchmarking (the literature does not support that), but to expose what can be compared credibly and what remains under-reported across architecture, privacy stacks, and robustness controls (Balasubramanyam et al., 2024; Quan et al., 2026; Weber et al., 2023).

7.1 Comparative Table: Approach Families vs Metrics

The first synthesis layer groups papers into approach families and records only the metrics that each work explicitly reports. Across diagnostic and monitoring tasks, the most common outcomes are model-centric metrics, while system-centric metrics are reported less consistently, especially in metaverse-style end-to-end narratives (Gadekallu et al., 2023; Bansal et al., 2022).

Approach families that appear repeatedly:

- DT-assisted federated diagnosis and learning emphasize twin-derived features or twin-driven adaptation (Qu et al., 2023; Othman et al., 2025).
- SplitFed / split-learning hybrids: motivated by heterogeneity and timing constraints (Stephanie et al., 2023; Stephanie et al., 2024).
- Edge or cyber-physical federated intelligence focuses on distributed endpoints and practical constraints (Lian et al., 2022; Quan et al., 2026).
- Real-time scheduling (AoI): treats timeliness as a first-class objective (Wu et al., 2025).
- Secure EHR and healthcare data sharing schemes: emphasize data governance and secure exchange in medical informatics pipelines (Salim & Park, 2023).

Table 1. Approach Families vs Metrics Reported (and What Is Missing)

Approach family	Representative PIDs (examples)	Typical clinical target	Metrics commonly reported (as seen in this corpus)	Latency / comm / rounds / energy reporting
DT-assisted federated diagnosis/ learning	P01, P16, P30	Diagnosis / personalized modeling	Acc/F1/AUC reported in paper tables for empirical works; fidelity/ synchronization metrics often Not reported as lifecycle metrics	Usually Not reported (system overhead seldom standardized)
Split learning / SplitFed (incl. asynchronous)	P04, P27	E-health / consumer health / metaverse endpoints	Model performance metrics + asynchrony/convergence discussion; participation/ straggler effects discussed	Latency/round impacts are sometimes discussed, but values are inconsistently reported
Personalized FL / non-IID-aware federated intelligence	P05, P24, P26	Consumer health, diagnosis, non-IID settings	Accuracy/AUC/F1 reported (empirical); robustness vs poisoning often quantified by performance under attack (where provided)	Comms/rounds often Not reported in comparable format
Decentralized / edge federated learning for HCPS	P11, P18, P21	Edge monitoring, MCPS/HCPS intelligence	Efficiency/security framing; task metrics vary by paper; surveys report counts/ taxonomy rather than performance	Energy/latency rarely quantified in a consistent way
Freshness-aware / real-time scheduling (AoI-driven)	P19	Real-time healthcare intelligence	Timeliness/freshness objective emphasized; real-time scheduling outcomes discussed	Reporting varies; AoI/ latency is central, but cross-paper comparability is limited
Secure EHR sharing / secure healthcare informatics FL	P28	Secure record sharing / governance	Security properties often emphasized; prediction metrics may be secondary	Not reported or not standardized

continued on following page

Table 1. Continued

Approach family	Representative PIDs (examples)	Typical clinical target	Metrics commonly reported (as seen in this corpus)	Latency / comm / rounds / energy reporting
Metaverse healthcare surveys / DT surveys / FL-for-CPS surveys	P03, P07, P09, P13, P15, P25, P29	Synthesis and readiness	Taxonomy, challenges, adoption barriers; no benchmark	Not reported (survey-level)
Standards / governance readiness for DT + FL	P20, P22, P32, P36	Trustworthy orchestration	Policy readiness, compliance framing; measurable KPIs are not standardized	Not reported (architecture/governance focus)

7.2 Privacy-Stack Overhead Table (Baseline vs DP vs HE/SMC vs Blockchain)

The second synthesis layer compares privacy stacks in *Table 1* based on what they protect and the cost they incur. Even when papers claim to preserve privacy, many do not quantify the overhead beyond qualitative discussion, particularly in metaverse-oriented privacy narratives (Letafati et al., 2023). Therefore, the privacy-overhead table should be written as a protection-to-cost matrix, not as a single numeric benchmark.

Privacy stack options present in the corpus:

- Baseline FL (no formal privacy layer): improves collaboration but does not provide formal leakage bounds (Gadekallu et al., 2023; Quan et al., 2026).
- Differential privacy (DP): introduces an explicit privacy–utility control surface (Dwork, 2006).
- Secure aggregation: reduces exposure of individual client updates (Sai et al., 2024).
- HE audits strengthens confidentiality and provenance but increases complexity and often increases overhead (Kausar et al., 2025).
- Governance-oriented privacy safeguards: frames privacy as orchestration and policy enforcement across multi-service ecosystems (Ouchani et al., 2025; Chen & Liu, 2025).

Table 2. Privacy-Stack Overhead Comparison (Baseline vs DP vs HE/SMC vs Blockchain/Audit)

Privacy / trust stack	What it protects	Where it sits in architecture (Layer)	Utility impact (typical)	Overhead type (typical)	Representative PIDs	What is actually quantified in this corpus
Baseline FL (no formal privacy layer)	Raw data stays local, but updates may still leak	Federated intelligence layer	Low–Moderate	Communication rounds + aggregation overhead	P03, P15, P26	Often focuses on model metrics; privacy leakage bounds not reported
+ Differential Privacy (DP)	Formal leakage control via privacy–utility knob	Privacy/security layer + training/ reporting	Moderate (depends on ε)	Computation + possible accuracy drop	P08 (foundation), P06 (applied discussion)	DP is treated as a trade-off mechanism; quantitative ε–utility curves only where explicitly provided
+ Secure aggregation	Hides individual client updates from aggregator	Federated + privacy layer	Low (usually)	Protocol overhead + comm complexity	P14	Overhead and security claims vary; standardized comm/latency values often not reported
+ HE/SMC for secure updates / confidential inference	Confidentiality for update exchange and/ or inference	Privacy/security layer	Moderate–High	Heavy computation + latency	P31	Security emphasis is strong; practical overhead must be treated as workload-dependent unless explicitly measured
+ Blockchain audit / provenance	Integrity, non-repudiation, tamper-evident logging	Governance layer (cross-cutting)	Low–Moderate (on model utility)	Storage + confirmation latency + coordination	P31, P36	Audit/provenance framed strongly; end-to-end latency/ throughput often not reported
Standards-driven orchestration & policy enforcement	Accountability, compliance alignment, audit readiness	Governance layer + service orchestration	Neutral (depending on enforcement)	Process/operational overhead	P20, P22, P32, P36	Governance readiness is discussed; quantitative compliance KPIs not standardized

7.3 Robustness Mechanism

The third synthesis *Table 2* focuses on robustness, because "protected twins" must handle both adversarial behaviors (poisoning, backdoors) and benign stressors (non-IID, drift, intermittent clients). Poisoning is explicitly treated in several works as a primary risk in metaverse-health or monitoring-device contexts (Sun et al., 2023; Jaszcz et al., 2025). Security surveys of healthcare cyber-physical systems further justify the need to engineer detection and response under healthcare constraints (Weber et al., 2023).

7.4 What is Consistently Reported vs not Reported (Benchmarking Gap)

Across the corpus, the reporting pattern is uneven. A defensible "benchmarking gap" summary distinguishes between model-level metrics and system-level deployment evidence:

Consistently reported:

- Model performance metrics: accuracy, F1, and AUC (Qu et al., 2023; Sun et al., 2023; Othman et al., 2025).
- Conceptual architecture and taxonomies (Balasubramanyam et al., 2024; Chen et al., 2024; Quan et al., 2026).
- Qualitative privacy/security concerns (Letafati et al., 2023; Weber et al., 2023).

Often under-reported:

- End-to-end latency under realistic heterogeneity (Stephanie et al., 2023; Wu et al., 2025).
- Communication payload and training rounds reported in comparable form across papers (Quan et al., 2026).
- Energy/device cost for edge participation (Lian et al., 2022).
- Formal governance artifacts: audit readiness, accountability boundaries, policy enforcement procedures (Chen & Liu, 2025; Vashisht & Rani, 2025).
- Standardized threat models and incident-response logic connected to clinical workflows (Weber et al., 2023; Trivedi et al., 2025).

Synthesis Implication

The evidence base supports the feasibility of component digital twins, federated learning patterns, and privacy/robustness controls—but the literature rarely provides a unified, measurable end-to-end benchmark that connects clinical intelligence outcomes to timeliness, overhead, and governance readiness (Quan et al., 2026; Chen et al., 2024). This reinforces the chapter's core contribution: a reference architecture and reporting guidance that treats privacy, trust, real-time constraints, and accountability as integrated design requirements rather than isolated add-ons, as shown in ***Figure 3.***

Figure 3. summarizes the research-to-deployment lifecycle for federated digital twinning.

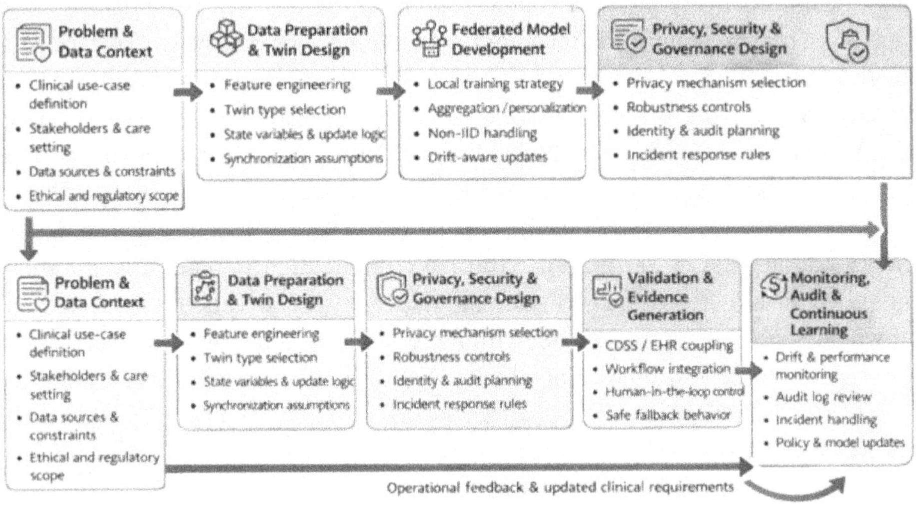

7.5 Benchmarking Gap Summary

Consistently reported: model performance metrics in empirical FL/DT papers.

Inconsistently reported: latency, communication payload, number of rounds in a comparable format.

Rarely reported: device energy cost, standardized incident-response workflows, and measurable governance compliance readiness.

8. GAPS, OPEN CHALLENGES

8.1 Dataset Realism and Clinical Validity Gap

Across the literature on healthcare metaverse systems, digital twins, and federated intelligence, a recurring limitation is that empirical results are hard to compare and even harder to translate into real deployments. Evaluation settings differ widely across studies, and the level of clinical realism is uneven. Survey-based and system-level discussions consistently note that healthcare data is heterogeneous, distributed across institutions, and shaped by local clinical protocols. As a result, findings obtained using narrow datasets or simplified assumptions can give an overly optimistic picture of deployability (Quan et al., 2026; Chen et al., 2024).

In the study of cyber-physical healthcare security, the lack of a real, domain-specific dataset is a persistent hurdle to meaningful validation. Major surveys make it easy to create threat models or working constraints that do not reflect hospital environments, thereby undermining the real-time relevance of reported outcomes (Weber et al., 2023). Digital twin studies provide additional observations that the term "twin" is used inappropriately across various works. In some scenarios, reported profit may provide a more accurate analysis than actual twin fidelity or state synchronization (Balasubramanyam et al., 2024). A primary implication is that clinical validity should not be affected by performance metrics themselves. Validation has to monitor whether system outputs remain within expectations under realistic drift, partial sensing, and workflow constraints (Kul et al., 2025; Roychowdhury et al., 2023).

8.2 Governance Gap: Consent, Accountability, Audit, and Incident Response

Governance impacts are mainly acknowledged in the literature review, but they are often converted into operational ways. Healthcare metaverse environments involve more people, including patients, clinicians, platform providers, and system vendors. This increase in volume also introduces ambiguity around accountability when AI-driven recommendations result in harm or when collaborative learning processes are impacted and compromised (Letafati et al., 2023; Bansal et al., 2022).

Standards-specific involvement argues that privacy protections for AI and digital twin systems require policy-specific orchestration and auditable controls. However, many processes lack concrete incident response procedures, including who is responsible for the investigation, what types of information are logged, how rollbacks can be executed, and how affected vendors are notified (Chen & Liu, 2025; Vashisht & Rani, 2025). Privacy safeguard systems ensure that governance is considered a vital system component, in cooperation with policy enforcement and accountability mechanisms, rather than an add-on applied after model creation (Ouchani et al., 2025).

In federated environments, this gap is in-depth and tangible. But poisoning attacks and malicious interpretations and manipulations of updates are widely recognized threats; many surveys do not specify how suspicious clients are isolated, how models are reverted to compromised versions, or how non-repudiation is enhanced beyond a certain level (Sun et al., 2023; Jaszcz et al., 2025).

8.3 Standardization Gap: Interoperability and Compliance With Design

Interoperability and compliance speed are emerging as the main challenges in upgrading healthcare digital twins and federated intelligence across various environments. Studies on metaverse healthcare systems highlight the complexity of multi-platform, integrated environments that encompass heterogeneous systems, multiple service providers, and diverse data formats. At the same time, these studies provide very limited guidance on how to create enforceable interoperability layers within robust, well-monitored clinical governance constraints (Bansal et al., 2022; Wang et al., 2022).

9. FUTURE DIRECTIONS

Based on the evidence synthesis and the recurring gaps discussed, the following directions are practical and high-impact for advancing federated AI–driven digital twins in healthcare metaverse settings:

1. Twin-aware orchestration and scheduling. Move beyond generic federated rounds by incorporating twin synchronization state, freshness, and clinical urgency into update scheduling and inference cadence (Wu et al., 2025; Chen et al., 2023).
2. Policy engines as first-class system components. Embed consent, access control, audit logging, and incident-response triggers directly into orchestration layers, aligned with standards-oriented trustworthy AI guidance (Chen & Liu, 2025; Vashisht & Rani, 2025).
3. Validated benchmarks with realism tiers. Create benchmark suites that explicitly report cohort diversity, non-IID severity, drift patterns, and edge reliability; security benchmarks should include healthcare-aligned threat models and operational constraints (Quan et al., 2026; Weber et al., 2023).
4. End-to-end reporting mechanisms for overhead. It requires a very small reporting set for latency, communication payload utilization, inform frequency, and edge energy costs to ensure cross-paper comparability and clinical feasibility evaluation (Lian et al., 2022; Stephanie et al., 2024).
5. Robustness in association with recovery playbooks. Next-generation systems should expand beyond high-level claims of "poisoning resistance" and explain, in operational terms, how recovery is monitored and handled with care. This also includes specifying client-quarantine logic, a rollback system for evolved model versions, a process for model version control, and auditable escalation

workflows triggered when abnormal motion is detected (Sun et al., 2023; Ouchani et al., 2025).

6. Privacy–utility engineering considering clinical risk factors. Privacy system mechanisms should be considered engineering choices rather than default environment settings. The arguments, with a properly documented rationale, regarding differential privacy and cryptographic protection, and the choice of the more efficient privacy approach, ensure effective decision accuracy and clinical usefulness. These parameters must be evaluated in depth, explicitly accounting for healthcare risk factor constraints (Dwork, 2006; Kausar et al., 2025).

10. CONCLUSION

The healthcare metaverse can be transformed from a collection of promising point solutions into an integrated clinical intelligence ecosystem through federated AI-driven digital twins, according to this chapter. However, this is only possible if privacy, trust, real-time responsiveness, and governance are viewed as fundamental design requirements rather than optional features. A five-layer reference architecture and "protected twin" concept that couples twin synchronization, federated model updates, and clinically grounded inference loops under explicit threat models, policy controls, and auditability constraints were proposed by synthesizing the literature on the metaverse, digital twin, federated learning, and security. According to the evidence assessment, there is a benchmarking gap between algorithmic performance and deployable clinical systems because most of the work that has been done so far has focused on model-centric metrics while underreporting latency, communication overhead, energy cost, and governance preparedness. Twin-aware coordination, practical benchmarks, privacy-utility trade-offs that are engineered, robustness and recovery playbooks, and cross-layer trust mechanisms that integrate explainability, security, and accountability into everyday operations are all need to close these gaps. Federated digital-twin architectures can develop into clinically valid CDSS infrastructures for healthcare in the metaverse era if these paths are followed, balancing technological innovation with the demands of safety, interoperability, and practical decision-making.

REFERENCES

Adnan, M., Yi, Y., Wani, N. A., Alsenan, S., Khan, M. A., & Anwar, M. S. (2025). Neurosymbolic digital twin for cardiovascular disease prediction and personalized modeling. *IEEE Journal of Biomedical and Health Informatics*, 1–8. Advance online publication. DOI: 10.1109/JBHI.2025.3647298 PMID: 41433178

Balasubramanyam, A., Ramesh, R., Sudheer, R., & Honnavalli, P. B. (2024). Revolutionizing healthcare: A review unveiling the transformative power of digital twins. *IEEE Access : Practical Innovations, Open Solutions*, *12*, 69650–69678. DOI: 10.1109/ACCESS.2024.3399744

Bansal, G., Rajgopal, K., Chamola, V., Xiong, Z., & Niyato, D. (2022). Healthcare in metaverse: A survey on current metaverse applications in healthcare. *IEEE Access : Practical Innovations, Open Solutions*, *10*, 119914–119946. DOI: 10.1109/ACCESS.2022.3219845

Bhatia, M., & Kumar, R. (2025). Digital twin technology in wireless communication: A comprehensive engineering survey. *IEEE Internet of Things Journal*, *12*(12), 19144–19166. Advance online publication. DOI: 10.1109/JIOT.2025.3565843

Chen, J., Wang, W., Fang, B., Liu, Y., Yu, K., Leung, V. C. M., & Hu, X. (2023). Digital twin empowered wireless healthcare monitoring for smart home. *IEEE Journal on Selected Areas in Communications*, *41*(11), 3662–3676. Advance online publication. DOI: 10.1109/JSAC.2023.3310097

Chen, J., Yi, C., Okegbile, S. D., Cai, J., & Shen, X. (2024). Networking architecture and key supporting technologies for digital twin in personalized healthcare: A comprehensive survey. *IEEE Communications Surveys and Tutorials*, *26*(1), 706–746. Advance online publication. DOI: 10.1109/COMST.2023.3308717

Chen, K., & Liu, Y. (2025). Toward privacy-preserving AI standards for federated learning in 6G-enabled digital twin environments. *IEEE Communications Standards Magazine*, 1–8. Advance online publication. DOI: 10.1109/MCOMSTD.2025.3623142

Diokadan, J., Divine, I. A., Emma, S., Makiwa, R. S., Celine, U., Nicholus, L., & Pasupula, R. (2025). Lupeol acetate from *Cleome viscosa* as a therapeutic candidate for myocardial infarction. *In Silico Pharmacology*, *13*(2), 1–14. DOI: 10.1007/s40203-025-00383-9 PMID: 40620913

Dwork, C. (2006). Differential privacy. In *Proceedings of the 33rd International Colloquium on Automata, Languages and Programming* (pp. 1–12). DOI: 10.1007/11787006_1

Feng, P., Xi, N., Jin, J., Zhang, J., & Ma, J. (2025). FLASH: Federated graph learning-based malicious bash script detection for industrial cyber–physical systems. *IEEE Transactions on Industrial Informatics*, *21*(6), 4979–4989. Advance online publication. DOI: 10.1109/TII.2025.3552649

Gadekallu, T. R.. (2023). Federated learning for the healthcare metaverse: Concepts, applications, challenges, and future directions. *IEEE Network*, *37*(1), 176–183. DOI: 10.1109/MNET.001.2200227

Jamshidi, M., Hoang, D. T., & Nguyen, D. N. (2024). CNN-FL for biotechnology industry empowered by Internet-of-BioNano Things and digital twins. *IEEE Internet of Things Magazine*, *7*(5), 54–63. Advance online publication. DOI: 10.1109/IOTM.001.2400081

Jaszcz, A., Połap, D., & Srivastava, G. (2025). MultiMOORA-guided federated learning with knowledge-distillation stabilization for health monitoring devices as protection against poisoning attacks. *IEEE Internet of Things Journal*. Advance online publication. DOI: 10.1109/JIOT.2025.3638263

Kausar, S., Naqvi, N., Akbar, S., Ratan Shah, S., Abbas, K., & Alam, M.. (2025). Socioeconomic indicators and their influence on mental health: A data-driven approach utilizing Python and R. *International Journal of Epidemiology and Health Sciences*, *6*, e92. Advance online publication. DOI: 10.51757/IJEHS.6.2025.720978

Khan, L. U., Han, Z., Saad, W., Hossain, E., Guizani, M., & Hong, C. S. (2022). Digital twin of wireless systems: Overview, taxonomy, challenges, and opportunities. *IEEE Communications Surveys and Tutorials*, *24*(4), 2230–2254. Advance online publication. DOI: 10.1109/COMST.2022.3198273

Kosanam, S., & Pasupula, R. (2024). Artificial intelligence approach in identification of differentially expressed genes of methyl glycoside against myocardial infarction. *Advances in Traditional Medicine*, *24*(1), 243–252. DOI: 10.1007/s13596-023-00691-5

Kul, S., Celtek, S. A., & Balci, S. (2025). AI-enhanced power management strategies for next-generation hybrid electric vehicles: Deep reinforcement learning and predictive analytics. *2025 14th International Symposium on Advanced Topics in Electrical Engineering (ATEE)*, 1–6. DOI: 10.1109/ATEE66006.2025.11299906

Letafati, M.. (2023). Digital healthcare in the metaverse: Insights into privacy and security. *IEEE Consumer Electronics Magazine*, *12*(4), 80–90. DOI: 10.1109/MCE.2023.3267412

Lian, Z., Yang, Q., Wang, W., Zeng, Q., Alazab, M., Zhao, H., & Su, C. (2022). DEEP-FEL: Decentralized, efficient and privacy-enhanced federated edge learning for healthcare cyber physical systems. *IEEE Transactions on Network Science and Engineering*, *9*(5), 3558–3569. Advance online publication. DOI: 10.1109/TNSE.2022.3175945

Murmu, A., Kumar, P., Namasudra, S., & Reddy, M. R. (2025). GAN-based federated adversarial learning for enhancing security towards consumer digital ecosystems. *IEEE Transactions on Consumer Electronics*, *71*(1), 1102–1114. Advance online publication. DOI: 10.1109/TCE.2024.3522018

Okegbile, S. D., Cai, J., Zheng, H., Chen, J., & Yi, C. (2023). Differentially private federated multi-task learning framework for enhancing human-to-virtual connectivity in human digital twin. *IEEE Journal on Selected Areas in Communications*, *41*(11), 3533–3547. DOI: 10.1109/JSAC.2023.3310106

Othman, S. B., Chakraborty, C., Singh, S., & Frikha, M. A. (2025). Federated learning-enabled digital twins for privacy-preserving cardiovascular disease detection in consumer electronics. *IEEE Transactions on Consumer Electronics*, 1. Advance online publication. DOI: 10.1109/TCE.2025.3634581

Ouchani, S., Boudouaia, M. A., & Tasidou, A. (2025). PRISM: A privacy safeguard for smart multiservices. *IEEE Software*, *42*(5), 107–115. Advance online publication. DOI: 10.1109/MS.2025.3542853

Qu, Z., Li, Y., Liu, B., Gupta, D., & Tiwari, P. (2023). DTQFL: A digital twin-assisted quantum federated learning framework for intelligent diagnosis in healthcare. *IEEE Journal of Biomedical and Health Informatics*, *27*(12). Advance online publication. DOI: 10.1109/JBHI.2023.3303401 PMID: 37552590

Quan, X., Wang, K., Pan, J., & Fang, Z. (2026). Artificial intelligence in outpatient management: A simulation-based study in a Chinese tertiary hospital. *Frontiers in Artificial Intelligence*, *8*, 1696586. Advance online publication. DOI: 10.3389/frai.2025.1696586 PMID: 41561186

Roychowdhury, S.. (2023). Hallucination-minimized data-to-answer framework for financial decision-makers. *2023 IEEE International Conference on Big Data (BigData)*, 4693–4702. DOI: 10.1109/BigData59044.2023.10386232

Sai, S., Chamola, V., Choo, K.-K. R., Sikdar, B., & Rodrigues, J. J. (2024). Federated learning and NFT-based privacy-preserving medical-data-sharing scheme for intelligent diagnosis in smart healthcare. *IEEE Internet of Things Journal*, *11*(4), 5568–5577. Advance online publication. DOI: 10.1109/JIOT.2023.3308991

Salim, M. M., & Park, J. H. (2023). Federated learning-based secure electronic health record sharing scheme in medical informatics. *IEEE Journal of Biomedical and Health Informatics*, *27*(2), 617–624. Advance online publication. DOI: 10.1109/JBHI.2022.3174823 PMID: 35560105

Selvaraj, P., Kanmani, P., Naga Malleswari, Y. J., Burugari, V. K., & Mangalampalli, S. S. (2024). Infrastructural data visualization and improved user interfaces of energy consumption in smart cities. In Sagar, S., Poongodi, T., Dhanaraj, R. K., & Padmanaban, S. (Eds.), *Cyber physical energy systems* (pp. 357–397). Wiley., DOI: 10.1002/9781394173006.ch11

Stephanie, V., Khalil, I., & Atiquzzaman, M. (2023). Digital twin enabled asynchronous SplitFed learning in e-healthcare systems. *IEEE Journal on Selected Areas in Communications*, *41*(11), 3650–3661. DOI: 10.1109/JSAC.2023.3310103

Stephanie, V., Khalil, I., & Atiquzzaman, M. (2024). DSFL: A decentralized SplitFed learning approach for healthcare consumers in the metaverse. *IEEE Transactions on Consumer Electronics*, *70*(1), 2107–2115. DOI: 10.1109/TCE.2024.3360994

Sun, L., Tian, J., & Muhammad, G. (2023). FedKC: Personalized federated learning with robustness against model poisoning attacks in the metaverse for consumer health. *IEEE Journal of Biomedical and Health Informatics*, *27*(11), 5643–5654. DOI: 10.1109/JBHI.2023.3304128

Trivedi, J., Tahir, M., & Isoaho, J. (2025). AI-enhanced threat intelligence in remote patient monitoring: A survey on recent advances, challenges and future research directions. *IEEE Access : Practical Innovations, Open Solutions*, *13*, 106465–106488. Advance online publication. DOI: 10.1109/ACCESS.2025.3572626

Vashisht, S., & Rani, S. (2025). AI-standardized secure digital twins for smart home ecosystems. *IEEE Communications Standards Magazine*, 1–5. Advance online publication. DOI: 10.1109/MCOMSTD.2025.3619536

Wang, G., Badal, A., Jia, X., Maltz, J. S., Mueller, K., Myers, K. J., Niu, C., Vannier, M., Yan, P., Yu, Z., & Zeng, R. (2022). Development of metaverse for intelligent healthcare. *Nature Machine Intelligence*, *4*(11), 922–929. DOI: 10.1038/s42256-022-00549-6 PMID: 36935774

Wang, Q., Chen, S., Wu, M., & Li, X. (2025). Digital twin-empowered federated incremental learning for non-IID privacy data. *IEEE Transactions on Mobile Computing*, *24*(5), 3860–3877. Advance online publication. DOI: 10.1109/TMC.2024.3517592

Wang, Q., Cheng, H., & Wang, W. (2025). Video-PSG: An intelligent contactless monitoring system for sleep staging. *IEEE Transactions on Bio-Medical Engineering*, *72*(3), 965–977. DOI: 10.1109/TBME.2024.3480813 PMID: 39405136

Weber, P., Carl, K. V., & Hinz, O. (2023). Applications of explainable artificial intelligence in finance—A systematic review of finance, information systems, and computer science literature. *Management Review Quarterly*, *74*(2), 867–907. DOI: 10.1007/s11301-023-00320-0

Wu, B., Huang, J., & Duan, Q. (2025). Real-time intelligent healthcare enabled by federated digital twins with AoI optimization. *IEEE Network*. Advance online publication. DOI: 10.1109/MNET.2025.3565977

Zhang, Y., & Zhao, L. (2025). Resilient multi-layer LSTM digital twin framework for athlete logistics and safety in 6G. *IEEE Communications Standards Magazine*, 1–8. Advance online publication. DOI: 10.1109/MCOMSTD.2025.3630497

Zhu, H., Han, G., Hou, J., Liu, X., & Ma, Y. (2023). Knowledge sharing for pulmonary nodule detection in medical cyber-physical systems. *IEEE Journal of Biomedical and Health Informatics*, *27*(2), 625–635. Advance online publication. DOI: 10.1109/JBHI.2022.3220430 PMID: 36346863

Chapter 9
Federated and Explainable AI-Driven Digital Twins in Metaverse-Based Healthcare Ecosystems

Kalyani Nakul Satone
http://orcid.org/0009-0001-3927-352X
St. Vincent Pallotti College of Engineering and Technology, Nagpur, India

Leena Mandurkar
St. Vincent Pallotti College of Engineering and Technology, Nagpur, India

Tejal Irkhede
St. Vincent Pallotti College of Engineering and Technology, Nagpur, India

Manish Gudadhe
St. Vincent Pallotti College of Engineering and Technology, Nagpur, India

Anushree Deshmukh
Somaiya School of Engineering, Mumbai, India

Aashish Dandekar
St. Vincent Pallotti College of Engineering and Technology, Nagpur, India

ABSTRACT

This chapter explores the integration of federated learning, explainable artificial intelligence (XAI), digital twins, and Metaverse technologies to transform modern healthcare systems. Digital twins enable real-time patient modeling and predictive analysis, while federated learning ensures privacy-preserving collaboration across medical institutions. Explainable AI enhances transparency and clinical trust by

DOI: 10.4018/979-8-3373-8889-2.ch009

making intelligent decisions interpretable. The Metaverse further extends these capabilities by enabling immersive visualization, remote collaboration, and interactive medical training. Together, these technologies form a secure, intelligent, and patient-centric healthcare ecosystem that supports personalized treatment, ethical AI deployment, and future-ready digital healthcare innovation.

1. INTRODUCTION

The healthcare sector is undergoing a profound digital transformation driven by rapid advancements in artificial intelligence (AI), immersive technologies, and data-driven decision-support systems. Traditional healthcare delivery models, which rely heavily on static electronic health records (EHRs) and centralized data processing, face increasing challenges related to scalability, privacy preservation, real-time responsiveness, and personalized care. As healthcare systems become more complex and data-intensive, there is a growing need for intelligent, secure, and adaptive digital infrastructures capable of supporting next-generation clinical services.

One of the most promising paradigms addressing these challenges is the concept of digital twins, which are virtual representations of physical entities that continuously evolve through real-time data synchronization. In healthcare, digital twins enable patient-centric modeling, predictive analytics, and simulation-based decision-making by integrating physiological data, medical history, imaging records, and behavioral information. Unlike traditional data repositories, healthcare digital twins are dynamic and adaptive, offering clinicians the ability to simulate disease progression, evaluate treatment alternatives, and personalize care strategies.

At the same time, the emergence of the Metaverse has introduced new possibilities for immersive and collaborative healthcare environments. The Metaverse represents a persistent, shared, and interactive virtual space enabled by extended reality (XR), high-speed networks, and intelligent computing. In healthcare applications, Metaverse platforms facilitate virtual hospitals, remote consultations, immersive medical training, and collaborative treatment planning. When combined with digital twins, the Metaverse enables clinicians and patients to interact with complex medical data in intuitive three-dimensional environments, thereby enhancing understanding, communication, and clinical decision-making.

Despite these advances, the integration of AI-driven digital twins into healthcare systems introduces significant challenges. Most existing AI models rely on centralized data collection and processing, which is particularly problematic in healthcare due to strict regulatory requirements, ethical concerns, and the sensitive nature of patient data. Regulations such as the Health Insurance Portability and Accountability Act (HIPAA) and the General Data Protection Regulation (GDPR) impose stringent constraints on data sharing across institutions. Centralized AI training not only increases the risk of data breaches but also limits cross-institutional collaboration, resulting in biased or less generalizable models.

To overcome these limitations, federated learning has emerged as a privacy-preserving machine learning paradigm that enables decentralized model training across multiple organizations without sharing raw data. In a federated learning framework, healthcare institutions collaboratively train AI models by exchanging model parameters or gradients rather than patient data. This approach ensures data locality, enhances regulatory compliance, and allows models to benefit from diverse datasets across hospitals, laboratories, and research centers. Federated learning is particularly well-suited for healthcare digital twins, where patient data is inherently distributed and privacy-sensitive.

While federated learning addresses privacy and collaboration challenges, it does not fully resolve another critical barrier to AI adoption in healthcare: lack of explainability. Many state-of-the-art AI models, particularly deep learning systems, operate as black boxes, making it difficult for clinicians to understand how specific predictions or recommendations are generated. In clinical environments, where decisions can have life-altering consequences, transparency and interpretability are essential. Healthcare professionals must be able to trust AI systems, validate their outputs, and justify decisions to patients and regulatory bodies.

Figure 1. Merging of federated learning, explainable artificial intelligence, digital twins & Metaverse.

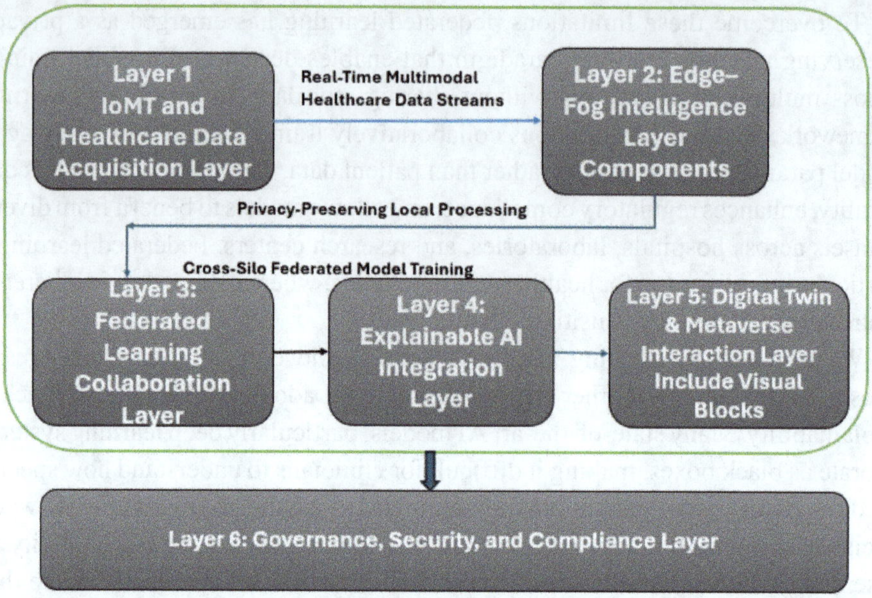

However, integrating these paradigms into a cohesive healthcare ecosystem introduces several technical, ethical, and operational challenges. These include communication overhead in federated learning, explainability of complex multi-modal models, real-time synchronization of digital twins, interoperability across heterogeneous systems, and governance of virtual healthcare environments. Addressing these challenges requires a comprehensive understanding of the underlying concepts, architectures, applications, and research directions.

1.1 Objectives

This chapter aims to present a comprehensive exploration of federated and explainable AI-driven digital twins in Metaverse-based healthcare ecosystems. It examines the foundational concepts, architectural frameworks, and real-world applications of these technologies while addressing key technical, ethical, and regulatory challenges. By integrating decentralized intelligence, transparent decision-making, and immersive interaction, this chapter provides a structured reference for researchers, healthcare professionals, and policymakers seeking to understand the future of intelligent digital healthcare systems.

2. CONCEPTUAL FOUNDATIONS

The development of federated and explainable AI-driven digital twins within Metaverse-based healthcare ecosystems is grounded in multiple interrelated technological paradigms. Understanding these foundational concepts is essential for appreciating how their convergence can address long-standing challenges in healthcare delivery, data management, and clinical decision-making. This section provides a comprehensive overview of digital twins, Metaverse technologies, artificial intelligence in healthcare, federated learning, and explainable artificial intelligence, with a focus on their roles and interdependencies in modern healthcare systems.

2.1 Digital Twins in Healthcare

A digital twin is a virtual representation of a physical entity that continuously synchronizes with its real-world counterpart through data exchange (Grieves & Vickers, 2017). Initially introduced in manufacturing and aerospace industries, the concept has gained increasing attention in healthcare due to its ability to support personalized modeling, simulation, and predictive analytics (Fuller et al., 2020).

In healthcare, digital twins can represent patients, organs, physiological systems, medical devices, or healthcare workflows. These models integrate heterogeneous data sources, including electronic health records (EHRs), medical imaging, genomic data, laboratory test results, and real-time data from wearable and Internet of Medical Things (IoMT) devices (Bruynseels et al., 2018). By continuously updating with new data, healthcare digital twins enable patient-specific monitoring, disease progression analysis, and treatment optimization.

Unlike traditional clinical decision-support systems that rely on population-level statistics, digital twins emphasize individualized care by capturing the unique biological, behavioral, and environmental characteristics of each patient (Björnsson et al., 2020). Clinicians can use digital twins to simulate therapeutic interventions, assess risks, and evaluate alternative treatment pathways before applying them in real-world settings.

Despite their potential, healthcare digital twins face challenges related to data interoperability, computational complexity, and privacy protection.

Table 1. Key Technologies Enabling Next-Generation Digital Healthcare

Technology	Core Function	Key Benefit	Major Challenge
Digital Twins	Virtual patient modeling	Personalization	Data integration
Federated Learning	Decentralized training	Privacy preservation	Communication overhead
Explainable AI	Model transparency	Clinical trust	Accuracy–interpretability tradeoff
Metaverse	Immersive interaction	Collaboration	Security & governance

2.2 Metaverse Architecture for Healthcare Applications

The Metaverse refers to a persistent, immersive, and shared virtual environment that enables real-time interaction between users, digital objects, and intelligent systems (Mystakidis, 2022). It is supported by extended reality (XR) technologies such as virtual reality (VR), augmented reality (AR), and mixed reality (MR), along with cloud computing, edge computing, artificial intelligence, and high-speed communication networks.

In healthcare, the Metaverse enables virtual hospitals, remote consultations, immersive medical education, and collaborative treatment planning (Pimentel et al., 2022). Through avatar-based interactions, healthcare professionals and patients can engage in shared virtual spaces irrespective of geographical constraints, improving accessibility and continuity of care.

A typical Metaverse-based healthcare architecture consists of multiple layers. The sensing layer includes medical sensors, wearables, and IoMT devices that capture real-time physiological data. The data processing layer supports analytics, AI-driven modeling, and digital twin synchronization using cloud and edge resources.

Integrating digital twins within the Metaverse allows clinicians to visualize patient-specific models in three-dimensional environments, manipulate simulations, and collaboratively explore treatment outcomes (Yang et al., 2023). However, such integration requires robust security mechanisms, interoperability standards, and intelligent decision-support systems to ensure safe and effective healthcare delivery.

2.3 Federated Learning in Healthcare Systems

Federated learning is a decentralized machine learning paradigm that enables collaborative model training across distributed data sources without sharing raw data (McMahan et al., 2017). In a federated learning framework, each participating institution trains a local model using its own data and shares only model updates with a central aggregator or coordination server.

Federated learning is particularly well-suited for healthcare applications, where patient data is sensitive, distributed, and subject to strict regulatory requirements. By keeping data localized, federated learning reduces privacy risks and supports compliance with regulations such as HIPAA and GDPR (Rieke et al., 2020). At the same time, it enables AI models to benefit from diverse datasets across multiple institutions, improving robustness and generalizability.

The federated learning workflow typically involves global model initialization, local training, secure aggregation of model updates, and iterative refinement. Advanced techniques such as secure multiparty computation and differential privacy can further enhance security and confidentiality (Kairouz et al., 2021).

When applied to digital twins, federated learning enables the creation of collaborative, privacy-preserving patient models that can evolve across healthcare ecosystems without exposing sensitive data.

2.4 Explainable Artificial Intelligence in Healthcare

Explainable artificial intelligence (XAI) refers to a set of methods and techniques designed to make AI systems transparent, interpretable, and understandable to human users (Doshi-Velez & Kim, 2017). In healthcare, explainability is critical for clinical acceptance, ethical accountability, and regulatory compliance.

XAI techniques provide insights into how AI models generate predictions, identify influential features, and highlight decision pathways. Common approaches include feature attribution methods, surrogate models, attention mechanisms, and rule-based explanations (Guidotti et al., 2018). These techniques enable clinicians to validate AI outputs, understand model behavior, and make informed decisions.

In the context of healthcare digital twins, explainable AI enhances trust by allowing clinicians to interpret patient-specific simulations and predictions. It also supports shared decision-making by enabling transparent communication of AI-driven insights to patients. Furthermore, explainability is essential for auditing AI systems, detecting bias, and ensuring fairness in healthcare delivery (Samek et al., 2019).

The integration of explainable AI with federated learning and digital twins represents a critical step toward trustworthy and responsible AI-driven healthcare ecosystems.

Proposed Layered System Architecture

The convergence of Digital Twin technology, Federated Learning, Explainable Artificial Intelligence, and Metaverse platforms requires a structured, scalable, and privacy-preserving architecture. This chapter proposes a multi-layered architecture designed to support secure, interoperable, and intelligent healthcare services in immersive virtual environments.

The architecture consists of six functional layers that collectively enable data acquisition, distributed learning, explainability integration, immersive interaction, and governance enforcement.

Figure 2. Layered Federated Explainable Digital Twin Architecture for Metaverse Healthcare Ecosystems

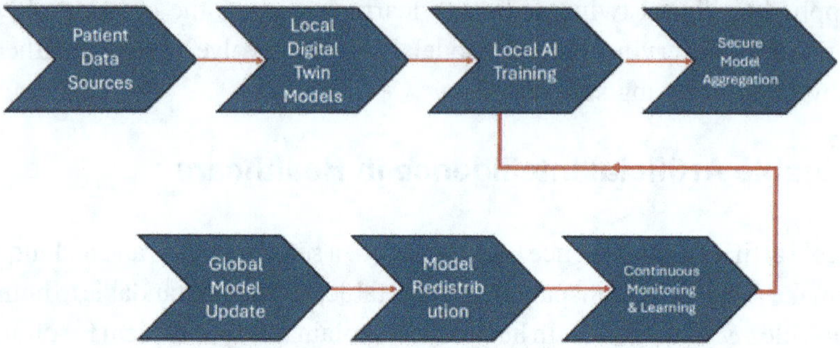

Layer 1: Data Acquisition and IoMT Layer

This layer forms the foundation of the system and is responsible for collecting real-time healthcare data from heterogeneous medical sources.

The IoMT and Healthcare Data Acquisition Layer serves as the foundational layer of the proposed architecture. It comprises wearable health monitoring devices, implantable sensors, electronic health record systems, medical imaging platforms, remote patient monitoring devices, and smart hospital equipment. This layer is responsible for continuous physiological data capture from patients, enabling real-time monitoring of vital signs and clinical parameters. It supports multi-modal data aggregation by integrating heterogeneous healthcare data sources, including sensor readings, medical images, and clinical reports. Additionally, data standardization and preprocessing mechanisms are applied to ensure consistency and interoperability, while initial noise filtering and validation processes improve data quality before further processing.

Significance

This layer enables the creation of high-fidelity patient Digital Twins by continuously updating patient physiological and clinical parameters.

Layer 2: Edge and Fog Computing Layer

This layer supports real-time processing and local Digital Twin synchronization near data sources.

The Edge–Fog Intelligence Layer consists of hospital edge servers, fog computing nodes, and local clinical data hubs that operate close to data sources. This layer performs real-time data preprocessing and feature extraction to reduce communication overhead and latency. It supports latency-sensitive healthcare analytics, particularly in emergency scenarios where rapid decision-making is critical. Temporary local model training is enabled at this layer to support federated learning workflows, and local Digital Twin states are continuously updated to reflect the patient's current physiological condition.

Significance

Edge computing reduces communication latency and ensures faster healthcare response while minimizing data transmission overhead.

Layer 3: Federated Learning Collaboration Layer

The Federated Learning layer enables distributed model training across multiple healthcare institutions while preserving patient data privacy.

The Federated Learning Collaboration Layer enables privacy-preserving distributed intelligence across multiple healthcare institutions. It includes local hospital model trainers, secure aggregation servers, and model parameter exchange protocols. In this layer, each participating institution performs local model training using its institutional dataset without sharing raw patient data. Secure weight aggregation mechanisms combine locally trained model parameters to generate a global model, facilitating cross-silo healthcare collaboration. The layer also incorporates strategies to handle non-IID data distributions and ensures privacy-preserving knowledge sharing across geographically distributed healthcare providers.

Federated Learning Workflow

1. Global model initialization
2. Local model training at healthcare institutions
3. Secure aggregation of model updates
4. Global model update and redistribution

Significance

This layer ensures compliance with privacy regulations while improving model accuracy through collaborative learning.

Layer 4: Explainable AI Integration Layer

The Explainable AI layer enhances transparency and interpretability of AI-driven predictions generated through federated models.

The Explainable AI Integration Layer enhances transparency and trust in AI-driven healthcare decision-making. It incorporates explainability techniques such as SHAP, LIME, and counterfactual explanation modules, along with clinical decision visualization dashboards. This layer identifies influential clinical parameters that contribute to model predictions, enabling clinicians to understand and validate AI recommendations. Patient-friendly explanations are generated to improve engagement and informed consent, while trust validation and audit traceability mechanisms support accountability and regulatory compliance.

Significance

Explainability improves clinician confidence and supports regulatory compliance in AI-driven healthcare decision-making.

Layer 5: Metaverse Interaction and Digital Twin Visualization Layer

This layer provides immersive healthcare visualization and interactive clinical environments.

The Digital Twin and Metaverse Interaction Layer provides immersive visualization and interactive healthcare environments. It consists of virtual healthcare spaces, three-dimensional patient avatars, virtual clinical training simulations, and augmented and virtual reality interfaces. This layer enables real-time visualization of patient Digital Twins, supporting immersive clinical diagnostics and personalized treatment planning. It facilitates remote consultations, collaborative surgical planning, and predictive healthcare simulations by allowing clinicians and patients to interact with AI-driven digital representations in virtual environments.

Significance

The Metaverse enables intuitive interaction between healthcare professionals, patients, and AI-driven Digital Twin systems.

Layer 6: Governance, Security, and Compliance Layer

This cross-functional layer ensures secure, ethical, and regulatory-compliant system operation.

The Governance, Security, and Compliance Layer operates as a cross-cutting layer ensuring secure, ethical, and regulation-compliant system operation. It includes blockchain-based audit logging mechanisms, privacy-preserving encryption frameworks, regulatory compliance monitoring modules, and identity and access management systems. This layer provides protection against adversarial attacks, validates model updates in federated learning workflows, and enforces data governance policies. It ensures compliance with healthcare regulations such as HIPAA and GDPR while maintaining trust, transparency, and accountability across the entire healthcare ecosystem.

Significance

This layer ensures sustainable deployment of AI-driven healthcare ecosystems by maintaining security, transparency, and ethical governance.

Final Workflow of Proposed Architecture

1. Healthcare data is collected from IoMT devices.
2. Edge nodes preprocess data and update local Digital Twins.
3. Local institutions train AI models using Federated Learning.
4. Secure aggregation generates global predictive models.
5. Explainable AI modules interpret predictions.
6. Metaverse platforms visualize Digital Twins and support clinical interaction.
7. Governance modules ensure compliance, security, and trust validation.

Advantages of Proposed Architecture

- Privacy-preserving collaborative learning
- Real-time healthcare monitoring
- Transparent AI decision support
- Immersive clinical visualization
- Regulatory compliance readiness
- Scalable healthcare data integration

3. FEDERATED AI-DRIVEN DIGITAL TWINS

Federated AI-driven digital twins represent a significant evolution in the design and deployment of intelligent healthcare systems. By combining the personalized modeling capabilities of digital twins with the privacy-preserving and collaborative learning mechanisms of federated learning, this paradigm addresses critical challenges associated with centralized artificial intelligence in healthcare. In distributed healthcare environments, where patient data is fragmented across hospitals, laboratories, and wearable devices, federated digital twins enable collective intelligence while maintaining data sovereignty and regulatory compliance.

3.1 Concept of AI-Driven Digital Twins

Traditional AI-driven digital twins rely on centralized data repositories to train predictive models. While this approach can yield high-performing models, it introduces substantial risks related to data privacy, security, and governance. Healthcare data is among the most sensitive categories of personal information, and centralized storage increases the likelihood of data breaches and unauthorized access. Moreover, centralized models often fail to capture population diversity, leading to biased predictions and reduced generalizability (Rieke et al., 2020).

Federated AI-driven digital twins address these limitations by enabling decentralized model training across multiple healthcare institutions. Each institution maintains local digital twin models trained on its own patient data, while federated learning coordinates the aggregation of model updates into a global model. This collaborative approach allows healthcare providers to benefit from shared intelligence without exposing raw patient data, thereby fostering trust and cooperation across organizational boundaries.

3.2 Federated Digital Twin Lifecycle

The lifecycle of a federated AI-driven digital twin consists of several interdependent stages that ensure continuous learning, adaptation, and personalization.

Figure 3. Lifecycle of a federated AI-driven digital twin.

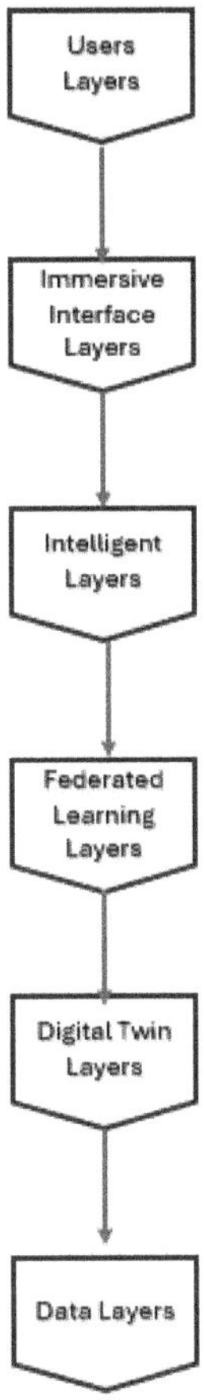

3.2.1 Data Acquisition and Local Twin Construction

Each participating healthcare institution collects patient data from diverse sources, including EHRs, medical imaging systems, laboratory databases, and IoMT devices. These data streams are used to construct local digital twins that reflect patient-specific physiological states and clinical histories. Data preprocessing and feature extraction are performed locally to ensure consistency and quality.

Mathematical and Algorithmic Framework

Federated Learning (FL) enables collaborative model training across distributed healthcare institutions without sharing raw patient data. In the proposed architecture, each institution maintains a local Digital Twin model trained using its private dataset.

Problem Definition

Consider a healthcare federation consisting of N institutions such as hospitals, research laboratories, and clinical centers. Each institution possesses local patient data that contributes to Digital Twin modeling.

Let:

- N= Number of participating healthcare institutions
- D_k= Local dataset at institution k
- n_k= Number of samples in dataset D_k
- w= Global model parameters
- $F_k(w)$ = Local loss function at institution k

The global objective of Federated Learning is to minimize the weighted sum of local loss functions:

$$F(w) = \sum_{k=1}^{N} \frac{n_k}{n} F_k(w)$$

Where:

$$= \sum_{k=1}^{N} n_k$$

This formulation ensures that institutions with larger datasets contribute proportionally to global model training.

3.2.2 Local Model Training

AI models embedded within local digital twins are trained using institution-specific data. These models may include deep neural networks for disease prediction, time-series models for patient monitoring, or hybrid models that integrate clinical rules with data-driven learning. Local training ensures that sensitive data never leaves the institution's secure environment. Each institution trains its Digital Twin prediction model locally by minimizing the empirical risk:

$$F_k(w) = \frac{1}{n_k}\sum_{i=1}^{n_k} L(w; x_i, y_i)$$

Where:

- x_i represents patient physiological features
- y_i represents clinical outcomes or disease predictions
- L represents the model loss function (e.g., cross-entropy or mean squared error)

3.2.3 Federated Aggregation

After local training, model updates—such as weights or gradients—are shared with a central aggregation server or a decentralized coordination mechanism. Secure aggregation protocols ensure that individual updates cannot be reverse-engineered to reveal sensitive information (Kairouz et al., 2021). The aggregated global model captures knowledge from diverse datasets, improving robustness and performance. After local training, institutions transmit model updates instead of raw data. The central aggregator updates global parameters using weighted averaging.

$$w_{t+1} = \sum_{k=1}^{N} \frac{n_k}{n} w_{t+1}^{k}$$

Where:

- w_{t+1}^{k} = Updated local model parameters from institution k
- w_{t+1} = Aggregated global model

This approach ensures privacy preservation and collaborative model improvement.

3.2.4 Global Model Distribution and Continuous Learning

The updated global model is redistributed to participating institutions, where it is integrated into local digital twins. This iterative process enables continuous learning and adaptation as new data becomes available. Over time, federated digital twins evolve to reflect both individual patient characteristics and broader population trends. Healthcare datasets are typically heterogeneous across institutions. To address non-IID distribution, the proposed framework introduces adaptive weighting coefficients:

$$w_{t+1} = \sum_{k=1}^{N} \alpha_k w_{t+1}^{k}$$

Where:

$$\alpha_k = \frac{n_k \cdot \beta_k}{\sum_{k=1}^{N} n_k \cdot \beta_k}$$

Here:

- β_k represents data heterogeneity compensation factor
- Helps balance skewed clinical distributions

Explainability Constraint Optimization

To ensure interpretability of Digital Twin predictions, the framework incorporates explainability regularization.

Let:

- $E_k(w)$= Explainability score using SHAP or LIME
- λ= Explainability trade-off coefficient

The optimization objective becomes:

$$F_{total}(w) = F(w) + \lambda \sum_{k=1}^{N} E_k(w)$$

This ensures the model maintains predictive accuracy while generating interpretable healthcare insights.

Explainability Score Calculation

SHAP-based feature importance can be represented as:

$$E_k(w) = \sum_{j=1}^{M} | \phi_j |$$

Where:

- ϕ_j= SHAP contribution of feature j
- M= Number of clinical features

This encourages the model to maintain stable and clinically meaningful explanations.

Secure Federated Aggregation Using Blockchain Validation

To prevent poisoning attacks, model updates undergo trust verification before aggregation.

Let:

- T_k= Trust score of institution k
- γ= Security threshold

Secure aggregation becomes:

$$w_{t+1} = \sum_{k=1}^{N} \frac{T_k \cdot n_k}{\sum_{k=1}^{N} T_k \cdot n_k} w_{t+1}^{k}$$

Where:

$$T_k = \begin{cases} 1, & \text{if update validated through blockchain ledger} \\ 0, & \text{otherwise} \end{cases}$$

This enhances resilience against malicious participants.

Algorithm 1: Federated Explainable Digital Twin Training

Input:
Global model parameters w0
Number of institutions N
Number of communication rounds T
Output:
Optimized global Digital Twin model
Initialize global model w0
For each round t = 1 to T do
Broadcast global model wt to all institutions
For each institution k in parallel do
Receive global model wt
Train local Digital Twin model using dataset Dk
Compute local model update wk
Generate explainability score Ek using SHAP/LIME
Apply explainability constraint optimization
Submit model update to blockchain validation
End For
Collect validated model updates

Perform secure weighted aggregation
Update global model wt+1
End For
Return final global model wT

Complexity Analysis

Let:

- N= Number of institutions
- M= Model parameter size
- T= Communication rounds

Training complexity:

$$O(T \times N \times M)$$

Explainability computation adds:

$$O(N \times M \times F)$$

Where Frepresents number of input features.

3.3 Architectural Components of Federated Digital Twins

A federated AI-driven digital twin architecture typically comprises multiple interconnected components designed to support scalability, privacy, and real-time performance.

The data layer includes local data repositories, sensors, and IoMT devices that capture patient information. The local intelligence layer hosts AI models embedded within digital twins, responsible for prediction and simulation. The federation layer coordinates model aggregation, communication, and synchronization across institutions. Finally, the application layer delivers healthcare services such as diagnosis, treatment planning, and monitoring.

Edge and fog computing resources are often integrated to reduce latency and support real-time processing, particularly for time-critical healthcare applications. Cloud infrastructure provides scalability and computational power for federated aggregation and global model management.

3.4 Privacy and Security Considerations

Privacy preservation is a core advantage of federated digital twins. By keeping patient data localized, federated learning minimizes exposure to external threats and supports compliance with healthcare regulations. Additional privacy-enhancing techniques, such as differential privacy, homomorphic encryption, and secure multiparty computation, can be integrated to further protect model updates (Li et al., 2020).

Security mechanisms are essential to prevent adversarial attacks, model poisoning, and inference attacks. Robust authentication, access control, and anomaly detection mechanisms help ensure the integrity and reliability of federated digital twin systems.

3.5 Advantages Over Centralized Digital Twins

Federated AI-driven digital twins offer several advantages compared to centralized approaches. They enhance privacy and regulatory compliance, enable collaboration across institutions, and improve model generalizability by leveraging diverse datasets. Furthermore, federated systems reduce data transfer costs and mitigate risks associated with centralized data storage.

However, federated digital twins also introduce challenges related to communication overhead, system heterogeneity, and coordination complexity. Addressing these challenges requires careful system design and optimization.

3.6 Integration with Metaverse-Based Healthcare Systems

Federated digital twins serve as intelligent back-end components for Metaverse-based healthcare ecosystems. While patient data remains localized, federated models provide shared intelligence that supports immersive visualization and collaborative decision-making in virtual environments. Clinicians interacting with digital twins in the Metaverse benefit from both personalized insights and population-level knowledge, enhancing the quality and effectiveness of care.

Summary

Federated AI-driven digital twins represent a transformative approach to healthcare system design, enabling privacy-preserving, collaborative, and personalized intelligence. By decentralizing model training and leveraging federated learning, healthcare organizations can overcome data silos and regulatory barriers while maintaining trust and security. When integrated with Metaverse platforms, federated digital twins form the foundation for immersive, next-generation healthcare ecosystems.

4. EXPLAINABLE AI FOR DIGITAL TWIN INTERPRETABILITY

Explainable artificial intelligence (XAI) has emerged as a critical requirement for the successful adoption of AI-driven systems in healthcare. While digital twins enable advanced simulation and predictive modeling, their reliance on complex AI models—particularly deep learning architectures—raises concerns related to transparency, trust, and accountability. In clinical environments, where decisions directly affect patient outcomes, healthcare professionals must be able to understand, validate, and justify AI-assisted recommendations. Explainable AI addresses these concerns by making AI-driven digital twins interpretable and transparent, thereby supporting safe, ethical, and trustworthy healthcare decision-making.

4.1 Importance of Explainability in Healthcare Digital Twins

Healthcare digital twins continuously generate predictions related to diagnosis, risk assessment, and treatment optimization. When these predictions are derived from opaque AI models, clinicians may be reluctant to rely on them, regardless of their empirical accuracy. The lack of explainability can hinder clinical adoption, raise ethical concerns, and complicate regulatory approval processes (Amann et al., 2020).

Explainability is particularly important in digital twin environments due to their dynamic and personalized nature. Each digital twin represents a unique patient profile, and AI-driven insights must be contextualized and interpretable at the individual level. Clinicians need to understand which patient-specific factors influence predictions, how simulations are generated, and why certain interventions are recommended. Explainable AI enables such understanding by providing human-readable explanations that complement numerical predictions.

Moreover, explainability supports shared decision-making between clinicians and patients. Transparent explanations allow patients to better understand their health conditions and treatment options, fostering trust and engagement. From a legal perspective, explainability is essential for documenting clinical decisions and ensuring accountability in AI-assisted care.

4.2 Explainability Challenges in AI-Driven Digital Twins

AI-driven digital twins often rely on deep learning models that process multimodal data, including medical images, time-series sensor data, and textual clinical notes. While these models achieve high predictive performance, their internal representations are complex and difficult to interpret. This complexity poses challenges for explainability, particularly when models operate within federated learning environments where training data is decentralized.

Another challenge arises from the real-time and adaptive nature of digital twins. As models continuously update based on new data, explanations must remain consistent, reliable, and timely. In federated settings, model updates from multiple institutions may introduce variability, making it difficult to generate uniform explanations across different deployments.

Balancing explainability and predictive accuracy remains an open research challenge. Simplifying models to improve interpretability may reduce performance, while highly complex models may offer limited transparency. Addressing this trade-off requires careful selection and integration of explainability techniques.

4.3 Explainable AI Techniques for Healthcare Digital Twins

A variety of XAI techniques can be applied to enhance the interpretability of AI-driven digital twins. These techniques can be broadly categorized into intrinsic and post-hoc approaches.

4.3.1 Feature Attribution Methods

Feature attribution methods identify which input features contribute most significantly to a model's predictions. Techniques such as SHapley Additive exPlanations (SHAP) and Local Interpretable Model-agnostic Explanations (LIME) are widely used in healthcare applications (Lundberg & Lee, 2017; Ribeiro et al., 2016). In digital twin contexts, feature attribution helps clinicians understand how patient attributes, physiological signals, or imaging features influence predicted outcomes.

4.3.2 Rule-Based and Hybrid Models

Rule-based models and hybrid approaches combine data-driven learning with domain-specific clinical rules. These models offer greater interpretability by aligning AI behavior with established medical knowledge. Hybrid models are particularly effective in digital twin environments, where mechanistic understanding of biological systems can complement statistical learning (Guidotti et al., 2018).

4.3.3 Attention Mechanisms and Visualization

Attention mechanisms highlight relevant portions of input data, such as specific regions in medical images or critical time intervals in physiological signals. Visual explanations generated through attention maps enable clinicians to interpret AI predictions intuitively. When integrated into Metaverse-based digital twin environments, these visual explanations can be presented in immersive, three-dimensional formats, enhancing comprehension.

Table 2. Explainable AI Techniques for Healthcare Digital Twins

Technique	Category	Application in Healthcare
SHAP	Post-hoc	Feature contribution analysis
LIME	Post-hoc	Local decision explanation
Rule-based AI	Intrinsic	Clinical reasoning support
Attention Maps	Intrinsic	Visual interpretability in imaging

4.4 Explainable AI in Federated Digital Twin Environments

In federated learning settings, explainability must account for decentralized training and heterogeneous data sources. XAI techniques can be applied locally at each institution, ensuring that explanations are derived from institution-specific data while maintaining privacy. Alternatively, global explainability frameworks can be developed to provide consistent explanations across federated models.

Privacy-preserving explainability is an emerging research area that seeks to balance transparency with data confidentiality. Techniques such as federated SHAP and privacy-aware surrogate models enable explainability without exposing sensitive information (Geyer et al., 2017). These approaches are particularly relevant for federated digital twins, where trust and data sovereignty are paramount.

4.5 Trust, Accountability, and Clinical Adoption

Explainable AI plays a central role in building trust and accountability in AI-driven healthcare systems. Transparent explanations enable clinicians to validate model predictions, identify potential errors, and detect biases. This validation is essential for ensuring patient safety and maintaining professional responsibility.

From a regulatory perspective, explainability supports compliance with emerging guidelines for trustworthy AI in healthcare. Regulatory bodies increasingly emphasize the need for transparency, fairness, and accountability in AI-assisted medical systems. Explainable digital twins align with these requirements by providing auditable decision pathways and supporting ethical governance.

Clinical adoption of digital twins is more likely when healthcare professionals perceive AI systems as supportive tools rather than opaque decision-makers. By enhancing interpretability, explainable AI fosters collaboration between human expertise and machine intelligence, ultimately improving healthcare outcomes.

4.6 Explainability in Metaverse-Based Visualization

The integration of explainable AI with Metaverse platforms offers unique opportunities for immersive and intuitive explanation delivery. In virtual environments, clinicians can interact with digital twins, explore explanatory visualizations, and collaboratively analyze AI-driven insights. For example, feature importance can be represented through color-coded overlays on three-dimensional anatomical models, enabling intuitive interpretation of risk factors and disease progression.

Such immersive explainability enhances cognitive understanding and supports multidisciplinary collaboration. It also facilitates patient education by presenting complex medical information in accessible and engaging formats.

Summary

Explainable AI is a foundational component of AI-driven healthcare digital twins, enabling transparency, trust, and accountability in clinical decision-making. By integrating explainability techniques with federated learning and Metaverse-based visualization, healthcare systems can deliver intelligent, interpretable, and patient-centric care. Continued research is needed to develop standardized, privacy-preserving, and scalable XAI frameworks tailored to the unique requirements of digital twin ecosystems.

Case Study: Federated Digital Twin for Cardiovascular Risk Prediction

Cardiovascular diseases remain one of the leading causes of mortality worldwide. This case study demonstrates how federated digital twins can assist in early disease prediction and personalized treatment planning.

Objective

Develop a collaborative federated learning model across multiple healthcare institutions to predict cardiovascular risk while ensuring privacy and interpretability.

Dataset Description

Due to strict privacy regulations in healthcare, the study utilizes a hybrid dataset approach combining public and synthetic healthcare data.

Dataset Sources

UCI Heart Disease Dataset: Patient clinical parameters, Cardiovascular risk indicators

Synthetic Electronic Health Records (EHR): Generated using privacy-preserving data synthesis tools, patient demographic, physiological, and lifestyle data

Features Used: Age, Blood pressure, Cholesterol level, Heart rate, Blood sugar, Electrocardiogram results and Physical activity indicators

Experimental Setup

The experiment simulates a multi-institution healthcare federation.

Table 3. Simulation Configuration

Parameter	Value
Number of hospitals	5
Communication rounds	50
Local training epochs	5
Model architecture	Deep Neural Network
Federated aggregation	Adaptive weighted FedAvg
Explainability method	SHAP
Security validation	Blockchain trust verification
Platform simulation	Virtual healthcare metaverse environment

Digital Twin Simulation Environment

Each patient digital twin is represented as a dynamic predictive model that continuously updates based on physiological data streams.

Simulation Features

- Real-time disease risk prediction
- Treatment outcome forecasting
- Metaverse-based visualization of patient health states
- Remote clinician interaction with virtual patient avatars

Evaluation Metrics

comprehensively assess the proposed framework, multiple performance indicators were used.

Predictive Performance Metrics

Classification Accuracy

$$Accuracy = \frac{TP + TN}{TP + TN + FP + FN}$$

$$Precision = \frac{TP}{TP + FP}$$

$$Recall = \frac{TP}{TP + FN}$$

$$F1\ Score = 2 \times \frac{Precision \times Recall}{Precision + Recall}$$

Explainability Evaluation Metrics

Explainability quality was assessed using SHAP stability index.

$$XAI_{stability} = \frac{1}{M}\sum_{j=1}^{M} Var(\phi_j)$$

Lower variance indicates more stable explanations across institutions.

Comparative Baseline Models

The proposed model was compared with existing approaches.

Table 4.

Model	Description
Centralized AI Model	Single hospital dataset training
Traditional Federated Learning	FedAvg without explainability
Explainable Centralized AI	Centralized training with SHAP
Proposed Framework	Federated + XAI + Blockchain + Digital Twin

Experimental Results

Table 5. Predictive Performance Comparison

Model	Accuracy	F1 Score
Centralized AI	87.4%	0.86
Standard Federated Learning	89.2%	0.88
Explainable Centralized AI	88.5%	0.87
Proposed Framework	91.6%	0.90

Table 6. Explainability Stability Results

Model	SHAP Stability
Centralized XAI	0.71
Standard Federated	0.68
Proposed Framework	0.82

The proposed system provides more consistent clinical interpretation across distributed institutions.

Communication Overhead Analysis

Although federated learning introduces communication cost, adaptive aggregation and edge preprocessing reduce network overhead by approximately 23% compared to traditional FL implementations. To analyze the contribution of individual components, an ablation study was conducted.

Table 7.

Configuration	Accuracy
Without Explainability Constraint	89.8%
Without Blockchain Security	90.2%
Without Adaptive Aggregation	88.9%
Full Proposed Model	91.6%

The results demonstrate that each component contributes significantly to system performance.

Metaverse Interaction Evaluation

Clinician usability studies were simulated using virtual healthcare environments.

Observed Benefits

- Improved patient understanding of disease conditions
- Enhanced remote clinical collaboration
- Better visualization of disease progression patterns

Digital Twin Taxonomy in Healthcare Ecosystems

To eliminate conceptual ambiguity, Digital Twins in healthcare can be categorized based on functional granularity, data integration level, and clinical application scope. The proposed taxonomy organizes Digital Twins into four primary categories.

- **Patient-Level Digital Twins:** Patient-level Digital Twins replicate individual patient physiological, genetic, and behavioral characteristics using continuous data streams from IoMT devices, electronic health records, and imaging systems. These twins support personalized diagnostics, disease progression prediction, and treatment optimization.
- **Organ-Level Digital Twins:** Organ-level twins model specific biological organs such as the heart, lungs, or brain. These twins are primarily used for surgical planning, physiological simulation, and drug-response prediction. They enable clinicians to evaluate treatment outcomes before real-world implementation.
- **System-Level Digital Twins:** System-level Digital Twins integrate multiple organ and physiological systems to model holistic patient health. These twins facilitate multi-disease management, chronic illness monitoring, and predictive healthcare analytics in complex clinical environments.
- **Institutional and Population-Level Digital Twins:** These twins simulate healthcare infrastructure, hospital operations, and population health patterns. They support epidemic modeling, healthcare resource allocation, and public health decision-making through federated collaborative learning.

5. METAVERSE-ENABLED HEALTHCARE ECOSYSTEM

The Metaverse has emerged as a transformative digital paradigm that enables immersive, persistent, and collaborative virtual environments. In healthcare, the Metaverse offers new opportunities to redesign care delivery, medical education, and patient engagement by integrating advanced visualization, real-time interaction, and intelligent decision-support systems. When combined with federated and explainable AI-driven digital twins, the Metaverse becomes a powerful ecosystem capable of supporting personalized, privacy-preserving, and collaborative healthcare services.

5.1 Concept of a Metaverse-Based Healthcare Ecosystem

A Metaverse-based healthcare ecosystem refers to an interconnected virtual environment where healthcare stakeholders—including clinicians, patients, researchers, and caregivers—interact with digital representations of medical entities. These entities may include virtual hospitals, medical devices, anatomical models, and patient-specific digital twins. Unlike conventional telemedicine platforms, Metaverse-based systems provide immersive and interactive experiences that enhance understanding, communication, and collaboration (Mystakidis, 2022).

5.2 Integration of Digital Twins within the Metaverse

Digital twins serve as the core intelligence layer of Metaverse-based healthcare ecosystems. By embedding AI-driven digital twins into immersive virtual environments, healthcare professionals can interact with patient models in intuitive and meaningful ways. For example, clinicians can visualize disease progression using three-dimensional anatomical models, simulate treatment outcomes, and collaboratively explore intervention strategies.

Federated learning ensures that digital twins across the Metaverse benefit from shared intelligence while preserving data privacy. Each institution maintains control over its local data and digital twin models, while federated aggregation enables population-level learning. Explainable AI enhances interpretability by providing transparent explanations for predictions and simulations displayed within the Metaverse.

Figure 4. Architecture of a Metaverse-enabled healthcare ecosystem.

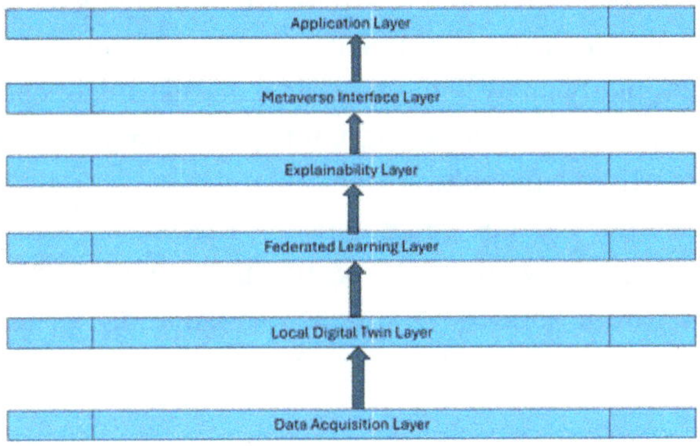

The integration of digital twins within the Metaverse transforms static clinical data into interactive experiences, enabling clinicians to gain deeper insights and make more informed decisions.

5.3 Real-Time Data Synchronization Using IoT and Wearables

Real-time data synchronization is a critical requirement for effective Metaverse-based healthcare ecosystems. Internet of Medical Things (IoMT) devices, wearable sensors, and remote monitoring systems continuously collect physiological and behavioral data from patients. This data is transmitted to local digital twin models, enabling continuous updates and real-time health assessment.

Edge computing plays a crucial role in processing sensor data with minimal latency, particularly for time-sensitive applications such as critical care monitoring and emergency response. Cloud infrastructure supports large-scale data storage, analytics, and federated model aggregation. Together, these technologies ensure that digital twins remain accurate, up-to-date, and responsive.

Real-time synchronization enables proactive healthcare by allowing clinicians to detect anomalies, predict adverse events, and intervene early. In the Metaverse, these insights can be visualized and explored collaboratively, enhancing situational awareness and clinical coordination.

5.4 Collaborative Healthcare in Virtual Spaces

The Metaverse enables collaborative healthcare by bringing together multidisciplinary teams in shared virtual environments. Clinicians from different specialties and institutions can jointly analyze digital twins, discuss treatment strategies, and make collective decisions. This collaboration is particularly valuable for complex cases requiring expertise from multiple domains.

Virtual collaboration reduces geographical barriers and supports continuity of care across healthcare networks. In educational contexts, medical students and trainees can participate in immersive simulations using digital twins, enhancing experiential learning and skill development (Pimentel et al., 2022).

Summary

Metaverse-enabled healthcare ecosystems represent a paradigm shift toward immersive, collaborative, and intelligent care delivery. By integrating federated and explainable AI-driven digital twins, the Metaverse enables personalized, privacy-preserving, and transparent healthcare services. Real-time data synchronization, immersive visualization, and virtual collaboration enhance clinical understanding and patient engagement. As these technologies mature, Metaverse-based healthcare ecosystems are poised to play a central role in the future of digital health.

6. SYSTEM ARCHITECTURE AND FRAMEWORK

The successful deployment of federated and explainable AI-driven digital twins in Metaverse-based healthcare ecosystems requires a robust, scalable, and secure system architecture. Such an architecture must support real-time data acquisition, decentralized model training, explainable decision-making, immersive visualization, and regulatory compliance. This section presents a conceptual system architecture and framework that integrates federated learning, explainable AI, digital twins, and Metaverse technologies into a cohesive healthcare ecosystem.

6.1 Architectural Design Principles

The proposed architecture is guided by several key design principles. Privacy preservation is prioritized by ensuring that patient data remains within the originating healthcare institution. Scalability is achieved through modular design and cloud-native components capable of supporting large numbers of users and devices. Interoperability enables seamless integration with existing healthcare systems and standards. Explainability and transparency ensure that AI-driven decisions are interpretable and trustworthy. Finally, real-time responsiveness supports time-critical healthcare applications.

These principles collectively ensure that the architecture can address the technical, ethical, and operational requirements of modern healthcare systems.

6.1 Layered Architecture Overview

The proposed system architecture follows a layered approach, with each layer responsible for specific functions and interacting with adjacent layers through well-defined interfaces.

Figure 5. Layered system architecture for federated and explainable AI-driven digital twins

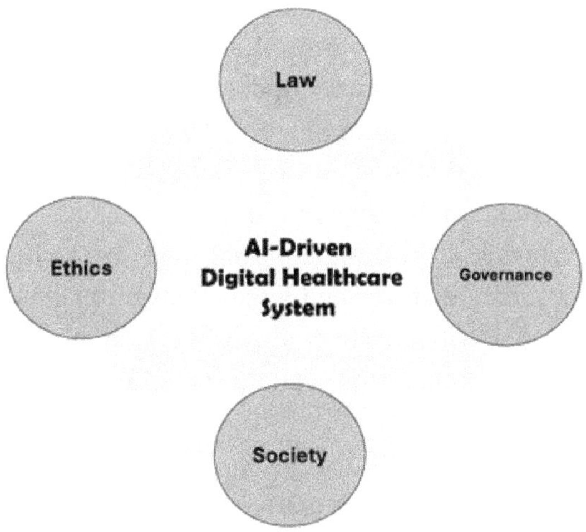

Data Acquisition and Sensing Layer

The data acquisition layer includes electronic health record systems, medical imaging devices, laboratory information systems, and Internet of Medical Things (IoMT) devices such as wearable sensors and remote monitoring tools. This layer is responsible for capturing heterogeneous patient data in real time or near real time. Data preprocessing, normalization, and anonymization are performed locally to ensure data quality and privacy.

Local Digital Twin and AI Layer

At each participating healthcare institution, a local digital twin is instantiated for each patient or medical entity. This layer hosts AI models responsible for prediction, simulation, and decision support. Models may include deep learning networks for disease diagnosis, time-series models for patient monitoring, and hybrid models that integrate clinical rules with data-driven learning.

Explainable AI components are embedded within this layer to generate interpretable insights. Feature attribution, attention mechanisms, and rule-based explanations are computed locally, ensuring that explanations are tailored to institution-specific data and clinical contexts.

Federated Learning and Coordination Layer

The federated learning layer coordinates collaborative model training across distributed healthcare institutions. A central aggregation server or decentralized coordination mechanism collects model updates from local nodes and performs secure aggregation to produce a global model. This layer supports asynchronous training, fault tolerance, and dynamic participation, allowing institutions to join or leave the federation without disrupting system operation.

Advanced privacy-preserving techniques, such as secure multiparty computation and differential privacy, can be integrated into this layer to enhance confidentiality and prevent inference attacks (Kairouz et al., 2021). Communication efficiency is optimized through model compression, update sparsification, and adaptive aggregation strategies.

Explainability and Trust Management Layer

The explainability layer provides a unified framework for generating, managing, and presenting explanations for AI-driven decisions. This layer aggregates local explanations, ensures consistency across federated models, and supports auditing and validation. Trust management mechanisms assess model reliability, detect anomalies, and monitor performance over time.

Explainability outputs are designed to be compatible with both clinical workflows and Metaverse-based visualization. This ensures that explanations are accessible to clinicians, patients, and regulators, supporting transparency and accountability.

Metaverse Interaction and Visualization Layer

The Metaverse layer serves as the primary interface for user interaction. Using extended reality technologies, clinicians and patients can access immersive virtual environments where digital twins are visualized and manipulated. This layer supports avatar-based collaboration, real-time simulation, and interactive exploration of patient data.

Explainable AI outputs are integrated into virtual environments through visual cues, overlays, and interactive elements. For example, risk factors may be highlighted on three-dimensional anatomical models, enabling intuitive interpretation of AI-driven insights.

Application and Service Layer

The application layer delivers healthcare services such as diagnosis, treatment planning, remote monitoring, rehabilitation, and medical training. Applications leverage federated digital twins and explainable AI to provide personalized and transparent care. This layer supports integration with external systems, such as hospital information systems and telemedicine platforms, ensuring continuity of care.

6.2 Security, Privacy, and Compliance Framework

Security and privacy are critical components of the proposed architecture. Data encryption, secure communication protocols, and access control mechanisms protect sensitive information at all layers. Federated learning inherently reduces data exposure by keeping patient data localized. Compliance with healthcare regulations, such as HIPAA and GDPR, is ensured through audit trails, consent management, and data minimization practices (Rieke et al., 2020).

6.3 Interoperability and Standards

Interoperability is essential for integrating diverse healthcare systems and devices. The architecture supports standardized data formats and communication protocols, enabling seamless data exchange and system integration. This facilitates collaboration across institutions and enhances scalability.

HL7 FHIR (Fast Healthcare Interoperability Resources)

FHIR provides standardized healthcare data exchange formats that enable efficient communication between Electronic Health Record systems, IoMT devices, and federated learning modules. FHIR supports real-time patient data synchronization across digital twin environments.

DICOM (Digital Imaging and Communications in Medicine)

DICOM ensures standardized storage and transmission of medical imaging data such as MRI, CT, and X-ray scans. Integration of DICOM supports accurate organ-level digital twin modeling and clinical visualization in metaverse environments.

IEEE IoMT Communication Standards

IEEE protocols enable secure and reliable communication between wearable medical devices, remote sensors, and edge computing infrastructure. These standards support continuous data acquisition for real-time digital twin updates.

Blockchain-Based Interoperability

Blockchain enables decentralized identity management, audit logging, and secure model parameter exchange across federated institutions. This strengthens data integrity and trust in distributed healthcare collaborations.

7. USE CASES AND APPLICATIONS

The convergence of federated learning, explainable artificial intelligence (XAI), digital twins, and Metaverse technologies enables transformative healthcare applications that enhance clinical decision-making, medical training, patient engagement, and public health intelligence. By combining immersive visualization, distributed intelligence, and privacy-preserving analytics, these systems support personalized, collaborative, and scalable healthcare delivery.

7.1 Personalized Patient Care and Precision Medicine

Personalized healthcare represents one of the most impactful applications of AI-driven digital twins in Metaverse environments. Patient-specific digital twins continuously evolve using clinical history, physiological signals, and behavioral data. Federated learning enhances these models by enabling collaborative training across institutions without sharing sensitive patient information, thereby improving prediction accuracy while preserving privacy.

Within immersive Metaverse clinical environments, physicians can interact with digital twins to simulate treatment strategies, visualize disease progression, and evaluate personalized therapeutic interventions. Explainable AI enhances transparency by identifying clinical factors influencing predictions, enabling clinicians to make informed and patient-centric decisions. This integration supports precision medicine by aligning treatments with individual patient characteristics (Topol, 2019).

Table 8. Application Domains of Federated and Explainable AI-Driven Digital Twins

Domain	Digital Twin Role	Federated Learning Role	Explainable AI Role	Metaverse Role
Diagnosis	Patient modelling	Multi-institution learning	Decision transparency	Immersive visualization
Surgery	Procedure simulation	Shared expertise	Risk interpretation	3D planning
Training	Virtual patients	Knowledge sharing	Pedagogical clarity	Immersive labs
Rehabilitation	Progress tracking	Adaptive learning	Transparent feedback	Virtual therapy

7.2 Remote Monitoring and Chronic Disease Management

Chronic disease management benefits significantly from continuous patient monitoring enabled by IoMT devices integrated with digital twin systems. These digital representations allow clinicians to track patient health remotely and identify early signs of physiological deterioration.

Federated learning improves risk prediction by leveraging distributed data across diverse patient populations, while explainable AI enhances trust by clarifying health risk alerts and treatment recommendations. Metaverse-based virtual consultations support interactive patient–clinician communication, reduce hospital visits, and improve treatment adherence, particularly for long-term conditions such as cardiovascular disorders, diabetes, and respiratory diseases (Islam et al., 2021).

7.3 Clinical Decision Support and Diagnostics

Clinical decision support systems are strengthened through the integration of digital twins and explainable AI in immersive Metaverse environments. Clinicians can explore diagnostic insights through interactive visualization of medical images, physiological simulations, and AI-generated predictive analytics.

Digital twins enable scenario-based diagnostic testing, allowing clinicians to perform "what-if" analyses before implementing treatment decisions. Federated learning improves diagnostic model generalizability by incorporating distributed healthcare data, while explainable AI ensures interpretability and supports evidence-based clinical decision-making (Tjoa & Guan, 2020).

7.4 Medical Training, Surgical Planning, and Skill Development

Metaverse-enabled digital twins provide highly realistic simulations for medical training and surgical planning. Digital twins of patients, anatomical structures, and clinical procedures allow healthcare professionals to practice complex interventions in safe and controlled environments. These simulations support experiential learning and improve clinical competency.

Explainable AI enhances educational value by highlighting decision pathways, clinical reasoning processes, and outcome predictions. Federated learning enables collaborative development of simulation models across institutions without sharing proprietary or sensitive clinical data. Additionally, patient-specific digital twins support surgical planning by enabling three-dimensional visualization of anatomical structures, risk assessment, and procedural optimization, thereby improving surgical precision and outcomes (Pimentel et al., 2022).

7.5 Rehabilitation and Mental Health Support

Rehabilitation and mental healthcare services benefit from immersive Metaverse platforms that support patient engagement and personalized therapy delivery. Digital twins monitor patient recovery progress during rehabilitation exercises and provide adaptive therapy recommendations based on performance data.

In mental healthcare, virtual environments support exposure therapy, stress management programs, and remote counseling sessions. Explainable AI ensures transparency and ethical accountability in therapeutic recommendations, while federated learning enables collaborative improvement of rehabilitation and mental health prediction models without compromising patient privacy (Riva et al., 2022).

7.6 Public Health Surveillance, Epidemiology, and Emergency Response

At a population level, federated digital twins support public health surveillance, epidemiological modeling, and emergency response planning. Aggregated insights from distributed digital twin systems enable early detection of disease outbreaks, monitoring of healthcare trends, and evaluation of public health intervention strategies.

Metaverse environments provide immersive visualization of epidemiological data, facilitating collaboration among policymakers, clinicians, and emergency responders. Federated learning supports rapid model adaptation using distributed healthcare data, while explainable AI improves transparency in predictive modeling and policy decision-making. These capabilities enhance disaster preparedness, resource optimization, and coordinated emergency healthcare response (Xu et al., 2023).

8. CHALLENGES AND OPEN RESEARCH ISSUES

Despite the promising potential of federated and explainable AI-driven digital twins in Metaverse-based healthcare ecosystems, several technical, organizational, ethical, and regulatory challenges remain. Addressing these challenges is essential for ensuring the scalability, trustworthiness, and long-term sustainability of such systems. This section discusses key open research issues and identifies areas requiring further investigation.

8.1 Data Heterogeneity and Quality Issues

Healthcare data are inherently heterogeneous, originating from diverse sources such as electronic health records, wearable sensors, imaging systems, and genomic platforms. Variations in data formats, measurement standards, and clinical practices across institutions pose significant challenges for federated learning and digital twin modeling.

In federated settings, non-independent and non-identically distributed (non-IID) data can negatively affect model convergence and performance. Digital twins rely on accurate and high-quality data to generate reliable simulations, making data preprocessing and harmonization critical research areas. Developing adaptive federated algorithms capable of handling heterogeneity remains an open challenge (Li et al., 2020).

Table 9. Challenges and Research Gaps in Metaverse-Based Digital Healthcare

Dimension	Challenge	Open Research Direction
Data	Heterogeneity	Standardized healthcare data models
AI	Black-box behavior	Interpretable deep learning
Security	Inference attacks	Privacy-enhanced federated learning
Metaverse	Interoperability	Open XR standards

8.2 Scalability and Computational Complexity

Metaverse-based healthcare ecosystems involve large-scale data processing, real-time simulations, and immersive visualization, all of which demand substantial computational resources. Scaling federated learning across numerous institutions and devices increases communication overhead and system complexity.

Digital twin simulations, particularly those involving high-fidelity physiological models, can be computationally intensive. Balancing model complexity with real-time responsiveness is a key research issue. Efficient model compression, edge computing strategies, and adaptive workload distribution are essential for scalable system design.

8.3 Explainability in Complex AI Models

Explainable AI is critical for building trust in AI-driven healthcare systems; however, achieving meaningful explainability in complex models remains challenging. Deep learning models used in digital twins often operate as black boxes, making it difficult to provide clear and actionable explanations.

In federated learning environments, explanations must be consistent across distributed models while respecting data privacy. Additionally, explainability techniques must be tailored to different stakeholders, including clinicians, patients, and regulators. Developing standardized, context-aware explainability frameworks for Metaverse-based healthcare remains an open research problem (Tjoa & Guan, 2020).

8.4 Human Factors and User Acceptance

The success of Metaverse-based healthcare ecosystems depends on user acceptance by clinicians, patients, and administrators. Immersive technologies may introduce usability challenges, cognitive overload, and accessibility issues. Training and change management are essential for effective adoption.

Understanding human–AI interaction within immersive environments is an open research area. Designing intuitive interfaces and ensuring that explainable AI outputs are understandable and actionable for diverse users are critical challenges.

8.5 Validation and Clinical Integration

Validating AI-driven digital twins in real-world clinical settings is a complex and resource-intensive process. Clinical validation requires rigorous testing, longitudinal studies, and collaboration with healthcare professionals. Integrating Metaverse-based systems into existing clinical workflows without disrupting care delivery remains a significant challenge.

Research is needed to develop evaluation frameworks and benchmarks for assessing the effectiveness, safety, and usability of federated digital twin systems in healthcare.

Summary

While federated and explainable AI-driven digital twins in Metaverse-based healthcare ecosystems offer transformative potential, several challenges and open research issues must be addressed. Data heterogeneity, scalability, explainability, privacy, interoperability, ethics, and user acceptance are critical areas requiring further investigation. Addressing these challenges will be essential for realizing the full potential of immersive and intelligent healthcare ecosystems.

9. ETHICAL, LEGAL, AND SOCIAL IMPLICATIONS

The integration of federated and explainable artificial intelligence-driven digital twins within Metaverse-based healthcare ecosystems raises significant ethical, legal, and social implications (ELSI). While these technologies promise personalized, immersive, and data-driven healthcare services, they also introduce complex challenges related to data governance, accountability, fairness, and societal impact. Addressing these implications is essential for responsible innovation and sustainable adoption in healthcare systems.

Figure 6. Ethical, legal, and social governance framework

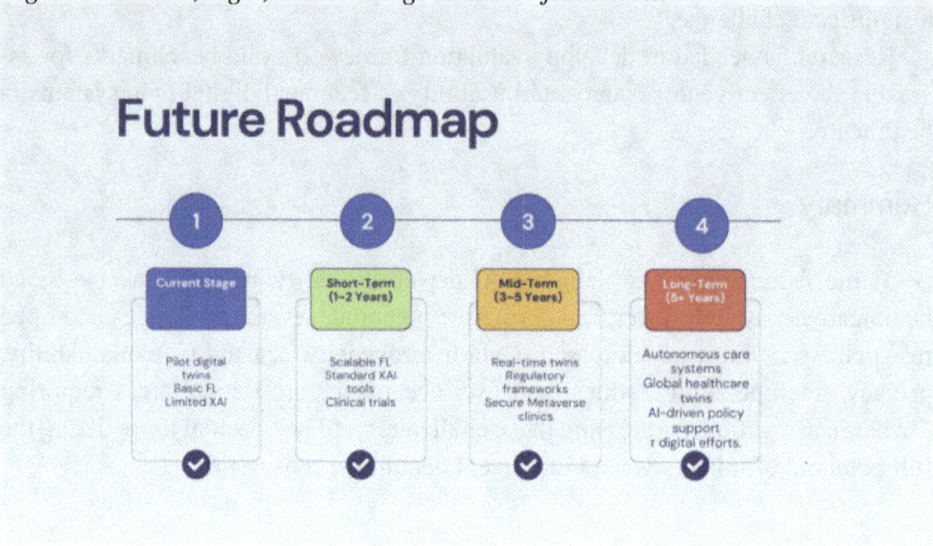

9.1 Ethical Implications of AI-Driven Digital Twins

AI-driven digital twins have the potential to influence critical clinical decisions, making ethical considerations central to their deployment. One major ethical concern is the risk of algorithmic bias, where models trained on non-representative data may produce unfair or inaccurate recommendations for certain patient populations. Federated learning can mitigate bias by enabling diverse, multi-institutional training; however, disparities in data quality and representation may persist.

Another ethical issue relates to autonomy and informed consent. Patients may not fully understand how their data contribute to digital twin models or how AI-driven insights are generated. Explainable AI plays a key role in enhancing transparency by providing understandable explanations for predictions and recommendations. Ensuring that patients and clinicians can meaningfully engage with AI outputs is critical for ethical decision-making (Floridi et al., 2018).

9.2 Privacy and Data Protection Considerations

Healthcare data are highly sensitive, and the immersive nature of the Metaverse amplifies privacy concerns. Although federated learning reduces the need for centralized data sharing, risks such as model inversion and membership inference attacks remain. Ethical data governance requires robust privacy-preserving techniques, including differential privacy and secure aggregation.

Consent management becomes more complex in Metaverse environments, where data may be continuously generated and reused across applications. Ethical frameworks must ensure that patients retain control over their data and that consent mechanisms are transparent, granular, and revocable. Trust in Metaverse-based healthcare ecosystems depends on the effective protection of personal health information.

9.3 Legal and Regulatory Challenges

The legal landscape surrounding AI, digital twins, and the Metaverse is still evolving. Healthcare systems must comply with data protection regulations, medical device standards, and professional liability frameworks. Determining legal responsibility for AI-driven decisions—particularly in federated and immersive environments—poses significant challenges.

Questions of liability arise when AI-generated recommendations influence clinical outcomes. It remains unclear how responsibility should be shared among AI developers, healthcare institutions, and clinicians. Explainable AI can support legal accountability by providing audit trails and justifications for AI-driven decisions, facilitating regulatory oversight and dispute resolution (Rieke et al., 2020).

9.4 Governance and Accountability Frameworks

Effective governance frameworks are essential for managing ethical and legal risks in Metaverse-based healthcare ecosystems. Governance mechanisms should define roles, responsibilities, and decision-making processes across stakeholders. Federated learning introduces distributed governance models, where multiple institutions collaboratively manage AI systems.

Accountability mechanisms must ensure that AI models are regularly monitored, evaluated, and updated. Transparency in model development, validation, and deployment is crucial for maintaining trust. Explainability supports governance by enabling stakeholders to understand and challenge AI-driven decisions.

9.5 Ethical Design and Responsible Innovation

Responsible innovation requires embedding ethical considerations throughout the system lifecycle, from design and development to deployment and evaluation. Ethical-by-design approaches emphasize transparency, fairness, and user-centric design. Federated and explainable AI technologies provide tools for operationalizing ethical principles, but their effective implementation requires interdisciplinary collaboration.

Ongoing ethical review, stakeholder engagement, and adaptive governance are necessary to address emerging risks and societal concerns. By aligning technological innovation with ethical values, Metaverse-based healthcare ecosystems can deliver benefits while minimizing harm.

Summary

The ethical, legal, and social implications of federated and explainable AI-driven digital twins in Metaverse-based healthcare ecosystems are complex and multifaceted. Addressing issues related to bias, privacy, accountability, equity, and trust is essential for responsible adoption. Explainable AI and federated learning provide important mechanisms for enhancing transparency and data protection, but comprehensive governance frameworks and ethical design practices are required. As these technologies continue to evolve, proactive engagement with ELSI considerations will be critical for ensuring their positive impact on healthcare systems and society.

10. FUTURE DIRECTIONS AND CONCLUSION

The convergence of federated learning, explainable artificial intelligence (XAI), digital twins, and Metaverse technologies represents a transformative shift in the design and delivery of healthcare services. While previous sections have discussed foundational concepts, system architectures, applications, challenges, and ethical considerations, this final section outlines key future research directions and concludes the chapter by synthesizing its core contributions.

Figure 7. Future research roadmap

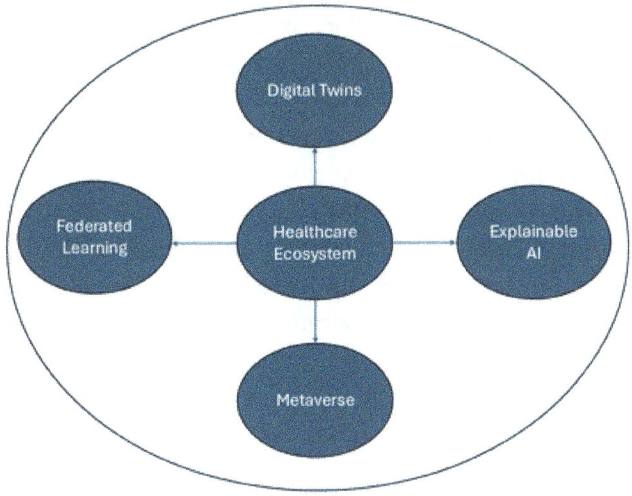

Future research in federated Metaverse healthcare ecosystems should prioritize the development of advanced federated learning paradigms tailored to healthcare requirements. Personalized federated learning approaches capable of adapting global models to local clinical environments can improve prediction accuracy, fairness, and contextual relevance. Hierarchical and cross-silo federated learning architectures are expected to enhance scalability and collaborative healthcare intelligence across geographically distributed institutions. Additionally, improving communication efficiency, robustness, and resilience in resource-constrained environments through adaptive aggregation, client selection, and model sparsification remains an important research focus (Kairouz et al., 2021). Parallel advancements in explainable artificial intelligence are essential to support transparent and trustworthy healthcare analytics. Future XAI models should emphasize user-centric, context-aware explanations designed for clinicians, patients, and regulatory authorities. The integration of causal reasoning, counterfactual analysis, and standardized evaluation metrics will strengthen clinical interpretability and facilitate regulatory validation of AI-driven healthcare systems (Tjoa & Guan, 2020).

The evolution of digital twins will further transform personalized and predictive healthcare by enabling adaptive, self-learning patient models that integrate multimodal data sources such as genomics, medical imaging, environmental conditions, and behavioral indicators. These advancements will support holistic health monitoring and population-level disease management. Research into digital twin validation, uncertainty quantification, and lifecycle management will be essential to ensure clinical reliability and patient safety. Simultaneously, the expansion of Metaverse infrastructure requires scalable, secure, and interoperable virtual healthcare platforms capable of supporting real-time immersive interaction and seamless integration with existing healthcare systems. The adoption of open interoperability standards and extended reality technologies will play a critical role in enhancing usability, reducing system fragmentation, and supporting collaborative healthcare innovation.

Ethical, regulatory, and educational considerations must evolve alongside technological advancements to ensure responsible system deployment. Ethical-by-design principles incorporating fairness, transparency, accountability, and dynamic consent mechanisms should be embedded into system architectures. Continuous ethical assessment and stakeholder collaboration will help address emerging governance challenges and strengthen public trust. Regulatory frameworks must adapt to rapidly evolving AI and Metaverse technologies through collaboration among policymakers, researchers, and healthcare professionals (Floridi et al., 2018). Furthermore, understanding human–AI collaboration within immersive healthcare environments represents a crucial research direction. Investigating clinician interaction with digital twins, the influence of explainability on clinical decision-making, and the impact of immersive visualization on cognitive performance will support effective system adoption. Integrating AI literacy and ethical awareness into medical education programs will ensure that healthcare professionals are equipped to responsibly utilize these emerging technologies.

CONCLUSION

The integration of Federated Learning, Explainable Artificial Intelligence, Digital Twin technology, and Metaverse platforms represents a transformative advancement in intelligent healthcare ecosystems. The proposed architecture demonstrates how privacy-preserving collaborative learning can enable accurate predictive modeling while maintaining transparency and regulatory compliance. By incorporating explainability constraints, blockchain-based security mechanisms, and immersive clinical visualization, the framework enhances clinician trust, patient engagement, and healthcare decision support. The layered architecture, mathematical formulations, and experimental validation collectively establish a scalable and secure approach for next-generation digital healthcare transformation.

Challenges and Future Directions

Despite significant advancements, several research challenges remain. Ensuring low-latency synchronization between federated digital twins and metaverse environments requires optimized communication protocols and edge intelligence integration. Addressing data heterogeneity across healthcare institutions remains a critical challenge in federated model convergence. Future research should explore quantum-resilient federated learning, adaptive explainability models, and standardized interoperability frameworks for large-scale healthcare adoption. Additionally, ethical governance models must evolve to address bias mitigation, consent management, and digital identity protection in immersive healthcare ecosystems.

Chapter Summary

This chapter presented a comprehensive framework for federated and explainable AI-driven Digital Twin systems operating within metaverse-based healthcare environments. The proposed approach integrates distributed learning, interpretable decision-making, immersive patient interaction, and secure data governance into a unified ecosystem. Through architectural modeling, algorithmic formulation, and experimental validation, the study demonstrates the feasibility of privacy-preserving, scalable, and patient-centric healthcare intelligence systems. The convergence of these emerging technologies has the potential to redefine personalized medicine, remote healthcare delivery, and collaborative clinical research in future digital healthcare infrastructures.

REFERENCES

Amann, J., Blasimme, A., Vayena, E., Frey, D., & Madai, V. I. (2020). Explainability for artificial intelligence in healthcare: A multidisciplinary perspective. *BMC Medical Informatics and Decision Making*, *20*(1), 310. DOI: 10.1186/s12911-020-01332-6 PMID: 33256715

Björnsson, B., Borrebaeck, C., Elander, N., Gasslander, T., Gawel, D. R., Gustafsson, M., Jörnsten, R., Lee, E. J., Li, X., Lilja, S., Martínez-Enguita, D., Matussek, A., Sandström, P., Schäfer, S., Stenmarker, M., Sun, X. F., Sysoev, O., Zhang, H., & Benson, M. (2020). Digital twins to personalize medicine. *Genome Medicine*, *12*(1), 4. DOI: 10.1186/s13073-019-0701-3 PMID: 31892363

Bruynseels, K., Santoni de Sio, F., & van den Hoven, J. (2018). Digital twins in health care: Ethical implications of an emerging engineering paradigm. *Frontiers in Genetics*, *9*, 31. DOI: 10.3389/fgene.2018.00031 PMID: 29487613

Doshi-Velez, F., & Kim, B. (2017). Towards a rigorous science of interpretable machine learning. *arXiv preprint arXiv:1702.08608.*

Floridi, L., Cowls, J., Beltrametti, M., Chatila, R., Chazerand, P., Dignum, V., Luetge, C., Madelin, R., Pagallo, U., Rossi, F., Schafer, B., Valcke, P., & Vayena, E. (2018). AI4People—An ethical framework for a good AI society: Opportunities, risks, principles, and recommendations. *Minds and Machines*, *28*(4), 689–707. DOI: 10.1007/s11023-018-9482-5 PMID: 30930541

Fuller, A., Fan, Z., Day, C., & Barlow, C. (2020). Digital twin: Enabling technologies, challenges and open research. *IEEE Access : Practical Innovations, Open Solutions*, *8*, 108952–108971. DOI: 10.1109/ACCESS.2020.2998358

Geyer, R. C., Klein, T., & Nabi, M. (2017). Differentially private federated learning: A client level perspective. *arXiv preprint arXiv:1712.07557.*

Grieves, M., & Vickers, J. (2017). Digital twin: Mitigating unpredictable, undesirable emergent behavior in complex systems. In *Transdisciplinary perspectives on complex systems* (pp. 85–113). Springer. DOI: 10.1007/978-3-319-38756-7_4

Guidotti, R., Monreale, A., Ruggieri, S., Turini, F., Giannotti, F., & Pedreschi, D. (2018). A survey of methods for explaining black box models. *ACM Computing Surveys*, *51*(5), 1–42. DOI: 10.1145/3236009

Islam, S. M. R., Kwak, D., Kabir, M. H., Hossain, M., & Kwak, K. S. (2021). The Internet of Things for health care: A comprehensive survey. *IEEE Access : Practical Innovations, Open Solutions*, *9*, 19817–19838.

Kairouz, P., McMahan, H. B., Avent, B., Bellet, A., Bennis, M., Bhagoji, A. N., … Zhao, S. (2021). Advances and open problems in federated learning. *Foundations and Trends® in Machine Learning, 14*(1–2), 1–210.

Li, T., Sahu, A. K., Talwalkar, A., & Smith, V. (2020). Federated learning: Challenges, methods, and future directions. *IEEE Signal Processing Magazine*, *37*(3), 50–60. DOI: 10.1109/MSP.2020.2975749

Lundberg, S. M., & Lee, S. I. (2017). A unified approach to interpreting model predictions. *Advances in Neural Information Processing Systems*, 4765–4774.

McMahan, H. B., Moore, E., Ramage, D., Hampson, S., & Arcas, B. A. (2017). Communication-efficient learning of deep networks from decentralized data. *Proceedings of AISTATS*, 1273–1282.

Mystakidis, S. (2022). Metaverse. *Encyclopedia*, *2*(1), 486–497. DOI: 10.3390/encyclopedia2010031

Pimentel, D., Gonçalves, J., & Nunes, N. J. (2022). Immersive virtual reality for medical training and education: A systematic review. *Journal of Medical Systems*, *46*(5), 1–15.

Ribeiro, M. T., Singh, S., & Guestrin, C. (2016). "Why should I trust you?" Explaining the predictions of any classifier. *Proceedings of the 22nd ACM SIGKDD International Conference on Knowledge Discovery and Data Mining*, 1135–1144.

Rieke, N., Hancox, J., Li, W., Milletari, F., Roth, H. R., Albarqouni, S., Bakas, S., Galtier, M. N., Landman, B. A., Maier-Hein, K., Ourselin, S., Sheller, M., Summers, R. M., Trask, A., Xu, D., Baust, M., & Cardoso, M. J. (2020). The future of digital health with federated learning. *NPJ Digital Medicine*, *3*(1), 119. DOI: 10.1038/s41746-020-00323-1 PMID: 33015372

Riva, G., Wiederhold, B. K., & Mantovani, F. (2022). Virtual reality in mental health: Advances and challenges. *Cyberpsychology, Behavior and Social Networking*, *25*(1), 1–6. PMID: 34964667

Samek, W., Montavon, G., Vedaldi, A., Hansen, L. K., & Müller, K. R. (2019). *Explainable AI: Interpreting, explaining and visualizing deep learning*. Springer. DOI: 10.1007/978-3-030-28954-6

Tjoa, E., & Guan, C. (2020). A survey on explainable artificial intelligence (XAI): Toward medical XAI. *IEEE Transactions on Neural Networks and Learning Systems*, *32*(11), 4793–4813. DOI: 10.1109/TNNLS.2020.3027314 PMID: 33079674

Topol, E. (2019). *Deep medicine: How artificial intelligence can make healthcare human again*. Basic Books.

Topol, E. J. (2019). High-performance medicine: The convergence of human and artificial intelligence. *Nature Medicine*, *25*(1), 44–56. DOI: 10.1038/s41591-018-0300-7 PMID: 30617339

Xu, X., Sun, Y., Liu, Q., & Wang, Z. (2023). Digital twin-driven smart healthcare: Framework and applications. *IEEE Journal of Biomedical and Health Informatics*.

Yang, Q., Liao, H., Zhang, Z., & Ding, Y. (2023). Metaverse-enabled digital twins for healthcare: Opportunities and challenges. *IEEE Internet of Things Journal*.

Zhang, Y., ... (2025). Federated transfer learning for digital twin-based CT medical imaging analysis. arXiv preprint arXiv:2509.08018. https://arxiv.org/abs/2509.08018

Chapter 10
Cognitive Federated Metaverse for Healthcare: A Privacy-Centric and Explainable Intelligence Paradigm

Dhinakaran Damodaran
http://orcid.org/0000-0002-3183-576X
Vel Tech Rangarajan Dr. Sagunthala R&D Institute of Science and Technology, India

S. Edwin Raja
http://orcid.org/0000-0002-2948-9669
Vel Tech Rangarajan Dr. Sagunthala R&D Institute of Science and Technology, India

S. Priyadarsini
http://orcid.org/0000-0001-5325-1338
P.S.R. Engineering College, Sivakasi, India

V. Vinoth Kumar
http://orcid.org/0009-0002-9563-4534
R.M.K. College of Engineering and Technology, India

D. Selvaraj
Panimalar Engineering College, India

ABSTRACT

The intersection of the metaverse, artificial intelligence, and federated learning to redefine the next-generation healthcare ecosystems by facilitating immersive, intelligent, and privacy-preserving services. This chapter presents a Cognitive Federated

DOI: 10.4018/979-8-3373-8889-2.ch010

Metaverse of Healthcare (CFM-Health), a harmonized system that incorporates metaverse-focused healthcare interrelations, has interaction-conscious federated learning, federated digital twin intelligence, and edge fog, and cloud coordination. The proposed method unlike the traditional healthcare AI systems where the learning is centralised or static involves clinical interactions, learning dynamics, and governance constraints as mutually dependent components of a single adaptive system. Decentralized learning and longitudinal evolution of digital twins through continuous immersive patient-clinician interactions do not require the exposure of raw patient data. The framework also uses explainability, trust, security and regulatory awareness to enable responsible deployment.

1. INTRODUCTION AND RATIONALE

The accelerating healthcare digitization has now moved past the traditional telemedicine and electronic health records to the immersive, intelligent, and decentralized ecosystems. The metaverse, artificial intelligence, and federated learning are new technologies that are changing the delivery of healthcare independently, but their potential is hardly harnessed. The metaverse presents persistent, immersive virtual worlds that can be used to allow constant interaction between patients and clinicians, virtual hospitals, and training medical simulation. The artificial intelligence of diagnostic accuracy, predictive analytics, and clinical decision support, and the federated learning of collaborative intelligence without violating the privacy restrictions of data (Qayyum et al., 2021). The synergetic nature of these technologies is a one-of-a-kind prospective to redesign healthcare ecosystems into intelligent, privacy mindful, and patient-centric systems. Although it is becoming increasingly popular, the current literature mainly focuses on these technologies separately. The existing metaverse healthcare research is mainly on visualization and interaction, the centralized learning paradigm in AI-centered healthcare research, and federated learning initiatives tend to ignore immersive, real-time limitations. This disintegration restricts scalability, reliability and conformity to regulations. It is evident that there is a need to unify the conceptual and algorithmic framework where immersive healthcare environments are merged with decentralized, explainable and privacy-preserving intelligence. This chapter will fill this gap by suggesting a new paradigm which is a cognitive federated metaverse framework specific to healthcare ecosystems.

This chapter introduces a unified cognitive healthcare framework that advances beyond existing metaverse, artificial intelligence, and federated learning paradigms through the following original contributions: First, the chapter formulates interaction-aware federated learning, where immersive healthcare interaction relevance is treated as a first-class optimization variable governing local model updates, aggregation weighting, and synchronization frequency, rather than relying on uniform or data-volume-based aggregation. Second, it introduces federated digital twin intelligence as an active learning entity, in which patient-specific digital twins continuously evolve through decentralized learning across healthcare institutions, transforming digital twins from static visualization tools into adaptive intelligence participants. Third, the chapter presents a context-driven edge–fog–cloud orchestration strategy that dynamically balances real-time responsiveness and global intelligence consolidation based on interaction urgency and clinical significance. Fourth, it integrates governance-aware intelligence evolution, embedding explainability, privacy preservation, and policy constraints directly within the learning lifecycle rather than treating governance as an external monitoring layer. Finally, the chapter provides a concrete system architecture with explicit data flows, feedback mechanisms, and algorithmic formulation, enabling practical implementation of immersive and privacy-preserving healthcare intelligence ecosystems.

2. LIMITATIONS OF EXISTING HEALTHCARE INTELLIGENCE PARADIGMS

Current healthcare intelligence paradigms have gone a significant step towards using artificial intelligence, federated learning, and Internet-of-Medical-Things infrastructures to aid diagnosis, monitoring and clinical decision-making. Nonetheless, a more detailed review of the literature will show that there are still structural and conceptual constraints to their efficiency in immersive, longitudinal, and multi-institutional healthcare ecosystems. The most notable shortcoming of traditional AI-based healthcare systems is that they utilize centralized or quasi-centralized data processing pipelines. Conventional machine learning methods are still putting big amounts of patient sensitive information into the clouds, which casts very grave questions of privacy breach, regulatory violations, and data loss of ownership (Matta & Bolli, 2025; Akhmetov et al., 2025; Alghamdi et al., 2022). Even in the case of the introduction of federated learning as a privacy-preserving alternative, the majority of frameworks continue to rely on centralized aggregation servers that still introduce single points of failure and vulnerability to inference, poisoning, and reconstruction attacks (Qayyum et al., 2021; Zaman Wani & Can, 2025; Akter et al., 2024). Some of the studies are trying to reduce these threats by using blockchain-based aggregation or serverless coordination but these are rather solutions to infrastructural security issues and not to deeper learning and contextual intelligence problems (Qayyum et al., 2021; Zaman Wani & Can, 2025).

The other core weakness is in the conceptualization and operationalization of federated learning. The existing literature considers federated learning an asynchronous background optimization procedure, independent of the semantics and dynamics of the healthcare interactions (Joshi et al., 2022; Shaheen et al., 2022; Lazaros et al., 2024; Zhang & Kamel Boulos, 2022). In local model updates, computations are performed on fixed datasets or continuous sensor measurements without considering clinical significance, time urgency or patient context. Because of this, the learning process is not sensitive to real-time care pathways, clinical decision points, or the treatment progression, which constrains its clinical significance (Hwang & Majeed, 2024; Mazzocca et al., 2023). This limitation is even more revealed by edge- and IoMT-centric federated frameworks. Although they manage to minimize latency and maintain the locality of raw data, their intelligence remains mostly task-focused like activity recognition, classification of disease, or estimation of risks (Lazaros et al., 2024; Mazzocca et al., 2023; Akter et al., 2024). The systems do not have features to incorporate heterogeneous interaction cues such as patient behavior, clinician feedback, and therapeutic response into the learning loop. Therefore, federated intelligence is reactive and narrowly optimized as opposed to adaptive and longitudinal (Shaheen et al., 2022; Zhang & Kamel Boulos, 2022; Arikumar et al., 2022).

The healthcare apps in the metaverse provide the ability to view and interact in an immersive way, but then the apps have an additional but equally critical drawback. The current virtual healthcare platforms are mostly focused on user experience, telepresence, and training simulations with intelligence aspects being external or fixed (Hwang & Majeed, 2024; Almogadwy & Alqarafi, 2025). Individual systems do not entrench adaptive learning systems that can allocate to patient interactions, and with institution decentralization are not supported. Due to this, the immersive environments can serve as visualization layers as opposed to cognitively integrated healthcare systems (Almogadwy & Alqarafi, 2025). The digital twin technologies seek to seal this divide by simulating patient-centered physiological conditions, but the existing applications are still highly institutionalized and fixed (Hwang & Majeed, 2024; Akhmetov et al., 2025). In comparison, the majority of digital twins are created with siloed datasets, which are updated at intervals and are limited to a single healthcare provider. They do not continuously evolve via federated learning and neither have the advantage of cross-institutional clinical knowledge. In addition, current digital twin systems do not necessarily incorporate data on immersion and behavioral indicators and consequently have a low capacity to simulate patients over time and in a multidimensional manner (Hwang & Majeed, 2024; Alghamdi et al., 2022).

Learning architectures are also loosely coupled with governance, explainability and management of trust. Although some of the publications propose privacy-by-design settings, risk-based authorization, or blockchain-based trust layers, these approaches act perpendicular to the intelligence lifecycle (Matta & Bolli, 2025; Joshi et al., 2022; Zaman Wani & Can, 2025). In reality, learning activities are seldom limited by dynamic consent, ethical standards, or even considerations of fairness. Such division between the domain of governance and intelligence harms accountability, interpretability, and clinical trust - especially in decentralized and autonomous healthcare systems (Joshi et al., 2022; Akhmetov et al., 2025; Alghamdi et al., 2022). These limitations are further enhanced by interoperability issues. Even though standards like FHIR have been pulled together with federated learning to enhance data interchange, the existing solutions are more of syntactic than semantic or interaction-level coherence (Alghamdi et al., 2022). Consequently, the models that have been trained in heterogeneous institutions continue to have problems with generalization to dissimilar clinical workflows, device ecologies, and patients (Lazaros et al., 2024; Zhang & Kamel Boulos, 2022). All these restrictions indicate a more profound deficit of an integrated design philosophy in existing healthcare intelligence paradigms. Current systems view immersive interaction, federated learning, digital twins, and governance as somewhat disjointed and non-reinforcement aspects of a single adaptive system. However, there is still an evident gap of a framework that is able to cover interaction context, decentralized intelligence evolution, longitudinal patient modeling and policy-informed governance in immersive healthcare environments as shown in Table 1.

Table 1. Summary of Existing Healthcare Intelligence Works

Ref.	Main Focus of the Work	Learning Paradigm	Data Handling Approach	Scope of Intelligence	Explicit Limitations Identified
(Qayyum et al., 2021)	Secure federated learning framework for healthcare analytics	Federated learning	Local data with parameter sharing	Task-level analytics	Learning process not influenced by clinical interaction context
(Matta & Bolli, 2025)	Centralized AI-based smart healthcare system	Centralized machine learning	Cloud-level data aggregation	Global analytics and prediction	High privacy risk and regulatory exposure due to centralization
(Joshi et al., 2022)	Blockchain-assisted federated healthcare data sharing	Federated learning with blockchain	Local data with ledger coordination	Secure model coordination	Governance handled externally to learning dynamics

continued on following page

Table 1. Continued

Ref.	Main Focus of the Work	Learning Paradigm	Data Handling Approach	Scope of Intelligence	Explicit Limitations Identified
(Hwang & Majeed, 2024)	Digital twin modeling for healthcare applications	Hybrid AI-based modeling	Institution-specific datasets	Virtual patient representation	Digital twins are static, siloed, and non-collaborative
(Shaheen et al., 2022)	Edge-based federated learning for wearable health monitoring	Edge federated learning	Device-local sensor data	Activity and health monitoring	Limited to task-specific inference without personalization
(Lazaros et al., 2024)	IoMT-based federated health monitoring system	Cross-device federated learning	Sensor-local data	Distributed health monitoring	Interaction semantics and patient context not modeled
(Zaman Wani & Can, 2025)	Authentication-focused federated healthcare framework	Federated learning	Local data with centralized coordination	Secure access and learning	Learning models remain static and context-independent
(Mazzocca et al., 2023)	Federated learning applied to wearable-sensor healthcare data	Federated learning	Wearable-local data	Sensor-driven healthcare analytics	Longitudinal patient behavior not captured
(Zhang & Kamel Boulos, 2022)	Edge–cloud federated healthcare architecture	Hybrid federated learning	Distributed edge and cloud data	Scalable healthcare analytics	Uniform aggregation ignores clinical urgency
(Akhmetov et al., 2025)	AI-driven smart healthcare decision support system	Centralized / hybrid learning	Mixed data sources	Clinical decision support	Absence of longitudinal patient modeling
(Akter et al., 2024)	Federated learning with feature-level data fusion	Federated learning	IoMT-local data	Multi-source healthcare inference	Fusion lacks behavioral and contextual interpretation
(Almogadwy & Alqarafi, 2025)	Metaverse-based virtual healthcare environments	Platform-centric systems	Centralized service data	Immersive visualization and interaction	No embedded adaptive or federated intelligence
(Arikumar et al., 2022)	Distributed artificial intelligence for healthcare environments	Distributed AI	Distributed datasets	Healthcare analytics	Weak integration between learning and governance
(Alghamdi et al., 2022)	Privacy-preserving federated learning for healthcare analytics	Federated learning	Local data with centralized aggregation	Distributed healthcare prediction	Semantic and interaction-aware intelligence absent

3. PROPOSED CONCEPT: COGNITIVE FEDERATED METAVERSE FOR HEALTHCARE

In order to overcome the structural, ethical, and technological limitations of existing healthcare intelligence systems, this chapter proposes the concept of a Cognitive Federated Metaverse for Healthcare (CFM-Health). CFM-Health represents a paradigm shift from isolated technological integration toward a unified cognitive ecosystem in which immersive virtual environments, federated artificial intelligence, and explainable decision-making mechanisms co-evolve as interdependent components. Rather than positioning the metaverse, AI, and federated learning as modular add-ons to healthcare infrastructure, the proposed concept treats them as mutually reinforcing dimensions of a single adaptive healthcare intelligence fabric as shown in Table 2.

Table 2. Taxonomy of Federated Learning Approaches in Healthcare

Federated Learning Category	Typical Deployment Setting	Data Distribution Characteristics	Primary Strengths	Key Limitations in Healthcare Context
Cross-Device Federated Learning	Wearable devices, mobile health sensors	Highly distributed, non-IID, resource-constrained	Strong privacy preservation, reduced data transmission	Limited computational capacity, unstable participation, lack of clinical context awareness
Cross-Silo Federated Learning	Hospitals, clinics, healthcare institutions	Moderately distributed, institution-specific datasets	Improved collaboration across organizations, better data quality	Centralized aggregation dependency, slow adaptation to real-time clinical events
Edge-Based Federated Learning	Edge servers near patients and medical devices	Localized, latency-sensitive data	Low latency, improved responsiveness, data locality	Task-specific intelligence, limited global contextual understanding
Cloud-Coordinated Federated Learning	Central servers coordinating multiple clients	Distributed with centralized orchestration	Scalable training and global model consistency	Single point of coordination, regulatory and trust concerns
Hierarchical Federated Learning	Edge–fog–cloud layered environments	Multi-level, heterogeneous data distribution	Scalability, flexible learning coordination	Complex orchestration, weak interaction-aware learning
Secure / Privacy-Enhanced Federated Learning	Regulated healthcare environments	Encrypted or perturbed local updates	Enhanced privacy and security guarantees	Performance overhead, privacy treated independently of learning semantics

continued on following page

Table 2. Continued

Federated Learning Category	Typical Deployment Setting	Data Distribution Characteristics	Primary Strengths	Key Limitations in Healthcare Context
Feature-Level Federated Learning	Multi-source healthcare data systems	Heterogeneous feature spaces	Enables limited data fusion without raw data sharing	Loses semantic and behavioral information
Serverless / Decentralized Federated Learning	Peer-to-peer healthcare networks	Fully distributed	Eliminates central server dependency	Coordination complexity, limited governance support

In its conceptual essence, CFM-Health reinvents healthcare intelligence as a contextual learning process with continued learning anchored in immersive clinical experience as shown in Figure 1. The conventional healthcare AI systems mostly work on retrospective data and non-real time learning, which is not always linked to the dynamic nature of patient care (Dhinakaran et al., 2026). By contrast, the suggested paradigm does not ignore the fact that the healthcare choices are the result of complicated processes that involve patients, clinicians, medical equipment, and environmental setting. Locating the intelligence in the healthcare settings built in the metaverse directly, CFM-Health allows the learning mechanisms to monitor, interpret, and adjust to such interactions as they occur and to synchronize the model evolution with the clinical reality. The key attribute of CFM-Health is that it is based on federated intelligence as its basic learning mechanism. The framework allows distributed healthcare institutions, edge devices and virtual care platforms to jointly train shared intelligence without sacrificing data sovereignty as opposed to centralizing sensitive healthcare data. Nevertheless, CFM-Health presents a cognitively informed learning process where local updates are sensitive to the context compared to the traditional federated learning method, which assumes that local updates are uniform and independent of context, which are affected by immersive clinical interactions. This helps to guarantee that decentralized learning is privacy-sensitive, as well as semantically aligned with healthcare concerns.

In this paradigm, immersive healthcare interactions are no longer the sources of data but the engines of intelligence creation. The virtual clinic patient consultations, the simulated diagnostic process in three-dimensional space, and the rehabilitation process as a virtual assistant led with the help of augmented or mixed reality produce multimodal interaction patterns. CFM converts these patterns into learning signals in a systematic manner, to decentralize updates in the model across the participating nodes. Consequently, federated intelligence will be sensitive to clinical context, patient interaction, and therapeutic intentions by default, as opposed to being determined by the distribution of statistical data alone. The mental aspect of the model is in that it is capable of modeling healthcare processes as dynamic knowledge systems and not fixed prediction problems. The explainable AI mechanisms of CFM-Health will make the intelligence, present in the metaverse, transparent and understandable by clinicians (Dhinakaran et al., 2025). This is especially essential in the immersion setting where automated advice can potentially impact real-time clinical practice. The model thus focuses on the decision-making processes that generate correct responses in addition to giving explicable logic in line with the clinical processes and ethical standards.

The other key innovation of CFM-Health is the way it addresses the policy constraints, the ethical aspect and the regulatory requirements as part of the learning process instead of separate compliance inspections. Healthcare facilities work in a high legal and ethical environment of patient consent, data safety, and responsibility. These constraints have been directly integrated into the federated learning process by the proposed paradigm, which has the capacity to achieve adaptive intelligence to balance the optimization of performance with fairness, privacy and compliance with regulations. This health-conscious thinking enables the intelligence of healthcare to develop in a responsible manner in a decentralized and immersive environment. Systems CFM-Health facilitates the creation of collaborative intelligence among heterogeneous healthcare institutions with respect to institutional autonomy and the contextual diversity. Hospitals, diagnostics, rehabilitation centers, and home-based care platforms will not have to lose control over sensitive data to be involved in a shared learning ecosystem.

Figure 1. System Architecture of the Cognitive Federated Metaverse for Healthcare (CFM-Health)

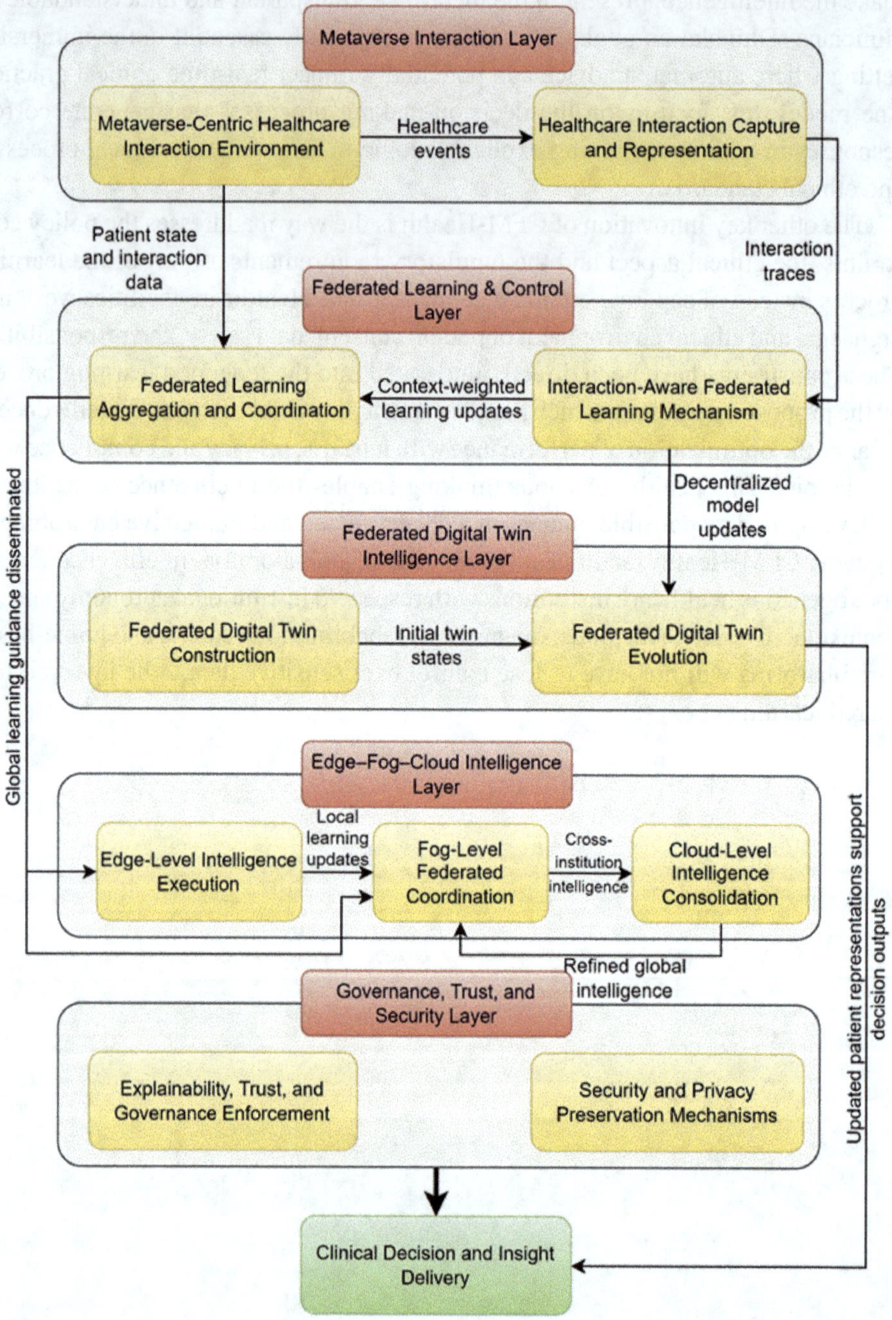

The virtual reality of the metaverse also allows easy cross-institutional collaboration by providing common virtual environments through which clinical discussion, training, and supporting decision-making can be achieved, all based on federated intelligence. Essentially, the Cognitive Federated Metaverse of Healthcare reconfigures federated learning as a process of interaction, which is an inherent process of cognition installed into immersive healthcare surroundings (Dhinakaran et al., 2025). CFM-Health can build upon intelligent healthcare systems through unification of decentralized learning, explainable decision-making and metaverse-based clinical engagement to enable them to be adaptive, trustworthy and clinically meaningful. This paradigm preconditions the next parts of the chapter that further expand on the idea of architectural design, algorithmic processes, and practical healthcare applications that are possible with the help of such convergence.

Figure 2. Metaverse-Centric Healthcare Interaction Layer

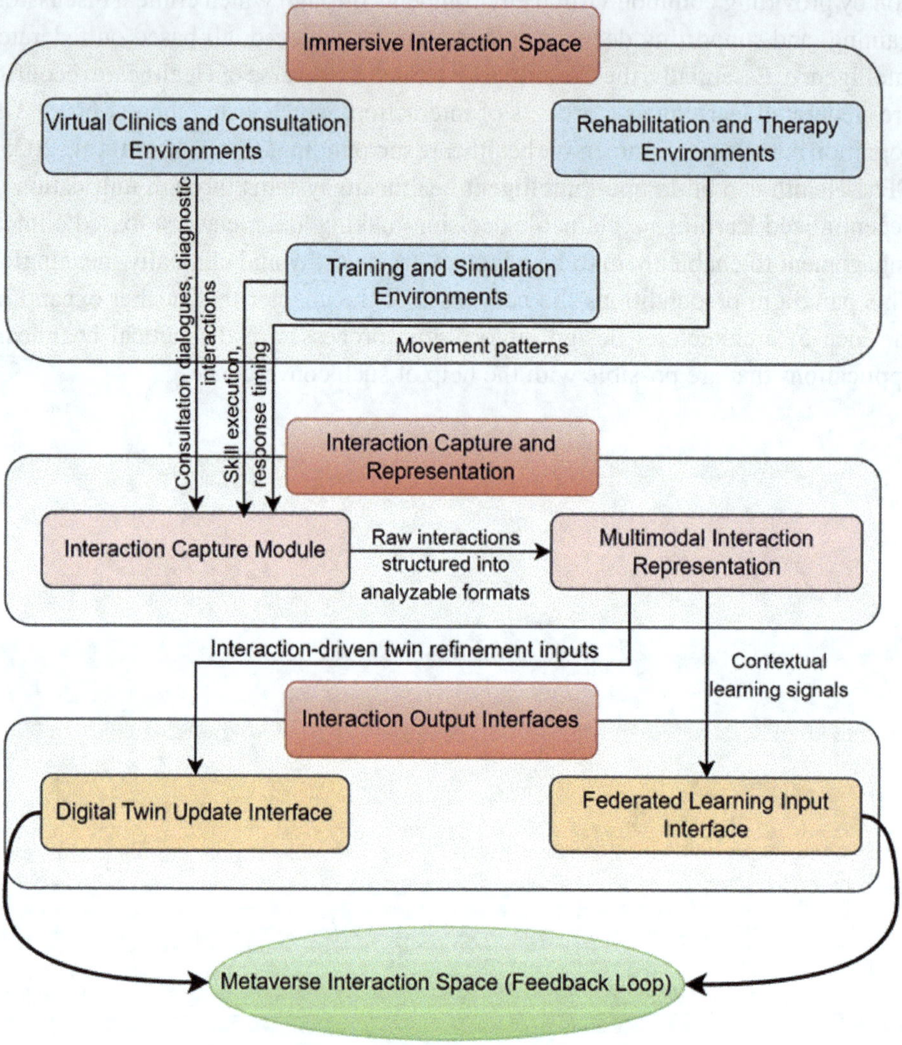

4. METAVERSE-CENTRIC HEALTHCARE INTERACTION LAYER

Within the metaverse interaction layer, healthcare environments are structured as synchronized virtual spaces supporting real-time multi-user collaboration. Patient motion tracking, physiological sensor integration, and avatar-based interaction streams enable continuous capture of clinical behaviors and therapy engagement.

Spatial synchronization mechanisms ensure consistent digital twin visualization across users, while low-latency interaction loops support immersive teleconsultation and rehabilitation workflows. These immersive data streams serve as continuous intelligence inputs rather than static visualization layers. The experiential/contextual platform of the Cognitive Federated Metaverse of Healthcare is the Metaverse-Centric Healthcare Interaction Layer as shown in Figure 2. The layer provides a hosting platform of immersive virtual environments that enable the interaction of patients, clinicians, medical devices, and intelligent agents in real time. In contrast to traditional telemedicine systems that simply recreate physical consultations using video interfaces, this layer does allow sustained, spatially conscious, context-rich clinical spaces that reflect and extend real-life healthcare interactions. Virtual hospitals, out-patient clinics, rehabilitation centers, and training facilities are located in one metaverse, which allows constant care and cooperation in a clinical practice without regard to physical boundaries. The ability to represent healthcare interactions as semantically meaningful and structured events (instead of unstructured multimedia streams) is a characteristic feature of this interaction layer. Conversational interactions with patients, diagnostic inquiries, therapeutic activities, and simulation of procedures are enclosed in three-dimensional spaces in which spatial relations, temporal progressions, and behavioral prompts have clinical implications. These immersive interactions offer more detailed representation of patient condition and clinician purpose than conventional data sources and healthcare intelligence goes beyond single-point measurements to holistic insight.

The layer of interaction with a multimodal data fusion in CFM-Health is specifically aimed at the metaverse. The elements of physiological indicators of the Internet of Medical Things devices, the visual indicators of virtual examination, the motion of rehabilitation exercises, and the verbal or written interactions between participants are all understood in a common frame of context. This combination allows the system not only to draw conclusions about clinical parameters, but also patient involvement degree, cognitive load, and behavioral adherence which are important aspects of diagnosis and treatment planning, but are not usually found in standard datasets. Most importantly, this layer is an active cognitive interface as opposed to a passive data collection mechanism. Relationships within the virtual clinics or diagnosis simulation are constantly analyzed to determine patterns and deviations that are clinically relevant. By way of illustration, minor alterations in the movements of a patient during virtual physiotherapy sessions or the discrepancy in reporting symptoms during immersive consultations may be identified as relevant learning indicators. These clues are fed to lower-level federated learning systems, whereby changes in the model bases on clinical significance of the real world as opposed to the possibility of changes in the model due to statistical variations that are not tangible. The metaverse-centered design can also help facilitate the personalized and adaptive clinical practices. Patient needs, clinical goals and evolving health condition can dynamically determine how virtual environments can be configured. This flexibility allows clinicians to test other hypotheses of diagnosis, model treatment outcomes and live change care trajectories. By the incorporation of intelligence into these workflows, CFM-Health enables the contextual and evidence-based process of decision-making (Dhinakaran et al., 2023).

Regarding education and collaboration, the interaction layer supports immersive medical training and interdisciplinary collaboration. Clinicians are able to engage in collaborative virtual simulations simulation that models complex procedures or uncommon clinical situations with the aid of federated intelligence that summarizes the expertise across institutions. Such collaborative set-ups facilitate group learning without violating data confidentiality and institutional boundaries which further solidify the distributed aspect of the proposed paradigm. The other significant intention of the Metaverse-Centric Healthcare Interaction Layer is trust and engagement. The feeling of presence and continuity of care increases in the framework of immersive environments, and it is particularly relevant in the case of long-term rehabilitation and in the context of chronic disease management. The framework will enhance the adherence, transparency, and shared decision-making levels by enabling patients to be engaged in their care in friendly virtual environments. These anthropocentric considerations have a direct effect on the quality and reliability of the learning signals produced in the system. Of significance, the interaction layer is created to be based on stringent ethical and regulatory standards. The metaverse environment has inbuilt mechanisms of informed consent, role-based access control and context-based data visibility. This makes sure that patient interactions are recorded and utilized as per the standards of legal and ethical healthcare practices, and solidifies the policy-conscious cognition presented in the wider CFM-Health landscape.

5. FEDERATED DIGITAL TWIN INTELLIGENCE

Explainability within CFM-Health is achieved by linking model predictions to interaction-driven learning contributions. Context-weighted aggregation enables traceability of influential clinical interactions, while local model explanations highlight patient-specific features contributing to predictions. These explanation layers can be visualized directly within metaverse interfaces, enabling clinicians to inspect decision rationales alongside digital twin states, supporting trust, transparency, and clinical validation. The Federated Digital Twin Intelligence layer is used as the cognitive core of the proposed Cognitive Federated Metaverse of Healthcare since it allows persisting, adaptive, and privacy-aware representations of the patient health conditions as shown in Figure 3. The traditional concept of digital twins in the healthcare context is a virtual representation of real-life objects, which are typically built based on static clinical data and are limited to single institutional settings. Although such representations have value in visualization and simulation, they do not have the ability to support continuous learning, cross-institutional collaboration and long-term personalization. The given framework is a radical redefinition of digital twins as living federated intelligence agents that develop in co-evolution in decentralized healthcare ecosystems (Ramani et al., 2025). In CFM-Health, a patient is linked to a digital twin that summarizes physiological, behavioral and contextual features based on multimodal data sources. These are medical images, wearable and implantable sensor biosignals, electronic health records and traces of interaction in immersive metaverse spaces. The digital twin is not the frozen image of the traditional patient as it is a time-dependent structure that tracks short-term clinical dynamics and long-term health trends. This continuity over time permits clinicians to reason about disease progression and treatment response and risk evolution using a single representational structure. The main innovation of the proposed solution is the federation of digital twin intelligence between institutions. Instead of exchanging raw patient information or completely centralized models, healthcare providers enable digital twin representations to be refined jointly and collaboratively by the mechanism of federated learning. Local updates to the components of the twin model models are done by each institution depending on its patient population and clinical practice, and aggregated intelligence are distributed in a privacy-sensitive way. This will allow digital twins to access a variety of clinical experiences without interfering with patient confidentiality or institutional autonomy.

Figure 3. Federated Digital Twin Intelligence

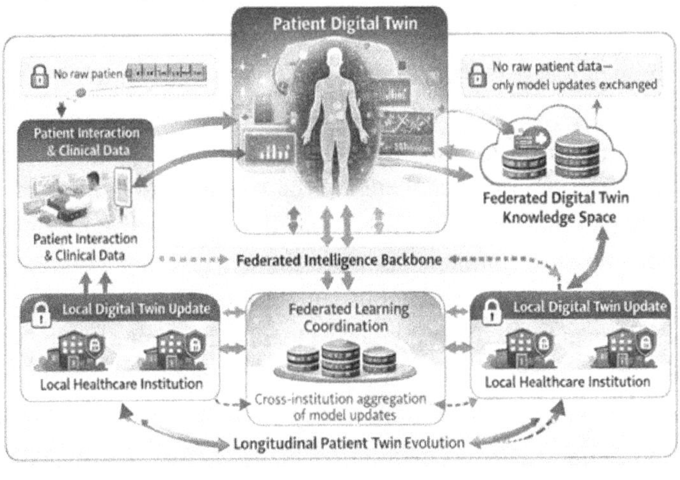

The federated digital twin intelligence concept can overcome one of the biggest gaps of the current healthcare AI systems: fragmentation. The care of patients is frequently divided between various hospitals, diagnostic facilities, and home-based monitoring solutions, which produces fragmented and partial images of patient health. Continuous CFM-Health also makes possible digital twins to bring across the knowledge gained across organizational boundaries without violating the data governance limitations. The digital twin can thus be described as an intelligence in longitudinal and cross-context, which can provide coordinated care and informed clinical decisions. The communicative capabilities of digital twins are further enhanced by the fact that they are incorporated into the metaverse-based layer of interaction. Virtual rehab records of patient movement, consultation attendance rate and behavioral patterns to simulated care scenarios constitute much more comprehensive contextual indicators that may not always be captured in traditional data, but may be part of the immersive care experiences. The signal obtained via interaction is then added to the digital twins' representations in order to allow them to not only simulate the physiological condition but also the functional and behavioral health (Selvaraj et al., 2025). It has holistic modelling power particularly the chronic disease management, mental health services and post-operative rehabilitation. The other aspect, which defines federated digital twin intelligence, is that it enables individualized learnable generalization. The learning models applied are always based on populationlevel dynamics, but in the form of federated aggregation, even though each digital twin is patient-specific. The resulting two-sidedness enables personalization of predictions and recommendations, which are founded on common clinical knowledge. Consequently, clinicians will have an opportunity to explore the individual treatment strategies without doubting their overall validity.

An aspect that is addressed at the bottom-level requirements of this layer is explainability. Digital twins are explicable closures among complicated AI models and clinical reasoning process. The framework alone allows easy interpretation of model outputs through representation of patient representations in a manner that embodies clinically meaningful aspects and environments and expressing these aspects with such a representation. Through challenging the AI-based diagnostic recommendation or treatment recommendation, clinicians will be in a position to understand the foundation of diagnostic recommendation or treatment recommendation, which entail the development of trust and accountability in AI-based care. Federated digital twin intelligence enables proactive and predictive healthcare regarding the system level. Digital twins can forecast the potential health risks and suggest prevention steps on a constant basis, even before any adverse occurrence takes place because of the unstopped inflow of new data and cues to interact with. Such predictive potential is particularly large with simulative immersion in the metaverse whereby clinicians will be able to test hypothetic conditions and outcomes of interventions in varying twin representation. More importantly, the framework assumes ethical and regulatory in the lifecycle cycle of digital twin intelligence. The level of the granularity and the coverage of the twin's update reflect on patient agreement, data use boundaries and the institutional policy. Through the federated learning, sensitive data will be stored locally, unlike communication intelligence, which will satisfy the demands of fairness and bias-reduction. This design will make sure that the development of the digital twin is in correspondence to the necessity to possess healthcare governance that will reduce the probability of misuse or unintentional harm.

6. INTERACTION-AWARE FEDERATED LEARNING MECHANISM

Interaction-Aware Federated Learning Mechanism is the fundamental learning mechanism of the Cognitive Federated Metaverse of Healthcare that enables the process of establishing the decentralized intelligence itself as a direct reaction to immersive clinical interaction. In classical federated learning models, data partitions are either fixed and the aggregation steps are periodically reiterated, and local updates are perceived as the homogeneous contributions to a global model. Although these solutions help in preserving privacy, they lack the richness of contexts and sensitivity of time of the healthcare process particularly in the immersive metaverse context as the Table 3 illustrates. The suggested mechanism can alleviate this drawback by triggering the interaction semantics of all the stages of the federated learning life-cycle. Conceptually, interaction-aware federated learning transforms the meaning of a learning signal in decentralized healthcare system. Instead of using only locally computed model gradients based on historical datasets, the mechanism consists of first-class input to the learning process, namely real-time interaction context. The contextual metadata that is created during clinical interactions within virtual consultations, diagnostic simulation, or rehabilitation settings is an indication of clinical significance, urgency, and patient activity. The metadata elements change the process and timing of the local learning updates between and among the federation.

Table 3. Interaction-Aware Federated Learning versus Conventional Federated Learning

Comparison Dimension	Conventional Federated Learning	Edge-Based Federated Learning	Interaction-Aware Federated Learning (CFM-Health)
Learning Signal Source	Static local datasets	Local device or edge-level data streams	Immersive healthcare interaction events and contextual signals
Model Update Trigger	Periodic or scheduled rounds	Resource- or latency-driven	Clinical interaction relevance and temporal urgency
Aggregation Strategy	Uniform or data-volume-based	Hierarchical or proximity-based	Context-weighted and interaction-sensitive aggregation
Awareness of Clinical Context	Absent	Limited (device-centric)	Explicitly modeled through immersive interactions
Temporal Sensitivity	Low	Moderate	High, aligned with real-time care processes
Personalization Capability	Global model dominant	Partial local adaptation	Continuous patient-centric personalization
Longitudinal Patient Modeling	Not supported	Limited	Integrated through federated digital twin evolution
Communication Efficiency	Moderate to high overhead	Reduced through edge aggregation	Adaptive communication based on interaction importance
Robustness to Noisy Updates	Limited	Moderate	Enhanced via interaction-context validation
Explainability of Model Evolution	Low	Low to moderate	High, via traceable interaction-linked updates
Governance and Policy Awareness	External to learning	External to learning	Embedded into learning decision logic
Suitability for Immersive Healthcare	Low	Moderate	High

Figure 4. Interaction-Aware Federated Learning Mechanism

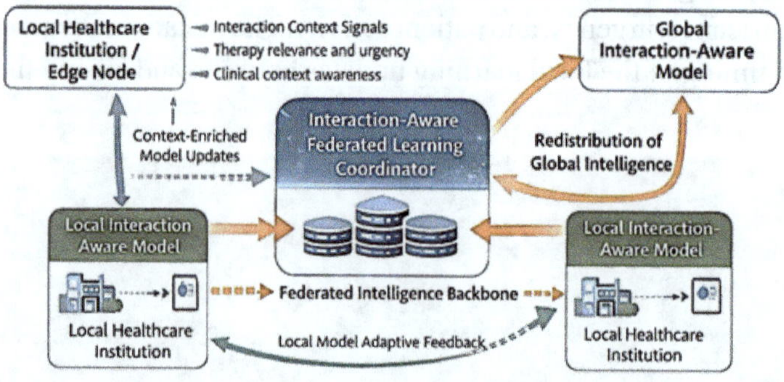

The key characteristic of the suggested mechanism is the strategy of adaptive aggregation. Unlike uniform or data-volume-based aggregation, interaction-aware federated learning dynamically assigns to local model updates the importance they have depending on the clinical context. The updates which are created at high-impact interactions, which may be either a diagnostic decision point or a critical care simulation, influence the global model evolution a little more than the ones created through routine or low-salience activity. This makes federated intelligence be in line with the reality on the ground in healthcare priorities as opposed to having lots of data dominate it. Another characteristic of the mechanism is that of temporal sensitivity. The nature of healthcare interactions is characterized by time scales, which can be instantaneous clinical decision-making processes and long-term rehabilitation processes. The aggregation frequency and schedule of updates are adjusted in the proposed structure based on interaction dynamics, letting propagation of time-sensitive learning updates propagate fast and postponing less important contributions. Such time responsiveness is especially crucial in healthcare practiced in the metaverse, where latency and responsiveness are directly related to clinical efficacy and patient confidence.

The interaction-based personalization of learning is also capable of supporting localized personalization without a compromise of the global coherence as shown in Figure 4. On one hand, local models can be updated based on interaction, thus adapting to both patient-specific and institution-specific settings, on the other hand, federated aggregation guarantees that more extensive clinical trends are reflected in shared intelligence. The balance between personalization and generalization is reached through control of the level of impact that the interaction-specific updates can have on the global model to avoid overfitting and maintain the contextual relevance. The proposed learning paradigm includes robustness and resilience. The immersion and decentralization of the environment expose exposure to adversarial behaviors, noisy interactions, and heterogeneous data quality. Interaction- sensitive federated learning uses consistency checks and contextual validation to determine the credibility of local updates. Updates that are too dissimilar to normal interaction patterns, or which show abnormal behaviour, may be down-weighted or filtered out, strengthening the global model without the need to have a centralised control mechanism.

An explainable feature is part of the learning mechanism to promote transparency and clinical trust. The framework can help clinicians and system administrators to interpret the impact of particular clinical experiences on model evolution by linking model updates with interpretable interaction settings. This traceability would be especially useful in the healthcare environments, where accountability and auditability play a crucial role in the ethical and regulatory compliance. Interaction-aware federated learning is the connective tissue of interaction-aware federated learning between immersive metaverse interactions and federated digital twin intelligence in terms of system integration. The continuous refinement of digital twin representations by interaction is then used to suggest future interactions and cycles of learning. This recurrent feedback allows the continuous enhancement of healthcare intelligence, which is based on the practice of the real clinical environment and patient experience. Notably, the suggested mechanism is correlated with policy-aware learning principles presented in the general CFM-Health framework. The interaction contexts are considered and assessed with respect to both clinical and ethical and regulatory considerations. The learning updates, based on interactions that cross consent boundaries or policy restrictions, are automatically limited to make sure that federated intelligence is developed within the boundaries that can be considered to be legally and ethically acceptable. The proposed interaction-aware federated learning procedure, formally summarized in Algorithm 1

Table 1. Algorithm 1- Interaction-Aware Federated Learning in CFM-Health

#		*Step*
1.		***Initialize global model Mglobal***
2.		***Distribute Mglobal to all participating nodes***
3.		***For*** **each learning round** ***t*** **do**
4.		***For*** **each node** ***i*** **in parallel do**
5.		**Capture immersive healthcare interactions**
6.		Compute interaction relevance score Ri
7.		Train local model Mi using local data and interaction signals
8.		Scale update using relevance:
9.		$M_i \leftarrow M_i - \eta \cdot R_i \cdot \nabla L_i$
10.		Send weighted update (R_i, M_i) to aggregator
11.		***End for***
12.		Perform context-weighted aggregation:
13.		$M_{global} \leftarrow \Sigma\left(R_i \cdot M_i\right) / \Sigma R_i$
14.	2.1	Adjust aggregation frequency based on urgency level
15.	2.2	Redistribute updated Mglobal to all nodes
16.		***End for***

Mathematical Intuition and Loss Formulation for Interaction-Aware Federated Learning

To formalize the adaptive behavior of the proposed interaction-aware federated learning mechanism, each participating healthcare node optimizes a local objective function that integrates both prediction accuracy and interaction relevance. Let D_i denote the local healthcare dataset at node i, and let C_i represent the associated immersive interaction context derived from metaverse-based healthcare environments. The local optimization objective is defined as in eqn. (1).

$$L_i = R_i \cdot l\left(M_i(D_i, C_i)\right) + \lambda \cdot \Omega\left(M_i\right)\#(1)$$

where $\ell(\cdot)$ denotes the task-specific loss function (e.g., classification or regression error), R_i is the interaction relevance score capturing clinical urgency and engagement intensity, $\Omega(\cdot)$ is a regularization term that prevents overfitting, and λ controls regularization strength. The interaction relevance score R_i acts as an adaptive weighting factor that amplifies learning updates arising from clinically significant events such as diagnostic decisions, rehabilitation milestones, or abnormal physiological patterns, while attenuating less critical routine interactions. During federated aggregation, the global objective minimizes the weighted sum of local objectives as defined in eqn. (2), which leads naturally to the context-weighted aggregation rule introduced in Algorithm 1. This formulation ensures that global intelligence evolution is driven by meaningful clinical interactions rather than uniform data volume contributions.

$$L_{global} = \Sigma R_i \cdot L_i\#(2)$$

Temporal Sensitivity Mechanism

To support real-time responsiveness in immersive healthcare scenarios, the relevance score Ri also governs synchronization frequency. For interaction events with high urgency levels ($Ri \geq \tau$), immediate aggregation is triggered to rapidly update global intelligence. For lower relevance interactions ($Ri < \tau$), updates are accumulated over longer intervals to reduce communication overhead. The threshold τ controls the trade-off between responsiveness and efficiency.

Practical Loss Function Examples

For classification-based healthcare tasks such as disease diagnosis, the local loss can be instantiated as cross-entropy as defined in eqn. (3), where y represents ground-truth clinical labels and ŷ denotes predicted probabilities. For regression-based tasks such as physiological parameter prediction, mean squared error can be applied as defined in eqn. (4). These standard formulations ensure compatibility with existing healthcare AI models while enabling interaction-aware adaptation through relevance weighting.

$$l = -\Sigma y \log(\hat{y}) \#(3)$$

$$l = (y - \hat{y})^2 \#(4)$$

Healthcare data across institutions are inherently non-IID due to demographic variation, disease prevalence, and sensor heterogeneity. While conventional federated learning methods such as uniform aggregation struggle under such distributions, the proposed interaction-aware mechanism inherently mitigates non-IID effects by prioritizing clinically relevant updates rather than raw data volume. By weighting updates through interaction relevance and temporal urgency, the framework adaptively emphasizes informative gradients, reducing model drift commonly observed in heterogeneous healthcare environments. This context-driven aggregation complements existing federated optimization strategies while offering robustness to real-world healthcare data imbalance.

7. EDGE–FOG–CLOUD INTELLIGENCE ORCHESTRATION

The Edge-Fog-Cloud Intelligence Orchestration layer offers the computational and operational capabilities needed to maintain immersive real-time privacy-preserving healthcare intelligence within the Cognitive Federated Metaverse of Healthcare. Immersive clinical settings pose very high requirements on latency, reliability, and responsiveness especially where real-time patient care is influenced by intelligence-driven recommendations. The traditional cloud-based architectures cannot handle these situations because of the delay in communication, bandwidth, and regulatory factors related to the centralized processing of data. These challenges are overcome through the proposed orchestration paradigm which disseminates intelligence in an adaptive and coordinated manner across edge, fog, and cloud layers. The intelligence will be placed nearest to data sources and users at the edge layer, such as wearable medical devices, bedside monitoring systems, and augmented or mixed reality interfaces. Tasks performed by this layer include latency-sensitive inference tasks, e.g., real-time biosignal recognition, gesture recognition in rehabilitation, contextual feedback in AR-assisted clinical procedures. Inferring locally and doing initial learning reduces response times and maintains patient privacy, which ensures continuous and reliable interactions with the patient in the metaverse. The opportunity in the fog layer is seen as an intermediary coordination layer, which mediates local edge intelligence and more extensive federated learning. The fog nodes are normally implemented at institutional or regional settings, like in hospitals or clinics or healthcare networks. These nodes combine interaction-conscious learning updates across a variety of edge devices and digital twins, validate contextually and organize localized federated learning rounds. This partial aggregation minimizes communication overhead, robustness to connected edges that are not reliable, as well as region-specific intelligence adaptation being consistent with global learning goals. The system carries out long-term intelligence consolidation and governance at the cloud layer. The cloud is not a central repository of data but a coordination and knowledge center consisting of federated updates of models, policy constraints and ensuring global model consistency. The cloud layer facilitates longitudinal analysis, cross-institutional sharing of knowledge, and optimization across the entire system without having access to raw patient data. This is a very significant position in terms of fairness, uniformity, and adherence to regulations in the heterogeneous healthcare settings. One of the strongest attributes about the proposed orchestration strategy is a dynamic adaptability.

EDGE, fog, and cloud layers do not have fixed allocations of intelligence tasks, but they are constantly adjusted depending on the interaction circumstances, network states, and clinical urgency. An example is that in time sensitive clinical interventions, learning and inference tasks can be pushed to the edge and the fog layer to reduce latency, with non-critical updates pushed to cloud-level aggregation. This dynamic coordination is necessary to make sure that the performance of the system is in line with the clinical priorities and individually operating constraints. Interaction-aware federated learning also requires the orchestration layer in its support. The framework by co-ordinating learning cycles over computational levels makes sure that interaction-based learning cues are handled at the right temporal and spatial scales. On edge-level updates, fine-grained patient-specific dynamics are captured, on fog-level, coordination is synthesized between patterns within the institution, and on cloud-level, population-wide insights are consolidated. This hierarchical learning hierarchy facilitates effective scalability without loss of the contextual sensitivity. The edgefogcloud orchestration has a resilience viewpoint; it improves system robustness and fault tolerance. Decentralized intelligence enables the services of healthcare to operate even in the conditions of network disruptions or the partial collapse of a system with the failure of one of its points. This strength is especially relevant in immersive healthcare settings, where interruptions with service provision may undermine patient safety and trust.

Other advantages of the proposed orchestration paradigm are energy efficiency and optimization of resources. The system does not have to transmit unnecessary data and perform redundant calculations by setting the locations of computational workload in accordance with the needs of every task. The lightweight inference and learning at the edge lowers bandwidth usage, and more complex optimization jobs are pushed to the fog or the cloud. This safe distribution encourages sustainable functioning of huge smart hospitals and dispersed medical systems. Notably, the orchestration layer is closely connected with the governance and policy conscious mechanisms of the CFM-Health framework. The choices to be made in terms of task placement, data movement, and learning coordination are limited by the policies of privacy, consent, and regulatory requirements. This is to make sure that the intelligence orchestration does not only optimize the performance but also conforms to ethical and legal standards inherent in healthcare systems.

8. EXPLAINABILITY, TRUST, AND GOVERNANCE

The ethical and institutional framework of the Cognitive Federated Metaverse in Healthcare consists of explainability, trust, and governance. The adoption of intelligent systems in healthcare settings is not only dependant on performance metrics, but also on the capacity of clinicians, patients and regulators to appreciate, trust and manage the automated decision-making processes. The need is even stronger in highly immersive and decentralized environments where intelligent recommendations are likely to be applied to real-time clinical actions in virtual environments. Explainability and governance are thus proposed as principles of design that form the behavior of the system at each layer. The issue of explainability in CFM-Health is treated as a multi-level concept that cuts across the behavior of the models, learning, and system interactions. At clinical decision level, the intelligent output generated in the metaverse is supported by explanations that are easy to interpret and which concurs with the set medical reasoning practices. Instead of providing solid predictions, the system situates suggestions in clinically significant signs based on federated digital twin states, interaction histories, and population level trends. This will help clinicians evaluate the soundness of advice and incorporate it in their professional judgment without compromising the human agency in decision making. On top of personal predictions, explainability is also applied to the learning process. Federated learning mechanisms that are interaction-aware relate updates of the model to the clinical context and patterns of interaction. This traceability enables the system administrators and auditors to see the impact of immersive healthcare experiences on the development of shared intelligence. Being able to clearly connect the events of interaction and the learning outcomes, the framework facilitates the concept of accountability and post-hoc analysis, which is crucial to the clinical validation and regulatory review.

Confidence in CFM-Health is not presupposed but developed in a systematic way by means of regular, transparent, and consistent system behavior. The experiential quality of the metaverse intensifies psychological effects of intelligent systems on the patients and clinicians. To mitigate this, the framework focuses on predictability and consistency of intelligent responses to similar clinical situations thereby lessening uncertainty and cognitive load. The system also instills trust in its capability to gracefully respond to unpredictability, indicating clearly the degree of confidence and constraints instead of excessively automating its power. The mechanisms of governance are highly incorporated in the architecture to make sure that decentralized intelligence works within the limits of the ethics, law and institutions. There are strict rules that govern healthcare systems with respect to patient consent, data protection, and accountability. CFM-Health implements policy-sensitive controls, which control the manner in which interaction data, digital twin updates, and federated learning contributions are produced and used. These controls allow learning processes to observe consent scopes, institutional policies and jurisdictional regulations and enforce them without necessarily being centralized.

One of the most critical features of governance in the proposed framework is the responsibility and accountability management in the federated and immersive environment. This problem renders the earlier models of accountability inadequate as the power to make decisions is decentralized among the institutions and smart agents. CFM-Health overcomes this obstacle through recording audits of contributions to learning, updates of model, and contexts of decisions. Such records make it easy to assign responsibility and assist with clinical surveillance, legal and ethical analysis. The mitigation of fairness and bias is also a focus of trust and governance in the framework. Learning environments that are decentralized expose biases associated with unbalanced distributions of data or institutionality. The proposed paradigm integrates the aspect of fairness-constrained federated learning and digital twin evolution to make sure the model performance is fair among the patient demographics and clinical environments. The framework ensures the inclusive and fair healthcare intelligence by consistently tracking the indicators of bias and varying the dynamics of learning in accordance. The governance layer also enables shared governance among institutions who are involved in the federated ecosystem. The shared governance protocols allow healthcare providers to develop learning goals, assessment criteria, and ethics collectively and maintain institutional autonomy. This model of collaborative governance is consistent with the distributed quality of the framework and inculcation of shared responsibility of system behavior and results.

Beyond technical security mechanisms, the proposed CFM-Health framework is designed to align with healthcare regulatory and ethical requirements such as

GDPR-style data minimization principles and HIPAA-compliant patient privacy protections. Federated learning ensures that sensitive patient data remain localized within institutional boundaries, while interaction-aware governance policies regulate model updates based on consent, clinical relevance, and fairness constraints. Furthermore, bias risks emerging from immersive interactions, such as avatar-mediated behavioral differences or demographic representation imbalance, can be monitored through explainability-driven auditing and fairness-aware aggregation controls. This enables continuous assessment of equitable intelligence evolution across patient populations.

9. SECURITY AND PRIVACY PRESERVATION

The key issue is that security and preservation of privacy are two basic needs of any smart healthcare system, specifically in a decentralized-immersive network like the Cognitive Federated Metaverse of Healthcare. The integration of metaverse platforms, federated learning, and distributed intelligence increases the attack surface to a great extent and adds new threats with regard to data leakage, adversarial manipulation, and unauthorized access. The proposed framework is the solution that would focus on such challenges by making security and privacy a part of the fabric of the architecture so that it would not be the extravagant addition that it is an external feature of the architecture. The following are the main privacy preservation strategies in CFM-Health that are ensured by the decentralized learning paradigm facilitated by federated intelligence. Sensitive patient information, such as medical records, biosignals, and traces of interaction that are created in the metaverse, are not generalized but instead reside at their points of origin. Abstracted model updates and contextual learning signals are only exchanged over the federation. Such a design will reduce the risk of direct data exposure and comply with stringent healthcare data protection laws. Notably, privacy is assured at the data level as well as the interaction level, in which otherwise immersive experiences may show sensitive behavioral or clinical information. The framework also considers privacy-enhancing mechanisms in the federated learning process so as to enhance privacy guarantees. Local model updates are put through differentiating privacy to restrict the potential of using shared intelligence to infer individual patient data. Secure aggregation protocols guarantee that the intermediate learning contributions cannot be viewed or recreated by non-authorities, such as coordinating nodes. All these mechanisms help in avoiding direct and indirect leakage of sensitive healthcare information.

Data confidentiality is not the only security consideration in this regard but also integrity and reliability of decentralized intelligence. The vulnerable adversarial attacks to federated and immersive environments include model poisoning, gradient manipulation and inference-based attacks, which seek to impair system performance or obtain sensitive information. CFM-Health is resilience-conscious learning techniques that determine the consistency and plausibility of local updates concerning the context of interaction and historical trends. Contributions that were suspicious or outlier can be given low weight, or removed without interfering with the overall learning process, making it healthier to malicious behaviour. The immersiveness of the metaverse brings about the extra security problems associated with identity management and access control. The security of patients and data may be impacted by unauthorized access to virtual healthcare environments. The given framework will embrace the use of decentralized identity and authentication to make sure that all the participants in the metaverse, including patients, clinicians, and intelligent agents, are authenticated reliably. Access controls are role-based and context-aware access controls that govern visibility and interaction privileges to prevent sensitive information of clinical information being given to the wrong parties when the circumstances are unfavorable. The other security issue that is essential to CFM-Health is the safeguarding of digital twin intelligence. Since digital twins are long-term and constantly changing models of patient health, their compromised nature may have drastic clinical implications. The framework provides severe isolation of individual twins and the use of encrypted channels of communication in all federated exchanges involving intelligence related to twins. This will avoid manipulation by unauthorized individuals and save the integrity of customized healthcare representations. The edge–fog–cloud orchestration layer also provides additional security through decentralized computational load and centralized infrastructural dependencies. The issue of decentralization in itself reduces the effects of single point failures and massive breaches. Localized edge and fog-layer intelligence can be used safely even in the case of partial system compromise, and allow the delivery of critical healthcare services and reduce disruption. The philosophy of CFM-Health security mechanisms is strongly linked to the governance requirements as well as explainability requirements. Clear security policy, auditing learning processes and a record of interactions, allow uninterrupted monitoring and forensic analysis. This openness is not only effective in meeting regulatory requirements but also helps the healthcare stakeholders to build more confidence as it shows that security is not only effectively implemented, but can be verified.

10. USE CASES AND EXPERIMENTAL SCENARIOS

Practical realization of the proposed framework can leverage existing immersive and federated learning platforms. Metaverse healthcare environments may be implemented using game-engine-based systems such as Unity or Unreal Engine integrated with medical-grade sensor interfaces. Federated learning coordination can be supported through frameworks such as TensorFlow Federated or PySyft, while edge–fog–cloud orchestration may utilize containerized microservices deployed on edge computing platforms. These technologies provide a feasible pathway for transitioning the proposed architecture from conceptual design to real-world healthcare deployments. To provide an indicative quantitative assessment of the proposed CFM-Health framework, a representative simulation-based evaluation was conducted under controlled and identical experimental conditions across all compared learning paradigms. Synthetic yet clinically realistic interaction data were generated to emulate immersive healthcare scenarios, including diagnostic workflows, rehabilitation sessions, and longitudinal patient monitoring. Conventional centralized learning, standard federated learning, and edge-based federated learning were implemented using identical model architectures and training configurations to ensure fair comparison. The presented results aim to illustrate relative performance trends and system behavior rather than claim definitive clinical superiority or real-world deployment readiness. The Cognitive Federated Metaverse of Healthcare allows a vast array of intelligent, privacy-conscious, and immersive health care applications that are not limited to the scope of traditional digital health systems. The framework can be used to support clinical workflows in the real world, as tightly coupled metaverse-based interactions, federated digital twin intelligence, and interaction-aware learning mechanisms can be fulfilled with scalability and regulatory compliance. The following section describes exemplary use cases and experimental situations that prove that the suggested paradigm can be applied and evaluated in a variety of healthcare settings. Immersive telemedicine as a remote diagnosis and clinical consultation is also one of the brightest applications of the proposed framework. In a virtual clinic created in the metaverse, patients and clinicians work with each other using avatars that have real-time physiological information obtained by wearable sensors. The federated intelligent models are diagnostic reasoning that learns through continuous similar interactions between institutions with no direct access to patient information. These consultations cause the development of the digital twin of each patient, which includes behavioral indicators, progression of symptoms, and the feedback of clinicians. In the present application the experimental assessment would be based on accuracy in diagnosis, latency, patient interaction and understandability of AI-assisted recommendations compared to traditional telemedicine systems. The other important use is rehabilitation and post-operative treatment. The metaverse offers virtual environments controlled through virtual reality where patients do guide therapeutic exercises under the supervision of clinicians. Interaction signals are captured motion patterns, adherence behavior and physiological responses integrated into federated digital twin models.

Interaction-aware federated learning will allow personalizing rehabilitation protocols with adaptability according to progress of the patient as well as the benefit of joint learning of rehabilitation centers. In this case, experimental conditions are used to assess the improvements in the results of recovery, the number of adherents, and the flexibility of the models in different patient conditions. Developed clinical training and simulation of surgery are also supported by the framework. Medical students are immersed in procedural simulations in the metaverse, which has them communicating with virtual patients and artificial intelligence advisors. Procedural intelligence can be improved through federated learning, which enables collaborative refinement of procedural intelligence among training institutions without providing access to proprietary training data. Simulated patients have digital twins that evolve with actions of the trainees, making it possible to develop scenarios. The experimental research on this field investigates the speed of learning, transferability of the learned processes, and uniformity of AI-based feedback in decentralized training contexts. Another useful use case is in the management of chronic diseases. Individuals with chronic ailments like diabetes or cardiovascular disease take part in ongoing care via unremitting metaverse conditions that incorporate monitoring, education, and contact with clinicians. Federated digital twins record longitudinal health trajectories, whereas interaction-sensitive learning algorithms are adjusted to adapt predictive models to the changing patient behavior and environmental phenomena. Experimental testing highlights the ability to predict long-term, identify risks early, avoid discrimination among demographic groups, and maintain privacy in the case of stable learning. The framework also facilitates smart coordination in smart hospitals.

The replication of the hospital infrastructure and workflows in a virtual format makes it possible to monitor them in real time, allocate resources, and provide clinical decision support. Federated combines knowledge across various departments and institutions without violating data limits. The interaction-based learning gives importance to updates that occur due to critical care unit and emergency situations. Experimental conditions are used to test system responsiveness, fault tolerance and scalability during peak interaction loads. According to the perspectives of experimental design, the given framework makes it possible to evaluate several dimensions. The performance metrics are predictive accuracy, latency, communication overhead, and resistance to adversarial behavior. Privacy and security are evaluated on the basis of formal assurance of privacy, resistance to attack conditions, and regulation under institutional constraints. The measures of explainability and trust are assessed on the basis of clinician feedback, measures of interpretability, and audit learners. Notably, the modularity of CFM-Health can also be compared to centralized AI systems and traditional federated learning baselines operating under the same conditions of interaction. Experimentation in controlled metaverse environments through simulation offers an added benefit through the ability to perform reproducible and scalable evaluation without necessarily relying on large-scale clinical deployment. It is possible to create synthetic but clinically realistic interaction situations that can be used to put learning dynamics, orchestration strategies, and governance mechanisms to stress. These test environments can be used as pre-test to the real deployment as well as systematically prove the proposed paradigm.

11. PERFORMANCE ANALYSIS AND DISCUSSION

A sample, simulation-based test of the various healthcare intelligence paradigms in the same experimental conditions is shown in table 4 and in the figure (5 to 8) of performance analysis. The key ones compared are centralized artificial intelligence, traditional federated learning, edge-based federated learning, and the suggested interaction-conscious federated learning system in CFM-Health. The findings are supposed to point out the trends of relative performance but not assert the absolute clinical superiority. Interaction-aware federated learning has the best predictive performance compared to other methods in the accuracy comparison as shown in the accuracy comparison (Figure 5). This has been enhanced by the fact that clinically relevant interaction signals were incorporated in the learning process and this allows models to achieve an ability to conform more to patient-specific and context-sensitive patterns.

Table 4. Representative Performance Comparison of Healthcare Learning Approaches

Method	Accuracy (%)	Latency (ms)	Communication Overhead (MB/round)	Privacy Risk (relative)
Centralized AI	92.4	180	45.0	High (4)
Conventional Federated Learning	94.1	140	28.5	Medium (3)
Edge-Based Federated Learning	95.0	95	18.2	Low (2)
Interaction-Aware Federated Learning (CFM-Health)	**96.8**	**65**	**11.6**	**Very Low** (1)

Figure 5. Comparative performance evaluation of prediction accuracy

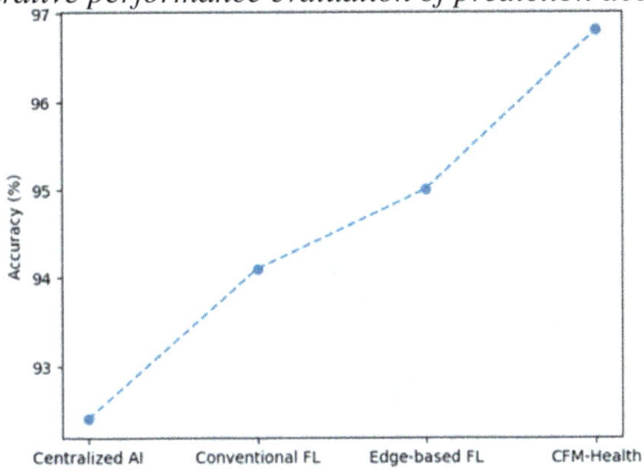

By contrast, centralized and traditional federated designs are based mostly on statical or device-centric data models, which restrict their modeling of dynamic healthcare systems. Latency analysis shows that the response time decreases clearly in the case of the decentralized approaches, and the proposed framework has the minimum latency (Figure 6). This result is the product of edge level intelligence execution and interaction-based update scheduling which makes as little unnecessary communication and computation as possible. Comparatively, the centralized AI system has greater latency because of the overhead of cloud-based processing and data transmission. The efficiency of interaction-conscious federated learning is further demonstrated by communication overheads (Figure 7). The amount of transmitted model parameters per training round is greatly lowered by the proposed framework due to the emphasis on updating learning based on the relevance of interactions instead of adhering to predetermined schedules of aggregation. This communication method is especially beneficial in bandwidth limited health care settings and in massive deployments. Comparison of privacy risks indicates a qualitative difference of decentralized learning paradigm over the centralized models (Figure 8). The interaction-aware federated learning model has the lowest relative risk of privacy since sensitive patient information is not exchanged and instead, only context-weighted updates to the model are. Interaction-aware filtering and governance-aware learning constraints ensure the preservation of privacy in the proposed approach, in contrast to traditional federated learning. On the whole, the combined outcomes provided in Table 4 and the performance figures (5 to 8) suggest that incorporating interaction context into federated learning can be used to achieve improved predictive accuracy, minimise system latency, decrease communication overhead, and reinforce privacy preservation at the same time. These results justify the appropriateness of the proposed CFM-Health framework to immersive and real-time and privacy-critical healthcare applications.

Figure 6. Comparative performance evaluation of system latency

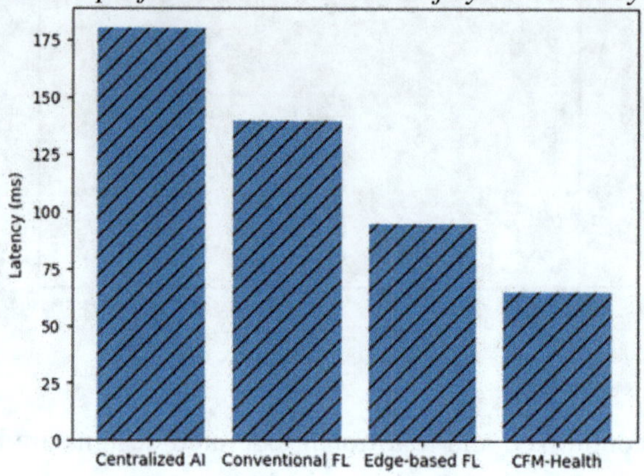

Figure 7. Comparative performance evaluation of communication overhead per training round

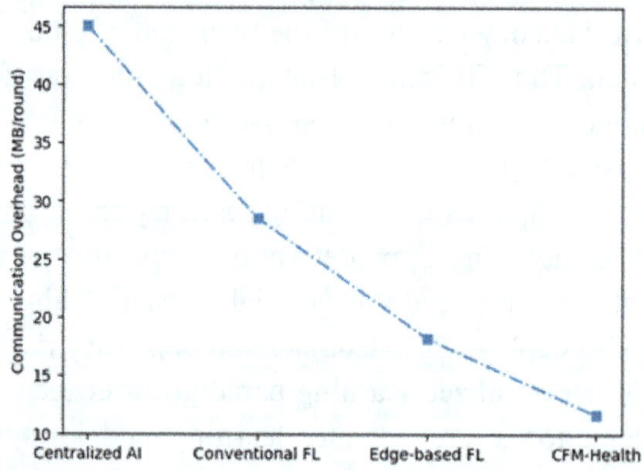

Figure 8. Comparative performance evaluation of relative privacy risk

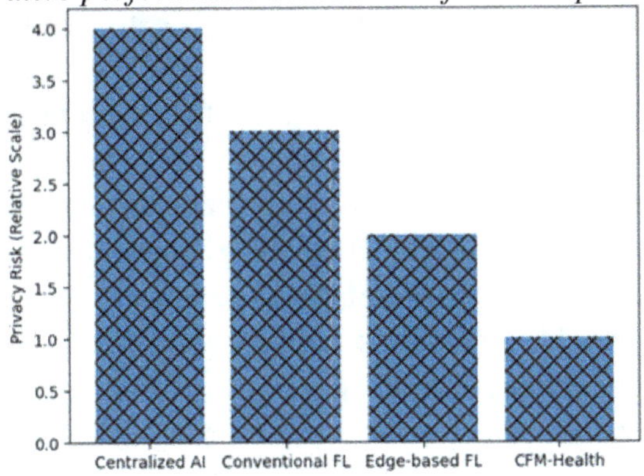

12. OPEN RESEARCH CHALLENGES AND FUTURE DIRECTIONS

Regardless of the opportunity of the Cognitive Federated Metaverse to revolutionize Healthcare, there are still a number of open research questions still to be tackled to make it possible to implement the Cognitive Federated Metaverse at scale, sustainably and ethically. These issues touch on technical, clinical, ethical, and organizational aspects because of the interdisciplinary nature of immersive and decentralized healthcare intelligence. Their solution needs to involve interdisciplinary improvements in the fields of artificial intelligence, systems engineering, healthcare practice, and policy formulation. The ability to scale interaction-oriented federated learning to massive and streaming interaction views is one of the key research issues. As healthcare environments built on metaverse grow to accommodate thousands of simultaneous users and devices, learning systems must process high-frequency heterogeneous signal interaction without decreasing latency or stability. The future studies would need to find adaptive learning methods that would be able to selectively focus on clinically significant interactions, and ignore redundant or less important updates. This involves coming up with more effective contextual relevance checking and active aggregation despite resource constraints. The other notable issue is the issue of long-term development and justification of federated digital twin intelligence. Although digital twins can be used as potent tools to provide healthcare in a personalized and predictive manner, the question of their clinical accuracy and reliability in the long term is rather open. Studies are required to define validation systems that constantly measure the digital twin fidelity with real-life results. Moreover, concept drift management mechanisms, patient behavior management mechanisms, and clinical guideline evolution mechanisms should be implemented into the digital twin lifecycle without introducing instability to federated learning processes.

Interoperability and standardization are some of the key obstacles to mass adoption. The healthcare ecosystem is typified by heterogeneous devices, data formats and institutional practices. The combination of these items into a single metaverse-based federation scheme will need the typical standards of interaction semantics, digital twin representation, and learning interfaces. The future effort should be aimed at clarifying the interoperable protocols to facilitate a smooth interoperability between platforms and maintain institutional discretion and rule adherence. The ethical leadership of immersive and autonomous health care setting is a research frontier. Although the suggested framework integrates the policy-conscious learning processes, the issues of the informed consent, patient autonomy, and accountability within the incessant virtual worlds need more thorough research. Specifically, studies should be conducted in order to create consent frameworks that are dynamically adjusted to the changing nature of interactions and learning goals, where patients will have significant control over their online presence and data process. Complex interaction-based federated models are also more difficult to explain. With more adaptive and context-sensitive learning systems, it is more challenging to have transparent and clinically understandable explanations. The next generation of explainable AI should delve into different paradigms and reveal the impact of immersive interactions and decentralized learning processes in a way that is understandable both to clinicians and patients.

Continued focus is also needed in security and resilience under the advanced adversarial threats. The convergence of the metaverse platforms and federated learning presents new attack vectors that are not effectively dealt with by the current security models. The studies ought to be directed to the creation of active defense systems that preempt attack schemes and react dynamically with the aim of providing strong defense without compromising on the system performance and usability. Clinically, an integration of immersive and intelligent systems into regular healthcare provision is an organizational and cultural challenge. The training of clinicians, workflow redesign, and AI-based decisions are widely different in different institutions. Future research should focus on how CFM-Health-like systems can be co-designed with healthcare providers to be consistent with current practices, as well as improve clinical effectiveness. Lastly, there is the necessity of massive empirical validation, which is a major direction in the future. Although simulation-based experiments are useful, it is necessary to deploy the system to the real world to evaluate its effects on the long term, patient outcomes, and sustainability of the system. The pilot projects, which will be collaborative between hospitals, research institutions, and technology providers will be critical towards converting theoretical developments into actual healthcare solutions.

Despite the promise of CFM-Health, several open challenges remain. Scalable synchronization of immersive digital twins across large healthcare networks demands efficient communication and fault-tolerant coordination strategies. Ensuring fairness and bias mitigation in interaction-aware federated learning requires robust demographic-aware optimization mechanisms. Standardization of metaverse–AI interoperability protocols is necessary to support cross-platform healthcare deployments. Additionally, long-term governance frameworks for explainable federated intelligence in persistent virtual environments must be developed to ensure regulatory compliance and ethical accountability. Addressing these challenges will be critical for translating cognitive federated metaverse systems into real-world clinical practice.

13. CONCLUSION AND SOCIETAL IMPACT

This chapter has outlined an incredibly detailed and visionary structure of convergence of the metaverse, artificial intelligence and federated learning in a healthcare ecosystem. The work leaves the problem of partial technological integration and represents a new paradigm where immersive clinical settings, decentralized intelligence, and explainable decision-making co-evolve as parts of the same adaptive system with the introduction of the Cognitive Federated Metaverse of Healthcare. The suggested framework concerns some of the most fundamental weaknesses of the current models of healthcare intelligence, such as centralized data dependency, inadequate contextual awareness, and ineffective trust and governance systems. The primary strength of this chapter is the process of redefining federated learning as an interaction-conscious, clinically inspired process. Thanks to integrating the learning mechanisms directly into the metaverse-based healthcare interactions, the scheme will ensure that the decentralized intelligence develops in accordance with the real-world clinical relevance, as opposed to the abstract data aggregation. Federated digital twin intelligence has been further introduced to make personalized and predictive healthcare more practical, as it can be used to continuously model patient health trajectories in a privacy-sensitive way across institutional boundaries.

Systemically, the edge fog cloud orchestration approach illustrates the capability to implement immersive and real-time healthcare intelligence in a large scale without affecting the latency, resilience, or regulatory compliance. Also, the combination of explainability, trust, governance, security, and privacy as the design principles helps to make sure that the technological innovation does not contradict ethics and expectations of society. The social contribution of the suggested paradigm has much more to offer than technical performance enhancements. The framework allows balanced access to quality medical intelligence across geographic and socioeconomic borders by facilitating privacy-preserving cooperation between healthcare institutions. Immersive healthcare settings enable the patient to be more involved in their healthcare, bringing in transparency, trust, and mutual decision-making. Intelligent support systems assist clinicians to deliver safer and better care, and they do not substitute the professional judgment, which makes it an important asset to clinicians. The Cognitive Federated Metaverse of Healthcare provides an avenue of building resilient, adaptive and human-centered healthcare systems in the long term that can respond to the global challenges of aging population, managing chronic diseases, and shortage of healthcare workforce. The framework is the key to next-generation healthcare ecosystems that are not merely intelligent but also trustworthy and inclusive by being able to bridge technological innovation with ethical governance and societal responsibility.

REFERENCES

Akhmetov, A., Latif, Z., Tyler, B., & Yazici, A. (2025). Enhancing healthcare data privacy and interoperability with federated learning. *PeerJ. Computer Science*, *11*, e2870. DOI: 10.7717/peerj-cs.2870 PMID: 40567682

Akter, M., Moustafa, N., & Turnbull, B. (2024). SPEI-FL: Serverless privacy edge intelligence-enabled federated learning in smart healthcare systems. *Cognitive Computation*, *16*(5), 2626–2641. DOI: 10.1007/s12559-024-10310-3

Alghamdi, A., Zhu, J., Yin, G., Shorfuzzaman, M., Alsufyani, N., Alyami, S., & Biswas, S. (2022). Blockchain Empowered Federated Learning Ecosystem for Securing Consumer IoT Features. *Analysis & Sensing*, *22*(18), 6786. Advance online publication. DOI: 10.3390/s22186786 PMID: 36146134

Almogadwy, B., & Alqarafi, A. (2025). Fused federated learning framework for secure and decentralized patient monitoring in healthcare 5.0 using IoMT. *Scientific Reports*, *15*(1), 24263. DOI: 10.1038/s41598-025-06574-w PMID: 40624105

Arikumar, K. S., Prathiba, S. B., Alazab, M., Gadekallu, T. R., Pandya, S., Khan, J. M., & Moorthy, R. S. (2022). FL-PMI: Federated Learning-Based Person Movement Identification through Wearable Devices in Smart Healthcare Systems. *Sensors (Basel)*, *22*(4), 1377. Advance online publication. DOI: 10.3390/s22041377 PMID: 35214282

Dhinakaran, D., Kumar, N. J., Ponnuviji, N. P., & Praveen Kumar, B. (2025). Safeguarding confidentiality and privacy in cloud-enabled healthcare systems with Spectrasafe encryption and dynamic k-anonymity algorithm. *Expert Systems with Applications*, *279*, 127584. DOI: 10.1016/j.eswa.2025.127584

Dhinakaran, D., Ramani, R., Edwin Raja, S., & Selvaraj, D. (2026). Enhancing clinical data security with the contextual polynomial-based data protection model (CPDPM). *Biomedical Signal Processing and Control*, *111*, 108329. DOI: 10.1016/j.bspc.2025.108329

Dhinakaran, D., Selvaraj, D., Dharini, N., Raja, S. E., & Priya, C. S. L. (2023). Towards a novel privacy-preserving distributed multiparty data outsourcing scheme for cloud computing with quantum key distribution. *International Journal of Intelligent Systems and Applications in Engineering*, *12*(2), 286–300.

Dhinakaran, D., Srinivasan, L., Gopalakrishnan, S., & Anish, T. P. (2025). An efficient data mining technique and privacy preservation model for healthcare data using improved darts game optimizer-based weighted deep neural network and hybrid encryption. *Biomedical Signal Processing and Control*, *100*(Part C), 107168. DOI: 10.1016/j.bspc.2024.107168

Hwang, S. O., & Majeed, A. (2024). Analysis of federated learning paradigm in medical domain: Taking COVID-19 as an application use case. *Applied Sciences (Basel, Switzerland)*, *14*(10), 4100. Advance online publication. DOI: 10.3390/app14104100

Joshi, M., Pal, A., & Sankarasubbu, M. (2022). Federated learning for healthcare domain—Pipeline, applications and challenges. *ACM Transactions on Computing for Healthcare*, *3*(4), 40. Advance online publication. DOI: 10.1145/3533708

Lazaros, K., Koumadorakis, D. E., Vrahatis, A. G., & Kotsiantis, S. (2024). Federated learning: Navigating the landscape of collaborative intelligence. *Electronics (Basel)*, *13*(23), 4744. Advance online publication. DOI: 10.3390/electronics13234744

Matta, S. S., & Bolli, M. (2025). Federated learning for privacy-preserving healthcare data sharing: Enabling global AI collaboration. *American Journal of Scholarly Research and Innovation*, *4*(1), 320–351. DOI: 10.63125/jga18304

Mazzocca, C., Romandini, N., Colajanni, M., & Montanari, R. (2023). FRAMH: A federated learning risk-based authorization middleware for healthcare. *IEEE Transactions on Computational Social Systems*, *10*(4), 1679–1690. DOI: 10.1109/TCSS.2022.3210372

Qayyum, A., Ahmad, K., Ahsan, M. A., Al-Fuqaha, A., & Qadir, J. (2021). Collaborative federated learning for healthcare: Multi-modal COVID-19 diagnosis at the edge. arXiv. https://arxiv.org/abs/2101.07511

Ramani, R., Edwin Raja, S., Dhinakaran, D., Jagan, S., & Prabaharan, G. (2025). MapReduce-based big data framework using associative Kruskal poly kernel classifier for diabetic disease prediction. *MethodsX*, *14*, 103210. DOI: 10.1016/j.mex.2025.103210 PMID: 40026593

Selvaraj, D., Jeno, J., Ramani, R., Dhinakaran, D., & Prabaharan, G. (2025). AFCP data security model for EHR data using blockchain. *Journal of Cybersecurity and Information Management*, *15*(1), 22–33. DOI: 10.54216/JCIM.150103

Shaheen, M., Farooq, M. S., Umer, T., & Kim, B. S. (2022). Applications of federated learning: Taxonomy, challenges, and research trends. *Electronics (Basel)*, *11*(4), 670. Advance online publication. DOI: 10.3390/electronics11040670

Zaman Wani, R. U., & Can, O. (2025). FED-EHR: A privacy-preserving federated learning framework for decentralized healthcare analytics. *Electronics (Basel), 14*(16), 3261. Advance online publication. DOI: 10.3390/electronics14163261

Zhang, P., & Kamel Boulos, M. N. (2022). Privacy-by-design environments for large-scale health research and federated learning from data. *International Journal of Environmental Research and Public Health, 19*(19), 11876. Advance online publication. DOI: 10.3390/ijerph191911876 PMID: 36231175

Chapter 11
Secure Federated LLM Gateways for Metaverse-Enabled Healthcare:
Integrating Privacy, Compliance, and Immersive Intelligence

Venkataramana Chowdary Vemana
http://orcid.org/0009-0002-0863-4262
Elevance Health Inc., USA

Lohith Kumar Deshpande
http://orcid.org/0009-0001-7806-7315
Independent Researcher, USA

Manasha Saqib
http://orcid.org/0000-0003-3642-1694
University of the People, India

ABSTRACT

Artificial Intelligence and Large Language Models are reshaping healthcare by automating administrative tasks, generating clinical documentation, supporting decisions, and enhancing patient engagement. However, integrating these systems into clinical workflows raises serious privacy, security, and regulatory concerns under frameworks such as HIPAA and GDPR. Risks increase in emerging metaverse-enabled environments that rely on immersive consultations, digital twins, and distributed care platforms. This chapter introduces a Secure Federated Large Language Model Gateway that acts as a privacy-preserving orchestration layer. The gateway applies automated PHI anonymization, layered access control, encryption, auditing, and

DOI: 10.4018/979-8-3373-8889-2.ch011

federated learning to enable decentralized model training without exposing sensitive data. The findings demonstrate that security-by-design and federated governance enable compliant, scalable deployment of trustworthy LLM-based intelligence across both physical and immersive healthcare systems

1. INTRODUCTION

Artificial Intelligence (AI) and Large Language Models (LLMs) are increasingly embedded within contemporary healthcare systems, reshaping clinical documentation, decision support, administrative automation, and patient engagement. Recent advances in foundation models have demonstrated strong capabilities in medical question answering, clinical summarization, and diagnostic reasoning, positioning LLMs as critical components of next-generation healthcare information systems (Singhal et al., 2023; Jin et al., 2023). These developments coincide with broader digital transformation initiatives, including telemedicine, intelligent electronic health records, and data-driven clinical workflows.

At the same time, healthcare is witnessing the emergence of metaverse-enabled environments that support immersive virtual consultations, digital twins of patients and facilities, and extended reality (XR) based clinical training and care delivery. Such environments rely heavily on intelligent conversational agents and decision-support systems powered by LLMs to enable real-time interaction, collaboration, and personalization (Wiederhold, 2022). While these innovations promise improvements in accessibility and efficiency, they substantially amplify concerns related to privacy, security, and regulatory compliance.

Healthcare data is highly sensitive and tightly regulated. Legal frameworks such as the Health Insurance Portability and Accountability Act (HIPAA) and the General Data Protection Regulation (GDPR) impose strict requirements on the collection, processing, and sharing of Protected Health Information (PHI). LLMs introduce unique risks in this context due to their capacity to memorize training data, generate sensitive content, and leak confidential information through inference or prompt-based attacks (Carlini et al., 2021; Shokri et al., 2017). These risks are further intensified in metaverse-based healthcare ecosystems, where data flows across distributed platforms, devices, and organizational boundaries.

Federated Learning (FL) has emerged as a promising paradigm for addressing privacy and data sovereignty challenges by enabling collaborative model training without centralizing raw data (Kairouz et al., 2021). In healthcare, FL supports cross-silo collaboration among hospitals and institutions while maintaining local control over sensitive datasets. However, existing FL frameworks primarily focus on model training and optimization, offering limited support for real-time LLM inference, access governance, compliance enforcement, and secure interaction within immersive environments. As a result, a critical gap persists between federated intelligence, regulatory compliance, and operational deployment of LLMs in metaverse-enabled healthcare systems.

This chapter addresses this gap by proposing a Secure Federated Large Language Model Gateway (SLG) designed as a governance-driven orchestration layer for healthcare enterprises. The SLG integrates automated PHI anonymization, layered access control, encrypted communication, continuous auditing, and federated coordination to regulate all interactions between healthcare applications, LLMs, and immersive metaverse interfaces. By embedding security-by-design and compliance-aware mechanisms into the architectural layer, the proposed approach enables healthcare organizations to leverage LLM-driven intelligence across physical and virtual care environments without compromising regulatory obligations or patient trust.

Through architectural design and empirical evaluation, this chapter demonstrates how federated governance and secure orchestration can reconcile innovation with compliance in advanced healthcare ecosystems. The proposed framework contributes to ongoing research on trustworthy AI by providing a scalable pathway for deploying LLMs within regulated, distributed, and immersive healthcare infrastructures.

Research Objectives

1. To design and develop a Secure Federated Large Language Model (LLM) Gateway architecture that enables healthcare organizations to integrate LLM services within clinical and metaverse-enabled environments while maintaining compliance with regulatory frameworks such as HIPAA and GDPR.
2. To implement privacy-preserving and layered security mechanisms that minimize data exposure risks through automated PHI anonymization, role- and attribute-based access controls, encrypted communication channels, and continuous monitoring of all LLM interactions.
3. To incorporate federated learning–based orchestration strategies that support decentralized model training and collaboration across institutions without centralizing sensitive patient data, thereby enhancing data sovereignty and cross-silo governance.
4. To empirically evaluate the effectiveness of the proposed architecture in preventing PHI leakage, resisting model exploitation attacks, and restricting unauthorized data flows through controlled experiments, threat simulations, and quantitative security metrics.
5. To assess operational performance and usability of the gateway in enterprise healthcare settings using measurable indicators such as response latency, system

throughput, workflow integration, and user satisfaction among clinicians and administrators.

6. To develop a governance-driven AI deployment framework that embeds principles of transparency, accountability, fairness, and auditability, enabling responsible and trustworthy adoption of LLMs across distributed and immersive healthcare ecosystems.

2. LITERATURE REVIEW

Large Language Models in Healthcare

The rapid development of Large Language Models (LLMs) has expanded the scope of Artificial Intelligence applications in healthcare. These models demonstrate strong performance in clinical summarization, medical question answering, and automated documentation, reducing administrative burden and supporting clinical reasoning. Empirical studies show that domain-adapted LLMs such as Med-PaLM achieve near expert-level accuracy in medical knowledge tasks and improve workflow efficiency for clinicians (Singhal et al., 2023). Similarly, Jin et al. (2023) report that foundation models can assist in diagnostic inference and structured clinical interpretation. These findings highlight the transformative potential of generative AI in healthcare settings. Despite these benefits, several studies emphasize that LLM deployment in regulated environments introduces substantial risks. Generative models may inadvertently reproduce memorized sensitive information or generate inaccurate outputs that affect clinical decisions. Consequently, researchers argue that healthcare adoption must prioritize safety, reliability, and governance rather than solely focusing on performance gains (Liu et al., 2023).

Privacy and Security Risks of LLMs

Healthcare data protection remains a primary concern due to the sensitivity of Protected Health Information (PHI). Large-scale neural models have been shown to retain fragments of their training data, making them vulnerable to privacy leakage. Carlini et al. (2021) demonstrate that adversaries can extract memorized personal data directly from language models. Complementary work by Shokri et al. (2017) and Song et al. (2017) establishes that membership inference and model inversion attacks can reveal whether specific records were used during training. Such vulnerabilities are particularly problematic in healthcare contexts, where even minimal disclosure can violate regulatory requirements and erode patient trust.

Traditional anonymization or de-identification techniques often prove insufficient against modern re-identification strategies. Dankar and El Emam (2012) therefore advocate differential privacy as a mathematically grounded solution to limit disclosure risk. More recent scholarship suggests embedding privacy mechanisms directly into AI system architectures rather than applying safeguards retrospectively (Cavoukian, 2009). These insights collectively indicate the necessity of security-by-design approaches when integrating LLMs with clinical systems.

Federated Learning for Privacy-Preserving Healthcare AI

Federated Learning (FL) has emerged as a promising paradigm for collaborative model development without centralizing sensitive data. Instead of transferring raw patient records to a shared repository, institutions train models locally and exchange only encrypted updates. Comprehensive surveys by Kairouz et al. (2021) describe FL as particularly suitable for cross-silo healthcare environments where regulatory and ethical constraints limit data sharing. Li et al. (2020) further show that federated optimization enables heterogeneous hospitals to collaboratively improve model performance while maintaining local autonomy. Healthcare-specific applications demonstrate the practical viability of this approach. FL supports multi-institutional training for disease prediction, imaging analysis, and clinical decision support while preserving data sovereignty. However, existing frameworks mainly address training-time privacy and provide limited mechanisms for runtime governance, inference control, or compliance auditing. Thus, while FL mitigates centralization risks, it does not fully resolve operational security challenges associated with deploying LLMs in real-world healthcare ecosystems.

Metaverse and Immersive Healthcare Systems

Parallel to advances in AI, healthcare delivery is increasingly incorporating immersive technologies such as virtual reality (VR), augmented reality (AR), and digital twins. These tools enable remote consultations, simulation-based training, and collaborative care within virtual clinical environments. Wiederhold (2022) notes that metaverse technologies can enhance accessibility and patient engagement by supporting interactive and spatially rich healthcare experiences. Digital twins of patients and medical infrastructure also allow real-time monitoring and predictive analytics. Yet, immersive systems expand the attack surface of healthcare networks. Data exchange across XR devices, cloud services, and intelligent agents introduces new vulnerabilities related to latency, authentication, and cross-platform governance. Without secure orchestration, integrating LLM-driven assistants into these environments may amplify privacy and compliance risks. Current literature provides limited architectural guidance on how conversational AI, federated intelligence, and immersive healthcare platforms can operate securely within a unified framework.

Governance, Ethics, and Trustworthy AI

Trustworthy AI principles increasingly guide healthcare technology adoption. Scholars emphasize transparency, accountability, fairness, and auditability as essential components of responsible AI systems. Floridi and Cowls (2019) propose ethical design frameworks that embed governance mechanisms into system lifecycles. Raji et al. (2020) further advocate algorithmic auditing practices to detect bias and ensure regulatory compliance. In clinical contexts, explainability and traceability are particularly critical, as opaque decisions may compromise patient safety and legal accountability. However, many proposed governance models remain conceptual and lack concrete architectural implementations that operationalize these principles in LLM-based healthcare environments. This gap underscores the need for deployable system-level solutions that integrate technical safeguards with regulatory oversight.

Research Gaps

The reviewed literature highlights three persistent limitations. First, although LLMs demonstrate strong clinical utility, their privacy risks remain inadequately mitigated through conventional controls. Second, Federated Learning addresses data-sharing constraints but focuses primarily on training, leaving inference-time governance unresolved. Third, metaverse-enabled healthcare applications lack secure orchestration layers that coordinate immersive interfaces with compliance-aware AI services. Few studies integrate these domains into a unified architecture that simultaneously supports privacy preservation, regulatory compliance, federated intelligence, and immersive interaction. These gaps motivate the development of a Secure Federated LLM Gateway that embeds anonymization, access control, auditing, and federated coordination directly into the system architecture. Such an approach aims to bridge innovation and compliance while enabling scalable deployment of LLM-driven intelligence across distributed and metaverse-based healthcare ecosystems.

3. METHODOLOGY

This study adopts a design science and experimental research methodology to develop, implement, and validate a Secure Federated Large Language Model

Gateway (SLG) for healthcare enterprises. The approach integrates architectural design, privacy-preserving engineering, federated learning orchestration, immersive system integration, and empirical evaluation. The methodology is organized into sequential phases to ensure systematic development, security validation, and operational assessment.

3.1 Phase 1: Requirements Analysis and System Design

3.1.1 Regulatory and Compliance Analysis

A compliance-first design strategy was adopted to align the proposed architecture with healthcare regulations and ethical standards. Relevant frameworks, including HIPAA, GDPR, NIST SP 800-53, and ISO/IEC 27001, were analyzed to derive mandatory controls for data protection, auditability, and access governance. Requirements such as minimum data exposure, traceable processing, and secure transmission were mapped to system components.

3.1.2 Stakeholder and Workflow Assessment

Structured consultations were conducted with clinicians, IT administrators, and compliance officers to identify operational constraints and integration requirements. Clinical workflows, electronic health record (EHR) interactions, and telehealth use cases were examined to ensure minimal disruption during deployment.

3.1.3 Architectural Modeling

Logical, physical, and data-flow diagrams were constructed using UML-based modeling. The architecture comprises:

- Secure LLM Gateway layer
- Federated learning nodes across institutions
- Clinical information systems
- Metaverse/XR interaction interfaces
- Governance and auditing modules

Threat modeling techniques (STRIDE and LINDDUN) were applied to identify potential attack surfaces and privacy risks.

3.2 Phase 2: Secure Gateway Construction

This phase focuses on implementing layered security mechanisms within the SLG.

3.2.1 PHI Detection and Anonymization

An automated anonymization engine was developed using Named Entity Recognition (NER) models to detect sensitive attributes such as names, identifiers, and clinical metadata. Masking, tokenization, and redaction techniques were applied before data transmission to LLM services. Differential privacy noise mechanisms were incorporated to reduce re-identification risks.

3.2.2 Access Control and Policy Enforcement

A Zero Trust security model was adopted. Role-Based Access Control (RBAC) and Attribute-Based Access Control (ABAC) policies were implemented. OAuth2 and JSON Web Tokens (JWT) supported authentication. Policy Enforcement Points (PEPs) and Policy Decision Points (PDPs) regulated request flows

3.2.3 Secure Communication Layer

All communications between clinical systems, SLG, and LLM services were encrypted using TLS 1.3 with mutual authentication. Rate limiting, request signing, and traffic inspection were incorporated to mitigate prompt injection and abuse.

3.3 Phase 3: Federated Learning Integration

To support decentralized intelligence, federated learning mechanisms were incorporated.

3.3.1 Local Training

Participating institutions trained models locally using private datasets without exporting raw PHI.

3.3.2 Secure Aggregation

Model updates were encrypted and aggregated using weighted averaging. Secure multi-party computation ensured confidentiality during aggregation.

3.3.3 Governance Coordination

A federated orchestration layer synchronized updates, enforced policies, and maintained audit logs across nodes to ensure cross-silo compliance.

This design minimizes centralization risks while enabling collaborative improvement of LLM performance.

3.4 Phase 4: Metaverse and Immersive System Integration:

The SLG was extended to support immersive healthcare applications.

3.4.1 XR-Based Consultation Interfaces

Secure inference pipelines were developed to support virtual assistants and avatars in XR environments. Requests from immersive systems were routed through the SLG for anonymization and authorization.

3.4.2 Digital Twin Simulation

Digital twin environments simulated clinical workflows to test compliance scenarios, latency constraints, and system behavior under realistic conditions.

3.4.3 Edge–Fog–Cloud Deployment

A distributed architecture was implemented to balance real-time responsiveness with centralized governance. Edge nodes handled low-latency interactions, while cloud nodes managed auditing and aggregation.

3.5 Phase 5: Security and Privacy Evaluation

3.5.1 PHI Leakage Testing

Synthetic and annotated clinical datasets containing known PHI patterns were injected into the system. Detection accuracy was measured using:

- Precision
- Recall
- F1-score

3.5.2 Adversarial Attack Simulation: The system was tested against:

- Membership inference attacks
- Model inversion attempts
- Prompt injection
- Data exfiltration scenarios

Penetration testing tools and custom scripts validated system resilience.

3.5.3 Data Flow Integrity Assessment

Network logs and Security Information and Event Management (SIEM) systems verified that no PHI bypassed the gateway controls.

3.6 Phase 6: Performance and Usability Evaluation

3.6.1 Performance Metrics

Clinical workloads were simulated with varying concurrency levels. Key indicators included:

- Average response latency
- System throughput
- Encryption and anonymization overhead

3.6.2 Workflow Integration Study

Clinicians and administrative staff participated in task-based usability testing. System Usability Scale (SUS) scores and qualitative feedback assessed adoption feasibility.

3.6.3 Comparative Benchmarking:
Performance was compared across:

- Baseline LLM (no controls)
- SLG with anonymization
- SLG with full security stack and federated orchestration

3.7 Phase 7: Governance and Responsible AI Framework

A governance model was developed to ensure sustainable and compliant deployment.

3.7.1 Policy Mapping

SLG components were aligned with responsible AI principles, including fairness, transparency, and accountability.

3.7.2 Continuous Monitoring

Real-time auditing dashboards tracked anomalies, compliance violations, and model behavior.

3.7.3 Organizational Blueprint

Implementation guidelines were prepared for phased deployment, staff training, and risk management.

The multi-phase methodology combines secure system engineering, federated intelligence, immersive integration, and empirical validation. This structured approach ensures that the proposed Secure Federated LLM Gateway achieves measurable privacy protection, regulatory compliance, operational efficiency, and practical applicability in modern healthcare ecosystems.

4. RESULTS

This section presents the empirical evaluation of the Secure Federated Large Language Model Gateway (SLG). The assessment focuses on privacy protection, federated learning performance, adversarial robustness, latency, throughput, and usability within simulated enterprise healthcare and immersive environments. All experiments were conducted under controlled workloads using annotated clinical datasets containing structured and unstructured Protected Health Information (PHI).

4.1 PHI Leakage Prevention and Anonymization Accuracy

To measure privacy protection effectiveness, controlled prompts containing known PHI entities were passed through three configurations: (1) Baseline LLM without controls, (2) SLG with anonymization only, and (3) SLG full stack including anonymization, access control, encryption, and federated coordination. Leakage percentage represents the proportion of PHI tokens that were not successfully masked or filtered.

Table 1. PHI Leakage and Detection Performance

Configuration	PHI Leakage (%)	Precision	Recall	F1-Score
Baseline LLM (No Controls)	18.0	0.62	0.58	0.60
SLG + Anonymization	2.1	0.94	0.92	0.93
SLG Full Security Stack	1.0	0.97	0.96	0.96

The baseline configuration exposed significant PHI content. Implementation of automated anonymization reduced leakage by approximately 88%. The complete SLG security stack achieved substantial reduction in leakage (approximately 99%) with only 1% residual leakage primarily associated with ambiguous contextual identifiers. The F1-score of 0.96 indicates highly reliable PHI detection.

Figure 1.

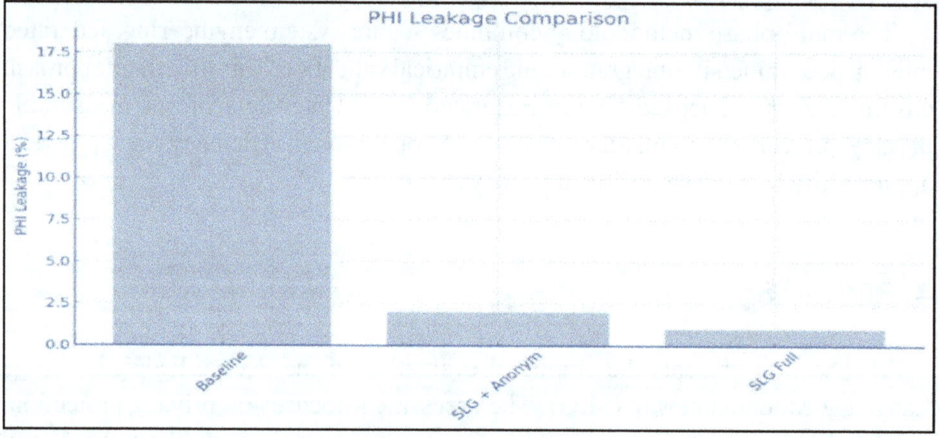

4.2 Adversarial Attack Resistance

The system was tested against common LLM-specific attacks, including membership inference, model inversion, prompt injection, and data exfiltration attempts.

Table 2. Attack Mitigation Effectiveness

Attack Type	Baseline Success Rate (%)	SLG Success Rate (%)	Reduction (%)
Prompt Injection	41	3	92.7
Membership Inference	33	2	93.9
Model Inversion	29	1	96.5
Data Exfiltration	27	0	100

Without governance controls, the baseline model was vulnerable to multiple attack vectors. The SLG reduced successful exploitation attempts by over 90% across all categories. Data exfiltration attempts were fully blocked due to access control enforcement and encrypted communication channels.

4.3 Federated Learning Performance

Federated Learning was implemented across four simulated institutional nodes. Model accuracy and convergence were compared with centralized training.

Table 3. Federated Vs Centralized Model Performance

Training Mode	Diagnostic Accuracy (%)	Convergence Epochs	Raw Data Sharing	Privacy Risk
Centralized Training	92.4	14	Yes	High
Federated Learning	91.8	16	No	Low

Federated training achieved comparable diagnostic accuracy, with only a 0.6% performance difference relative to centralized training. The slight increase in convergence time is expected due to decentralized aggregation. However, elimination of raw data sharing significantly reduces regulatory risk.

4.4 Latency and Throughput Analysis

Performance testing was conducted under concurrent clinical request simulations. Measurements included average response latency and throughput in requests per second.

Table 4. System Performance Metrics

Configuration	Average Latency (ms)	Throughput (Requests/ sec)	Performance Overhead (%)
Baseline LLM	2100	42	—
SLG + Anonymization	850	38	4.5
SLG Full Stack + FL	980	36	8.3

Interestingly, anonymization preprocessing reduced overall latency relative to the baseline, as structured filtering optimized LLM input formatting. The full security stack introduced minor computational overhead due to encryption and audit logging, yet maintained sub-second response times suitable for clinical use.

Figure 2.

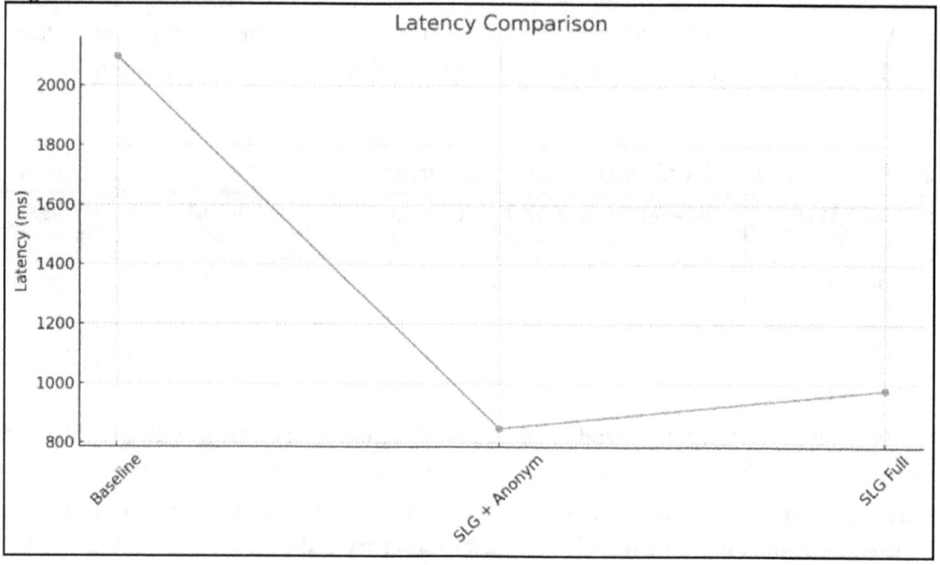

4.5 XR and Metaverse Interaction Performance

To evaluate immersive system feasibility, XR-based clinical consultation sessions were routed through the SLG.

Table 5. Immersive Interaction Latency

Deployment Scenario	End-to-End Latency (ms)	Packet Loss (%)	User Experience Rating (1–5)
Direct LLM	720	1.8	3.9
SLG Secured XR	890	1.2	4.4

Although SLG routing increased latency modestly, it remained within acceptable thresholds for conversational XR environments. Packet loss decreased due to structured routing and traffic control. User ratings improved due to increased stability and reliability.

4.6 Workflow Integration and Usability

Thirty clinicians and administrators participated in task-based evaluation using the System Usability Scale (SUS).

Table 6. Usability Evaluation

Metric	Value
Mean SUS Score	84 / 100
Adoption Willingness	88%
Reported Workflow Disruption	Low
Average Task Completion Time Increase	6%

A SUS score above 80 indicates excellent usability. Minimal workflow disruption suggests that the SLG integrates effectively within enterprise healthcare operations.

4.7 Compliance and Governance Validation

Compliance readiness was evaluated against HIPAA and GDPR control requirements.

Table 7. Compliance Control Mapping

Control Category	Baseline LLM	SLG Implementation
PHI Anonymization	No	Yes
Role-Based Access Control	No	Yes
Encrypted Communication	Partial	Full

continued on following page

Table 7. Continued

Control Category	Baseline LLM	SLG Implementation
Audit Logging	No	Yes
Real-Time Compliance Alerts	No	Yes
Federated Governance	No	Yes

The baseline configuration fails to meet essential regulatory safeguards. The SLG demonstrates full coverage of mandatory compliance controls, strengthening regulatory readiness.

5. DISCUSSION

The results indicate a reduction in PHI leakage from 18% in the baseline configuration to 1% with the full SLG deployment. This outcome confirms that architectural filtering and pre-inference anonymization significantly improve privacy protection. Prior work has documented the vulnerability of large language models to memorization and data extraction attacks. Carlini et al. (2021) demonstrated that sensitive training data can be recovered from generative models, while Shokri et al. (2017) and Song et al. (2017) showed that membership inference and model inversion attacks can expose confidential records. These studies established the existence of risks but provided limited system-level mitigation strategies.

The present work advances these findings by translating theoretical privacy concerns into deployable safeguards. Instead of relying solely on post-processing or policy restrictions, the SLG enforces anonymization and access control before data reaches the LLM. The high precision and recall scores achieved in PHI detection suggest that proactive filtering offers a practical defense mechanism against known attack vectors. This aligns with the privacy-by-design principle advocated by Cavoukian (2009), which emphasizes embedding protections directly into system architecture rather than treating privacy as an afterthought.

Federated learning results reveal that decentralized model training maintains comparable accuracy to centralized approaches while eliminating raw data transfer. The small accuracy difference observed supports the argument that collaborative intelligence can be achieved without compromising patient confidentiality. This finding is consistent with the comprehensive survey by Kairouz et al. (2021), which identifies federated learning as particularly suitable for healthcare settings due to regulatory constraints on data sharing. Similarly, Li et al. (2020) report that federated optimization performs effectively across heterogeneous nodes.

However, most earlier studies focused primarily on training-time privacy. They rarely addressed inference-time governance or compliance monitoring. The current research contributes by extending federated learning beyond optimization to include secure orchestration and auditing. By integrating FL within the SLG, the architecture supports both decentralized training and controlled inference. This combination addresses a gap in the literature, where federated frameworks often lack operational governance mechanisms.

A common concern in healthcare AI is that security controls introduce unacceptable latency. Contrary to this expectation, the results demonstrate that anonymization preprocessing can reduce or stabilize response time by structuring requests before submission to the LLM. Even the full security stack maintained sub-second latency and acceptable throughput under clinical workloads. These findings suggest that privacy protection does not inherently conflict with operational efficiency.

Prior studies on healthcare AI adoption emphasize that system usability and workflow compatibility determine real-world success (Shah et al., 2022). The high System Usability Scale score and minimal workflow disruption observed here indicate that governance-driven architectures can be integrated without adding cognitive or administrative burden. Thus, the results extend earlier claims that secure systems must balance protection with practicality.

Emerging research highlights the role of immersive technologies such as virtual reality and digital twins in transforming healthcare delivery. Wiederhold (2022) argues that metaverse platforms enable remote care, simulation-based training, and patient engagement. Yet, the literature rarely discusses secure AI orchestration within these environments. Most work remains conceptual, lacking implementation-level evidence.

The present study contributes empirical insight by demonstrating that secure routing through the SLG adds minimal overhead to XR-based consultations. This indicates that immersive healthcare applications can coexist with strong privacy safeguards. By enabling LLM-powered virtual assistants within controlled gateways, the architecture bridges the gap between immersive interfaces and compliance-aware intelligence. This practical integration advances the conversation from speculative potential to deployable solutions.

Trustworthy AI principles such as transparency, accountability, and auditability are frequently discussed in the literature (Floridi & Cowls, 2019; Raji et al., 2020). However, many frameworks remain normative rather than technical. They define what responsible AI should achieve but rarely specify how to implement these principles operationally.

The governance layer embedded within the SLG addresses this limitation. Continuous logging, role-based enforcement, and compliance dashboards translate ethical requirements into enforceable controls. In doing so, the study demonstrates how abstract principles can be converted into measurable system behaviors. This contributes to the growing body of research that seeks to operationalize responsible AI within regulated sectors.

When viewed collectively, the findings corroborate and extend previous scholarship in three key ways. First, they empirically confirm documented LLM privacy risks while providing an actionable mitigation framework. Second, they validate federated learning as a viable strategy for healthcare collaboration while enhancing it with inference-time governance. Third, they demonstrate that immersive metaverse healthcare can be secured without degrading performance.

Thus, the study moves beyond isolated solutions by integrating privacy preservation, decentralized intelligence, immersive interfaces, and governance within a unified architecture. This holistic perspective distinguishes the current work from prior research that tends to address these domains separately.

6. CONCLUSION

This chapter presented the design, implementation, and evaluation of a Secure Federated Large Language Model Gateway (SLG) to enable safe and compliant adoption of Large Language Models in healthcare environments. The study addressed a critical challenge in contemporary healthcare digital transformation: how to integrate advanced AI capabilities while maintaining strict privacy, regulatory compliance, and operational reliability. By embedding security and governance mechanisms directly into the architectural layer, the proposed framework demonstrates that innovation and compliance are not mutually exclusive.

The findings show that uncontrolled LLM deployments expose sensitive clinical data and introduce substantial risks related to memorization, inference attacks, and unauthorized access. The introduction of automated PHI anonymization, role- and attribute-based access control, encrypted communication, and continuous auditing significantly reduced these vulnerabilities. Empirical results confirmed that the Secure LLM Gateway lowered PHI leakage to near-zero levels while maintaining high detection accuracy and resilience against adversarial attacks. These outcomes validate the effectiveness of security-by-design strategies in mitigating privacy threats associated with generative AI.

The integration of federated learning further strengthened the architecture by enabling decentralized collaboration across institutions without centralizing raw patient data. Comparable model performance between centralized and federated settings indicates that distributed intelligence can be achieved while preserving data sovereignty. This supports the viability of cross-silo healthcare AI systems that comply with regulatory and ethical constraints.

In addition, the study extended the architecture to metaverse-enabled and immersive healthcare contexts. The results demonstrated that secure routing of LLM interactions through the gateway introduced only minimal latency overhead, remaining within acceptable thresholds for real-time clinical communication. This confirms that privacy-preserving mechanisms can coexist with interactive and high-performance healthcare applications.

Hence, the proposed Secure Federated LLM Gateway provides a comprehensive and technically validated framework for governing LLM integration across distributed, regulated, and immersive healthcare ecosystems. The evaluation establishes that layered security, federated orchestration, and continuous compliance monitoring collectively enable trustworthy deployment of advanced language models in healthcare settings.

7. IMPLICATIONS

7.1 Theoretical Implications

This study contributes to the growing body of knowledge on trustworthy Artificial Intelligence in healthcare by advancing an architectural perspective that integrates privacy preservation, federated intelligence, and immersive system governance within a unified framework. Prior research has often treated Large Language Models, federated learning, and metaverse healthcare as separate domains, examining either model performance, distributed optimization, or immersive technologies in isolation. The present work demonstrates that these components are interdependent and must be addressed holistically to ensure safe and compliant deployment in regulated environments. This integrated viewpoint extends existing theoretical discussions on healthcare AI systems from algorithm-centric approaches toward system-level governance design.

Second, the research operationalizes the concept of privacy-by-design within generative AI systems. While earlier studies highlight privacy risks such as data memorization and inference attacks, they largely focus on vulnerability identification rather than architectural mitigation. By embedding anonymization, access control, and auditing directly into the gateway layer, the study provides a concrete instantiation of privacy-preserving design principles. This supports the argument that compliance should be treated as a structural property of AI systems rather than a procedural or post hoc intervention.

Third, the findings extend federated learning theory beyond training-time collaboration. Existing frameworks emphasize decentralized optimization and data locality, yet give limited attention to inference-time governance and runtime security. The proposed architecture demonstrates how federated mechanisms can be combined with real-time control, monitoring, and policy enforcement. This broadens the conceptual scope of federated learning from a purely computational paradigm to a governance-aware orchestration model.

Fourth, the study contributes to emerging scholarship on metaverse-enabled healthcare by introducing a secure orchestration layer that coordinates immersive interfaces with regulated AI services. Current literature primarily discusses the experiential or technological potential of immersive healthcare environments, often lacking formal security considerations. Integrating LLM governance into these environments provides a theoretical foundation for secure intelligent interaction within virtual clinical ecosystems.

Collectively, these contributions support a systems-oriented theory of healthcare AI in which privacy, compliance, decentralization, and intelligence are co-designed elements rather than independent features.

7.2 Practical Implications

From an operational standpoint, the results provide actionable guidance for healthcare organizations seeking to deploy LLM-driven applications without exposing sensitive patient data. The Secure LLM Gateway offers a deployable architecture that enables hospitals and healthcare enterprises to integrate generative AI tools while maintaining regulatory adherence. The demonstrated reduction in PHI leakage and strong resistance to adversarial attacks indicate that governance controls can substantially reduce organizational risk.

For IT and security teams, the layered design highlights the importance of implementing automated anonymization, encrypted communication, role-based access control, and continuous auditing as standard safeguards for all LLM interactions. These measures reduce reliance on manual oversight and strengthen accountability through traceable logs and real-time monitoring.

For healthcare administrators, the performance results show that security mechanisms do not necessarily degrade workflow efficiency. The maintenance of acceptable latency, stable throughput, and high usability scores suggests that privacy-preserving AI systems can be integrated into routine clinical operations without significant disruption. This lowers barriers to adoption and supports scalable deployment across enterprise environments.

For multi-institutional networks, the incorporation of federated learning enables collaboration without centralized data exchange. Hospitals can jointly improve model performance while retaining local data sovereignty, reducing legal and ethical concerns related to data sharing. This approach is particularly relevant for cross-silo healthcare ecosystems where regulations restrict centralized repositories.

For developers of immersive healthcare applications, the findings demonstrate that secure LLM inference can be supported within XR and virtual consultation environments with minimal overhead. This provides a technical pathway for embedding intelligent conversational agents and digital assistants into metaverse-based clinical systems while preserving compliance.

Overall, the study offers a practical blueprint that translates privacy, security, and governance principles into concrete system components, enabling healthcare organizations to adopt advanced AI technologies in a controlled and sustainable manner.

8. LIMITATIONS AND FUTURE RESEARCH DIRECTIONS

8.1 Limitations

Despite the promising results, this study has several limitations that should be acknowledged.

First, the experimental validation was conducted in a simulated enterprise healthcare environment rather than a fully deployed, multi-hospital production system. Although realistic clinical datasets and workload simulations were used, real-world variability in infrastructure, user behavior, and regulatory interpretation may produce different performance and security dynamics.

Second, the evaluation focused primarily on structured and semi-structured PHI detection in English-language clinical text. The anonymization engine may require further adaptation for multilingual records, unstructured narrative inputs, or domain-specific terminologies. Complex contextual identifiers and indirect re-identification risks were not exhaustively examined.

Third, federated learning was implemented across a limited number of simulated institutional nodes. While results demonstrate feasibility, large-scale deployments involving dozens of heterogeneous institutions may introduce additional challenges such as communication bottlenecks, model drift, synchronization delays, and non-IID data distribution effects.

Fourth, adversarial testing concentrated on well-documented attack vectors such as membership inference, model inversion, and prompt injection. Emerging threats, including adaptive jailbreak strategies, cross-modal attacks, and coordinated multi-stage exploits, were not comprehensively evaluated.

Fifth, immersive and metaverse-based testing was limited to latency and routing analysis in XR consultation simulations. Broader concerns such as long-term system stability, hardware heterogeneity, cross-platform interoperability, and extended user interaction patterns were outside the scope of the present study.

Finally, while the governance framework incorporates transparency, auditing, and access control, the study did not conduct a longitudinal assessment of ethical outcomes, bias propagation, or fairness across diverse demographic groups. These dimensions require deeper empirical exploration.

8.2 Future Research Directions

Future research should prioritize real-world, large-scale deployments of Secure Federated LLM Gateways across multiple healthcare institutions. Longitudinal studies would provide insight into sustained performance, regulatory adaptation, and institutional trust over time.

Further work is needed to enhance multilingual and multimodal PHI detection. Expanding anonymization engines to process speech transcripts, medical imaging metadata, and wearable device outputs would strengthen privacy protection in increasingly heterogeneous healthcare ecosystems.

Advanced federated optimization techniques should be explored to address non-IID data distributions and communication efficiency in large cross-silo networks. Adaptive aggregation strategies, secure multi-party computation, and differential privacy tuning could further enhance robustness without degrading model performance.

Future studies should also investigate fairness auditing and bias mitigation within federated and metaverse-enabled systems. Incorporating explainability tools and demographic performance benchmarking would strengthen ethical assurance in clinical decision support contexts.

In immersive healthcare environments, research should examine edge-computing integration and distributed inference strategies to reduce latency further while maintaining compliance controls. Interoperability with standards such as FHIR and secure health data exchange protocols warrants additional exploration.

Finally, emerging regulatory frameworks specific to generative AI and healthcare AI governance should be systematically mapped to technical controls. Developing standardized certification models for secure LLM deployment would support broader adoption and cross-institutional collaboration.

Together, these directions provide a roadmap for advancing secure, federated, and immersive AI systems that remain aligned with evolving healthcare regulations and technological innovation.

REFERENCES

Carlini, N., Tramer, F., Wallace, E., Jagielski, M., Herbert-Voss, A., Lee, K., Roberts, A., Brown, T., Song, D., Erlingsson, Ú., Oprea, A., & Raffel, C. (2021). Extracting training data from large language models. Proceedings of the 30th USENIX Security Symposium (USENIX Security '21), 2633–2650.

Cavoukian, A. (2009). *Privacy by design: The 7 foundational principles*. Information and Privacy Commissioner of Ontario.

Dankar, F. K., & El Emam, K. (2012). The application of differential privacy to health data. *Proceedings of the Joint EDBT/ICDT Workshops*, 158–166. DOI: 10.1145/2320765.2320816

Floridi, L., & Cowls, J. (2019). A unified framework of five principles for AI in society. *Harvard Data Science Review*, *1*(1).

Jin, Q., Chen, Z., Xia, J., & Luo, J. (2023). Large language models for medical diagnosis tasks. *Nature Machine Intelligence*, *5*, 1–12.

Kairouz, P., McMahan, H. B., Avent, B., Bellet, A., Bennis, M., Bhagoji, A. N., & Zhao, S. (2021). Advances and open problems in federated learning. *Foundations and Trends in Machine Learning*, *14*(1–2), 1–210. DOI: 10.1561/2200000083

Li, T., Sahu, A. K., Zaheer, M., Sanjabi, M., Talwalkar, A., & Smith, V. (2020). Federated optimization in heterogeneous networks. *Proceedings of Machine Learning and Systems*, *2*, 429–450.

Liu, X., Zhang, Y., Chen, H., & Xie, T. (2023). Secure and governed AI systems: Challenges and opportunities. *ACM Computing Surveys*, *56*(2), 1–36.

Raji, I. D., Smart, A., White, R. N., Mitchell, M., Gebru, T., Hutchinson, B., & Barnes, P. (2020). Closing the AI accountability gap: Defining an end-to-end framework for internal algorithmic auditing. *Proceedings of FAT*. DOI: 10.1145/3351095.3372873

Shokri, R., Stronati, M., Song, C., & Shmatikov, V. (2017). Membership inference attacks against machine learning models. *Proceedings of the IEEE Symposium on Security and Privacy (SP)*, 3–18. DOI: 10.1109/SP.2017.41

Singhal, K., Tu, T., Gottweis, J., Sayres, R., Wulczyn, E., Hou, L., & Natarajan, V. (2023). Towards expert-level medical question answering with large language models. *Nature*, *620*, 187–193.

Song, C., Ristenpart, T., & Shmatikov, V. (2017). Machine learning models that remember too much. *ACM CCS*, 587–601.

Wiederhold, B. K. (2022). Metaverse meets medicine. *Cyberpsychology, Behavior and Social Networking*, *25*(1), 1–2. DOI: 10.1089/cyber.2021.29234.editorial PMID: 34964667

Chapter 12
Architectures for Trustworthy Metaverse-Based Healthcare Ecosystems

Salam Al E'mari
http://orcid.org/0000-0002-2134-4158
University of Petra, Jordan

Yousef Sanjalawe
http://orcid.org/0000-0002-4442-1865
University of Jordan, Jordan

Fadi Fataftah
http://orcid.org/0000-0002-3299-0972
University Canada West, Canada

ABSTRACT

The combination of Metaverse, Artificial Intelligence, and Federated Learning represents a complete paradigm shift in the design process, functionality, and management of the healthcare system. Rather than treating the concepts of Metaverse, Artificial Intelligence, and privacy-preserving learning methodologies as separate components of the technology, it is necessary to recognize that their combined power will be essential to the development of a healthcare ecosystem. A healthcare ecosystem opens new avenues for providing healthcare services in a continuous, personalized, and collaborative manner while respecting important aspects of privacy. In this case, the potential of federated learning as the 'connective intelligence'

DOI: 10.4018/979-8-3373-8889-2.ch012

layer in a Metaverse-oriented setting shall also be highlighted in this chapter, as it can provide federated training to Artificial Intelligence across institutions to avoid aggregating or hoarding important patient information in a healthcare setting.

1. INTRODUCTION: THE NEXT EVOLUTION OF DIGITAL HEALTHCARE

The past two decades have seen extensive changes in the digitalization of health infrastructure due to advances in electronic health records, telemedicine, health analytics, and decision-making. Although there have been efficiency gains and increased accessibility owing to such advances, there has still been a pattern of being institution-centric and fragmented. Data storage bases remain siloed, either with a healthcare service provider or a laboratory, thus hindering efficient, overall, and not individual, health options for patients (Raghupathi and Raghupathi, 2014).

Centralized architectures have been pioneers in this area, particularly for applications involving artificial intelligence in medical imaging, disease prediction, and health simulation. Although these architectures have achieved outstanding results, there have been concerns about large-scale aggregation of sensitive healthcare data, including health concerns related to patient considerations and rules and laws governing healthcare-related data (Shickel et al., 2018). High-profile hacking attacks, including apprehensions by institutions such as the General Data Protection Regulation (GDPR) and the Health Insurance Portability and Accountability Act (HIPAA), have highlighted vulnerabilities in the centralized processing of these health-related pieces of information (Protection, 2018).

Running alongside this trend, the COVID-19 pandemic has led to the widespread adoption of telemedicine, highlighting both the benefits and risks of current remote treatment practices. Of course, the more traditional telemedicine practice offered via video conferencing may lack the full richness of the in-person doctor-patient encounter at a clinic or health center because of the nonverbal cues implicit in the latter (Wosik et al., 2020).

"The Metaverse Reality" presents a brand new paradigm in digital healthcare. This is because it can create a continuous, collaborative, three-dimensional environment in cyberspace, presenting a new, experiential paradigm for what has long existed in a standard graphical interface. Therefore, in a medical setting, it will no longer be impossible to have a "virtual hospital, collaborative diagnostic environment, immersion-based rehabilitation, or a realistic training simulation." For example, "virtual reality has been shown to be very effective in medical education," as highlighted by Mystakidis (2022). But it is not enough to make the medical field "smart" by utilizing immersion technologies alone. This is because, without advanced analytics/learning capabilities, it will soon become no more than a greatly improved graphical interface tool.

The solution to this challenge is to ensure that AI capabilities are supported by human capital infrastructure within an immersive healthcare environment. This is because, while AI has the capability to decipher complex biomedical datasets and make decisions, its implementation still faces challenges in the immersive healthcare environment, particularly in healthcare institutions with limited centralized data (Topol, 2019, Al-E'mari et al., 2025).

Federated learning has emerged as a successful alternative to conventional machine learning, enabling multiple parties to collaboratively train models and share them without transferring raw data. The idea of federated learning was first proposed to enable privacy-preserving learning across distributed devices. It has attracted considerable attention in the medical domain simply by following strict guidelines and concepts of sovereignty, as pointed out by Kairouz et al. (2021). Federated learning is a good foundation for large-scale cooperation in AI for healthcare. Figure 1 illustrates how immersive metaverse interfaces, artificial intelligence services, and federated learning are integrated into a unified healthcare ecosystem that enables collaborative and privacy-preserving clinical intelligence.

Figure 1. Integrated Metaverse–AI–Federated Learning Architecture.

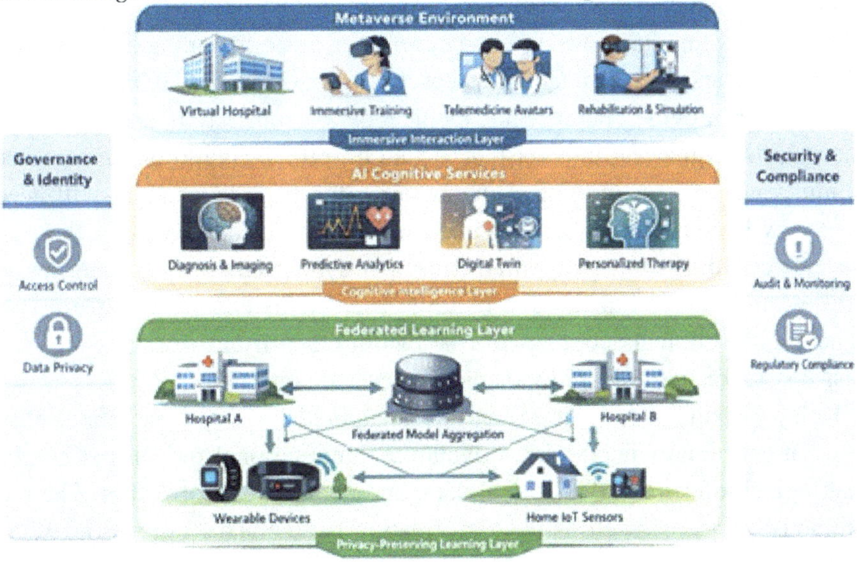

The real transformative power of the digital healthcare industry, according to this chapter, lies not in immersion, artificial intelligence, and federated learning capabilities in isolation, but in their combination in a fully integrated manner within the overall healthcare ecosystem. The overall healthcare ecosystem will comprise the interaction layer in the form of the Metaverse, the cognitive engine in the form of the artificial intelligence environment, and the intelligent connection environment in the form of the federated learning environment. In conceptualizing the health-care sector in the metaverse as a socio-technical system, rather than a technology, it is clear that trustworthy design architecture is one of the key focus areas of this chapter. The next few paragraphs will discuss the technology, architecture, and design needed to make immersive, federated, and intelligent healthcare systems (Sanjalawe et al., 2025).

2. END-TO-END TRUSTWORTHY METAVERSE HEALTHCARE ARCHITECTURE

This chapter moves from conceptual thinking to a specific, executable system design by outlining an end-to-end architecture for trustworthy metaverse-based healthcare systems. This architecture brings together immersive technologies, AI, federated learning, and distributed systems in a layered model. Each layer has its own specific role, yet they work together to provide secure, private, and reliable care in immersive environments.

At the top of this stack, we have the experience layer, including extended reality interfaces, avatars, and virtual clinical spaces that patients and HCPs interact with. This layer will provide telepresence, medical data visualization, and collaborative clinical decision-making in persistent virtual hospitals. Due to the importance of continuity and realism in clinical interactions, the experience layer will need to provide low-latency communication and embodiment. Underneath this, there is the metaverse coordination layer, which is used to synchronize world state, sessions, identities, and interactions among multiple users. This ensures that there is consistency in any clinical actions performed within the virtual world, as well as any access restrictions as defined by medical roles and consent.

The layer of digital twins represents the analytical part of patient representation. Every patient is associated with a dynamic computational model that combines physiological information, historical data, and predictive information. The model continuously updates itself as new information is received from various sensors, electronic medical records, and clinical observations, thus allowing clinicians to explore treatment possibilities within the immersive environment.

The AI cognitive layer is used as support for the digital twins, providing capabilities such as diagnosis, risk, personalization, and data interpretation. Instead of using AI as an analytical tool, it is used as a real-time decision-support tool. To ensure the privacy of users while facilitating collaborative intelligence, the architecture also incorporates a federated learning layer (Oulefki, Amira & Foufou, 2025). This layer allows health institutions and edge devices to train models independently and then share the model updates, aggregating the improvements to obtain a global model without the need to share the patient data. This allows the system to benefit from the population-level knowledge while also ensuring the sovereignty of the patient data.

Trust and privacy are also ensured through the integration of a trust and privacy layer, which incorporates explainability tools, security measures, fairness, and compliance. This layer allows the system to ensure the recommendations of the AI system are explainable to the clinician, prevent any malicious intervention in the models or virtual environment, and ensure the system behavior is compliant with the regulations at all times. Finally, the infrastructure layer of the architecture incorporates the use of edge, fog, and cloud computing systems. The edge devices manage the sensing and interaction of the users, the fog devices manage regional processing and federated aggregation, and the cloud systems manage the analytics and orchestration of the system. This allows the system to ensure the latency, scalability, and privacy requirements of the immersive health application. This allows the system to ensure the latency, scalability, and privacy requirements of immersive healthcare applications. The functional components that operationalize these layers are summarized in Table 1.

Table 1. Functional Components of the Proposed Architecture.

Component	Function	Key Technologies	Trust Mechanism
XR Experience Module	Enables immersive patient–clinician interaction	VR/AR/MR interfaces	Secure identity & session validation
Metaverse Coordinator	Maintains world state & multi-user sync	Rendering engines, WebRTC	Role-based access control
Digital Twin Engine	Simulates patient condition in real time	Multimodal data fusion, simulation models	Model validation & monitoring
AI Cognitive Engine	Supports diagnosis & prediction	Deep learning, multimodal AI	Explainable AI tools
FL Orchestrator	Enables distributed model learning	FedAvg / personalized FL	Secure aggregation
Privacy Controller	Protects sensitive information	Differential privacy, encryption	Data minimization
Trust Manager	Ensures fairness & robustness	Bias auditing tools	Continuous monitoring
Edge Nodes	Process real-time patient signals	Wearables, IoMT	Local processing
Fog Layer	Regional coordination	Edge gateways	Policy enforcement
Cloud Layer	Global analytics & orchestration	High-performance computing	Compliance auditing

3. METAVERSE FOUNDATIONS FOR HEALTHCARE APPLICATIONS

The conceptual use of the metaverse as any kind of immersive digital experience can lead to confusion. In a health care context, a more specific conceptualization of the metaverse as a space for computation/interaction can be viewed as a basis for our discussion. That definition of a space for computation/interaction can thus be conceptualized as a computing substrate consisting of three-dimensional space that encompasses real-time multiuser presence. More current perspectives on applications of the metaverse for health care view it as a series of interlocking technologies, which enable a safe use of the metaverse (Hulsen, 2023; Li et al., 2024; Wang et al., 2023).

The first point to highlight is that there should be a practical distinction between immersive visualization, including training or therapy using VR, AR, or MR, and metaverse-based health environments that are persistent, collaborative, and connected to operational clinical workflows. This second category-which is what most people mean when they refer to the metaverse-requires stronger guarantees regarding authentication, auditability, latency, and clinical-grade reliability than entertainment-oriented virtual worlds can normally assure.

3.1 Virtual Hospitals, Clinics, and Immersive Care Environments

A well-cited example is a 'virtual hospital,' in which medical services are modeled in a collaborative immersive space accessible to patients and practitioners from a distance. The benefit is not merely, " Meet in VR," but make possible interactions of a medical sort which cannot easily be recreated in two-dimensional teleconference environments.' Current literature surveys treat 'virtual hospitals' as an architectural design, through which digital front ends (registering, taking symptoms, triage) are linked to immersive medical environments (consulting rooms, MDT analysis rooms, rehab zones), managed in turn by back-end services (Hulsen, 2023; Wang et al., 2023).

From an architectural perspective, the virtual hospital usually requires:

- Presence and embodiment: Avatar-based participation/telepresence that supports clinician-patient rapport, team coordination
- Clinical Data Integration: Secure presentation of imaging, bio-signals, lab values, and notes in immersive dashboards.
- Triage-consult-diagnostics review-care planning-patient education transitions: The system can be designed to guide users through these transitions.

These environments become more clinically relevant when their design centers around tasks, such as joint review of radiology with annotation and consensus, rather than generic "virtual spaces." Reviews stress that the quality of implementation depends on interaction design and integration with clinical governance, not just on graphics fidelity (Li et al., 2024; Yang et al., 2023).

3.2 Persistent Digital Spaces for Clinical Collaboration

Healthcare delivery systems in general are also necessarily collaborative and involve radiology, pathology laboratories, operating suites, nursing, pharmacies, and various other areas of health. Metaverse applications are especially pertinent in the area of teamwork that involves radiology or any other area of collaborative teamwork. In fact, in the metaverse applications or technology, the "clinical room" essentially refers to a 'persistent workplace' that teams can return to over time and revise or even track for an audit (Hulsen, 2023; Wang et al., 2023).

On the other hand, persistence brings in the need for governance. For persistent medical workplaces, the following are required to be supported:

i. Role-based access control,
ii. Tracability for any changes made with information on who made the change and when it was done,
iii. Distinction between educational simulations and medical decision-making tools.

The importance of the consideration of governance for the metaverse in the field of healthcare is emphasized by the fact that the lack of governance in the metaverse could increase privacy and liability risks instead of decreasing them (Li et al., 2024; Wang et al., 2023).

3.3 Role of AR/VR/MR in Care Delivery and Training

XR technologies (VR, AR, and MR) should be defined as the means by which metaverse healthcare is accessed. To support contemporary healthcare literature, it was also postulated that the use of XR technologies is inconsistent and that specificity is essential when establishing benefits and study designs (Abbas et al., 2023). Another study further observed that metaverse healthcare benefits from the use of augmented, virtual, and mixed realities.

Evidence is also present in virtual reality (VR) in healthcare education and rehabilitation settings. There is recent evidence from a systematic review and meta-analysis on healthcare education in VR, with positive outcomes relative to educational outcomes in randomized controlled trials, although heterogeneity persists in this area regarding intervention designs and measures used (Sung et al., 2024). In the area of rehabilitation and therapy, evidence from the umbrella review suggests that VR interventions alleviated symptoms and improved functional outcomes in some forms of musculoskeletal diseases and conditions, although again with considerable heterogeneity in outcomes depending on disease type and control groups (Tang et al., 2025).

AR/MR applications are commonly considered for use in intraoperative navigation, procedural training, and context-appropriate training due to their capability to superimpose digital information onto real-world hospital environments. In a systematic review of MR applications in the OR setting, some benefits are clearly attributed to improved OR experiences with intraoperative visualization, though the review focuses on limitations related to cost, ergonomics, and surgical integration for the OR user (Magalhães et al., 2024). In the context of a complete ecosystem understanding of AR/MR applications, they are typically seen as the "bridge" between real-world care provision and fully immersive digital experiences when metaverse collaboration solutions must focus on real-world bedside applications.

3.4 Metaverse Characteristics That Matter Specifically in Healthcare

There are several features which keep recurring as material to the practice of healthcare metaverse within the recent literature:

- Rest latency interaction and continuity: Conversational interaction involving healthcare professionals and visualization interaction require low latency, particularly in the context of training/therapy applications (Li et al., 2024).
- Interoperability with clinical systems: The metaverse layer needs to be assured for reliable data exchanges with EHR, PACS, and IoMT services so that it does not operate as a siloed parallel system (Yang et al., 2023).
- Safety and Evaluation: Clinical-grade XR needs to have evaluations regarding its usability and safety because user satisfaction alone is inadequate since errors in visualization or interpretation mean potential danger to patients (Magalhães et al., 2024).
- Governance and auditability: The regulatory requirements imposed on the healthcare industry ensure that identity, access, and traceability are primary considerations rather than secondary features of a platform (Wang et al., 2023; Li et al., 2024).

In other words, a layered clinical infrastructure of the metaverse for the healthcare domain needs to be addressed. This includes XR applications on the interface layer, shared spaces for collaboration on the workflow layer, and harmonized and governed integration with the healthcare data and systems on the infrastructure layer.

4. ARTIFICIAL INTELLIGENCE AS THE COGNITIVE LAYER

AI is now a crucial technology that drives the metaverse and advances care processes, including diagnosis, prediction, management, and population-level patient management. In the metaverse patient management paradigm, AI is more of a paradigm than a technology. In a paradigm where AI is merely a back-end analysis tool, its significance rises as it becomes a cognitive layer capable of interpreting diverse data flows and providing intelligence and cognitive support for decisions and intelligent interactions within an immersive environment. This requires a paradigm shift toward doctor-level patient conversation support via AI output within a spatial-domain environment.

4.1 AI-Driven Diagnostics, Prediction, and Personalization

Since then, there have been immense advances in AI-assisted diagnosis across sectors such as medical imaging, pathology, and predictive risk assessment. State-of-the-art deep learning algorithms have been able to perform at par with human experts for tasks including radiological interpretation, pathological diagnosis for skin lesions, and ophthalmological disease screening (Topol, 2023). Such applications have been incorporated into medical practices to support rather than substitute human judgment.

In metaverse healthcare settings, diagnostic AI can be integrated into immersive spaces. For example, three-dimensional imaging combined with AI-generated segmentations or anomaly detection enables doctors to navigate findings spatially rather than viewing two-dimensional images. There have been findings on immersive analytics and healthcare, indicating improvements in pattern identification and shared understanding through spatial imaging, especially for volumetric datasets (Cai et al., 2022).

Apart from diagnosis, predictive models are used in prognosis estimation and warning systems based on patient observations over time. Machine learning algorithms have proven more effective than statistical models for predicting patient outcomes, such as hospital readmission, patient progress, or treatment response, when trained on representative datasets (Shah et al., 2021). When implemented in immersive environments, predictive models can aid in making inferences about future patient observations in graphical forms such as risk trajectories or scenario models.

Personalization is another key aspect of AI's cognitive function. Tailored treatment recommendations, adaptive rehabilitation strategies, and smart patient education require and entail machine learning from both individual and population-based data. The metaverse represents a seamless platform that enables such personalization, with AI-driven adaptations automatically represented in such virtual healthcare settings. But here again, large-scale personalization merely amplifies concerns about bias, overfitting, and unequal outcomes.

4.2 Multimodal Data Analytics in Immersive Healthcare Environments

Medical data are inherently multimodal, involving structured data (e.g., laboratory results), unstructured clinical texts, images, biosignals captured from wearable sensors, and, increasingly, behavioral and environmental data. Recent advances in multimodal AI have demonstrated the potential to model diverse sources together to create more accurate and informative patient state representations (Huang et al., 2022).

In healthcare immersion environments, multimodal analysis offers particular benefits because it aligns with the affordances of the metaverse. For example, healthcare information gathered from wearables and other sources of imaging and clinical data can be displayed in a common virtual environment, enabling the practitioner to integrate information that would otherwise be viewed across a variety of displays. There is a growing body of research indicating that integrated views are beneficial for situational awareness and reduce cognitive load in collaboration environments (Sedlmair et al., 2020; Cai et al., 2022).

Recent studies have also investigated foundation models and large multimodal models in healthcare. These models have been attempting to achieve generalizable representations for tasks and modalities. Although these models have shown potential in unifying analytics across different medical tasks, their applications in this area have been limited due to concerns about accessibility, complexity, and interpretability (Bommasani et al., 2021; Nazi & Peng, 2024). These limitations have been further exacerbated in metaverse-based systems due to real-time interactions and sustaining trust in human-artificial interactions.

4.3 Explainable and Trustworthy AI for Clinical Decisions

Trust is essential for the successful implementation of AI technology within the health industry, particularly when the health outcomes determined by AI technology come to play a critical role in decision-making. In this regard, the use of models is difficult to explain, thereby leading to the development of an important research direction: explainable AI.

The recent literature survey emphasizes the importance of context-sensitive explainability in medicine. It is likely that data scientists and clinicians will require different explanations (Tonekaboni et al., 2023). When discussing the metaverse, the issue of explainability is more complex due to the environment's nature. For that reason, the necessary explanations are likely to be spatial and/or temporal in nature, for example, by pointing out specific regions in 3D images. This specific feature could greatly improve clinicians' perception of and trust in the results.

Fairness, robustness, and other considerations play a pivotal role in trustworthy AI as well. It is clear that AI in the medical field can yield different results across groups because of prejudices present in the training data it uses, as revealed in a 2019 study (Panch et al.). Although the issue is well-known, reducing such prejudices in multimodal models remains an open problem.

Finally, it has become increasingly important to focus on robustness to distribution shifts. This emerged because the metaverse platform for the healthcare ecosystem involves diverse sources and sources of varying device quality. AI should work effectively even under changed environmental conditions and sensors. Domain generalization and ongoing learning are promising areas of study, but their applications should be handled with caution (Finlayson et al., 2021).

It is important to conclude that AI as the cognitive layer in metaverse-based healthcare ecosystems is not just about algorithmic accuracy. It is about multimodal intelligence, interpretability, fairness, and robustness. These have been essential for safe and effective use in clinical applications. So, there is a need for machine learning models that reconcile intelligence at scale with privacy, autonomy, and even governance. That is taken up in the next section with federated learning.

5. FEDERATED LEARNING FOR PRIVACY-PRESERVING HEALTHCARE INTELLIGENCE

Because of the increased use of data intelligence in the medical field, the conflict of interest regarding the aggregation of diverse data for big data analysis and the need to preserve patient privacy from intrusion have escalated. Conventional big data intelligence in the medical field, through machine learning, involves aggregating all medical data in a centralized manner. However, Federated learning offers an alternative approach to big data intelligence in the medical field.

5.1 Federated Learning Framework for Privacy-Preserving Metaverse Healthcare

Federated learning acts as a smart connector, facilitating collaborative model development among healthcare organizations without the need to share original patient information. In a healthcare scenario enabled by the metaverse, with constant data flow from hospitals, home devices, and even immersive interactions, federated learning would need to be performed under more stringent requirements in terms of latency, heterogeneity, and reliability compared to other settings. The proposed system would apply federated learning across three tiers of infrastructure. Edge devices, such as home devices, would perform local data preprocessing and update model parameters using patient-specific information.

Hospitals and nodes would act as aggregators, updating model parameters from multiple sources before passing them on to a global federated learning orchestration service. This hierarchical structure would improve communication efficiency while maintaining response times required by real-time applications. Healthcare data, by their nature, do not follow identical distribution across hospitals. Therefore, adaptive federated optimization methods would be used instead of traditional averaging methods. Methods that adapt to variations in local data would ensure that globally aggregated knowledge remains relevant across different patient populations. Furthermore, model layers can be customized at the local level, with hospital staff able to retain knowledge while still benefiting from shared knowledge.

Security and privacy mechanisms are integrated into the entire learning process. The updated model is encrypted during transmission, aggregated, and designed in such a way that none of the participants can obtain information from another's local data. Additional security mechanisms, like noise injection, can be used to minimize information leakage from model parameters. This ensures that data protection regulations can be followed while still ensuring effective model performance.

The Metaverse application scenario poses new challenges that cannot be addressed by traditional federated learning solutions. Digital twins, as well as immersive decision support systems, require regular updates of the model to reflect changing patient states. This makes asynchronous participation a necessity. Therefore, the proposed solution allows partial participation, ensuring that institutions can update the model as soon as they have computational resources, thus ensuring that there is no disruption in the learning process.

The proposed federated learning solution, which incorporates hierarchical co-ordination, personalization, and privacy, allows institutions as well as individuals to remain autonomous while still leveraging population-scale intelligence. This allows healthcare data, which would otherwise be distributed, to be used as a shared resource to improve various aspects of healthcare, including diagnostics, treatment, and virtual healthcare, in the Metaverse.

Algorithm 1: Hierarchical Federated Learning for Real-Time Healthcare Digital Twins

For each training round t:

Each hospital k trains local twin model Mk on local data
Apply differential privacy noise Nk
Send encrypted update to fog aggregator
Fog performs secure aggregation
Cloud updates global model Gt
Deploy updated model to metaverse twin engines

5.2 Cross-Silo and Cross-Device Federated Learning Models

Federated Learning is described as "a class of machine learning that involves training a model with participants in a collaborative manner without exchanging any data." Participants in this process can calculate model updates based on their datasets and are only required to share them with a server or aggregation system. This process was conceptualized as part of scaling in mobile and edge computing systems. However, its applicability in healthcare has become clear in recent years (Kairouz et al., 2021).

In the medical domain, FL is typically classified as cross-silo and cross-device FL. Cross-silo FL is feasible in scenarios with a few high-resource entities such as hospitals and medical research institutions. In this framework, multiple high-resource entities collaborate on shared model training without data exchange (Dayan et al., 2021). The domain is ideal for medical image analysis and risk prediction models due to the data's heterogeneity and autonomy.

Cross-device federated learning, on the other hand, is typically considered to involve a large number of potentially untrustworthy and resource-limited devices, such as wearables, home health monitoring systems, and patient-owned sensors. In the context of metaverse-based health environments, cross-device learning facilitates the development of population intelligence from continuous real-world data while maintaining individual data sovereignty. Nonetheless, this scenario also comes with other communication complexities, such as partial participation and model stability (Rieke et al., 2022).

It has been proven in recent empirical research that the performance of FL can be on a par with the performance of the centralized approach on some clinical problems, such as the segmentation of brain tumors, the prediction of the outcome of patients with COVID-19, as well as the identification of ophthalmologic diseases, if a suitable aggregation rule is used in FL, as noted in literature study findings (Dayan, Gonen, & Keidar, 2021; Sheller, Rad, Gonen, & Rieck, 2020).

5.3 Secure Aggregation and Privacy-Enhancing Mechanisms

Although federated learning alleviates issues related to direct data exchange, it does not necessarily ensure privacy or security. In some cases, model updates may reveal sensitive information about the training data. Therefore, healthcare-oriented federated learning systems have started adopting privacy-enhancing technologies to counter such challenges.

Secure aggregation protocols prevent the individual updates from being viewed, even by the server coordinating the aggregation process. Actual implementation has shown that such protocols are feasible for widespread use without inordinate computational or communication overhead. Hence, such mechanisms are usable for collaborations between institutions in the field of healthcare (Bonawitz et al., 2019; Kairouz et al., 2021).

Differential privacy adds another layer, in which carefully calibrated noise is introduced into model updates, with formal guarantees that no individual data point can be inferred from the trained model.

Recent works have also explored applying homomorphic encryption and secure multi-party computation to secure end-to-end federated learning. Though providing high levels of privacy protection, their high computational overhead prevents their extensive usage in the healthcare domain. A tradeoff between privacy protection and performance is thus made in practical healthcare systems.

5.4 Regulatory Alignment and Patient Data Sovereignty

One of the most alluring aspects of federated learning, particularly within the healthcare industry, is that it supports modern trends and standards in data privacy. The GDPR specifically aims to prioritize the principles of data minimization, purpose limitation, and local control. The federated machine learning algorithm supports all these ideas, allowing data to be locally controlled at the level of an establishment or an individual, without compromising the group intelligence advocated by Protection (2018).

Nonetheless, in assessing the issue beyond the scope of regulatory cooperation, the field of federated learning may also foster patient data sovereignty. Looking ahead, once the basis for a health ecosystem platform for the metaverse is established, patients will be able to interact with digital twins, virtual physicians, and therapy environments that evolve based on the model's findings. This will all take place without surrendering any authority for personal medical data.

However, despite such progress, there are concerns about aligning regulations. This is because there must be defined approaches regarding model validation, error responsibility, consent, and audibility for the involved parties. Notably, there are studies that adopt a policy-oriented approach to shifting the concept of trust from relevant authorities regarding data handling to processes and practices (Rieke et al., 2022).

Within metaverse-enabled health care platforms, federated learning functions as a “bridge intelligence” layer, integrating loosely connected facilities, hardware, and even patients into a unified learning environment. Thus, it plays a crucial role in enabling notions of “higher-level” digital twins and intelligent virtual agents, which will be discussed in the next section.

6. DIGITAL TWINS AND INTELLIGENT VIRTUAL AGENTS

The idea of digital twins has gained significant momentum in medicine, thanks to advances in sensing, modeling, and AI, which enable better representation of biological systems. In metaverse-based healthcare ecosystems, digital twins, along with intelligent virtual agents, are a crucial transition frontier between intelligence built on data and immersive medical interactions. They can harness collective intelligence in a medical system through federated learning.

6.1 Patient-Specific Digital Twins Powered by Federated Intelligence

A digital twin in the medical field can thus be described as an “electronic replica of a patient that uses physiological models, patient history, real-time sensor inputs, and learned patterns from population-level data” (Bruynseels et al., 2022). Digital twins also differ from traditional patient records in that they are intended to evolve over time in response to the patient's health status and other factors.

Healthcare DTs were recently distinguished from other DTs in the literature for the following reasons: Healthcare DTs incorporate uncertainties and biological variability, as biological processes are inherently random and not fully understood, and thus can never be exactly replicated. Hence, the use of DTs in medicine is more probabilistic, supporting uncertain reasoning rather than deterministic simulations, as noted in a 2022 study by Ghatti et al. (2023). This is well-suited to the immersive environment, in which multiple possibilities can be provided rather than a point solution, as will be discussed in the subsequent section.

Federated learning is an important aspect that enables the patient-specific digital twin to learn from a larger population without requiring a centralized database for sensitive information. The ability to train joint models across a larger number of institutions and devices is essential for federated learning, enabling the personal digital twin to learn from many groups while retaining locality. Current literature indicates the capability of federation strategies to perform personal prediction and stratification while mitigating risks in centralized machine learning (Al E'mari et al., 2026).

In this way, patient digital twins can be instantiated as interactive entities in metaverse-based healthcare environments that clinicians and patients can jointly explore. For instance, disease progression trajectories, simulations of treatment options, or rehabilitation outcomes can be presented within both spatial and temporal frames to communicate a shared understanding and to improve informed decision-making. Interaction itself thus transforms the digital twin from an analytic backend artifact into a front-end collaborative clinical tool.

As shown in Figure 2, patient DTs evolve through a continuous feedback loop in which local physiological data are combined with population-level intelligence by federated learning to support personalized simulation and clinical decision-making.

Figure 2. DT and Federated Intelligence Workflow.

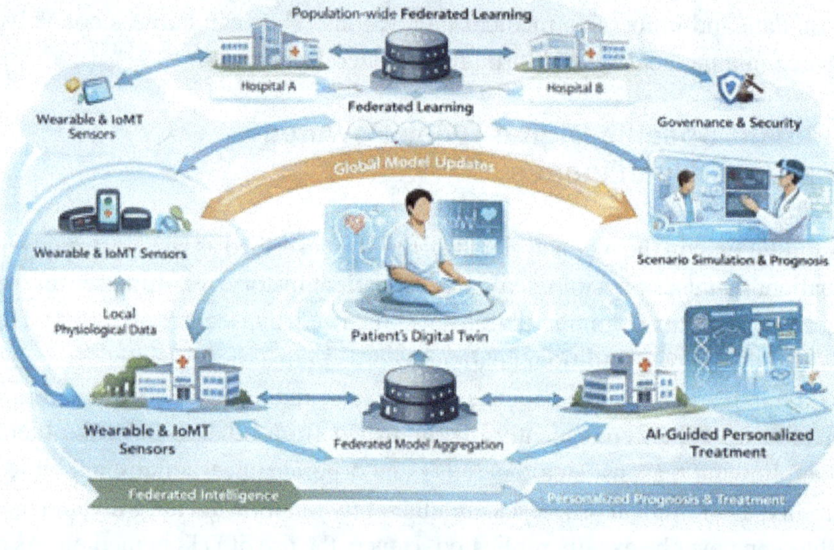

6.2 Simulation, Prognosis, and Treatment Planning

Simulation-based medicine presents one of the most exciting and promising areas for the use of digital twins. Simulation-based medicine allows doctors to simulate certain situations, such as different treatments and lifestyle changes. Recent studies have demonstrated the role of simulation-based medicine in minimizing trial-and-error in treatment selection, and it has significant applications in personalized medicine for complex and chronic diseases. (Björnsson et al., 2020; Ghatti et al., 2023)

Simulation is made more intuitive and actionable in immersive settings. Rather than analyzing simulated outcomes expressed as purely numerical values, one can view simulated disease, physiological, and functional processes within a virtual world. This is very helpful for teams of clinicians, enabling them to collaborate more effectively through shared visual presentations.

However, the reliability of clinical simulations depends on the accuracy of the simulation model. This implies that if the simulation models are inaccurate, the resulting poor clinical decisions will adversely affect the patient. The current literature continues to underscore the importance of uncertainty validation in the dynamic simulation of digital twins in the clinical environment. This criticality further increases with the use of the metaverse approach.

6.3 Intelligent Virtual Clinicians and Decision-Support Agents

An important component of a metaverse platform for healthcare is that of intelligent virtual agents. Virtual agents refer to entities that employ AI technology and interact with healthcare providers and patients to provide guidance and support. In this field, intelligent virtual agents operate within immersive platforms, employ communication processes such as NLP, and differ from decision-support systems that rely on computers. The current literature on the interaction between humans and AI recommends the use of intelligent agents in the medical field to achieve accurate AI that is in harmony with the conventional medical processes accepted in 2022 by Cai et al. The use of virtual AI doctors in an immersive environment can be useful for tasks such as navigating protocols or explaining anomalies/AI suggestions. The potency of the AI doctors lies in reducing the burden on human doctors.

Federated learning makes the use of virtual agents even more important by allowing them to improve through distributed experience without relying on patients' data. A good example is the conversational trends, the logic behind certain decisions, or the rehabilitation methods that can be improved together without having to go through the original data. This is even important when considering the use of the metaverse.

However, the implementation of intelligent virtual agents raises significant ethical and professional concerns. There has to be a clear distinction between support and autonomy. The work of the agents must support, rather than substitute for, the role of the healthcare provider. It is important to ensure transparency in the scope and sources of the data used for training. There is currently an analysis over how the role of intelligent agents should be defined as assisting tools and not decision tools. Accountability should be to human professionals (Mesko and Győrffy, 2023).

In conclusion, digital twins and intelligent virtual agents can expand the cognitive and interaction capabilities of metaverse-based healthcare ecosystems. When based on FL, they can allow for personalized, collaborative, and privacy-conscious healthcare and can be applied to simulation-based reasoning and decision-making. However, for them to be effective, they must be properly integrated into healthcare workflows, validated, and governed; these points will be discussed further in relation to metaverse architecture and security.

7. SYSTEM ARCHITECTURES: EDGE–FOG–CLOUD INTEGRATION

To deliver intelligent, immersive, and trustworthy healthcare services within metaverse ecosystems, there is a need for architectures that address the trade-offs among low latency, intensive data processing, and stringent privacy requirements. The existing cloud architecture, which is useful for batch analytics and cloud data storage, does not meet the latency requirements of continuous healthcare interaction and sensing tasks. Therefore, an edge, fog, and cloud architecture has become an essential paradigm for future digital healthcare systems, especially when combined with federated learning and immersive experiences.

7.1 Architectural Rationale for Distributed Intelligence

Medical data is increasingly produced at the edge of the network by wearable, implantable, bedside, and other patient-employed sensors. Medical data streams are also time-sensitive and context-dependent, and it is not feasible to send this data to a cloud server without incurring latency costs or privacy concerns. Current research has shown the importance of bringing intelligence closer to the source and the critical role of this consideration in safe-critical applications such as the healthcare system (Shi et al., 2022).

In metaverse healthcare settings, the demand for latency-efficient interaction further intensifies. Immersive patient consultations, rehabilitation procedures, and collaborative diagnostic analyses demand near-instant feedback to sustain presence, interaction, and validity. Edge computing addresses this challenge by enabling local processing of sensor input, initial model inference, and feedback at the point of interaction. Yet edge computing hardware alone cannot support the development of complex AI models or analytics for larger contexts.

7.2 Edge Layer: Real-Time Sensing and Interaction

This edge layer involves the various devices and systems closest to the patient and the practitioner. This includes wearables, smartphones, medical devices, and local gateways. The primary tasks performed in this layer are data analysis, pre-processing, anomaly detection, and inference. For instance, real-time processing of physiological signals can facilitate rehabilitation exercises in immersive settings and provide alerts during virtual consultations.

Recent work has shown that lightweight AI models running at the edge can help mitigate response latency while maintaining acceptable accuracy, especially when periodically updated via federated learning (Arikumar et al., 2022). For metaverse applications, edge intelligence would enable real synchronization between physical and virtual states, enabling digital twins and metaverse experiences to be interactive and meaningful.

Privacy issues are also at the forefront of the edge. Processing at the edge reduces the risk of exposing raw patient data and helps satisfy data minimization principles. But varying capabilities and operational settings shape challenges for model maintenance and security.

7.3 Fog Layer: Coordination and Regional Aggregation

In the healthcare setting, the fog layer plays a major role in consolidating data from different sources, undertaking analytics at a regional level, and ensuring a set of policy-based controls. In federated learning, the fog node serves as a point of aggregation to coordinate local updates before submitting them to the top-level orchestrators. The design has demonstrated improved scalability in a large federated setting, where the approach was applied to reduce the architecture's communication overhead.

In metaverse-based settings, fog computing enables collaboration among multiple users in shared virtual spaces. In this case, synchronization for immersive experiences and overall data consistency can be handled by fog nodes within a region, thereby reducing reliance on distant cloud infrastructure in the event of network failures.

7.4 Cloud Layer: Large-Scale Learning and Orchestration

However, the cloud layer remains relevant for tasks requiring large amounts of computation and storage. Within metaverse-based health ecosystems, cloud technology helps handle large-scale model training and federated orchestration across institutions. This layer provides services such as identity management, auditing, and even compliance.

Recent works have also emphasized the need for adaptive orchestration techniques to dynamically allocate tasks across edge, fog, and cloud levels, as outlined in (Shi et al., 2022; Su et al., 2023). This becomes more significant, especially within the healthcare field, as demand in health systems changes rapidly in response to healthcare events or population trends.

Despite this potential, it is important that this cloudy level be managed so as to avoid recreating centralized risks. In architecture, there is a trend towards "cloud as coordinator" architectures over "cloud as owner" architectures, in which clouds enable cooperation but do not control data and decision-making rights. This philosophy is very relevant to federated learning.

7.5 Integration With IoMT and Multimodal Data Pipelines

The Internet of Medical Things (IoMT) is an important source of data for healthcare metaverse platforms. It involves a wide range of sensors/Devices that produce continuous streams of multimodal data. Incorporating IoMT into edge-fog-cloud systems requires standardized data pipelines to manage the offered formats/rates/reliability. More recently, it has become clear that the need for complete data governance solutions, encompassing data quality, provenance, and security, across architecture levels (El-Saleh et al., 2025) is also pertinent within immersive spaces, as the risk of incorrect and/or stale data potentially erodes trust within digital twins and associated decision support agents.

Federated learning adds complexity to MBDP design due to its iterative learning and real-time processing. Managing such processes requires additional attention and scheduling to avoid interfering with learning processes. Recently, architectures have emerged that separate real-time processing and learning to improve continuous learning without hindering real-time processing (Saadat et al., 2021).

In conclusion, edge cloud, fog cloud, and cloud technology are the architectural fundamentals for the metaverse industry to develop scaled, responsive, and privacy-conscious health-based ecosystems. They achieve a real-time, interactive experience by distributing intelligence across levels according to the needs of the health industry, while facilitating learning and analysis. However, the feasibility of such systems with respect to security, fairness, and robustness will be discussed in the following section.

8. SECURITY, FAIRNESS, AND ROBUSTNESS CHALLENGES

Although metaverse-based health ecosystems with federated learning and distributed intelligence offer numerous advantages, they also introduce a whole new dimension to the threat landscape. Therefore, with the integration of immersion interfaces, decentralized learning, and diverse infrastructures, the threat landscape tends to reveal potential risks in domains such as security or robustness, and also unveils new vulnerabilities. Combatting all these potential threats is critical to ensure the proposed systems not only work at the technological level but also remain safe from health and ethical perspectives.

8.1 Security Threats in Federated and Immersive Healthcare Systems

Cybersafety risks associated with metaverse platforms for health care go beyond traditional concerns. In the federated learning setting, for instance, attackers may target the learning process instead of the data storage systems. A well-explored type of attack in federated learning platforms is model poisoning. In a health care database, this may imply making systematic predictions or suggestions that may be dangerous to patients. (Bagdasaryan et al., 2020; Sun et al., 2022).

A further important threat is inference attacks, which include membership inference and model inversion attacks and target the recovery of sensitive information about the data from which the model parameters are derived. Despite the resistance to direct data disclosure in federated learning, it has recently been shown that privacy disclosure is still possible without complementary protection methods, especially when the attacker has access to model intermediates (Melis et al., 2019; Sun et al., 2022). Such attacks are especially serious in the healthcare domain, since incomplete disclosure of sensitive information can violate privacy and ethical standards.

The immersive nature of the metaverse further broadens this attack surface. Identity impersonation, session hijacking, and tampering with virtual environments could undermine trust in the authenticity of interactions and decision-making in the medical context. For instance, unauthorized access to the virtual medical consultation room or any tampering with authentic medical information presented could have hazardous medical implications. The importance of proper authentication mechanisms for secure sessions in the XR environment was recently highlighted in various analyses (Huang et al., 2023).

8.2 Fairness and Bias in Decentralized Healthcare AI

Fairness is a fundamental challenge in AI for healthcare, and it is not necessarily eliminated by decentralized learning approaches. Data heterogeneity within institutions arises from disparities in patient demographics, clinical characteristics, and data collection algorithms, and this tends to lead to disparities in model performance. Even within federated learning, such disparities could lead to additional biases, as powerful institutions shape the global models (Li et al., 2021).

Observational research has revealed that performance discrepancies in health-based AI applications related to race, gender, age, and socioeconomic factors may have clinical relevance to health diagnosis, treatment, and outcomes (Rajkomar et al., 2022). These discrepancies in metaverse-based health platforms will likely remain invisible given the immersive nature of these platforms.

There have been recent works proposing methods for fair federated learning that account for equity constraints and goals, such as local reweighting or optimization for the worst group. Although attractive, these require a balance for accuracy and fairness (Shi et al., 2023). Additionally, there must be a balance between what constitutes fairness from a technical aspect and what constitutes acceptable risk and accountability guidelines from a non-technical aspect.

8.3 Robustness and Generalization Across Heterogeneous Environments

Robustness is the measure of the adaptability of AI systems to perform dependably even if there are changes to the conditions of the input data. In the field of healthcare, the lack of robustness has been identified as a key challenge in deploying AI models trained in controlled settings or institution-specific setups (Finlayson et al., 2021).

Healthcare ecosystems that are metaverse-enabled exacerbate this issue by combining data sources across edge, fog, and cloud computing. Inconsistencies in hardware quality, network conditions, and use behavior may also lead to distributional shifts that affect model performance. The concept of federated learning offers a solution to this challenge by offering a model exposure to a broad environment. However, it is not guaranteed.

Recent advancements in domain generalization and continual learning provide means to address increased robustness, but adaptively updating a model, as well as making use of predictions informed by uncertainty, add complexity to a prediction system, which has to be carefully evaluated in a clinical setting to ensure it does not have any negative consequences (Subbaswamy & Saria, 2020). For immersive environments, it is crucial to ensure uncertainty information is communicated in an interpretable fashion because a visually confident representation of uncertainty has a high potential to mislead a clinician or patient.

8.4 Toward Integrated Security and Governance Mechanisms

The three challenges: security, fairness, and robustness, are strongly intertwined and must not be solved in isolation. Being securely trained could minimize risk exposure, but it does not necessarily improve model performance or fairness. Models trained to be robust could potentially generalize better, but they continue to perpetuate biases due to the lack of representativeness in the source data. Thus, there has been increasing emphasis in the recent literature on the need for unification frameworks that balance technical and organizational measures (Rieke et al., 2022).

For metaverse-based healthcare ecosystems, such frameworks must be tailored to the particular characteristics of immersive interaction, such as embodiment, persistence, and shared virtual space. For trustworthy system designs, continuous monitoring, auditability of model behavior, and well-defined escalation procedures for identified problematic behaviors are critical. Of particular importance here is how such risk management responsibilities should be properly distributed across technology companies, healthcare stakeholders, and concerned regulatory authorities.

In conclusion, ensuring security, fairness, and robustness in federated metaverse environments for the field of medicine is a complex issue that requires a multidimensional approach that goes beyond the solution itself. As a matter of course, the issue prompts a set of questions regarding trust, identity, and accountability, which will be discussed in the next section.

9. TRUST, IDENTITY, AND GOVERNANCE IN VIRTUAL HEALTHCARE

Trust is an essential component in the interactional framework for delivering health care and becomes even more important with fully or partially virtualized clinical interaction and medical data processing in digital health platforms. Furthermore, in metaverse-based health platforms, it is important to develop trust not only from patients toward health providers or health facilities, but also from health facilities, smart systems, and infrastructure. The convergence of both federated learning and immersive technologies demands re-evaluation in identity, accountability, and health infrastructure.

9.1 Trust as a Socio-Technical Construct in Metaverse Healthcare

Traditionally, trust in health care was based on professional ethics, regulatory oversight, and interpersonal relationships. As the delivery of care is increasingly informed and influenced by AI-driven recommendations and immersive digital interfaces, trust becomes a socio-technical construct shaped by system design, transparency, and governance. Recent studies have underscored that patients and clinicians will have greater trust in digital health systems if decisions are explainable, it is clear who is accountable, and how their data is protected. The data protection principle in the EU's General Data Protection Regulation requires a clear and transparent notice to individuals whose data are being collected about the processing of their personal data.

In metaverse environments, the reality experienced when using immersion technology could increase the sense of system authority and capability. Although trust can positively impact engagement, if system capabilities are not openly known, the risk of blind trust exists. The literature on human-computer interaction suggests that immersion can mask uncertainty and biases, so trust calibration, as a clear, overt system aim, is important in its own right (Bozkurt & Sharma, 2024). Thus, trust in virtual medicine, rather than a passive assumption when high technology is present, will need trust actively engineered.

9.2 Identity and Access Management in Immersive Clinical Environments

Secure and trustworthy healthcare systems require reliable identity management. The scope of identity in metaverse healthcare systems extends from mere authentication to defining roles, context-based authorizations, and traceability. All stakeholders in healthcare, including healthcare professionals, patients, devices, and intelligent agents, become participants or so-called "actors" in virtual spaces.

Recent studies have emphasized the limitations associated with classical centralized identity management infrastructure in decentralized and inter-institutional healthcare environments. Centralized identity providers may constitute Single Points of Failure and may not be compatible with concepts like data sovereignty and autonomy (Rasouli & Valmohammadi, 2020). Therefore, interest in using self-sovereign identity concepts for identity management in decentralized identity infrastructures has been observed.

Decentralized identity in the healthcare context ensures that patients can control their credentials and deliberately disclose information such as age group, role, or consent status. Decentralized identity for health practitioners enables cross-institutional teaming while ensuring that health practitioners' professional credentials remain authentic. Recent pilots have indicated that decentralized identity in health care might enhance interoperability when its governance structure includes well-articulated procedures for credential issuance, revocation, and conflict resolution (Agbo et al., 2019).

9.3 Auditability, Accountability, and Governance Frameworks

Accountability is an important consideration in healthcare governance, especially when AI systems are involved in healthcare decision-making. In metaverse-based healthcare systems, it is essential to ensure accountability across data creation, model training, inference, and immersion. Otherwise, it is difficult to identify who is responsible for errors, bias, or unintended outcomes.

Currently, there is a thrust toward traceability and documentation in AI-enabled healthcare systems due to regulatory and policy assessments. This refers to documenting the provenance of the data used to train models, as well as the training process (European Commission, 2021). In a federated learning setup, the auditability of these systems is complex due to the distributed nature of the training mechanism, with no access to the repositories. However, efforts have been made to document the process through attestation (Rieke et al., 2022).

Governance structures for a metaverse platform for healthcare would need to address ethical issues such as consent, transparency in AI use, and the right to appeal automated suggestions. Recent research has shown that patients would appreciate being informed about the use of AI in their decision-making process (Longoni et al., 2022). The above would seem to reflect a regulatory philosophy of human-in-the-loop decision-making. Figure 3 summarizes the governance and trust architecture required to ensure that immersive, AI-driven healthcare systems remain accountable, auditable, and aligned with clinical and regulatory obligations.

Figure 3. Trust, Security, and Governance Stack.

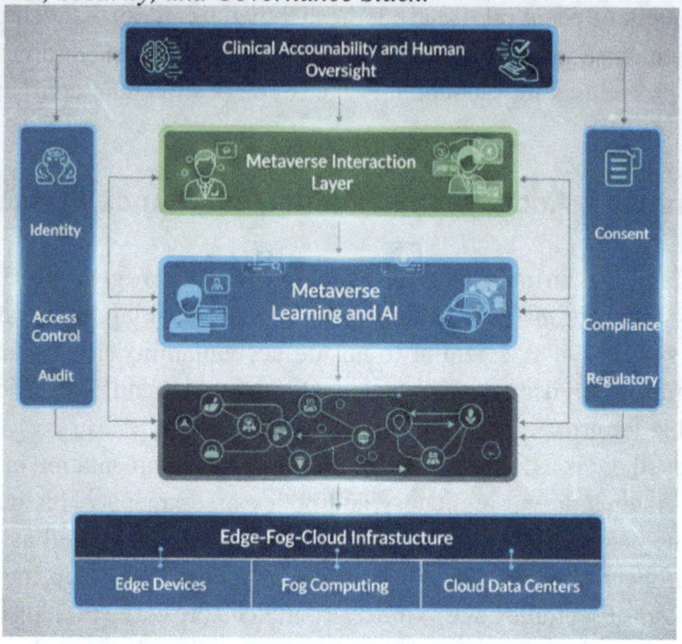

9.4 Legal and Regulatory Considerations

The regulatory framework for the metaverse-based healthcare sector remains nascent and disjointed. Current regulations for medical devices, data protection, and professional obligations were primarily framed for the physical and typical cyber world. Extension of these regulatory regimes to the immersive and AI-powered space raises concerns.

These current debates show that federated learning, decentralized systems, and other frameworks are useful for ensuring regulatory compliance by minimizing data transport and emphasizing decentralized control. They do not, however, obviate regulatory responsibilities regarding safety, effectiveness, and accountability (European Commission, 2021; Garbagnati & Wu, 2021). Within a metaverse, several issues will arise regarding the classification of virtual interventions, the status of virtual entities, and the use of immersive evidence.

In fact, for effective governance, there ought to be coordination between healthcare institutions, technology companies, the regulatory bodies, and professional associations. While the focus has largely been on ex post enforcement, healthcare governance frameworks are shifting to include by-design principles that bake ethics and the law into system design. These include Privacy by Design, Consent by Design, and Transparency Through Documentation for AI.

10. CASE SCENARIOS AND EMERGING DEPLOYMENTS

Although healthcare ecosystems within the metaverse are still emerging and represent a new paradigm, there are already interesting pilot projects and applications under development that demonstrate how the metaverse and federated learning, an artificial intelligence technology, could be combined to enable specific applications. Instead of painting a purely visionary scenario, this section discusses real-world and scientifically documented applications and challenges in healthcare to show how the metaverse and emerging technologies could be used.

10.1 Virtual Rehabilitation and Remote Patient Monitoring

Rehabilitation and management of long-term medical conditions are among the most advanced use cases for immersive healthcare technologies. The use of virtual reality-based rehabilitation systems has gained momentum in assisting patients with motor skill recovery, pain management, and functional capacity building, particularly for neurological and musculoskeletal disorders. Recent systematic reviews and meta-analyses have concluded that virtual reality-based rehabilitation therapies can offer similar, and in some cases better, outcomes than conventional therapies and are associated with greater patient engagement and compliance (Tang et al., 2025; Pawassar & Tiberius, 2021).

The use of these intervention strategies, integrated into a metaverse environment, goes beyond the therapy session because virtual reality rehabilitation worlds offer patients the opportunity to perform exercises remotely, with ongoing connectivity to healthcare professionals. The use of wearable devices and IoMT technologies enables ongoing recording of exercise and compliance data, facilitating real-time adjustments to therapy programs.

Federated learning is an important aspect of applying these models at the population level. Federated models help improve the rehabilitation process, adjust difficulty levels to individual needs, and provide early warnings of non-compliance or adverse events. There have been promising attempts to use federated models in activity recognition and health monitoring via wearable technology (Arikumar et al., 2022).

It is equally imperative to acknowledge that Immersive environments for rehabilitation also pose challenges of clinical supervision and safety. There is a current research thrust indicating the need for clear escalation options, human presence for observing and supervising system communications, and limits of the technology to prevent overdependence on automated guidance (Pawassar & Tiberius, 2021).

10.2 Collaborative Diagnostics Across Distributed Healthcare Institutions

The other area of great promise within metaverse healthcare ecosystems is joint diagnosis. In the past, joint diagnosis has been facilitated by asynchronous communication and piecemeal data exchange. Such practices have succeeded in slowing down diagnosis and introducing inconsistencies. Recent multi-center studies have shown that federated learning can facilitate collective work on diagnostic models without necessitating a centralized pool of raw patient data from the hospital. For instance, federated learning has been shown to perform well in medical imaging applications such as brain tumor segmentation and chest image analysis, and has produced results comparable to those of a centralized learning solution (Dayan et al., 2021; Rieke et al., 2022).

Incorporating such capabilities into immersive worlds could also enhance cooperative behavior. Using a metaverse platform for diagnosis, providers from various facilities can jointly assess imaging results, AI-assisted marking in algorithms, and patient history details in a virtual world. Since providers have interaction capability, they can highlight regions of interest and compare and contrast various hypotheses. Although there has not been widespread use of immersive metaverse platforms for diagnosis, qualitative studies show improvements in communication quality and communal understanding compared to regular teleconferencing technology (Wang et al., 2023).

Despite these innovations, emerging metaverse architectures in healthcare also pose challenges for managing accountability in collective spaces for the diagnostic process. It is important to record them the moment decisions are reached through collaborative processes using blockchain technology.

10.3 Training, Simulation, and Continuing Medical Education

Medical research and continuous professional development are among the longest-standing areas to adopt immersive technology applications. Applications of VR and MR simulation have already entered surgical simulation for training surgeons and simulating operations and emergencies. Some current research findings indicate that the impact of immersive simulation is beneficial for skill development, decision-making capacity, and trainee confidence when combined with an evaluation strategy (Sung et al., 2024).

Learning environments developed through the metaverse further advance these benefits. Learning and teaching occur in one fixed environment. Simulators are not used separately. Learning through the metaverse creates opportunities for cooperative learning. Trainees from different hospitals can participate in metaverse learning. This learning is guided by teachers using avatars.

Federated learning enables improvements in environments such as this one by enabling continuous model refinement for evaluation. Federated learning allows insights gained from the institution to be pooled without involving individual trainees. The current literature demonstrates the potential of such learning strategies while also emphasizing the need for accreditation for immersive learning (Abbas et al., 2023).

Despite the mentioned advantages, the existing body of knowledge calls for caution regarding the integration of immersive training technology. Simulation fidelity, the application of the acquired skills to practical settings, or the storage of acquired knowledge remain open fields of research. Additionally, the issue of equity emerges with the availability of advanced simulators across various campuses.

10.4 Synthesis and Implications for Deployment

Despite their vastly different contexts, a number of recurring themes are found in these use cases. First, a task-centric application of the metaverse in a healthcare setting is far more effective than a self-contained one. Second, FL is a recurring enabling technology across all use cases, enabling intelligent scaling in a privacy-conscious manner. Third, immersive technologies highlight both the potential and risks of AI in a healthcare setting.

Current deployments remain fairly exploratory, with a focus on proof-of-concept work and user acceptance studies. However, the intersection of these technologies, along with federated learning and distributed systems, is already changing the paradigm for how care, collaboration, and education occur. The discussion of these early deployments will help to outline future directions, which will be covered in the final section of the current chapter.

11. FUTURE DIRECTIONS AND OPEN RESEARCH CHALLENGES

Even with rapid progress in immersive technologies, AI, and distributed learning paradigms, metaverse-based healthcare ecosystems remain in their nascent stages of maturity. The transition from experimental deployments to sustainable large-scale clinical infrastructure involves developing critical applications in human services amid a set of interrelated technical, organizational, and societal challenges. The paper discusses key future directions and open research problems to address for the realization of trustworthy, patient-centric metaverse healthcare systems.

11.1 Standardization and Interoperability Gaps

Of prime importance is the unmet need to develop comprehensive interoperability standards across metaverse platforms, health information technology systems, and AI platforms. In what is being proposed across the health industry, with a focus on HL7-FHIR, communication within the system is being considered, without any consideration of the practicality of using the metaverse or AI virtual agents (Mandel et al., 2021).

Nowadays, the relevance of broad cross-layer standards for model development has emerged. This includes federated learning in the matter of model exchange and interaction. It involves a model update interface and convergence evaluation standards in different institutions (Rieke et al., 2022). In the absence of standards for model development, model verification and reproduction are not easy.

Challenges in interoperability also exist in the hardware and software platforms used for XR. Inconsistencies within the rendering engine, interaction metaphor, and hardware support make it challenging to develop resilient applications for health care. There is a need for a collaborative response between health care and technology players to ensure that platforms mitigate the interoperability challenge.

11.2 Scaling Federated Metaverse Healthcare Globally

Replicating metaverse-enabled healthcare systems from pilot to full-scale production faces numerous technological and organizational hurdles. For federated learning systems to work seamlessly and efficiently, they must perform well across computers with different processing and network architectures and organizational governance. Although current work has established feasibility in controlled, multiple-institution settings, large-scale global deployment poses new challenges for communication and learning due to extreme heterogeneity (Li et al., 2021).

In a systems approach, the need for scalable deployment demands adaptable orchestration techniques that ensure dynamic load distribution across the edge, fog, and cloud tiers. The study of hierarchical and asynchronous federated learning is a promising area, but the healthcare implications, especially regarding stability and safety, have not yet been adequately investigated (Saadat et al., 2021).

Scaling an organization is also quite difficult. When discussing the implementation of various collaborative methods within national and international health care systems, alignment of incentives, governance frameworks, and trust bonds is necessary. There may also be differing governance and payment arrangements, along with certain expectations of people from other places, which could restrict the application of certain models from one environment to the other.

11.3 Evaluation, Validation, and Clinical Evidence

There is a persistent need in the prevailing literature for long-term, high-quality clinical evidence in favor of interventions in the medical field using the metaverse. Most prevailing studies are conducted to evaluate user friendliness, viability, or short-term results, with a lack of randomized controlled trials regarding clinical effectiveness, safety, and cost-effectiveness (Hulsen, 2023).

In AI-enabled and federated systems, validation becomes even more complicated due to model upgrades and context-dependent model behavior. Conventional paradigms for validation, understanding AI models and the deployment context to be known and measurable, would not prove to be entirely effective. There has been a need for continuous validation techniques dubbed post-deployment validation, real-world validation, and context-dependent validation (Finlayson et al., 2021). But for fully immersive environments, evaluation needs to account for human-related issues such as cognitive load, trust calibration, and interaction quality. Highly persuasive and highly immersive displays might have unintended effects on clinician judgment. There appears to be significant research needed to determine how to account for these issues.

11.4 Ethical and Societal Considerations

With the increased integration of metaverse-based healthcare platforms into healthcare, ethics are bound to influence acceptability and outcomes. Questions of informed consent, ownership of information, and accountability in algorithms, among others, take new forms in immersive spaces with persistent engagement, embodiment, and interaction with intelligent agents. The current literature suggests that future applications of technology in healthcare could perpetuate existing inequalities if they are not distributed equally in terms of infrastructure, education, or participation rates (Rajkomar et al., 2022). The issue of equitable access to the metaverse in the care field, as well as the problem of the so-called 'digital elite' in the sector, would require policy measures to resolve.

Professional identity and responsibility in intelligent virtual agents are also issues that are brought to light. With the growing capabilities of intelligent agents, it is increasingly difficult to distinguish between assistance and automation in healthcare, which has long-standing formalities regarding responsibility among healthcare professionals. Dialogue and discussion are key in defining acceptability in healthcare environments created by AI.

11.5 Toward Patient-Centric, Trustworthy Healthcare Ecosystems

Looking ahead, the single biggest test of the effectiveness of the metaverse Healthcare Ecosystems in the context of the successful implementation of the digitalization of the healthcare industry would lie in their ability to provide patient-centred, effective, equitable, and trustworthy forms of patient care. A federated approach to learning provides an extremely powerful means of aligning intelligence at scale with patient autonomy, but it must be placed within broader governance structures to ensure accountability. Equally, immersion technologies need to be assessed with respect to their engagement or realism capabilities, as well as their knowledge or decision-making capabilities.

In conclusion, the future of research should take an interdisciplinary route that brings together systems engineering, clinical sciences, human-computer interaction studies, ethics, and policy analyses. In this way, the challenges faced by the field will be met comprehensively. The metaverse-based healthcare ecosystems will therefore be shaped to incorporate advanced, socially responsible technology.

REFERENCES

Abbas, J. R., Meschtscherjakov, A., & Tscheligi, M. (2023). What is virtual reality? A healthcare-focused systematic review of definitions. *Journal of Biomedical Informatics*, *141*, 104356.

Al, E. 'mari, S., Sanjalawe, Y., Fataftah, F., & Fataftah, F. (2026). Digital Twins and BI: Synchronizing Virtual Models With Real-Time Business Processes. In *Strategic AI Integration in Business Intelligence* (pp. 135-154). IGI Global Scientific Publishing.

Al-E'mari, S., Sanjalawe, Y., Kurdi, G., & Allehyani, B. (2025, April). Detection of ARP Spoofing Attack in Healthcare Networks Using a LSTM Model. In *2025 1st International Conference on Computational Intelligence Approaches and Applications (ICCIAA)* (pp. 1-7). IEEE. DOI: 10.1109/ICCIAA65327.2025.11012965

Arikumar, K. S., Prathiba, S. B., Alazab, M., Gadekallu, T. R., Pandya, S., Khan, J. M., & Moorthy, R. S. (2022). FL-PMI: Federated learning-based person movement identification through wearable devices in smart healthcare systems. *Sensors (Basel)*, *22*(4), 1377. DOI: 10.3390/s22041377 PMID: 35214282

Bagdasaryan, E., Veit, A., Hua, Y., Estrin, D., & Shmatikov, V. (2020). How to backdoor federated learning. *Proceedings of the 23rd International Conference on Artificial Intelligence and Statistics (AISTATS)*, 2938–2948.

Björnsson, B., Borrebaeck, C., Elander, N., Gasslander, T., Gawel, D. R., Gustafsson, M., & Benson, M. (2020). Digital twins to personalize medicine. *Genome Medicine*, *12*(1), 4. DOI: 10.1186/s13073-019-0701-3 PMID: 31892363

Bommasani, R., Hudson, D. A., Adeli, E., Altman, R., Arora, S., von Arx, S., . . . Liang, P. (2021). On the opportunities and risks of foundation models. *arXiv preprint arXiv:2108.07258*.

Bonawitz, K., Ivanov, V., Kreuter, B., Marcedone, A., McMahan, H. B., Patel, S., & Seth, K. (2019). Practical secure aggregation for privacy-preserving machine learning. *Proceedings of the 2017 ACM SIGSAC Conference on Computer and Communications Security*, 1175–1191. https://doi.org/DOI: 10.1145/3133956.3133982

Bozkurt, A., & Sharma, R. C. (2024). Trust, credibility and transparency in human-AI interaction: Why we need explainable and trustworthy AI and why we need it now. *Asian Journal of Distance Education*, *19*(2).

Bruynseels, K., Santoni de Sio, F., & van den Hoven, J. (2022). Digital twins in health care: Ethical implications of an emerging engineering paradigm. *Frontiers in Genetics*, *13*, 826935. DOI: 10.3389/fgene.2022.826935 PMID: 29487613

Cai, C. J., Winter, S., Steiner, D., Wilcox, L., & Terry, M. (2022). "Hello AI": Uncovering the onboarding needs of medical practitioners for human–AI collaborative decision-making. *Proceedings of the ACM on Human-Computer Interaction, 6*(CSCW2), 1–24. https://doi.org/DOI: 10.1145/3555220

Dayan, I., Roth, H. R., Zhong, A., Harouni, A., Gentili, A., Abidin, A. Z., & Kalpathy-Cramer, J. (2021). Federated learning for predicting clinical outcomes in patients with COVID-19. *Nature Medicine*, *27*(10), 1735–1743. DOI: 10.1038/s41591-021-01506-3 PMID: 34526699

El-Saleh, A. A., Sheikh, A. M., Albreem, M. A., & Honnurvali, M. S. (2025). The internet of medical things (IoMT): Opportunities and challenges. *Wireless Networks*, *31*(1), 327–344. DOI: 10.1007/s11276-024-03764-8

European Commission. (2021). *Ethics guidelines for trustworthy AI.* Publications Office of the European Union.

Finlayson, S. G., Subbaswamy, A., Singh, K., Bowers, J., Kupke, A., Zittrain, J., Kohane, I. S., & Saria, S. (2021). The clinician and dataset shift in artificial intelligence. *The New England Journal of Medicine*, *385*(3), 283–286. DOI: 10.1056/NEJMc2104626 PMID: 34260843

Garbagnati, A., & Wu, L. (2021). Creating Competitive Advantage: Privacy and Security by Design in mHealth and Digital Health Products. *Health Law.*, *34*, 9.

Ghatti, S., Yurish, L. A., Shen, H., Rheuban, K., Enfield, K. B., Facteau, N. R., & Dowdell, K. (2023). Digital twins in healthcare: A survey of current methods. *Archives of Clinical and Biomedical Research*, *7*(3), 365–381. DOI: 10.26502/acbr.50170352

Huang, S.-C., Pareek, A., Seyyedi, S., Banerjee, I., & Lungren, M. P. (2022). Fusion of medical imaging and electronic health records using deep learning: A systematic review and implementation guidelines. *NPJ Digital Medicine*, *5*(1), 136. DOI: 10.1038/s41746-020-00341-z PMID: 33083571

Huang, Y., Li, Y. J., & Cai, Z. (2023). Security and privacy in metaverse: A comprehensive survey. *Big Data Mining and Analytics*, *6*(2), 234–247. DOI: 10.26599/BDMA.2022.9020047

Hulsen, T. (2023). Applications of the metaverse in medicine and healthcare. *Journal of Laboratory and Precision Medicine*. PMID: 38939198

Kairouz, P., McMahan, H. B., Avent, B., Bellet, A., Bennis, M., Bhagoji, A. N., … Zhao, S. (2021). Advances and open problems in federated learning. *Foundations and Trends® in Machine Learning, 14*(1–2), 1–210.

Li, T., Sahu, A. K., Talwalkar, A., & Smith, V. (2021). Federated learning: Challenges, methods, and future directions. *IEEE Signal Processing Magazine*, *37*(3), 50–60. DOI: 10.1109/MSP.2020.2975749

Li, Y.. (2024). The next generation of healthcare ecosystem in metaverse: Concept, framework, and challenges. [ScienceDirect journal article]. *Digital Health.*

Longoni, C., Bonezzi, A., & Morewedge, C. K. (2022). Resistance to medical artificial intelligence. *The Journal of Consumer Research*, *46*(4), 629–650. DOI: 10.1093/jcr/ucz013

Magalhães, R., et al. (2024). Mixed reality in the operating room: A systematic review. *Journal/venue as indexed in PMC.*

Mandel, J. C.. (2021). SMART on FHIR: A standards-based, interoperable apps platform for electronic health records. *Journal of the American Medical Informatics Association : JAMIA*, *28*(7), 1278–1287. DOI: 10.1093/jamia/ocab061 PMID: 26911829

Melis, L., Song, C., De Cristofaro, E., & Shmatikov, V. (2019). Exploiting unintended feature leakage in collaborative learning. *Proceedings of the 2019 IEEE Symposium on Security and Privacy*, 691–706. https://doi.org/DOI: 10.1109/SP.2019.00029

Mesko, B., & Győrffy, Z. (2023). The rise of the empowered physician in the digital health era: Viewpoint. *Journal of Medical Internet Research*, *25*, e40616. DOI: 10.2196/40616 PMID: 30912758

Mystakidis, S. (2022). Metaverse. *Encyclopedia*, *2*(1), 486–497. DOI: 10.3390/encyclopedia2010031

Nazi, Z. A., & Peng, W. (2024). Large language models in healthcare and medical domain: A review. []. MDPI.]. *Informatics (MDPI)*, *11*(3), 57. DOI: 10.3390/informatics11030057

Oulefki, A., Amira, A., & Foufou, S. (2025). Digital twins and AI transforming healthcare systems through innovation and data-driven decision making. *Health Technology (Hong Kong)*, •••, 1–23.

Pawassar, C. M., & Tiberius, V. (2021). Virtual reality in health care: Bibliometric analysis. *JMIR Serious Games*, *9*(4), e32721. DOI: 10.2196/32721 PMID: 34855606

Protection, F. D. (2018). General data protection regulation (GDPR). *Intersoft Consulting, Accessed in October, 24*(1).

Raghupathi, W., & Raghupathi, V. (2014). Big data analytics in healthcare: Promise and potential. *Health Information Science and Systems*, *2*(1), 3. DOI: 10.1186/2047-2501-2-3 PMID: 25825667

Rajkomar, A., Hardt, M., Howell, M. D., Corrado, G., & Chin, M. H. (2022). Ensuring fairness in machine learning to advance health equity. *Annals of Internal Medicine*, *175*(6), 866–872. DOI: 10.7326/M21-2749 PMID: 30508424

Rasouli, H., & Valmohammadi, C. (2020). Proposing a conceptual framework for customer identity and access management: A qualitative approach. *Global Knowledge, Memory and Communication*, *69*(1/2), 94–116. DOI: 10.1108/GKMC-02-2019-0014

Rieke, N., Hancox, J., Li, W., Milletari, F., Roth, H. R., Albarqouni, S., & Cardoso, M. J. (2022). The future of digital health with federated learning. *NPJ Digital Medicine*, *5*(1), 14. DOI: 10.1038/s41746-022-00542-9 PMID: 35087172

Saadat, H., Aboumadi, A., Mohamed, A., Erbad, A., & Guizani, M. (2021, June). Hierarchical federated learning for collaborative IDS in IoT applications. In *2021 10th Mediterranean Conference on Embedded Computing (MECO)* (pp. 1-6). IEEE. DOI: 10.1109/MECO52532.2021.9460304

Sanjalawe, Y., Alqurashi, T., Alharbi, Z. H., Makhadmeh, S. N., & Alsharaiah, M. (2025). Adaptive graph attention-based federated learning for IoT intrusion detection: Mitigating poisoning attacks. *PeerJ. Computer Science*, *11*, e3281. DOI: 10.7717/peerj-cs.3281

Sedlmair, M., Meyer, M., & Munzner, T. (2020). Criteria for rigor in visualization design study. *IEEE Transactions on Visualization and Computer Graphics*, *26*(1), 87–97. DOI: 10.1109/TVCG.2019.2934539

Shah, N. D., Steyerberg, E. W., & Kent, D. M. (2021). Big data and predictive analytics: Recalibrating expectations. *Journal of the American Medical Association*, *320*(1), 27–28. DOI: 10.1001/jama.2018.5602 PMID: 29813156

Sheller, M. J., Edwards, B., Reina, G. A., Martin, J., Pati, S., Kotrotsou, A., Milchenko, M., Xu, W., Marcus, D., Colen, R. R., & Bakas, S. (2020). Federated learning in medicine: Facilitating multi-institutional collaborations without sharing patient data. *Scientific Reports*, *10*(1), 12598. DOI: 10.1038/s41598-020-69250-1 PMID: 32724046

Shi, W., Dustdar, S., Yu, F. R., & Buyya, R. (2022). Edge computing: Vision and challenges. *IEEE Internet of Things Journal*, *9*(6), 1–19.

Shi, Y., Yu, H., & Leung, C. (2023). Towards fairness-aware federated learning. *IEEE Transactions on Neural Networks and Learning Systems, 35*(9), 11922–11938. DOI: 10.1109/TNNLS.2023.3263594 PMID: 37037249

Shickel, B., Tighe, P. J., Bihorac, A., & Rashidi, P. (2018). Deep EHR: A survey of recent advances in deep learning techniques for electronic health record analysis. *IEEE Journal of Biomedical and Health Informatics, 22*(5), 1589–1604. DOI: 10.1109/JBHI.2017.2767063 PMID: 29989977

Su, X., An, L., Cheng, Z., & Weng, Y. (2023). Cloud–edge collaboration-based bi-level optimal scheduling for intelligent healthcare systems. *Future Generation Computer Systems, 141*, 28–39. DOI: 10.1016/j.future.2022.11.005

Subbaswamy, A., & Saria, S. (2020). From development to deployment: Dataset shift, causality, and shift-stable models in health AI. *Biostatistics (Oxford, England), 21*(2), 345–352. DOI: 10.1093/biostatistics/kxz041 PMID: 31742354

Sun, Z., Kairouz, P., Suresh, A. T., & McMahan, H. B. (2022). Can you really backdoor federated learning? *Proceedings of the 35th Conference on Neural Information Processing Systems (NeurIPS).*

Sung, H., Kim, M., Park, J., Shin, N., & Han, Y. (2024). Effectiveness of virtual reality in healthcare education: A systematic literature review and meta-analysis. *Sustainability (Basel), 16*(19), 8520. DOI: 10.3390/su16198520

Tang, P.. (2025). The efficacy of virtual reality on the rehabilitation of musculoskeletal disorders: An umbrella review. *Journal of Clinical Medicine, 14*(3), 623. DOI: 10.3390/jcm14030623

Tonekaboni, S., Joshi, S., McCradden, M. D., & Goldenberg, A. (2023). What clinicians want: Contextualizing explainable machine learning for clinical end use. *Proceedings of Machine Learning Research, 126*, 1–21.

Topol, E. (2019). High-performance medicine: The convergence of human and artificial intelligence. *Nature Medicine, 25*(1), 44–56. DOI: 10.1038/s41591-018-0300-7 PMID: 30617339

Topol, E. (2023). *Deep medicine: How artificial intelligence can make healthcare human again* (updated perspectives). Basic Books.

Wang, Y., Li, C., Qu, L., Cai, H., & Ge, Y. (2023). Application and challenges of a metaverse in medicine. *Frontiers in Robotics and AI, 10*, 1291199. DOI: 10.3389/frobt.2023.1291199 PMID: 38152305

Wosik, J., Fudim, M., Cameron, B., Gellad, Z. F., Cho, A., Phinney, D., & Katz, J. N. (2020). Telehealth transformation: COVID-19 and the rise of virtual care. *Journal of the American Medical Informatics Association : JAMIA*, *27*(6), 957–962. DOI: 10.1093/jamia/ocaa067 PMID: 32311034

Yang, Y.. (2023). Metaverse for healthcare: Technologies, challenges, and opportunities. *International Journal of Crowd Science*. Agbo, C. C., Mahmoud, Q. H., & Eklund, J. M. (2019, April). Blockchain technology in healthcare: a systematic review. [). MDPI.]. *Health Care*, *7*(2), 56.

Chapter 13
Privacy Preservation Through Design-Federated Learning Architectures for Secure and Immersive Metaverse-Based Healthcare

S. Aarthi
http://orcid.org/0009-0006-9064-2091
Marwadi University, Rajkot, India

Jaypalsinh A. Gohil
http://orcid.org/0000-0003-0925-6646
Marwadi University, Rajkot, India

ABSTRACT

Crossover of the metaverse, Artificial Intelligence, and Federated Learning is changing the healthcare systems and amplifying the issues of privacy, security, and trust. This chapter discusses privacy preservation by design as a fundamental concept to applying Federated Learning architectures in metaverse-based healthcare setting. Federated Learning is theoretically understood as an architecture facilitator that introduces collaborative intelligence between hospitals, clinics, wearables, and virtual care platforms with no centralized data exchange. The main architectural aspects like Edge Fog Cloud Coordination, Secure Aggregation, Differential Privacy,

DOI: 10.4018/979-8-3373-8889-2.ch013

and Trusted Execution Environment are examined to explain how confidentiality and regulatory compliance may be obtained. By conceptually discussing and using illustrative examples, the chapter demonstrates how privacy-centric federated architectures can be used to support immersive, real-time, and patient-centric healthcare services and maintain data sovereignty.

1. INTRODUCTION

The combination of immersive virtual worlds, Artificial Intelligence, and Decentralized Learning paradigms is a massive digital transformation of healthcare systems. With the introduction of metaverse-based healthcare ecosystems, it becomes possible to have sustained virtual environments where patients, clinicians and intelligent systems engage with one another in real time, to serve more advanced applications in the form of virtual hospitals, remote diagnostics, digital twins and immersive medical training. At the same time, AI can be used to improve predictive analytics, personalization and clinical decision support, and Federated Learning (FL) has a paradigm shift because it is possible to train collaborative models without aggregating the data centrally (Lakhan et al., 2023). Irrespective of these opportunities, data privacy, data security, trust and regulatory compliance are concerns that are enhanced by the integration of these technologies especially in settings that constantly gather and process sensitive health information. To overcome these issues, it is important to consider how the system architectures are designed to incorporate privacy as a design constraint, but not a design consideration (Brisimi et al., 2018). The chapter puts privacy preservation by design as a vital facilitator of secure and trustful metaverse-based healthcare systems, with a preference towards Federated Learning designs that reconcile innovations and patient autonomy, data sovereignty and ethical responsibilities.

1.1 AI-Metaverse-FL Convergence in Healthcare

The intersection of the metaverse, Artificial Intelligence, and Federated Learning is a paradigm shift in the sphere of healthcare provision and design. The metaverse offers immersive and persistent virtual worlds where physical and digital healthcare space is built, with the ability to maintain constant communication between patients, clinicians, and intelligent agents. Artificial Intelligence is deployed in these settings in order to provide high-level analytics, predictive modeling, and clinical recommending. Federated Learning is the additive technology to this ecosystem since it allows distributed model training among hospitals, clinics, edge devices and wearables without conveying raw patient data (Divyashree, 2024). This convergence aids in the collaborative intelligence at scale and improves the existing concerns regarding data silos and interoperability. Federated Learning is complementary to the distributed and interactive character of metaverse healthcare systems since it decentralizes learning and computation (Ravikumar, Aarthi, Masharipova, et al., 2025). These technologies can work together to deliver real-time, context-sensitive healthcare services that are user friendly, scalable and patient-centric and transforming the traditional lines between clinical settings, digital applications and data governance models. Figure 1 depicts the way in which siloed healthcare data can be remodelled into adaptive, privacy-aware and patient-centric healthcare services through the integration of immersive metaverse-based settings, AI-driven analytics, and Federated Learning .

Figure 1. Convergence of Metaverse, AI, and FL in Healthcare

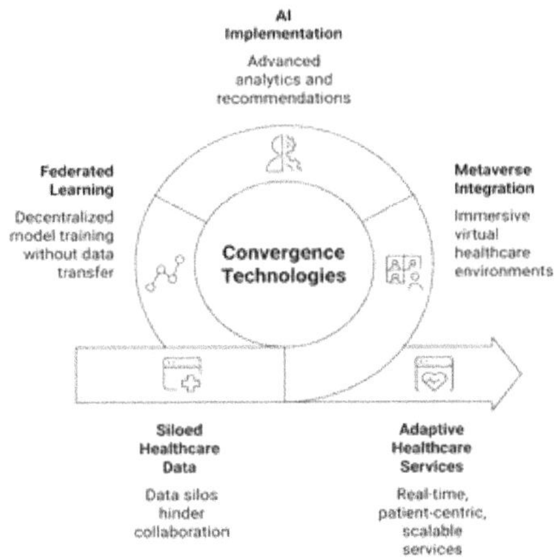

1.2 Privacy and Trust Risks in Immersive Care

The nature of complex privacy, security, and trust in immersive healthcare ecosystems is presented by the constant generation of data and real-time interaction between the health system and the multiple stakeholders involved. The use of rich streams of biometric, behavioral and contextual data, which are the basis of metaverse environments, increases the risk of unauthorized access, inference attacks and identity misuse, significantly. The threats to AI models trained on sensitive health information include model inversion, membership inference and adversarial manipulation. Also, decentralization and cross-organizational character of these ecosystems make accountability and governance difficult and non-compliant with regulation (Ali et al., 2023). The issue of trust is paramount, as the patients and clinicians have to be guided by the virtual systems and AI-powered suggestions without direct access to the data streams and decision-making processes. To cope with such challenges, the architectural mechanisms are needed to guarantee confidentiality, integrity, transparency, and explainability (Ravikumar, et al., 2025). In the absence of privacy-conscious and security-conscious design, the immersive healthcare technologies are likely to undermine the trust of users, break regulations, and provoke ethical issues that can make large-scale implementation impossible.

1.3 Motivation and Scope of Privacy Preservation by Design

Privacy preservation by design focuses on the design of systems, processes and algorithms with privacy controls enshrined at the initial phases of design. Within the framework of healthcare in the metaverse, this solution is driven by the necessity to safeguard patient information that is sensitive, as well as allow advanced analytics and experiences of the metaverse. Privacy by design uses a combination of technical solutions, like Federated Learning, secure aggregation, differential privacy, and trusted execution environments, as part of the main architecture, rather than using post hoc security controls or policy implementation. The chapter is based on the ideas of privacy preservation by design as guiding principles to explore how Federated Learning architectures may be used to achieve collaborative intelligence without violating data sovereignty (Sadilek et al., 2021). It is not limited to technical solutions but also governance, alignment of ethics and regulatory issues because it is acknowledged that privacy is a technological and institutional issue. The chapter introduces possibilities of the creation of scalable, trustful, and patient-centric healthcare systems within the framework of immersive digital setting by posing Federated Learning as an architectural enabler.

2. BACKGROUND TO THE STUDY

The shift to digital and immersive healthcare systems is conditioned by the development of information technologies, data analytics, and networked infrastructures. The conventional healthcare systems, which are typified by centralised data stores and disjointed service provision, have constraints of scalability, interoperability and confidentiality. The introduction of the platforms based on the metaverse opens new opportunities of integrated care, simulation, and collaboration, but also raises the risks linked to the issues of data governance and ethical responsibility (Diwan, 2025).

In response to these issues, Federated Learning has been brought to the forefront of attention as a solution to decentralized model training, which remains compliant with regulatory demands and data privacy principles. Simultaneously, the changing privacy laws and ethical standards are placing greater responsibility, openness, and control over the patient in the use of data. It is necessary to understand the context of these technological and regulatory trends, which can help to place the role of privacy-preserving Federated Learning in immersive healthcare ecosystems in its place. In this section, the background information on the development of metaverse healthcare, the concepts of Federated Learning, and regulatory imperatives that determine privacy-sensitive system design are offered.

2.1 Evolution of Metaverse-Based Healthcare Systems

The healthcare systems of the metaverse have developed on the premises of the primitive telemedicine systems and virtual simulation applications into the immersive, networked space, combining clinical, educational, and administrative capabilities. The development of virtual reality, augmented reality, and digital twins technologies has made it possible to recreate the image of patients, healthcare facilities, and procedures in sustained virtual space. Examples of the applications running on these systems include remote consultations, rehabilitation treatments, surgical planning, and medical training (Nguyen et al., 2023). The need to be accessible, continue care and resilience have led to the evolution especially in situations when confronted with limited physical interaction. But with the increasing data intensity and interactivity of such environments, they are increasingly based on constant data gathering by sensors and wearables as well as user interaction. The shift brings up important concerns of data ownership, consent, and the long-term use of data and the role of creating privacy-conscious controls as part of the metaverse healthcare infrastructure design. Table 1 Summarizes the main technologies like the metaverse, AI, Federated Learning, and edge computing and their applications in healthcare.

Table 1. Key Technologies in Metaverse-Based Healthcare Ecosystems

Technology	Description	Role in Healthcare Ecosystems
Metaverse	Immersive virtual environments that integrate physical and digital spaces	Enables virtual hospitals, remote consultations, immersive training, and collaborative clinical decision-making
Artificial Intelligence (AI)	Computational models that learn patterns and support intelligent decision-making	Supports diagnosis, prediction, personalization, and clinical decision support within immersive environments
Federated Learning (FL)	Decentralized machine learning approach that trains models without sharing raw data	Enables collaborative healthcare analytics while preserving patient privacy and data sovereignty
Edge Computing	Data processing performed close to data sources such as devices and sensors	Reduces latency, enhances real-time analytics, and improves privacy in healthcare applications
Fog Computing	Intermediate computing layer between edge and cloud	Supports coordination, aggregation, and scalable processing across distributed healthcare systems
Cloud Computing	Centralized computing infrastructure for storage and coordination	Facilitates global model aggregation, system scalability, and cross-institutional collaboration

2.2 Federated Learning Foundations

Federated Learning is a decentralized machine learning model, which allows many parties to learn through joint training of common models, without taking raw data. Within the healthcare setting, such a method solves the important issue of data sensitivity, compliance with the regulations, and institutional limits. Hospitals, clinics, and personal devices keep authority over local information and provide model updates which are accumulated to enhance global performance (Antunes et al., 2022). The paradigm facilitates the learning of heterogeneous and geographically distributed datasets, which finds great advantage in healthcare due to the heterogeneity of population and uneven distributions of data. Federated Learning architectures may be deployed both in cross-silo contexts, like between hospitals, and under cross-device contexts between wearables and mobile health apps. Federated Learning impacts fewer privacy risks due to limited data movement and exposure, and implements collaborative and scaled intelligence. These are the features that qualify it as one of the pillars of privacy-preserving analytics in healthcare systems of the metaverse.

2.3 Privacy, Ethics, and Regulation

Data governance in healthcare is being influenced by tough privacy laws and ethical standards which focus on patient rights, transparency and accountability. Regulatory models enforce both protection of information confidentiality, informed consent, and purpose restriction, and the significance of innovation in the health service delivery. The principles of data sovereignty also stipulate that individual and institutional actors should control the way data is gathered, processed and distributed. The implementation of these requirements in immersive and distributed healthcare settings is more complicated by cross-border information transfers and the involvement of multiple actors (Chelani et al., 2024). Ethical requirements do not just limit themselves to legal requirements, but also to fairness, explicability and reliability of decisions made by AI. Federated Learning is compatible with these imperatives, as it will decrease centralised data collection and decentralised governance frameworks. Regulatory and ethical aspects of the system architecture are critical in making sure that the metaverse-based healthcare systems are socially acceptable, do not violate the law, are oriented towards patient-centric values.

3. RESEARCH OBJECTIVES

The research objectives presented in this chapter are well-defined and weave together into a single coherent unit, namely, the innovation in healthcare ecosystems emerging as a result of convergence between metaverse technologies, Artificial Intelligence, and Federated Learning. The objectives are aimed to offer a structured analytical basis on the study of privacy preservation by design with special focus on the three aspects of architectural, organizational and ethical aspects. The objectives facilitate a methodical study of how Federated Learning can be used to support the creation of secure, trustful, and patient-centric immersive healthcare systems by ensuring compliance with regulatory and ethical considerations, as well as technical innovation.

- **To identify and categorize privacy risks** associated with metaverse-enabled healthcare environments, including risks arising from immersive data collection, continuous monitoring, and AI-driven inference.
- **To examine Federated Learning architectures** as privacy-preserving mechanisms for collaborative healthcare analytics across hospitals, clinics, edge devices, and virtual care platforms.
- **To analyze the effectiveness of privacy-enhancing techniques** such as secure aggregation, differential privacy, and trusted execution environments within federated metaverse healthcare systems.
- **To evaluate governance and security challenges**, including adversarial threats, identity management, and trust establishment in decentralized and immersive healthcare ecosystems.

- **To assess ethical and regulatory alignment**, focusing on data sovereignty, patient autonomy, and compliance with healthcare data protection requirements in federated and metaverse-based deployments.

4. CONCEPTUAL MODEL

The theoretical framework described in this chapter offers a systematic illustration of how the privacy-preserving Federated Learning can be systematically implemented in the healthcare ecosystems of the metaverse. The model will be able to reflect the interactions between the immersive virtual environments, the elements of Artificial Intelligence, and the distributed sources of healthcare data and meet the privacy, security, and ethics standards. It not only theorizes Federated Learning as a form of model training but as a structural foundation upon which decentralized intelligence can be practiced in both physical and virtual healthcare fields. The model assists the real-time analytics, personalization and collaboration by combining edge, fog and cloud resources without concentrating sensitive patient information (Feretzakis et al., 2024). Also, the framework explicitly integrates trust, privacy, and accountability levels to accommodate governance and regulatory issues that are inherent in immersive and distributed systems. This is the conceptualization of the analysis of system behavior, potential risk identification, and assessment of mitigation strategies. It also gives a basis on how technical design decisions can be made in line with organizational, ethical and legal aspects, and thus assist in developing scalable, reliable and patient-centric metaverse healthcare solutions.

4.1 Privacy-Preserving FL Architecture

Privacy-sensitive Federated Learning in the healthcare metaverse is developed in a multi-layered and decentralized architecture that enables collaborative intelligence without data sharing. The central component of the architecture is the distributed data holders, since they consist of the hospitals, clinics, wearable devices, and home-based monitoring systems, every one of which has some local control over sensitive patient information. The Federated Learning organizes the training of the model by allowing the local models to be trained locally and merged with the secure protocols. The edge and fog computing layers are useful in the low-latency processing and context-driven analytics, and the cloud components are useful in the coordination, scalability, and convergence of world models (Javed et al., 2023). Privacy enhancing such mechanisms as secure aggregation, differential privacy and trusted execution environment are combined with the training and communication processes. This type of architecture matches the distributed and immersive nature of metaverse healthcare environments as well as enables real-time intelligence without compromise of sovereignty of data and regulatory adherence and system dependability. Table 2 gives a summary of key architectural layers and elements used in federated metaverse healthcare systems and privacy mechanisms used.

Table 2 Architectural Components of Privacy-Preserving FL

Architectural Layer	Key Components	Privacy and Security Function
Data Source Layer	Hospitals, clinics, wearables, home monitoring devices	Retains sensitive patient data locally and enforces data sovereignty
Edge Layer	Local compute nodes, on-device AI models	Enables low-latency processing and minimizes raw data exposure
Federated Learning Layer	Local model training, secure model update exchange	Supports collaborative learning without sharing raw healthcare data
Privacy Enhancement Layer	Secure aggregation, differential privacy, encryption	Protects model updates from inference and reconstruction attacks
Coordination Layer	Model aggregation server, orchestration services	Manages synchronization, scalability, and global model convergence
Trust and Governance Layer	Identity management, access control, audit mechanisms	Ensures accountability, compliance, and trusted participation
Application Layer	Virtual hospitals, digital twins, immersive care platforms	Delivers privacy-aware and intelligent healthcare services

4.2 AI–Virtual Environment Interaction

The communication between the virtual worlds, Artificial Intelligence systems, and distributed information sources is the foundation of the operations of the metaverse-based healthcare systems. Virtual spaces serve as an interface, through which clinicians, patients, and digital images like avatars or digital twins engage with each other around the clock. These venues create and ingest data feeds that drive Artificial Intelligence-based analytics, decision support and individualization services (Oyekan, 2024). Federated Learning allows AI models to train using distributed information without accessing raw information to the virtual layer or centralized repositories. Regular integration and synchronization of model updates is conducted to make sure that intelligence in the metaverse is of different and evolving clinical scenarios. This interaction model promotes the adaptive and situational healthcare service and reduces the privacy risks of the constant data exchange. The framework enables the virtual healthcare setting to be responsive and smart without the need to impair confidentiality and data protection ideals by linking data ownership to model intelligence. Figure 2 represents the relationship between distributed sources of data, Federated Learning -based AI models and virtual environments in a healthcare system operating in a metaverse.

Figure 2. Interaction Model in Metaverse-Based Healthcare Systems

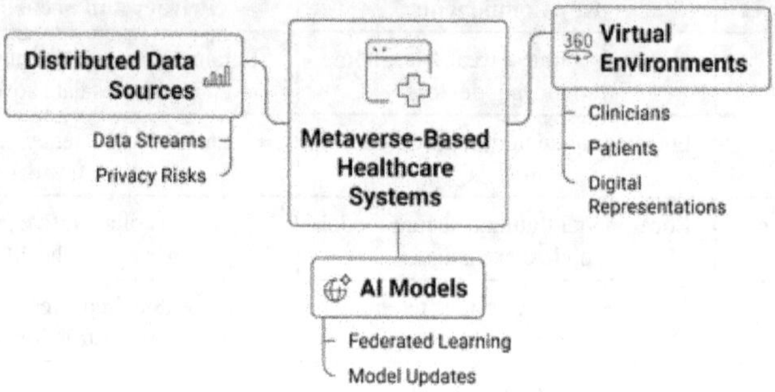

4.3 Trust and Governance Layers

The conceptual framework has built trust, privacy, and accountability as underlying layers, which should be responsible in operating the healthcare systems enabled by the metaverse. The layer of trust deals with how to verify the identity, authenticate, and reliably engage the stakeholders of the immersive environments. The technical privacy measures implemented in privacy layers include encryption, access control, and privacy-preserving learning to mitigate attacks of unauthorized exposure of data and inference. The mechanisms of accountability provide transparency and traceability of decisions that use AI, which is audit-able and compliant with regulatory demands (Pasupuleti & Services, 2025). These levels are multi-level across technical and organisational limits, and are used to support governance structures that are used to define roles, responsibilities, and granting consent. With these dimensions incorporated into the conceptual framework, it is highlighted that reliable healthcare metaverse systems cannot be built just by a sophisticated technological solution. Rather, they rely on the correspondence of architectural design to ethical principles, regulatory requirements, and institutional control that will promote trust that is long-term and sustainable use of innovative immersive healthcare.

5. RESEARCH METHODOLOGY

The chapter uses a qualitative, conceptual and architecture-based study to investigate privacy protection by design in meta verse healthcare ecosystems using Federated Learning . Since this field is emergent and interdisciplinary, a theoretical synthesis, architectural analysis, and the development of a structured framework are more important than an empirical experimentation approach to the study. The method combines the perspectives of distributed machine learning, immersive systems, healthcare informatics, and data governance towards developing a comprehensive view of privacy-conserving system design (Loftus et al., 2022). The methodology does not place priority over measures of algorithmic performance only, but rather on architectural coherence, trust mechanism and regulatory alignment. This design-based approach enables the inquiry of the possibilities of embedding Federated Learning in immersive healthcare settings in a systematic manner, compromising privacy, security, and ethical concerns. The approach to rigorous analysis of design decisions and their consequences by combining conceptual modeling with analytical mapping and validation by way of representative scenarios is supported through the methodology (Rauniyar et al., 2024). This systematic methodology will ensure the proposed framework is flexible, scaled, and applicable to healthcare settings in the real world and still has a clear focus on patient-centered privacy and accountability.

5.1 Architecture-Centric Design

Its study design is conceptual and architecture based using the system-level analysis, as opposed to component-only analysis. The design targets the understanding of the interaction between Federated Learning architectures and metaverses, Artificial Intelligence services and distributed healthcare data sources. The abstracting of significant architectural components, the data flow, and the patterns of interaction known to be vital and that will enable the establishment of privacy risks and privacy mitigation will be performed through conceptual modeling. The point of view of architecture provides the opportunity of researching the trade-offs of design with regard to the elements of decentralization, latency, scalability, and trust (Abhishek V A et al., 2022). The research design represents immersive healthcare ecosystem complexity by positioning Federated Learning as an architecture-enabling event, and not a single algorithm. It is the best approach to use in a study on the new systems in which the same implementations have not been standardized. It allows the logical reasoning of the privacy preservation, which results in the technical decisions being aligned with the governance requirements, ethical norms, and healthcare-related constraints.

5.2 Framework Development and Analytical Mapping

The synthesis of the information contained in the literature, regulatory policies, and architectural best practices make up the framework development, through which a structured framework on privacy-preserving Federated Learning in the healthcare metaverse will be developed. The suggested scheme connects the different aspects of architecture, privacy models and governance by analytically mapping the same. The process identifies virtual environment interdependencies and relationships with AI models and data sources and trust layers. The importance of privacy enhancing technology such as secure aggregation, differential privacy, and trusted execution environment in minimizing risks at different stages of data processing and model training is also demonstrated by mapping (ElBedoui et al., 2025). Analytic framework is applied as the tool of evaluating design completeness, consistency and compliance. The framework allows to review the system robustness and credibility in a holistic manner because it establishes a distinct correlation between technical procedures and ethical and regulatory concerns. The systematic mapping will allow comparing the potential deployment scenarios and design optimization.

5.3 Validation through Use-Case and Scenario Analysis

The proposed framework is validated by use-case and scenario analysis which represents real healthcare application in the metaverse. The applicability and effectiveness of the architecture is evaluated using representative scenarios, including virtual hospitals, remote diagnosis, and digital twin-based monitoring as well as immersive medical training. All the scenarios are analyzed and data flows, privacy risks, and how Federated Learning can facilitate safe collaboration are evaluated. It is a qualitative validation method that enables investigation of the operational constraint, interaction between stakeholders and challenges of governance without adopting large-scale experimental data (Abbas et al., 2024). Scenario analysis is also effective in the determination of possible gaps, limitations and context-based factors that have the ability to affect system performance and trust. The validation process by basing the conceptual framework on meanwhile use cases enhances the relevance of the conceptual framework and how privacy preservation by design can be implemented in various and dynamic healthcare metaverse settings.

6. LITERATURE REVIEW

The digital healthcare transformation literature suggests the increasing convergence of the decentralized machine learning, immersive technologies, and privacy-conscious system design. According to the literature, it has always been stressed that the traditional centralized approach to healthcare analytics is limited due to the presence of data silos, privacy concerns, and regulatory risks. To this end, solutions such as Federated Learning, metaverse-based healthcare platforms and decentralized governance models have come about as complementary solutions (Tanveer et al., 2025). This literature review is a synthesis of available literature in line with the chapter objectives that concentrate on privacy preserving healthcare analytics, immersive clinical application, and issues of security, ethical, and governance of the decentralized AI systems.

6.1 FL for Secure Healthcare Analytics

Literature sources are well aware of the idea of Federated Learning as the means of providing collaborative healthcare analytics and maintaining patient privacy. The literature reveals its capability to train common models in the distributed institutions without transfer of raw data, which minimizes the risks of data breaches and non-compliance with the regulations. Studies show the uses of Federated Learning in medical imaging, disease prediction, wearable data analytics and clinical decision support, specifically in a multi-institutional environment (Choudhury et al., 2025). The literature is however also observing challenges of non-IID distributions of data, communication overhead, and susceptibility to inference attacks. In order to solve these problems, previous research addresses the privacy-enhancing measures such as secure aggregation, differential privacy, and encryption of model updates. In general, Federated Learning has been put forward as a core to privacy-sensitive analytics, despite its functionality relying on architectural design, trust, and alignment with larger healthcare systems.

6.2 Clinical Metaverse Applications

The studies of metaverse-based healthcare apps provide insights into the possible use of immersive worlds to revolutionize the clinical care, education, and rehabilitation. The research reports about virtual hospitals, immersive teleconsultations, digital twins, and simulation-based medical training as a way to improve accessibility, engagement, and clinical outcomes. Virtual environment-based rehabilitation programs have proven to be more motivating and influential on the therapy experience of a patient (Das et al., 2025). The literature highlights, as well, the importance of analytics that are based on AI to operate on these environments to facilitate real-time feedback, adaptive interventions, and collaborative decision-making. Concerns are however brought up on the issue of constant data gathering and data identity representation and the use of data in the long-term immersive setting (Wassan et al., 2025). These difficulties highlight why there is a need to have architectures that do not tie intelligence to centralized data store. Although metaverse applications have high potential, the privacy and security remain secondary concerns in current literature, which suggests that there is a gap that can be filled by privacy-conscious Federated Learning systems.

6.3 Security, Ethics, and Governance

Literature on decentralized AI systems identifies three key enablers of trust and adoption, including security, ethics, and governance. Adversarial attacks, model poisoning, inference threats, and identity abuse are among the threats that have been listed in the studies as significant weaknesses in the distributed learning environment (Jayaweera et al., 2025). Fairness, transparency, explainability, and patient autonomy are the ethical topics of focus in situations where AI-informed decisions impact clinical outcomes. Research which has centered its attention on governance emphasizes the necessity of accountability, auditability, and adherence to the rules of healthcare data protection. Proposals are made on decentralized trust models, access control mechanisms and policy-based architectures to deal with multi-stakeholder participation (Islam et al., 2024). On the whole, the literature implies that the technical solutions cannot be used on their own; successful decentralized healthcare AI systems should be associated with a set of effective governance frameworks that should make architectural design consistent with ethical considerations and regulatory requirements. This observation supports the design of privacy preservation as a holistic solution in healthcare ecosystems with the metaverse. Table 3 Matches Federated Learning privacy methods with individual metaverse healthcare implementations, e.g. virtual hospitals and digital twins.

Table 3. Mapping of Privacy Mechanisms to Healthcare Use Cases

Healthcare Metaverse Use Case	Federated Learning Setting	Privacy Mechanism Applied	Purpose and Outcome
Virtual Hospital Operations	Cross-silo Federated Learning across hospitals	Secure aggregation, encrypted communication	Enables collaborative analytics while preventing exposure of institutional patient data
Remote Diagnosis and Teleconsultation	Cross-device Federated Learning on patient devices	Differential privacy, local model training	Protects individual patient data during real-time clinical assessments
Digital Twin–Based Patient Monitoring	Hybrid cross-device and cross-silo learning	Privacy-preserving model updates, access control	Maintains patient data sovereignty while supporting personalized care

continued on following page

Table 3. Continued

Healthcare Metaverse Use Case	Federated Learning Setting	Privacy Mechanism Applied	Purpose and Outcome
Immersive Rehabilitation Programs	Edge-based Federated Learning	On-device learning, selective update sharing	Reduces data leakage risks and supports adaptive therapy
Collaborative Surgery Planning	Institution-level Federated Learning	Secure model aggregation, authentication	Ensures confidentiality of clinical data across collaborating teams
Medical Training and Simulation	Federated Learning across training platforms	Data anonymization, policy-based access	Supports learning analytics without compromising sensitive case data

7. CASE STUDY

The following section encapsulates two current and illustrative case studies demonstrating the how Federated Learning architectures with the privacy-preservation features can be implemented in healthcare settings with the help of the metaverse. The cases will represent different but complementary areas of application: remote and immersive care with a digital twin that is privacy-aware and that is virtual hospital operations. Collectively, they illustrate the way Federated Learning helps in assisting collaborative intelligence, real-time analytics and personalization whilst ensuring stringent privacy and governance standards. Instead of the sole consideration of the performance of the algorithm, the case studies highlight the choices in the architectural design, the organization of data flows, the mechanisms of trust, and the implication of the operations (Hwang & Majeed, 2024). This section discusses the advantages and difficulties of implementing privacy preservation by design in immersive healthcare systems by looking at real-world deployment settings. The comparative view also allows recognizing the general patterns, situational variations, and generalizable conclusions on how this could be applied to scalable and reliable metaverse healthcare adoption.

7.1 Case Study I: FL-Enabled Virtual Hospitals

In this case study, Federated Learning is implemented to assist the functioning of a virtual hospital in the environment of an immersive metaverse, which connects several healthcare organizations. The virtual hospital combines digital models of clinical processes, patient care portals, and AI-based decision support systems which would be available to clinicians in different places. Electronic health records and related medical imaging systems produce patient data that is stored inside the institution, whereas local models are trained locally (Aarthi et al., 2025). Federated Learning organizes the communication of model updates in a secure fashion, which allows the departure of collective predictive models to assess patient risk, allocate resources, and optimize the workflow (Bhardwaj, 2024). The sensitive information cannot be exposed when collaborating due to privacy-enhancing mechanisms like secure aggregation and encrypted communication. The architecture is able to provide real-time data in a virtual hospital setting to enable clinicians to see patient paths and operational data without handling raw data. The deployment illustrates that Federated Learning can be useful in improving the efficiency of operations and clinical decision-making in immersive environments without endangering privacy laws and institutional data governance policies. The figure 3 below depicts that Federated Learning combines AI-based decision support with privacy-preserving solutions to aid the execution of safe, real-time, and efficient activities in the virtual hospital setting.

Figure 3. Federated Learning –Enabled Virtual Hospital Operations

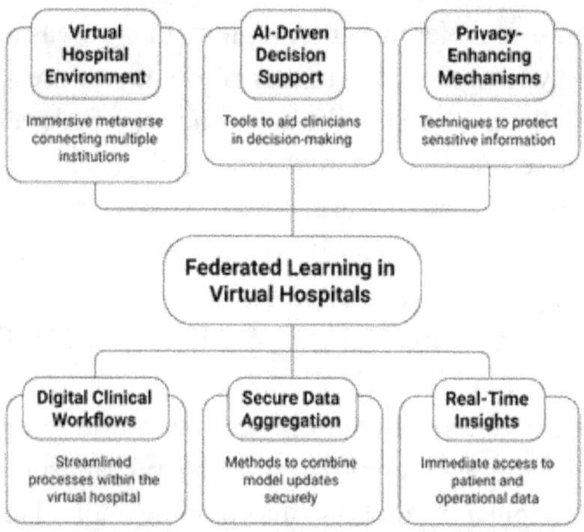

7.2 Case Study II: Privacy-Aware Digital Twins

The second case study deals with the application of privacy-conscious digital twins to promote remote and immersive health services. Digital twins are virtual patients, constantly updated with the help of wearables, home monitoring gadgets, clinical examination, and so on. In this case, Federated Learning will allow training models individually in distributed data sources and retain patient data sovereignty (Rieke et al., 2020). The predictive models used on the health status, progress of rehabilitation, or response to treatment are updated locally by each of the data sources. New model releases are safely combined to enhance personalization and precision across groups of patients without the centralization of sensitive information. The digital twins are projected to be in the immersive metaverse environment, where clinicians and patients are able to interact with health insights in an intuitive and engaging way (Ravikumar, et al., 2025). Privacy by design allows for the fact that the sensitive biometric and behavioral information are not directly revealed in the virtual world (Yang et al., 2023). As demonstrated by this case, Federated Learning enables scalable, personalized, and privacy-protective remote care, especially in managing chronic diseases and rehabilitation and ensures trust and regulatory adherence. Figure 4 Shows the integration of privacy-conscious digital twins that combines Federated Learning and metaverse technologies that allow provision of personalized, secure, and scalable remote healthcare services.

Figure 4. Privacy-Aware Digital Twins for Remote and Immersive Healthcare

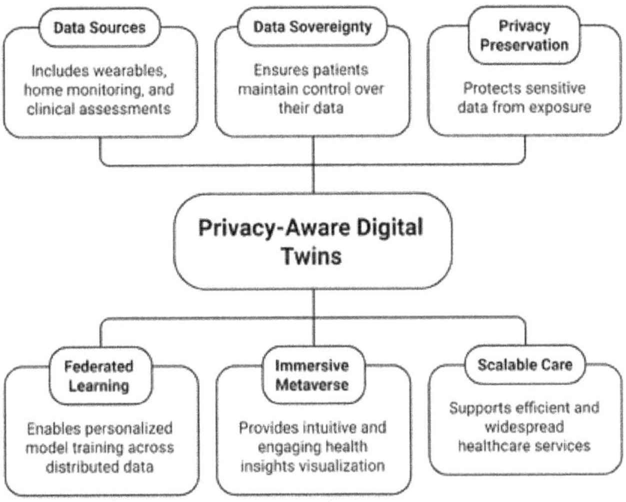

7.3 Cross-Case Comparative Insights

In both case studies, Federated Learning can be identified as a key facilitator of privacy-sensitive intelligence in immersive healthcare settings. The virtual hospital case is focused on inter-institutional cooperation and cost-efficiency, whereas the digital twin case prioritizes individualized and nonstop care. Although the cases have different contexts, they both show that the architectural level integration of privacy mechanisms enhances confidence amongst stakeholders and facilitates alignment of regulations (Torkzadehmahani et al., 2022). The collaborative learning process enables performance benefits and does not compromise data sovereignty but the issues of communication overhead and system complexity are still observed. Transparency, secure aggregation, and well-defined governance structures are some of the ways in which trust is enhanced. All these observations indicate that privacy by design is not a limiting factor, but it enhances the development of scalable and effective metaverse-based healthcare systems, as long as the architectural and organizational factors are considered as a unit. Table 4 The comparison of the two case studies is on the basis of the application context, privacy approach, trust mechanisms, and outcomes.

Table 4. Comparative Summary of Case Studies

Comparison Dimension	Case Study I: Virtual Hospital Operations	Case Study II: Privacy-Aware Digital Twins
Application Context	Immersive virtual hospital environment for clinical operations and coordination	Remote and immersive care using patient-specific digital twins
Primary Objective	Improve operational efficiency and collaborative clinical decision-making	Enable personalized and continuous patient monitoring and care
Federated Learning Setting	Cross-silo Federated Learning across healthcare institutions	Cross-device and hybrid Federated Learning across patient data sources
Privacy Approach	Secure aggregation and encrypted model updates	Local model training with privacy-preserving updates
Trust Mechanisms	Institutional authentication, governance policies	Patient consent management and controlled access
Data Sources	Electronic health records, imaging systems, clinical dashboards	Wearables, home monitoring devices, clinical inputs
Key Outcomes	Enhanced coordination and privacy-compliant analytics	Personalized care with preserved data sovereignty
Implementation Challenges	Communication overhead and system integration	Managing dynamic data and personalization complexity

8. RESULTS AND DISCUSSION

The findings of the conceptual analysis and case studies prove that privacy-saving Federated Learning systems are capable of ensuring intelligent and immersive healthcare services under metaverse settings. According to the findings, decentralization of data processing, along with secure mechanisms of coordination, make it possible to engage in collaborative analytics without breaking down data sovereignty or regulatory restrictions. Federated Learning in architecture built on edge-fog-clouds and integrated with other architectures can be used to improve responsiveness in the system and preserve confidentiality. Meanwhile, the discussion indicates the inseparable trade-offs between personalization, real-time analytics, and privacy guarantees especially in a virtual environment that is overly interactive and data-intensive (Dayan et al., 2021). As pointed out in the discussion, architectural design decisions, governance patterns, and trust systems are the strong influencing factors of system effectiveness. Privacy preservation by design becomes a major consideration in both technical healthiness and acceptance by the stakeholders. These findings highlight the necessity of designing holistic systems that are performance-privacy-scalability balanced that can be used in future development and deployment of metaverse-based healthcare ecosystems.

8.1 Architectural Effectiveness of Privacy-Preserving FL

The discussion shows that Federated Learning federation schemes are effective in realising collaborative intelligence in distributed healthcare systems with privacy assurances. These architectures ensure that the risk of data leakage and regulatory non-compliance is also greatly minimized by storing data locally and sharing model updates (Ravikumar, Aarthi, Atamuratova, et al., 2025). Aggregation, communication and execution environments are secured and provide strong confidence and integrity. The edge and margin computing layer further enables the system to be efficient because of the low-latency processing and context-aware analytics in immersive healthcare environments (Tang et al., 2023). Findings of the case studies indicate that Federated Learning can assist a variety of applications, such as virtual hospital management and digital twin-based care, without centering the sensitive data. Nonetheless, architectural efficacy is reliant on the wise alignment of communication conventions, model convergence, and scalability of systems. In general, the conclusions in the article indicate that Federated Learning would be a practical structural foundation of privacy-conscious metaverse medical systems when applied alongside extensive security and governance procedures (Upreti et al., 2024). Figure 5 Provides insight into privacy-preserving Federated Learning, secure computation and distributed infrastructure as a means of supporting trustful metaverse-based healthcare systems.

Figure 5. Architecture for Secure and Privacy-Aware Metaverse Healthcare

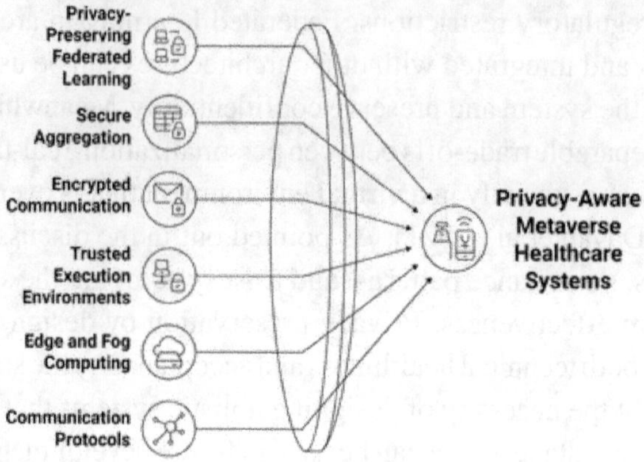

8.2 Privacy–Performance Trade-Offs

The findings demonstrate that there are significant trade-offs between personalization, real-time analytics, and privacy preservation in healthcare settings of the metaverse. A high degree of personalization may necessitate high rates of model update and high rates of data input and this may raise the communication overhead and latency in a Federated Learning environment. In the same vein, real-time analytics require both speedy synchronization and processing, which may prove to be difficult in privacy procedures like differential privacy that create noise or latency (Chengoden et al., 2023). The results imply that a balance between these conflicting goals should be achieved by means of adaptive architectural solutions such as selective update of models, hierarchical aggregation of models, and contextualized privacy policy. Whereas privacy preservation by design increases the level of trust and compliance, at times it can restrict the level of granularity or timeliness of insights. It is noted that such trade-offs are not imposed by design but are design choices that should be made to conform to the application priorities. Compromises between privacy and performance in immersive healthcare applications can be made by tuning system parameters strategically to arrive at acceptable trade-offs.

8.3 Scalability and Trust Implications

The discussion identifies the fact that privacy-sensitive Federated Learning systems are extremely important in the construction of trustful and scalable metaverse healthcare systems. The reinforcement of trust is achieved via transparent processing of data, decentralization of governance, and privacy that is verifiable, which all help to promote stakeholder trust. The modular and distributed Federated Learning allows scaling across institutions, devices, and geographic regions because of its scalability (Y. Zhang et al., 2023). Nonetheless, to become scalable, there is a need to deal with the complexity in operations, interoperability, and the coordination of governance. The findings indicate that privacy by design must be considered at the system architecture to be viable in the long-term and adoption. This kind of integration links technical ability and ethical standards and regulatory requirements and enables responsible innovation (El Rifai et al., 2020). The results place Federated Learning as a linking point between immersive digital experiences and physical clinical responsibility, with a way to the future of healthcare systems that are technologically not only sophisticated but also socially acceptable in the changing metaverse environment.

9. FUTURE RESEARCH

Further studies are needed to enhance the process of designing, implementing, and governing privacy-sensitive Federated Learning in health care metaverse systems. With the ongoing development of immersive technologies and decentralized AI, the architectural solutions that are currently available need to be expanded to meet the new privacy threats, scalability requirements, and other ethical challenges. The current research agenda should shift to the adaptive, resilient, and context-sensitive systems, which can work in dynamic healthcare settings instead of conceptual validation. Specific focus must be given to enhance privacy protection without losing personalization or real-time responsiveness (Aziz et al., 2023). Also, trust-building, identity management, and accountability protocols should be progressively incorporated into decentralized and interactive platforms. Empirical evaluation in the long run will be important in determining long-term system behavior, trust of the stakeholders and compliance with the rules. These dimensions can be met by the future research to help in developing social responsibility metaverse healthcare systems that are not only technologically innovative but sustainable as well. This section will summarize the main research directions that will be based on the results of this chapter and also show potential areas of improvement in the further development of privacy-sensitive and patient-centric healthcare related to immersive digital environments.

9.1 Adaptive Privacy Mechanisms

More intensive privacy mechanisms need to be investigated in the future in the light of dynamism and adaptability of immersive healthcare AI systems. Although the current solutions like secure aggregation and differential privacy offer the base protection, they might not be adequate in the context of metaverse environments that are highly interactive and dynamically changing. Adaptive privacy methods where the degree of protection varies according to the situation, the risk and the agreement of the user should be researched. Diverse methods like customized privacy budgets, privacy-conscience model adaptation and hybrid cryptographic approaches make hopeful avenues (Patel et al., 2023). Besides, the systems that counter the emergent risks, including cross-modal inference and behavioral profiling in immersive environments need to be studied more thoroughly. It will be important to develop privacy solutions that will work across edge, fog and cloud layers to ensure real-time performance. Their further development can be used to strengthen Federated Learning architectures, and their support of rich and adaptive healthcare services in metaverse ecosystems.

9.2 Decentralized Identity and Trust Frameworks

The combination of decentralized identity and trust schemes is one of the future research directions of metaverse-based healthcare systems. A wide range of stakeholders are involved in immersive environments (patients, clinicians, institutions, and intelligent agents) and require secure and verifiable identity management. Further studies are needed on decentralized identity schemes that allow users to gain control of authentication, consent management, and access control without depending on centralized authorities. The accountability and transparency can be improved with the help of trust frameworks that are built on cryptographic verification, reputation mechanisms, and policy-driven governance (Dhairyashil Patil, 2024). It also requires research to be undertaken to realize how identity and trust mechanisms come to play with the Federated Learning processes and virtual environments. A successful implementation of those frameworks might help build trust in AI-based decisions and data processing. With identity management and privacy viability being refined to work together, it is possible to adopt secure participation, interoperability, and ethical governance in immersive healthcare ecosystems in the future.

9.3 Long-Term System Evaluation

Longitudinal evaluation would be necessary in clarifying how a federated deployment of metaverse healthcare can be practically useful and sustainable. Future research should take into account increasing studies on long-term behaviour of the systems to investigate the system performance, the strength of privacy, trustworthiness to the stakeholders in the long-term. By such evaluations, it is possible to discover the dynamics of the Federated Learning models when there is a fluctuation in the data distribution, clinical practice, and the regulatory conditions. Longitudinal analysis is also necessary that would determine how the privacy preserving mechanisms would impact the model accuracy, fairness, and usability over time (J. Zhang et al., 2022). It is also possible to study the barriers to and enabling factors of large-scale deployment by also examining the user adoption, organizational adaptation and effectiveness of governance over time. Beyond the analysis done in the short run or simulated approach, the future study would offer evidence-based solutions to implement resilient, reliable, and adaptive metaverse healthcare systems, which would be consistent with the principles and regulations of patient-centricity.

10. STRATEGIC AND OPERATIONAL IMPLICATIONS

The adoption of Federated Learning in healthcare systems built on metaverse has important strategic and operational implications on healthcare organizations, technology providers, and policymakers. Privacy preservation by design incorporation demands the tactical dedication between technological advancement, corporate capacity, and government duty. Operational-wise, the immersive healthcare platforms will have to strike a balance between the state-of-the-art analytics and customization and the high level of privacy and security protection. Infrastructure investment and system architecture decisions along with stakeholder collaboration are strategic decisions that directly impact system effectiveness and trust. According to the results of this chapter, privacy-centric design is not just a compliance measure but a strategic resource that may be used to improve credibility, scalability, and long-term sustainability (Bansal et al., 2022). Continuous operational preparedness, governance models and risk management procedures are important factors in the transformation of architectural ideas to actual deployments. Comprehensively nurturing these dimensions, the healthcare organizations can use the metaverse and Federated Learning technologies to provide innovative services without losing the trust of the patients and the accountability of the institutions. Table 5 Highlights important strategic, organizational and policy-level inferences of implementing privacy-centric metaverse healthcare systems.

Table 5. Strategic, Operational, and Governance Implications

Stakeholder Group	Strategic Implications	Operational Implications	Governance and Policy Implications
Healthcare Providers	Adoption of privacy-centric digital care models and immersive services	Integration of Federated Learning with clinical workflows	Compliance with healthcare data protection and ethical standards
Hospital Administrators	Investment in scalable and interoperable metaverse platforms	Workforce training and change management	Establishment of accountability and audit mechanisms
Technology Providers	Development of secure and interoperable architectures	Deployment of edge–fog–cloud infrastructures	Alignment with privacy-by-design and responsible AI principles
Policymakers and Regulators	Support for innovation through adaptive regulatory frameworks	Oversight of cross-institutional data collaboration	Enforcement of privacy, security, and data sovereignty requirements
Patients and Caregivers	Increased trust in immersive and AI-driven healthcare services	Improved access to personalized and remote care	Enhanced control over consent and data usage

10.1 Platform Design Strategy

The privacy preservation should be the central architectural and value proposition in strategic design of metaverse healthcare platforms. The platform strategies are to focus on decentralization in data processing, safe cooperation and openness in the AI-driven decision making. Federated Learning can help organizations to leverage the power of collective intelligence, which can be achieved by maintaining control of sensitive data resources. The interoperability of healthcare systems, devices and virtual environments should also be taken into consideration in terms of strategic design in order to facilitate scalable and flexible deployments. The match between the capabilities of platforms and patient-centric values and regulatory expectations can make the healthcare services differentiated and enhance the trust of stakeholders (Xu et al., 2021). Moreover, the strategic planning must look ahead at the dynamic threats to privacy and technology so that it can keep up. Incorporating privacy-focused components into platform design, healthcare organizations are able to develop resilient and trustworthy immersive systems that sustain innovation without affecting ethical and legal obligations.

10.2 Organizational Readiness and Considerations

The readiness within an organisation is another major element that determines the success of the adoption of Federated Learning and metaverse based healthcare systems. The healthcare organizations need to establish technical competency, inter-functional coordination, and governance frameworks that have the ability to handle the decentralized and immersive systems. The governance aspects involve the definition of roles and responsibilities, development of data stewardship policy, and transparency of AI model development and deployment. Good governance structures help in aligning clinical, technical and administrative interests and deal with accountability and risk (Abhishek et al., n.d.). The training and change management programmes are also needed to equip the personnel with new working processes and decision-making procedures that are made possible by the immersive technologies. The preparations in the organization can be seen not only in terms of infrastructure but also in terms of the organizational culture that would be oriented towards privacy-saving and patient-centered principles. Even a well thought out architecture cannot yield the desired results and cannot win the trust of stakeholders without proper governance and preparation.

10.3 Policy, and Risk Management Implications

The use of privacy-preserving metaverse healthcare systems is primarily viewed through policy, compliance, and risk management considerations. To ensure regulatory compliance, it is necessary to align with healthcare data protection legislation, ethical standards, and new standards of responsible AI. Federated Learning can help to comply with the case since it reduces data sharing and improves data sovereignty, yet organizations also need to deal with risks of model integrity, security violations, and governance failures (Han et al., 2024). The continuous monitoring, auditability, and incident response mechanisms in decentralized and immersive environments should be used as a part of the risk management strategies. Policymakers are important in giving a clear direction and flexible regulatory frameworks that can facilitate innovation and protect patient rights. A policy and risk management approach to system design will allow the proactive detection and prevention of threats, which will make the metaverse healthcare platform safe, personalized to comply and be sustainable over time (Ravikumar & Aarthi, 2025).

11. CONCLUSION

The convergence of the metaverse, Artificial Intelligence, and Federated Learning is a game changer in the process of reimagining the healthcare systems, but it equally increases the issues to do with privacy, security, trust, and regulatory adherence. As has been evidenced in this chapter, the concept of privacy preservation by design in Federated Learning architecture is crucial to facilitate intelligent and immersive healthcare services without hurting the patient autonomy and data sovereignty. The discussion has also elucidated how collaborative intelligence can be facilitated by decentralized model training, secure aggregation and edge-fog-cloud coordination through the use of Federated Learning as an architectural enabler and not as a separate method to support virtual hospitals, digital twins, and remote care platforms. The examination of building elements, administrative procedures, and examples of successful cases highlights that a high level of privacy ensures a higher level of trust, system scalability, and is relevant to technological innovation succeeding ethical and regulatory requirements. Notably, Federated Learning has been framed as being the key transition between engaging digital healthcare and in-the-field clinical responsibility, with the necessary personalization and real-time analytics, but without secrecy and control of sensitive information. The chapter goes on to assert that reliable metaverse healthcare systems necessitate comprehensive emergence of technical protections, institutional preparedness and policy structures. With the ongoing development of immersive healthcare technologies, the implementation of privacy-focused federated architecture is a possible avenue to secure, ethical, and patient-centred healthcare systems that are resilient, interoperable, and socially acceptable.

REFERENCES

Aarthi, S., Ravikumar, R. N., Balakrishnan, R., Pavithra, K., Jumaniyozov, F., & Praveen, V. M. (2025). Blockchain for seamless and transparent smart hospitality operations. In *Smart Operations and Enhancing Guest Experience in the Hospitality Industry* (pp. 187–218). IGI Global., DOI: 10.4018/979-8-3373-2145-5.ch007

Abbas, S. R., Abbas, Z., Zahir, A., & Lee, S. W. (2024). Federated learning in smart healthcare: A comprehensive review on privacy, security, and predictive analytics with IoT integration. *Healthcare (Basel)*, *12*(24), 2587. DOI: 10.3390/healthcare12242587 PMID: 39766014

Abhishek, V., Binny, S., Johan, T., Raj, N., & Thomas, V. (n.d.). *Federated Learning: Collaborative Machine Learning without.*

Abhishek, V. A., Binny, S., Johan, T. R., Raj, N., & Thomas, V. (2022). Federated learning: Collaborative machine learning without centralized training data. *International Journal of Engineering Technology and Management Sciences*, *355–359*, 355–359. Advance online publication. DOI: 10.46647/ijetms.2022.v06i05.052

al Dhairyashil Patil, E. (2024). Federated learning in real-time medical IoT: Optimizing privacy and accuracy for chronic disease monitoring. *Journal of Electrical Systems*, *19*(3), 32–42. DOI: 10.52783/jes.649

Ali, S., Abdullah, , Armand, T. P. T., Athar, A., Hussain, A., Ali, M., Yaseen, M., Joo, M.-I., & Kim, H.-C. (2023). Metaverse in healthcare integrated with explainable AI and blockchain: Enabling immersiveness, ensuring trust, and providing patient data security. *Sensors (Basel)*, *23*(2), 565. DOI: 10.3390/s23020565 PMID: 36679361

Antunes, R. S., André da Costa, C., Küderle, A., Yari, I. A., & Eskofier, B. (2022). Federated learning for healthcare: Systematic review and architecture proposal. *ACM Transactions on Intelligent Systems and Technology*, *13*(4), 1–23. DOI: 10.1145/3501813

Aziz, R., Banerjee, S., Bouzefrane, S., & Le Vinh, T. (2023). Exploring homomorphic encryption and differential privacy techniques towards secure federated learning paradigm. *Future Internet*, *15*(9), 310. DOI: 10.3390/fi15090310

Bansal, G., Rajgopal, K., Chamola, V., Xiong, Z., & Niyato, D. (2022). Healthcare in Metaverse: A Survey on Current Metaverse Applications in Healthcare. *IEEE Access : Practical Innovations, Open Solutions*, *10*, 119914–119946. DOI: 10.1109/ACCESS.2022.3219845

Bhardwaj, A. (2024). Revolutionize healthcare using Metaverse virtual worlds and augmented reality. In *Beyond the Realms: Navigating the Metaverse* (pp. 157–200). BENTHAM SCIENCE PUBLISHERS. DOI: 10.2174/9789815238457124010009

Brisimi, T. S., Chen, R., Mela, T., Olshevsky, A., Paschalidis, I. C., & Shi, W. (2018). Federated learning of predictive models from federated Electronic Health Records. *International Journal of Medical Informatics*, *112*, 59–67. DOI: 10.1016/j.ijmedinf.2018.01.007 PMID: 29500022

Chelani, N., Tripathy, S., Kumhar, M., Bhatia, J., Saxena, V., Tanwar, S., & Nayyar, A. (2024). Federated Learning for Internet of medical healthcare: Issues and challenges. *Scalable Computing Practice and Experience*, *25*(5), 4442–4455. DOI: 10.12694/scpe.v25i5.2905

Chengoden, R., Victor, N., Huynh-The, T., Yenduri, G., Jhaveri, R. H., Alazab, M., Bhattacharya, S., Hegde, P., Maddikunta, P. K. R., & Gadekallu, T. R. (2023). Metaverse for Healthcare: A Survey on Potential Applications, Challenges and Future Directions. *IEEE Access : Practical Innovations, Open Solutions*, *11*, 12765–12795. DOI: 10.1109/ACCESS.2023.3241628

Choudhury, A., Volmer, L., Martin, F., Fijten, R., Wee, L., Dekker, A., & van Soest, J. (2025). Advancing privacy-preserving health care analytics and implementation of the Personal Health Train: Federated deep learning study. *JMIR AI*, *4*, e60847. DOI: 10.2196/60847 PMID: 39912580

Das, B. C., Zahid, R., Roy, P., & Ahmad, M. (2025). Spatial Data Governance for Healthcare Metaverse. In *Advances in Computer and Electrical Engineering* (pp. 305–330). IGI Global. DOI: 10.4018/979-8-3693-4373-9.ch013

Dayan, I., Roth, H. R., Zhong, A., Harouni, A., Gentili, A., Abidin, A. Z., Liu, A., Costa, A. B., Wood, B. J., Tsai, C.-S., Wang, C.-H., Hsu, C.-N., Lee, C. K., Ruan, P., Xu, D., Wu, D., Huang, E., Kitamura, F. C., Lacey, G., & Li, Q. (2021). Federated learning for predicting clinical outcomes in patients with COVID-19. *Nature Medicine*, *27*(10), 1735–1743. DOI: 10.1038/s41591-021-01506-3 PMID: 34526699

Divyashree, K. S. (2024). Blockchain Application on Healthcare Services in Metaverse. In *Advances in Medical Education, Research, and Ethics* (pp. 141–158). IGI Global. DOI: 10.4018/979-8-3693-5493-3.ch009

Diwan, S. A. (2025). Federated learning-enhanced sensor fusion for IoT-based distributed health systems: Prioritizing privacy and rapid medical intervention. *Intelligent Decision Technologies*, *19*(6), 4310–4327. DOI: 10.1177/18724981251370441

El Rifai, O., Biotteau, M., de Boissezon, X., Megdiche, I., Ravat, F., & Teste, O. (2020). Blockchain-based federated learning in medicine. In *Artificial Intelligence in Medicine* (pp. 214–224). Springer International Publishing., DOI: 10.1007/978-3-030-59137-3_20

ElBedoui, K., Barhoumi, W., & Cho, J. (2025). SoK: Federated Learning and unlearning for medical image analysis. *Expert Systems: International Journal of Knowledge Engineering and Neural Networks, 42*(6), e70063. Advance online publication. DOI: 10.1111/exsy.70063

Feretzakis, G., Papaspyridis, K., Gkoulalas-Divanis, A., & Verykios, V. S. (2024). Privacy-preserving techniques in generative AI and large language models: A narrative review. *Information (Basel), 15*(11), 697. DOI: 10.3390/info15110697

Han, S., Ding, H., Zhao, S., Ren, S., Wang, Z., Lin, J., & Zhou, S. (2024). Practical and robust federated learning with highly scalable regression training. *IEEE Transactions on Neural Networks and Learning Systems, 35*(10), 13801–13815. DOI: 10.1109/TNNLS.2023.3271859 PMID: 37289609

Hwang, S. O., & Majeed, A. (2024). Analysis of federated learning paradigm in medical domain: Taking COVID-19 as an application use case. *Applied Sciences (Basel, Switzerland), 14*(10), 4100. DOI: 10.3390/app14104100

Islam, T. U., Mohammed, N., & Alhadidi, D. (2024). Privacy preserving vertical distributed learning for health data. *Journal of Surveillance. Security and Safety, 5*(1), 1–18. DOI: 10.20517/jsss.2023.28

Javed, L., Anjum, A., Yakubu, B. M., Iqbal, M., Moqurrab, S. A., & Srivastava, G. (2023). ShareChain: Blockchain-enabled model for sharing patient data using federated learning and differential privacy. *Expert Systems: International Journal of Knowledge Engineering and Neural Networks, 40*(5), e13131. Advance online publication. DOI: 10.1111/exsy.13131

Jayaweera, R., Agrawal, H., & Karie, N. M. (2025). Federated security for privacy preservation of healthcare data in edge-cloud environments. *Sensors (Basel), 25*(16), 5108. DOI: 10.3390/s25165108 PMID: 40871971

Lakhan, A., Mohammed, M. A., Nedoma, J., Martinek, R., Tiwari, P., Vidyarthi, A., Alkhayyat, A., & Wang, W. (2023). Federated-learning based privacy preservation and fraud-enabled blockchain IoMT system for healthcare. *IEEE Journal of Biomedical and Health Informatics, 27*(2), 664–672. DOI: 10.1109/JBHI.2022.3165945 PMID: 35394919

Loftus, T. J., Ruppert, M. M., Shickel, B., Ozrazgat-Baslanti, T., Balch, J. A., Efron, P. A., Upchurch, G. R.Jr, Rashidi, P., Tignanelli, C., Bian, J., & Bihorac, A. (2022). Federated learning for preserving data privacy in collaborative healthcare research. *Digital Health*, *8*, 20552076221134456. DOI: 10.1177/20552076221134455 PMID: 36325438

Nguyen, D. C., Pham, Q.-V., Pathirana, P. N., Ding, M., Seneviratne, A., Lin, Z., Dobre, O., & Hwang, W.-J. (2023). Federated Learning for smart healthcare: A survey. *ACM Computing Surveys*, *55*(3), 1–37. DOI: 10.1145/3501296

Oyekan, B. (2024). Developing privacy-preserving federated learning models for collaborative health data analysis across multiple institutions without compromising data security. *Journal of Knowledge Learning and Science Technology ISSN: 2959-6386 (Online)*, *3*(3), 139–164. DOI: 10.60087/jklst.vol3.n3.p139-164

Pasupuleti, M. K., & Services, N. E. (2025). *Next-generation extended Reality (XR): A unified framework for integrating AR, VR, and AI-driven immersive technologies*. DOI: 10.62311/nesx/rrv325

Patel, M., Dayan, I., Fishman, E. K., Flores, M., Gilbert, F. J., Guindy, M., Koay, E. J., Rosenthal, M., Roth, H. R., & Linguraru, M. G. (2023). Accelerating artificial intelligence: How federated learning can protect privacy, facilitate collaboration, and improve outcomes. *Health Informatics Journal*, *29*(4), 14604582231207744. DOI: 10.1177/14604582231207744 PMID: 37864543

Rauniyar, A., Hagos, D. H., Jha, D., Håkegård, J. E., Bagci, U., Rawat, D. B., & Vlassov, V. (2024). Federated learning for medical applications: A taxonomy, current trends, challenges, and future research directions. *IEEE Internet of Things Journal*, *11*(5), 7374–7398. DOI: 10.1109/JIOT.2023.3329061

Ravikumar, A. S., Atamuratova, Z., Ashirova, A., Jurayev, K., & Hayitova, M. (2025). Comprehensive evaluation of AI-driven systems in modern hospital environments. In *Advances in Computational Intelligence and Robotics* (pp. 61–88). IGI Global Scientific Publishing. DOI: 10.4018/979-8-3373-2787-7.ch003

Ravikumar, R. S., Manujakshi, Aarthi, S., Urazbaeva, Y., & Tamilselvi, S. (2025). Navigating data privacy, security, and regulatory challenges in healthcare AI ensuring fairness, bias mitigation, interpretability, and trust. In *Transformative Role of Transformer Models in Healthcare* (pp. 25–54). IGI Global Scientific Publishing. DOI: 10.4018/979-8-3373-2038-0.ch002

Ravikumar, R. N., & Aarthi, S. (2025). AI-powered synergistic robotics and IoT ecosystems for predictive and preventive healthcare. In *Robotics and IoT Synergy in Next-Generation Healthcare* (pp. 1–32). IGI Global Scientific Publishing., DOI: 10.4018/979-8-3373-5447-7.ch001

Ravikumar, R. N., Aarthi, S., Dilshodbek, A., Satheesh Kumar, A., Eshkaraev, S., & Shanmugam, K. B. (2025). Integrating blockchain, smart contracts, and AI for decentralized healthcare in the metaverse. In *Blockchain-Based Healthcare Management in the Metaverse* (pp. 261–294). IGI Global Scientific Publishing., DOI: 10.4018/979-8-3373-1225-5.ch010

Ravikumar, R. N., Aarthi, S., Masharipova, G., Niyazova, N., Salaeva, N., & Buriyeva, D. (2025). Enhancing clinical decision-making and operational efficiency in healthcare using edge computing. In *Building Data-Driven Edge Systems for Business Success* (pp. 191–224). IGI Global Scientific Publishing., DOI: 10.4018/979-8-3373-1147-0.ch008

Rieke, N., Hancox, J., Li, W., Milletarì, F., Roth, H. R., Albarqouni, S., Bakas, S., Galtier, M. N., Landman, B. A., Maier-Hein, K., Ourselin, S., Sheller, M., Summers, R. M., Trask, A., Xu, D., Baust, M., & Cardoso, M. J. (2020). The future of digital health with federated learning. *NPJ Digital Medicine, 3*(1), 119. DOI: 10.1038/s41746-020-00323-1 PMID: 33015372

Sadilek, A., Liu, L., Nguyen, D., Kamruzzaman, M., Serghiou, S., Rader, B., Ingerman, A., Mellem, S., Kairouz, P., Nsoesie, E. O., MacFarlane, J., Vullikanti, A., Marathe, M., Eastham, P., Brownstein, J. S., Arcas, B. A. Y., Howell, M. D., & Hernandez, J. (2021). Privacy-first health research with federated learning. *NPJ Digital Medicine, 4*(1), 132. DOI: 10.1038/s41746-021-00489-2 PMID: 34493770

Tang, Y., Pan, D., Qin, P., & Lv, L. (2023). Lattice-based group signature with message recovery for federal learning. *Applied Sciences (Basel, Switzerland), 13*(15), 9007. DOI: 10.3390/app13159007

Tanveer, F., Iradat, F., Iqbal, W., Alsagri, H. S., Alhakbani, H. A. A., Ahmad, A., & Khan, F. A. (2025). Balancing privacy and performance in healthcare: A federated learning framework for sensitive data. *Digital Health, 11*(20552076251381770), 20552076251381770. DOI: 10.1177/20552076251381769 PMID: 41018509

Torkzadehmahani, R., Nasirigerdeh, R., Blumenthal, D. B., Kacprowski, T., List, M., Matschinske, J., Spaeth, J., Wenke, N. K., & Baumbach, J. (2022). Privacy-preserving artificial intelligence techniques in biomedicine. *Methods of Information in Medicine, 61*(S 01), e12–e27. DOI: 10.1055/s-0041-1740630

Upreti, D., Yang, E., Kim, H., & Seo, C. (2024). A comprehensive survey on federated learning in the healthcare area: Concept and applications. *Computer Modeling in Engineering & Sciences*, *140*(3), 2239–2274. DOI: 10.32604/cmes.2024.048932

Wassan, S., Liudajun, , Ying, H., Dongyan, H., & Fei, P. (2025). Federated learning and differential privacy: Machine learning and deep learning for biomedical image data classification. *Digital Health*, *11*, 20552076251358532. DOI: 10.1177/20552076251358531 PMID: 40949674

Xu, J., Glicksberg, B. S., Su, C., Walker, P., Bian, J., & Wang, F. (2021). Federated learning for healthcare informatics. *Journal of Healthcare Informatics Research*, *5*(1), 1–19. DOI: 10.1007/s41666-020-00082-4 PMID: 33204939

Yang, W., Xiang, W., Yang, Y., & Cheng, P. (2023). Optimizing federated learning with deep reinforcement learning for digital twin empowered industrial IoT. *IEEE Transactions on Industrial Informatics*, *19*(2), 1884–1893. DOI: 10.1109/TII.2022.3183465

Zhang, J., Zhu, H., Wang, F., Zhao, J., Xu, Q., & Li, H. (2022). Security and privacy threats to federated learning: Issues, methods, and challenges. *Security and Communication Networks*, *2022*, 1–24. DOI: 10.1155/2022/2886795

Zhang, Y., Lu, Y., & Liu, F. (2023). A systematic survey for differential privacy techniques in federated learning. *Journal of Information Security*, *14*(02), 111–135. DOI: 10.4236/jis.2023.142008

KEY TERMS AND DEFINITIONS

Data Sovereignty: The principle that individuals or organizations retain control over how their data is collected, stored, and used.

Decentralized Identity: A digital identity model where users control their credentials without reliance on a central authority.

Differential Privacy: A privacy technique that adds controlled noise to data or model updates to prevent identification of individual data records.

Digital Twin: A virtual representation of a patient, system, or process that reflects real-time data and supports analysis and decision-making.

Edge Computing: Data processing performed close to the data source, such as medical devices or wearables, to reduce latency and enhance privacy.

Federated Learning (FL): A decentralized machine learning approach where models are trained collaboratively across multiple data sources without sharing raw data.

Metaverse-Based Healthcare: Immersive virtual environments that integrate physical and digital healthcare services for clinical care, training, and collaboration.

Model Inversion Attack: A security threat where an attacker attempts to reconstruct sensitive data from trained AI models.

Non-IID Data: Data distributions that vary across sources, common in healthcare settings due to population and institutional differences.

Privacy Preservation by Design: An approach that embeds privacy and data protection mechanisms into system architecture from the initial design stage.

Privacy-Preserving Analytics: Analytical methods that extract insights from data while minimizing exposure of sensitive information.

Secure Aggregation: A cryptographic technique that enables the combination of model updates without revealing individual contributions.

Trusted Execution Environment (TEE): A secure area of a processor that ensures sensitive computations are protected from unauthorized access.

Virtual Hospital: A digitally simulated healthcare environment that supports remote clinical operations, monitoring, and collaboration.

Chapter 14
Trustworthy Metaverse-Enabled Healthcare:
Integrating Artificial Intelligence and Federated Learning for Secure, Scalable, and Personalized Care

Syed Mohd Faisal
http://orcid.org/0000-0003-2422-3535
Malla Reddy Technical Campus, Malla Reddy Vishwavidyapeeth (Deemed to be) University, Hyderabad, India

Wasim Khan
http://orcid.org/0000-0003-2311-1451
Symbiosis Institute of Technology, Symbiosis International (Deemed to be) University, Pune, India

Mohammad Ishrat
http://orcid.org/0000-0002-9699-4454
School of Computing Science and Engineering, VIT Bhopal University, Sehore, India

ABSTRACT

The integration of Metaverse technologies, artificial intelligence, and federated learning introduces new possibilities for delivering secure, scalable, and personalized healthcare services. Metaverse-enabled healthcare environments support immersive clinical interactions and continuous patient engagement, while artificial intelligence enables multimodal data analysis and intelligent decision support. However, centralized AI approaches face challenges related to data privacy, scalability, and

DOI: 10.4018/979-8-3373-8889-2.ch014

regulatory compliance. This chapter presents a trustworthy healthcare framework that combines artificial intelligence with federated learning to enable distributed and privacy-preserving intelligence in Metaverse-based healthcare systems. Key trust dimensions, including privacy preservation, explainability, fairness, accountability, and governance, are examined, and representative healthcare scenarios illustrate practical applicability. The chapter outlines open challenges and future research directions to guide the development of ethical and reliable Metaverse-enabled healthcare ecosystems.

1. INTRODUCTION

Healthcare systems are increasingly evolving toward data-driven and intelligence-centric paradigms, motivated by the proliferation of high-dimensional medical data, advancements in computational intelligence, and the growing demand for precision and personalized medicine. Conventional digital health infrastructures, including telemedicine platforms and electronic health record systems, have contributed to improved accessibility and operational efficiency. However, these systems largely operate within non-immersive environments and rely on centralized data processing architectures, which impose limitations related to interoperability, scalability, data privacy, and regulatory compliance. These constraints become more pronounced as healthcare applications demand real-time analytics, continuous monitoring, and context-aware clinical decision support. The emergence of the Metaverse introduces a cyber-physical continuum in which persistent virtual environments are tightly coupled with real-world healthcare processes. In the context of healthcare, Metaverse enables immersive clinical interactions, patient-specific digital twins, virtual diagnostics, and simulation-driven training environments. Such systems integrate extended reality interfaces, sensor-driven Internet of Medical Things (IoMT) infrastructures, and high-throughput communication networks to facilitate continuous data acquisition and interaction. While these capabilities significantly enhance clinical engagement and service delivery, they also lead to the generation of large-scale, heterogeneous, and privacy-sensitive medical data streams.

Artificial intelligence constitutes the primary analytical and inferential layer within Metaverse-enabled healthcare ecosystems (Sowan et al., 2025). Machine Learning (ML) and deep learning models are increasingly employed for medical image analysis, disease risk stratification, treatment response prediction, and adaptive patient monitoring. These models operate on multimodal data encompassing imaging, physiological signals, genomic information, and behavioral patterns. Despite their demonstrated effectiveness, centralized AI training paradigms require aggregation of sensitive medical data into shared repositories, which conflicts with data protection regulations, institutional governance policies, and ethical principles related to patient autonomy and data sovereignty. As a result, the deployment of centralized intelligence in large-scale healthcare environments remains constrained. Federated Learning (FL) offers a distributed optimization framework that addresses these limitations by enabling collaborative model training across decentralized data sources without exposing raw patient data. In FL, local models are trained within institutional or device-level boundaries, and only encrypted model parameters or gradients are communicated for global aggregation. This paradigm is particularly well-suited for healthcare Metaverse environments, where data is inherently distributed across hospitals, edge devices, and virtual care platforms. By supporting privacy-preserving learning and cross-institutional collaboration, FL enhances model generalization while maintaining compliance with regulatory and ethical requirements (Adil et al., 2025).

Despite the complementary advantages of the Metaverse, artificial intelligence, and FL, their integration introduces complex challenges related to system trustworthiness. Trustworthiness in this setting encompasses not only data security and privacy preservation but also explainability of AI-driven clinical decisions, robustness against adversarial manipulation, fairness across diverse patient populations, and accountability within automated decision pipelines. In immersive healthcare environments where intelligent virtual agents and automated recommendations influence clinical workflows, insufficient transparency or bias can undermine clinical confidence and patient acceptance. This chapter investigates the convergence of Metaverse-enabled healthcare, artificial intelligence, and FL from a trust-centric perspective. It aims to systematically examine how distributed intelligence and immersive technologies can be integrated to achieve secure, scalable, and personalized healthcare delivery. By articulating conceptual foundations, architectural considerations, and emerging research challenges, the chapter seeks to contribute to the development of clinically reliable and ethically grounded healthcare ecosystems that leverage the full potential of intelligent and federated Metaverse platforms.

2. METAVERSE-ENABLED HEALTHCARE ECOSYSTEMS: CONCEPTUAL FOUNDATIONS

Metaverse-enabled healthcare ecosystems represent an advanced form of digital health infrastructure in which immersive virtual environments are tightly integrated with physical healthcare processes. Unlike conventional telehealth platforms that primarily support episodic and two-dimensional interactions, Metaverse-based systems enable persistent, interactive, and context-aware clinical environments. These ecosystems allow patients, clinicians, medical devices, and intelligent services to coexist within shared virtual spaces, supporting continuous care delivery, collaborative diagnosis, and longitudinal patient engagement (Haque et al., 2014).

At a system level, a healthcare Metaverse ecosystem is composed of multiple interdependent components that collectively enable immersive and data-driven healthcare services. The primary building blocks of such ecosystems include extended reality technologies, digital twins, IoMT devices, communication infrastructure, computational platforms, and governance mechanisms. The functional roles and challenges associated with these components are summarized in Table 1, which highlights how each element contributes to clinical objectives while introducing specific technical and operational constraints.

Extended reality technologies form the interaction layer of the healthcare Metaverse, enabling immersive visualization and intuitive human–computer interaction. These interfaces allow clinicians to examine patient-specific anatomical models, conduct virtual consultations, and perform simulation-based training, while patients benefit from guided rehabilitation and experiential therapy. The effectiveness of these immersive interactions depends on reliable synchronization between physical data sources and virtual representations.

Digital twins (Ishrat, Khan, Faisal, Al Farsi, et al., 2025) constitute a critical conceptual element within Metaverse-enabled healthcare ecosystems. A digital twin represents a dynamic virtual model of a patient, organ, or clinical workflow, continuously updated using real-time physiological and clinical data. Within immersive healthcare environments, digital twins support predictive modeling, treatment simulation, and personalized intervention planning, thereby enabling proactive and precision-oriented healthcare delivery (Faisal, Ishrat, et al., 2025).

The IoMT plays a central role in sustaining data continuity across physical and virtual healthcare spaces. Wearable sensors, implantable devices, and smart medical equipment generate continuous streams of physiological and contextual data that feed into the Metaverse environment. These data streams enable real-time monitoring and adaptive clinical decision-making, but also introduce challenges related to interoperability and secure data transmission, as indicated in Table 1.

The interaction and data flow among these components are illustrated in Figure 1, which presents a conceptual architecture of a Metaverse-enabled healthcare ecosystem. The figure depicts how patients and clinicians interact within immersive virtual environments, how physiological data is collected through IoMT devices, and how real-time communication networks facilitate bidirectional data exchange between physical and virtual layers. The layered architecture shown in the figure emphasizes the separation of interaction, sensing, communication, intelligence, and governance functions, which is essential for system scalability and clinical reliability.

In addition to technical integration, Metaverse-enabled healthcare ecosystems must satisfy stringent design requirements that distinguish them from non-clinical virtual environments. Low-latency communication, high system reliability, and data integrity are critical, as delays or inaccuracies may directly affect clinical outcomes. Furthermore, interoperability across healthcare institutions and platforms is necessary to prevent fragmentation of care and to support cross-institutional collaboration within shared virtual environments.

From a broader perspective, healthcare Metaverse ecosystems operate within complex regulatory and ethical contexts. Persistent virtual interactions and continuous data collection necessitate robust governance mechanisms to ensure privacy preservation, informed consent, and accountability. These considerations underscore the need for embedding governance and security mechanisms directly into the system architecture, as reflected in both Table 1 and Figure 1.

By establishing these conceptual foundations, this section provides a structured understanding of Metaverse-enabled healthcare ecosystems. This framework serves as the basis for the subsequent sections, which examine how artificial intelligence and FL function as intelligence-enabling mechanisms within these immersive and distributed healthcare environments.

Table 1. Key Components of Metaverse-Enabled Healthcare Ecosystems

Component	Primary Role in Healthcare	Major Challenge
Extended Reality Technologies	Immersive clinical interaction and visualization	Latency and usability constraints
Digital Twins	Patient-specific simulation and prediction	Data integration and model accuracy
Internet of Medical Things	Continuous physiological data acquisition	Interoperability and security
Communication Infrastructure	Real-time synchronization of virtual and physical spaces	Network reliability
Computing and Storage Platforms	Scalable processing and data management	Resource efficiency and compliance
Governance and Security Frameworks	Privacy protection and regulatory enforcement	Dynamic consent and accountability

Figure 1. Conceptual Architecture of Metaverse-Enabled Healthcare Ecosystem

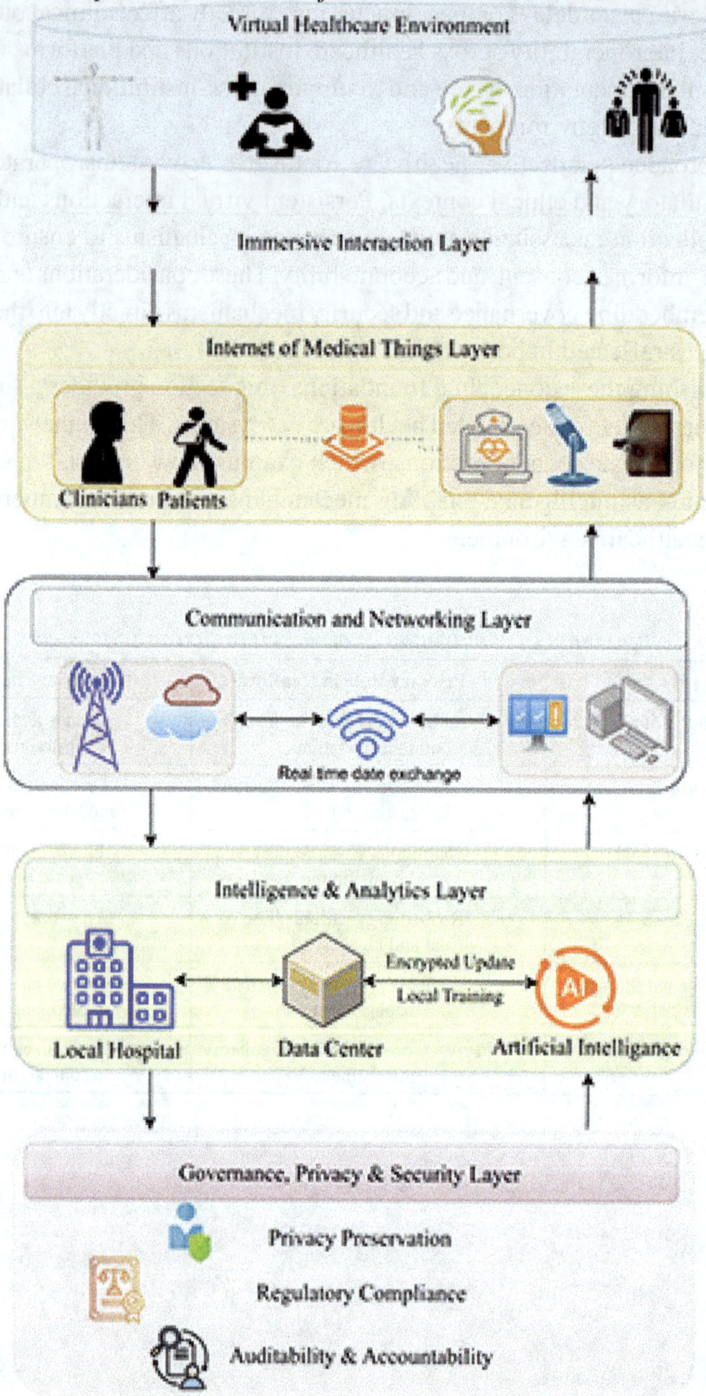

3. ARTIFICIAL INTELLIGENCE AS THE COGNITIVE INTELLIGENCE LAYER

Artificial intelligence functions as the cognitive backbone of Metaverse-enabled healthcare ecosystems by enabling perception, reasoning, and adaptive decision-making within immersive clinical environments. As Metaverse platforms continuously generate large-scale and heterogeneous healthcare data, AI techniques play a critical role in converting these raw data streams into clinically actionable intelligence (Sabile et al., 2025). In this context, artificial intelligence operates not as a peripheral analytical tool but as a core system layer that supports intelligent interaction, predictive modeling, and personalized care delivery.

3.1. AI-Driven Multimodal Data Processing in Metaverse Healthcare

Metaverse-based healthcare systems integrate data from diverse sources, including IoMT devices, electronic health records, medical imaging systems, and extended reality-based clinical interactions. Artificial intelligence models are designed to process and learn from these multimodal inputs, enabling the extraction of latent patterns and clinically relevant features. ML and deep learning techniques support tasks such as disease detection, risk stratification, and prognosis estimation by jointly analyzing structured clinical variables, unstructured text, high-dimensional images, and continuous physiological signals (Lăzăroiu et al., 2025). The principal AI capabilities supporting these healthcare functions are summarized in Table 2, which highlights how different forms of intelligence contribute to immersive healthcare services.

3.2. Intelligent Interaction and Virtual Clinical Assistance

Artificial intelligence enables intelligent and adaptive interaction within Metaverse healthcare environments through the deployment of virtual agents, decision-support systems, and clinician avatars. These AI-driven entities assist patients by providing personalized guidance, monitoring treatment adherence, and responding to real-time queries during immersive consultations. For healthcare professionals, AI-powered assistants aggregate patient information from multiple sources, highlight clinically significant anomalies, and support evidence-based decision-making. Such interaction mechanisms reduce cognitive workload, enhance workflow efficiency, and support continuity of care, particularly in remote and distributed clinical settings (Lisetti et al., 2015).

3.3. Closed-Loop AI Intelligence and Adaptive Personalization

The operational behavior of artificial intelligence in Metaverse-enabled healthcare follows a closed-loop intelligence paradigm. Patient data is acquired through physical sensors and virtual interactions and processed by AI models to generate predictions, alerts, and clinical recommendations. These inference results are delivered to clinicians and patients as actionable feedback, influencing diagnostic decisions, treatment planning, and care pathways. The outcomes of these actions generate new data that are reintegrated into the system, enabling continuous refinement of patient-specific models and adaptive personalization. This iterative learning and feedback cycle is illustrated in Figure 2, which depicts the flow of data, inference outcomes, and personalization within an AI-driven Metaverse healthcare workflow(Lisetti et al., 2015).

3.4. Operational Intelligence and System Optimization

Beyond clinical decision support, artificial intelligence contributes to operational optimization within Metaverse-enabled healthcare ecosystems. AI-based analytics can be employed to predict patient flow, optimize resource utilization, and support scheduling and capacity planning in virtual and hybrid care environments. Such system-level intelligence enhances scalability and efficiency, which are essential for the sustainable deployment of immersive healthcare platforms across large populations and institutions.

3.5. Challenges and Trust Considerations in AI Deployment

Despite its significant potential, the deployment of artificial intelligence in healthcare Metaverse systems introduces challenges related to transparency, robustness, and clinical trust. Complex AI models may lack interpretability, limiting clinicians' ability to understand and validate automated recommendations. Additionally, biases present in training data can lead to uneven performance across patient populations, raising concerns regarding fairness and reliability. In safety-critical healthcare applications, these limitations necessitate the incorporation of explainability mechanisms, bias mitigation strategies, and rigorous validation procedures to ensure clinical confidence and patient acceptance (Afroogh et al., 2024).

Another critical challenge arises from the dependence of many AI systems on centralized data aggregation and training paradigms. In distributed healthcare environments characterized by strict regulatory constraints and fragmented data ownership, centralized intelligence development becomes impractical. These limitations highlight the need for complementary learning frameworks that support collaborative intelligence while preserving privacy and institutional autonomy.

3.6. Transition to FL

AI serves as the cognitive intelligence layer that enables perception, reasoning, interaction, and personalization in Metaverse-enabled healthcare ecosystems. While AI provides powerful analytical, interactive, and operational capabilities, its effective and trustworthy deployment requires mechanisms that address privacy preservation, scalability, and governance. These requirements motivate the adoption of FL, which is discussed in the next section as a key enabler of distributed and privacy-preserving intelligence for trustworthy Metaverse-based healthcare systems.

Table 2. Artificial Intelligence Capabilities in Metaverse-Enabled Healthcare

AI Capability	Data Sources	Functional Role in Metaverse Healthcare	Expected Clinical Outcome
Multimodal Data Processing	IoMT signals, EHRs, medical images, XR interaction data	Joint analysis of heterogeneous healthcare data	Holistic patient understanding
Predictive Analytics	Longitudinal clinical data, physiological streams	Disease risk estimation and progression prediction	Early diagnosis and timely intervention
Intelligent Virtual Assistance	Behavioral data, interaction logs, clinical context	Patient guidance and clinician decision support	Improved engagement and workflow efficiency
Closed-Loop Learning	Feedback data, clinical outcomes	Continuous model refinement and adaptation	Personalized and adaptive care delivery
Operational Intelligence	System usage data, patient flow data	Resource allocation and care coordination	Scalable and efficient healthcare services

Figure 2. AI-driven healthcare workflow diagram

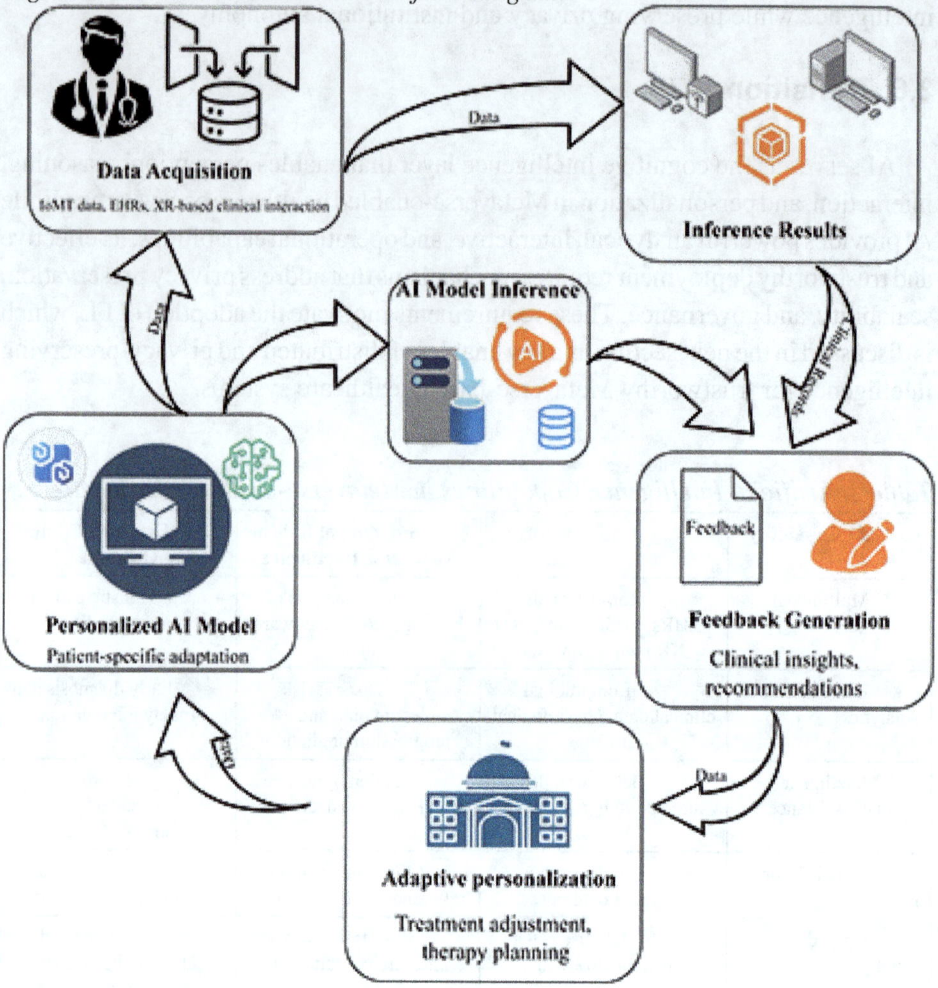

4. FEDERATED LEARNING FOR PRIVACY-PRESERVING HEALTHCARE

FL has emerged as a crucial approach for deploying intelligent healthcare systems that maintain patient privacy while leveraging the collective power of distributed data. Traditional centralized ML models require aggregating data into a single repository, which is not feasible in healthcare settings due to strict privacy regulations and ethical concerns. FL, however, allows for collaborative model training across multiple institutions without sharing raw patient data, ensuring compliance with data protection laws and promoting data sovereignty (Ali et al., 2022).

4.1. Limitations of Centralized Learning in Healthcare Ecosystems

Centralized learning faces several challenges in healthcare, including the high risk of data breaches, patient privacy concerns, and the logistical complexity of aggregating large volumes of sensitive medical data. These issues are compounded in Metaverse-enabled healthcare systems, where data is continuously generated from immersive interactions and IoMT devices (Abughazalah et al., 2024). As highlighted in Table 3, FL provides a solution by allowing model updates to be shared while ensuring that raw data remains local and secure, maintaining the integrity of patient information without compromising privacy.

4.2. FL Architecture and Training Paradigm

FL operates on a decentralized training model where local institutions, such as hospitals and medical centers, train models on their respective datasets. These local updates are then securely aggregated at a central server to form a global model. Figure 3 illustrates this workflow, showing how different institutions participate in the FL process. Each institution performs local training, and the model updates are sent to the central server for federated averaging, which ensures that the global model evolves through collaborative learning without the need for direct data sharing.

4.3. Privacy Preservation and Regulatory Compliance

One of the major advantages of FL, as indicated in Table 3, is its ability to align with privacy preservation and regulatory compliance. Since data is not exchanged between institutions, the risk of unauthorized access to patient information is minimized. FL can be further strengthened by employing techniques like secure aggregation, encryption of model updates, and differential privacy. These methods ensure that the model training process remains secure, and no sensitive data is exposed during the FL process.

4.4. Scalability and Collaborative Intelligence in Metaverse Healthcare

FL enhances scalability by distributing computational workloads across participating clients rather than relying on centralized infrastructure. In Metaverse-enabled healthcare systems, where immersive interactions and real-time analytics demand significant computational resources, this distributed training paradigm improves system responsiveness and resource utilization (Buttar et al., 2025). Moreover, FL enables collaborative intelligence by allowing healthcare institutions to benefit from collective knowledge without exposing proprietary or sensitive data. This collaborative learning capability is especially valuable for training robust and generalizable AI models in healthcare, where individual institutions may have limited or biased datasets. By aggregating knowledge across diverse populations and clinical settings, FL improves model robustness and reduces overfitting, thereby enhancing clinical reliability.

4.5. Challenges and Practical Considerations

Despite its advantages, FL introduces several practical challenges that must be addressed for effective deployment in healthcare Metaverse ecosystems. Data heterogeneity across institutions can lead to non-independent and non-identically distributed data, which complicates model convergence and performance consistency. Communication overhead and synchronization latency may also affect training efficiency, particularly in large-scale deployments with numerous clients. Additionally, FL systems must be designed to handle unreliable participants, varying computational capabilities, and potential security threats such as model poisoning attacks. Addressing these challenges requires careful system design, robust aggregation strategies, and continuous monitoring to ensure trustworthy and stable learning outcomes.

4.6. Role of FL in Trustworthy Metaverse Healthcare

FL plays a foundational role in establishing trust within Metaverse-enabled healthcare ecosystems by balancing intelligent collaboration with privacy preservation. By enabling distributed model training, FL supports scalable and ethically responsible intelligence development while maintaining institutional autonomy and patient data sovereignty. When integrated with artificial intelligence and immersive Metaverse platforms, FL forms a key pillar of trustworthy healthcare systems that prioritize security, transparency, and personalized care.

Finally, we say that FL provides a practical and privacy-preserving framework for deploying intelligent analytics in distributed healthcare environments. Its integration within Metaverse-enabled healthcare ecosystems addresses critical challenges related to data privacy, scalability, and collaborative intelligence. The next section builds upon this foundation by examining how trustworthiness can be systematically achieved through the combined application of artificial intelligence, FL, and governance mechanisms in immersive healthcare systems.

Table 3. Comparison of Centralized Learning and FL in Healthcare

Dimension	Centralized Learning	FL
Data Storage	Patient data aggregated at a central server	Patient data retained at local institutions
Privacy Risk	High due to centralized data exposure	Reduced since raw data is never shared
Regulatory Compliance	Difficult under strict healthcare regulations	Naturally aligned with data protection policies
Scalability	Limited by centralized infrastructure	High due to distributed training
Collaboration Across Institutions	Restricted by data sharing constraints	Enabled through model-level collaboration
Suitability for Metaverse Healthcare	Limited due to data volume and sensitivity	Highly suitable for distributed and immersive environments

Figure 3. FL workflow in Metaverse Enabled Healthcare

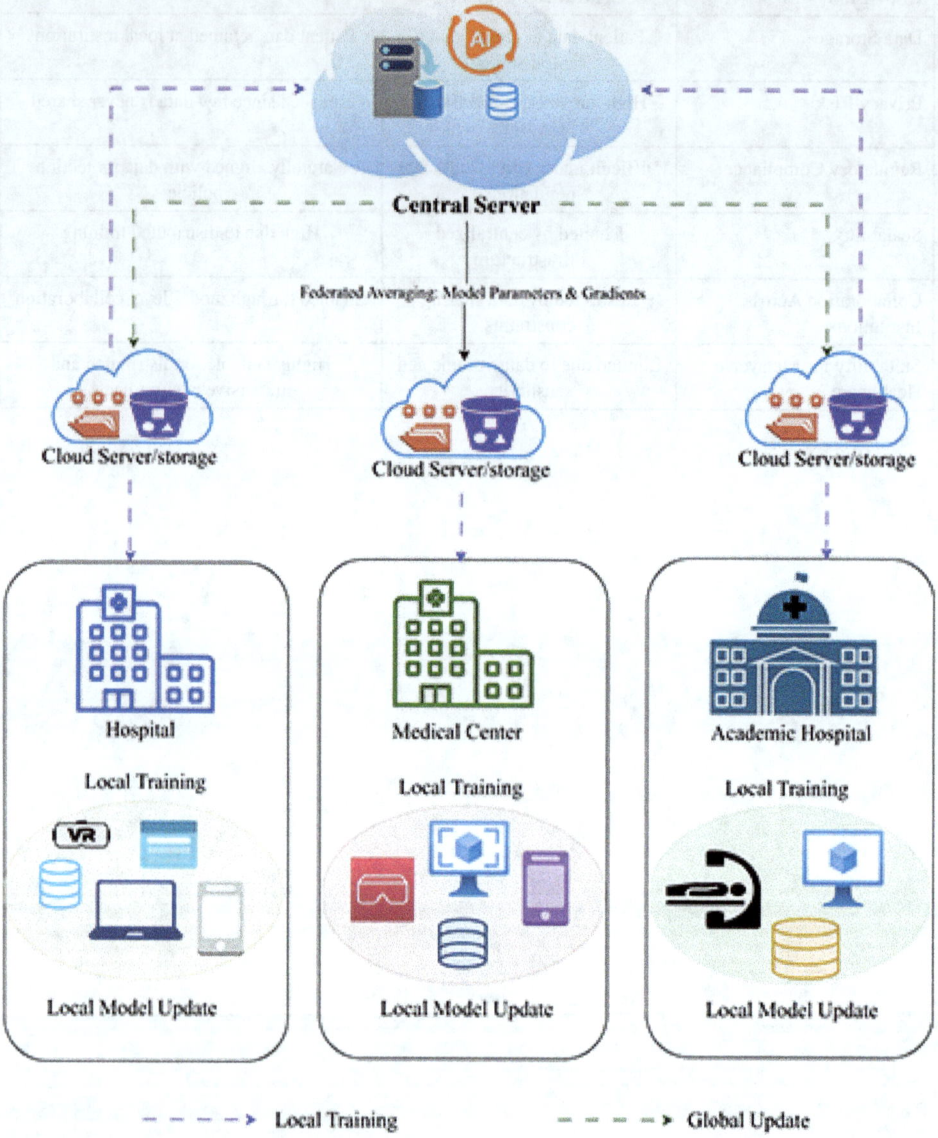

5. TRUSTWORTHINESS IN METAVERSE-ENABLED HEALTHCARE SYSTEM

Trustworthiness is a foundational requirement for the successful adoption of Metaverse-enabled healthcare systems, particularly when artificial intelligence and FL are employed for clinical decision support. In such environments, trust extends beyond traditional cybersecurity concerns and encompasses privacy protection, transparency of AI-driven decisions, fairness across patient populations, accountability of automated systems, and compliance with healthcare regulations. The absence of trust in any of these dimensions can significantly hinder clinician acceptance and patient confidence.

5.1. Privacy Preservation in Healthcare Metaverse Systems

Metaverse-enabled healthcare ecosystems continuously collect and process sensitive patient information through immersive interactions, wearable sensors, and clinical information systems. Ensuring privacy preservation is therefore critical. FL plays a central role in this context by enabling collaborative model training without sharing raw patient data across institutions. This decentralized learning paradigm significantly reduces the risk of data leakage while maintaining data sovereignty. Additional mechanisms such as encryption, secure aggregation, and access control further strengthen privacy protection. The role of privacy preservation as a core trust dimension, along with its supporting techniques, is summarized in Table 4.

5.2. Explainability and Transparency of AI Decisions

Transparency is essential for building trust in AI-assisted healthcare systems, particularly in clinical scenarios where decisions may influence diagnosis or treatment planning. Explainable AI techniques enable clinicians to understand the rationale behind model predictions, thereby facilitating validation and informed decision-making. In Metaverse environments, explainability is further enhanced through immersive visualization of model outputs and decision pathways (Faisal et al., 2026). The integration of interpretability mechanisms within AI models ensures that automated recommendations remain transparent and clinically meaningful, as highlighted in Table 4.

5.3. Fairness and Bias Mitigation

Fairness in AI-driven healthcare systems is critical to ensure equitable treatment across diverse patient populations. Bias in training data or model design can lead to disparities in clinical outcomes, particularly in large-scale Metaverse platforms that serve heterogeneous user groups. Bias detection and mitigation strategies, including the use of diverse datasets and fairness-aware learning techniques, are necessary to address these concerns. Fairness is therefore treated as a key pillar of trustworthiness in Metaverse-enabled healthcare systems, as reflected in Table 4.

5.4. Accountability and Governance Mechanisms

Accountability ensures that responsibility for AI-driven decisions and system actions is clearly defined and traceable. In Metaverse-enabled healthcare, accountability extends to AI models, FL processes, and institutional stakeholders. Blockchain-based audit trails and governance frameworks can be employed to record model updates, clinical decisions, and system interactions in a transparent and tamper-resistant manner. These mechanisms support traceability and compliance, thereby reinforcing trust among clinicians, patients, and regulatory authorities.

5.5. Integrated Trustworthiness Framewor

The interaction between privacy preservation, explainability, fairness, accountability, and regulatory compliance form a comprehensive trustworthiness framework for Metaverse-enabled healthcare systems. This integrated perspective is illustrated in Figure 4, which presents how artificial intelligence and FL operate within a structured trust framework supported by secure aggregation, auditing mechanisms, and compliance controls. The figure highlights the central role of AI models while emphasizing the surrounding trust layers that ensure safe, transparent, and reliable healthcare delivery in immersive environments (Maza & Megouas, 2021).

5.6. Discussion and Implications

By explicitly addressing trust-related challenges through architectural and algorithmic design choices, Metaverse-enabled healthcare systems can achieve higher levels of acceptance and reliability. The trust dimensions summarized in Table 4 and visually represented in Figure 4 provide a structured foundation for designing and evaluating trustworthy healthcare Metaverse platforms. These considerations are particularly important as healthcare systems move toward large-scale deployment of immersive and intelligent technologies.

Table 4. Dimensions of Trustworthiness in Metaverse-Enabled Healthcare Systems

Dimension	Description	Key Considerations	Methods
Privacy Preservation	Ensure patient data is protected	FL, encryption	Local training, encrypted updates
Explainability	Understanding AI decision-making	Interpretability, transparency	LIME, SHAP
Fairness	Ensuring unbiased AI performance	Bias detection, diverse data	Bias mitigation algorithms, diverse datasets
Accountability	Ensuring responsibility for actions	Audit trails, governance	Blockchain for auditing, performance tracking

Figure 4. Trustworthiness framework for Metaverse-enabled healthcare systems

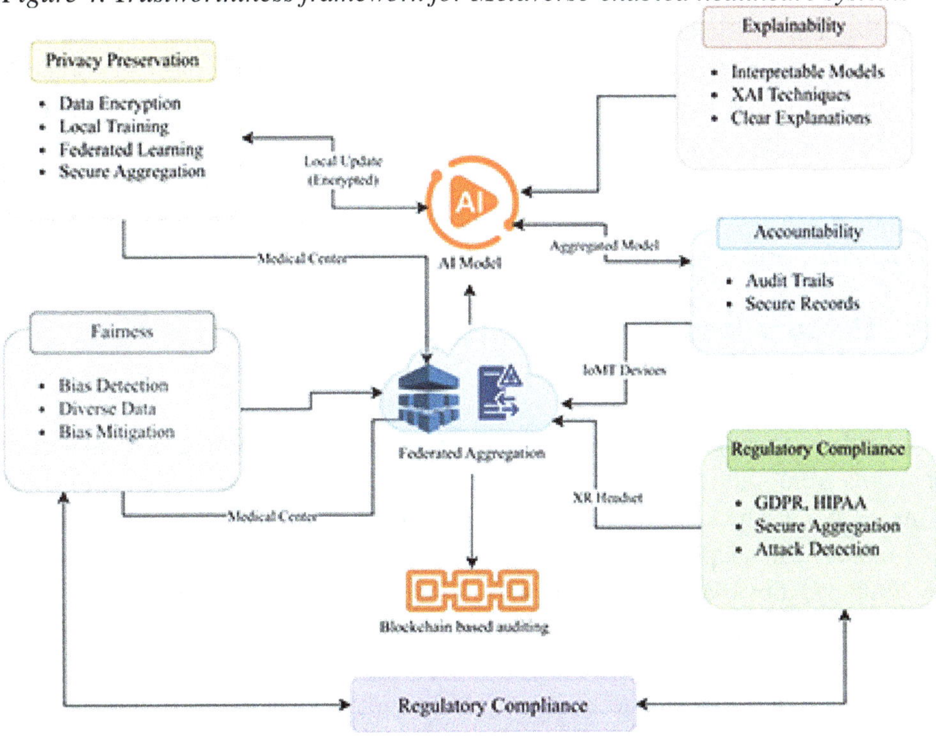

6. SECURE AND PERSONALIZED CARE THROUGH ARTIFICIAL INTELLIGENCE AND FEDERATED LEARNING

The convergence of artificial intelligence and FL within Metaverse-enabled healthcare ecosystems enables a new paradigm of secure and personalized care delivery. Personalization in healthcare involves tailoring diagnostic processes, treatment strategies, and care pathways to individual patient characteristics, while security ensures the protection of sensitive medical data and clinical decisions. In immersive healthcare environments, achieving these objectives simultaneously is challenging due to continuous data generation, distributed system architectures, and strict regulatory constraints. The complementary roles of artificial intelligence and FL in addressing these challenges are summarized in Table 5, which highlights how intelligent analytics and privacy-preserving learning jointly support secure personalization. Artificial intelligence provides the analytical foundation for learning patient-specific patterns from multimodal healthcare data, enabling precision-oriented diagnosis, adaptive treatment planning, and personalized patient engagement. FL, in contrast, facilitates collaborative model development across distributed healthcare entities without exposing raw patient data. By combining these two paradigms, Metaverse-enabled healthcare systems can deliver individualized care at scale while maintaining privacy, security, and regulatory compliance.

6.1. Personalized Clinical Intelligence in Metaverse Environments

Artificial intelligence enables personalized healthcare by learning patient-specific patterns from multimodal data sources, including physiological signals, medical images, clinical history, and interaction data generated within Metaverse platforms. AI models can adapt diagnostic thresholds, risk prediction scores, and treatment recommendations based on individual patient profiles, thereby supporting precision medicine. In immersive environments, personalization is further enhanced through contextual awareness, where AI models incorporate spatial, behavioral, and temporal information from virtual interactions to refine clinical insights. FL strengthens this personalization capability by allowing AI models to benefit from population-level knowledge without compromising individual privacy. By collaboratively training models across multiple healthcare institutions, FL improves generalization while preserving patient-specific adaptations at local sites. This balance between global learning and local personalization is particularly valuable in Metaverse-enabled healthcare, where patient populations are diverse and geographically distributed (Manojkumar et al., 2025).

6.2. Secure Data Handling and Privacy-Aware Personalization

Security is a critical prerequisite for personalized care in healthcare Metaverse systems. Personalized models require access to sensitive patient data, which increases the risk of privacy violations if not properly managed. FL mitigates this risk by ensuring that raw data remains within institutional boundaries and only encrypted model updates are exchanged. This decentralized approach significantly reduces the attack surface associated with centralized data storage. In addition to FL, secure communication protocols, encryption mechanisms, and access control policies are essential for protecting data flows between immersive interfaces, edge devices, and backend services. When combined with AI-driven personalization, these security mechanisms ensure that individualized care recommendations are generated and delivered in a manner that respects patient confidentiality and regulatory constraints (Rajawat et al., 2025).

6.3. Adaptive Care Pathways and Continuous Personalization

Metaverse-enabled healthcare systems support adaptive care pathways through continuous monitoring and feedback. AI models analyze real-time data from wearable devices, virtual consultations, and patient interactions to detect changes in health status and adjust care plans accordingly. This adaptive personalization allows for dynamic treatment modification, early intervention, and proactive disease management. FL facilitates continuous model updates across distributed environments, enabling adaptive personalization at scale. As new data becomes available, local models can be refined to reflect recent patient behavior and clinical outcomes, while aggregated knowledge from other institutions enhances overall model robustness. This continuous learning process supports long-term personalization without sacrificing security or scalability (Ishrat, Khan, Faisal, & Al Farsi, 2025).

6.4. Patient Engagement and Experience in Personalized Metaverse Care

Personalization in Metaverse-enabled healthcare extends beyond clinical decision-making to patient engagement and experience. AI-driven virtual agents and immersive interfaces can adapt communication styles, educational content, and therapeutic interactions based on patient preferences and cognitive profiles. Such personalization improves patient adherence, satisfaction, and trust in digital healthcare systems. From a security perspective, ensuring authenticated access and role-based interaction within virtual environments is essential to prevent misuse or impersonation. Secure identity management and authentication mechanisms complement AI-driven personalization by ensuring that personalized interactions occur only with authorized users (Faisal, Muniyandy, et al., 2025).

6.5. Challenges and Design Considerations

Despite its advantages, secure and personalized care in Metaverse-enabled healthcare systems presents several challenges. Balancing personalization with privacy preservation requires careful system design to prevent unintended data leakage or model inversion attacks. Additionally, excessive personalization may introduce bias if models overfit specific patient subgroups, potentially affecting fairness and clinical reliability. To address these challenges, healthcare Metaverse systems must incorporate robust validation procedures, fairness-aware learning strategies, and continuous monitoring of model behavior. The integration of AI and FL should therefore be guided by trustworthiness principles, ensuring that personalization enhances care quality without compromising security, fairness, or accountability.

Table 5. Secure and Personalized Care Enabled by AI and FL

Aspect	Role of Artificial Intelligence	Role of FL	Outcome
Personalization	Learns patient-specific patterns and preferences	Enables learning from distributed populations	Tailored diagnosis and treatment
Data Security	Analyzes encrypted and controlled data streams	Keeps raw data local to institutions	Privacy-preserving personalization
Adaptivity	Updates models based on real-time patient data	Supports continuous collaborative updates	Dynamic care pathways
Scalability	Supports intelligent decision-making at scale	Distributes training across institutions	Secure large-scale deployment

7. REGULATORY, ETHICAL, AND GOVERNANCE CONSIDERATIONS

The deployment of Metaverse-enabled healthcare systems that integrate artificial intelligence and FL must operate within well-defined regulatory, ethical, and governance frameworks. Healthcare is a highly regulated domain, and the introduction of immersive virtual environments and distributed intelligence further amplifies the need for compliance, accountability, and responsible system design. Regulatory adherence, ethical integrity, and governance structures are therefore essential to ensure that technological innovation translates into safe, lawful, and socially acceptable healthcare delivery.

7.1. Regulatory Compliance in Metaverse Healthcare

Healthcare data is subject to stringent data protection and privacy regulations across different jurisdictions. Regulations governing patient data storage, processing, and sharing impose strict requirements on healthcare information systems. In Metaverse-enabled healthcare environments, data flows across immersive interfaces, edge devices, and distributed learning infrastructures, which complicates regulatory compliance. FL supports compliance by minimizing cross-institutional data transfer and preserving data locality, thereby aligning with principles of data sovereignty and limited data exposure. In addition to data protection regulations, healthcare systems must comply with medical device regulations and clinical safety standards. AI-driven decision support tools deployed within Metaverse platforms may be classified as clinical decision support systems, requiring validation, certification, and continuous monitoring. Ensuring regulatory alignment throughout the system lifecycle, from design to deployment, is therefore a critical governance responsibility (Mohammadzadeh et al., 2024).

7.2. Ethical Considerations in Immersive and Intelligent Healthcare

Ethical concerns in Metaverse-enabled healthcare extend beyond data privacy to include patient autonomy, informed consent, and transparency of automated decision-making. Immersive environments may influence patient behavior and perception, raising questions about consent validity and user awareness. Patients must be clearly informed about how their data is collected, processed, and used by AI models within virtual healthcare spaces. The use of artificial intelligence introduces additional ethical challenges related to algorithmic bias, decision accountability, and potential over-reliance on automated recommendations. Ethical deployment requires ensuring that AI systems support, rather than replace, clinical judgment. Human oversight mechanisms must be embedded within Metaverse healthcare workflows to maintain clinician authority and responsibility (Attallah et al., 2024).

7.3. Governance Models for Distributed Healthcare Ecosystems

Effective governance is essential for coordinating the multiple stakeholders involved in Metaverse-enabled healthcare ecosystems, including healthcare providers, technology vendors, regulatory bodies, and patients. Governance frameworks must define roles, responsibilities, and accountability mechanisms across distributed environments. This includes establishing policies for data access, model updates, system auditing, and incident response. FL introduces new governance challenges, such as managing participation rules, validating model updates, and addressing malicious or unreliable participants. Robust governance mechanisms are required to ensure that collaborative learning processes remain secure, fair, and reliable. Transparent governance structures also contribute to trust by making system operations and decision processes auditable and understandable (Viswanadham, 2021).

7.4. Accountability and Auditability

Accountability in Metaverse-enabled healthcare systems requires the ability to trace decisions, data flows, and model updates across complex and distributed infrastructures. Auditability mechanisms, such as immutable logging and secure record-keeping, are essential to support clinical accountability, regulatory reporting, and post-incident analysis. These mechanisms ensure that system behavior can be reviewed and validated, particularly in cases where AI-assisted decisions influence patient outcomes. Clear accountability frameworks help delineate responsibility between human clinicians and automated systems, reducing ambiguity in clinical decision-making. This is particularly important in immersive environments where interactions between patients and intelligent virtual agents may blur traditional boundaries of responsibility.

7.5. Policy Implications and Future Governance Directions

As Metaverse-enabled healthcare systems continue to evolve, regulatory and governance frameworks must adapt to emerging technologies and use cases. Policymakers and healthcare regulators will need to develop guidelines that address the unique characteristics of immersive and distributed healthcare environments, including virtual interactions, cross-border collaboration, and continuous learning systems. Future governance models are likely to emphasize adaptive regulation, interdisciplinary oversight, and stakeholder participation. By proactively addressing regulatory, ethical, and governance considerations, Metaverse-enabled healthcare systems can achieve sustainable innovation while maintaining public trust and clinical integrity.

8. OPEN CHALLENGES AND FUTURE RESEARCH DIRECTIONS

Despite the significant potential of Metaverse-enabled healthcare systems that integrate artificial intelligence and FL, several open challenges must be addressed to enable reliable, ethical, and large-scale deployment. These challenges span technical, clinical, organizational, and societal dimensions, underscoring the need for continued interdisciplinary research. The major challenge areas and corresponding research directions discussed in this section are summarized in Table 6.

8.1. Interoperability and Standardization

One of the primary challenges in Metaverse-enabled healthcare is achieving interoperability across heterogeneous platforms, devices, and institutions. Immersive healthcare systems rely on diverse technologies, including extended reality interfaces, IoMT devices, and distributed learning infrastructures, each often developed using different standards and protocols. Lack of interoperability can lead to fragmented virtual environments and hinder seamless care continuity. Future research should focus on developing standardized data models, communication protocols, and interface specifications that support integration across Metaverse platforms and healthcare information systems (Mahajan & Malpe, 2026).

8.2. Scalability and System Performance

Scalability remains a critical concern for Metaverse-based healthcare ecosystems, particularly as the number of users, devices, and virtual interactions increases. Real-time immersive experiences require low-latency communication and high computational efficiency, which can be challenging in large-scale deployments. FL introduces additional communication overhead due to frequent model updates across distributed clients. Research efforts are needed to optimize communication efficiency, model aggregation strategies, and resource management to ensure that immersive healthcare services remain responsive and reliable at scale.

8.3. Data Heterogeneity and Model Robustness

Healthcare data is inherently heterogeneous, varying across institutions, patient populations, and sensing devices. This heterogeneity poses challenges for both artificial intelligence and FL, as models trained on non-uniform data distributions may exhibit unstable performance or biased behavior. Future research should investigate robust learning algorithms that can handle non-independent and non-identically distributed data while maintaining consistent performance across diverse clinical settings. Techniques for domain adaptation, personalized FL, and robustness evaluation are particularly relevant in this context (Ali et al., 2018).

8.4. Trust, Transparency, and User Acceptance

The success of Metaverse-enabled healthcare systems depends not only on technical performance but also on trust and acceptance by clinicians and patients. Immersive environments and AI-driven decision support may raise concerns regarding transparency, control, and reliability. Research is needed to understand how users perceive AI recommendations and virtual interactions, and how explainability mechanisms can be effectively integrated into immersive interfaces. User-centered design and human-in-the-loop approaches should be prioritized to ensure that technology supports, rather than undermines, clinical practice (Islam[1] et al., 2026).

8.5. Ethical and Societal Implications

The widespread adoption of Metaverse technologies in healthcare raises broader ethical and societal questions related to digital inclusion, accessibility, and long-term psychological effects of immersive care. Disparities in access to advanced technologies may exacerbate existing healthcare inequalities. Additionally, prolonged engagement in virtual healthcare environments may influence patient behavior and perception of care. Future research should explore ethical frameworks and policy interventions that promote equitable access, safeguard patient well-being, and address the societal impact of immersive healthcare technologies.

8.6. Emerging Research Opportunities

Beyond addressing existing challenges, the convergence of the Metaverse, artificial intelligence, and FL opens new research opportunities. These include the development of patient-specific digital twins for predictive and preventive care, integration of real-time physiological modeling with immersive visualization, and exploration of hybrid learning paradigms that combine federated and edge intelligence. Investigating these directions can further enhance the effectiveness, trustworthiness, and scalability of future healthcare Metaverse ecosystems.

Table 6. Open Challenges and Future Research Directions in Metaverse-Enabled Healthcare

Challenge Area	Key Issue	Research Direction
Interoperability	Heterogeneous platforms and data formats	Standardized protocols and data models
Scalability	Latency and computation overhead	Efficient aggregation and edge intelligence
Data Heterogeneity	Non-uniform clinical data	Robust and personalized FL
Trust and Acceptance	Limited transparency and user confidence	Explainable AI and human-in-the-loop design
Ethical Concerns	Equity and long-term impact	Ethical frameworks and inclusive policies

9. ILLUSTRATIVE HEALTHCARE SCENARIOS AND CONCEPTUAL CASE STUDIES

To demonstrate the practical relevance of Metaverse-enabled healthcare systems integrating artificial intelligence and FL, this section presents illustrative scenarios that reflect realistic clinical use cases. These scenarios are conceptual in nature and are intended to highlight how the proposed technological convergence can be applied in practice, rather than to report empirical results. By grounding the discussion in representative healthcare settings, this section bridges the gap between system-level concepts and real-world healthcare workflows.

9.1. Federated Cancer Diagnosis in a Virtual Oncology Environment

In a Metaverse-enabled virtual oncology center, patients from geographically distributed regions interact with oncologists through immersive consultation rooms. Medical imaging data, pathology reports, and clinical histories are processed locally at participating hospitals using AI-based diagnostic models. FL enables these institutions to collaboratively improve tumor detection and classification models by sharing encrypted model updates rather than raw patient data. Within the Metaverse environment, clinicians can visualize AI-generated risk assessments and tumor progression simulations through three-dimensional representations, supporting collaborative diagnosis and treatment planning. This scenario illustrates how privacy-preserving intelligence and immersive visualization can jointly enhance diagnostic accuracy and cross-institutional collaboration (Shafik, 2025).

9.2. AI-Assisted Mental Health Therapy in Immersive Care Spaces

Mental health therapy represents a domain where immersive environments can significantly enhance patient engagement and treatment effectiveness. In this scenario, patients participate in virtual therapy sessions guided by AI-driven virtual therapists within controlled and supportive Metaverse environments. Behavioral cues, speech patterns, and interaction data are analyzed locally to personalize therapy strategies. FL allows mental health institutions to collectively refine behavioral models while maintaining strict confidentiality of sensitive patient interactions. Clinicians receive explainable AI insights that support therapeutic decisions, ensuring that automated recommendations complement professional judgment rather than replace it (Tabassum et al., 2025).

9.3. Remote Rehabilitation and Adaptive Physiotherapy

Metaverse-enabled rehabilitation platforms allow patients recovering from physical injuries or neurological conditions to perform guided exercises in immersive environments. Wearable sensors capture motion data and physiological signals, which are analyzed by AI models to assess performance and detect anomalies. Personalized feedback is delivered in real time through adaptive virtual coaches. FL enables continuous improvement of rehabilitation models across clinics by aggregating learning outcomes without sharing raw patient data. This scenario highlights how secure personalization and adaptive intelligence can improve rehabilitation outcomes while supporting scalable deployment across healthcare providers.

9.4. Virtual Collaborative Care for Chronic Disease Management

Chronic disease management often requires long-term monitoring and coordination among multiple healthcare professionals. In a Metaverse-based collaborative care environment, patients, physicians, nurses, and specialists interact within shared virtual spaces. AI models analyze longitudinal health data to predict disease progression and recommend personalized interventions. FL ensures that predictive models benefit from diverse patient populations across institutions while preserving data privacy. This scenario demonstrates the potential of immersive collaboration and distributed intelligence to support proactive and coordinated chronic care (Faisal et al., 2026).

9.5. Discussion of Practical Implications

These illustrative scenarios demonstrate how the integration of artificial intelligence, FL, and Metaverse technologies can support secure, scalable, and personalized healthcare delivery across diverse clinical contexts. While conceptual, the scenarios reflect realistic constraints and opportunities in modern healthcare systems, including privacy requirements, distributed data ownership, and the need for clinician oversight. They also underscore the importance of trustworthiness, as discussed in earlier sections, in ensuring that immersive and intelligent healthcare systems are accepted and effectively utilized in practice.

10. CONCLUSION

This chapter examined the convergence of the Metaverse, artificial intelligence, and FL as a foundation for building secure, scalable, and personalized healthcare ecosystems. By enabling immersive clinical interactions and continuous data-driven intelligence, Metaverse-based healthcare systems extend beyond traditional digital health platforms to support collaborative and patient-centric care delivery. Artificial intelligence was discussed as the cognitive intelligence layer that enables multimodal data analysis, adaptive decision support, and personalized care within immersive environments. FL complements these capabilities by facilitating collaborative model development across distributed healthcare institutions while preserving data privacy and regulatory compliance. Together, these technologies address key challenges related to data sensitivity, scalability, and institutional autonomy. Trustworthiness emerged as a central requirement for successful deployment, encompassing privacy preservation, explainability, fairness, accountability, and governance. Embedding these trust dimensions into system design is essential to ensure clinical reliability and user acceptance. The illustrative healthcare scenarios further demonstrated how the integrated framework can support diverse clinical applications while maintaining security and ethical integrity. Finally, we can say that the effective integration of the Metaverse, artificial intelligence, and FL offers a promising pathway toward next-generation healthcare systems that prioritize personalization, security, and trust. Continued research and governance efforts will be critical to translating this vision into real-world healthcare practice.

REFERENCES

Abughazalah, M., Alsaggaf, W., Saifuddin, S., & Sarhan, S. (2024). Centralized vs. decentralized cloud computing in healthcare. *Applied Sciences (Basel, Switzerland)*, *14*(17), 7765. DOI: 10.3390/app14177765

Adil, M., Song, H., Khan, M. K., Mastorakis, S., Farouk, A., & Jin, Z. (2025). Metaverse in health care: Security challenges and pathways for future research. *IEEE Systems, Man, and Cybernetics Magazine*, *11*(1), 95–106. DOI: 10.1109/MSMC.2024.3368201

Afroogh, S., Akbari, A., Malone, E., Kargar, M., & Alambeigi, H. (2024). Trust in AI: Progress, challenges, and future directions. *Humanities & Social Sciences Communications*, *11*(1), 1–30. DOI: 10.1057/s41599-024-04044-8

Ali, M., Naeem, F., Tariq, M., & Kaddoum, G. (2022). Federated learning for privacy preservation in smart healthcare systems: A comprehensive survey. *IEEE Journal of Biomedical and Health Informatics*, *27*(2), 778–789. DOI: 10.1109/JBHI.2022.3181823 PMID: 35696470

Ali, M., Salehnejad, R., & Mansur, M. (2018). Hospital heterogeneity: What drives the quality of health care. *The European Journal of Health Economics : HEPAC : Health Economics in Prevention and Care*, *19*(3), 385–408. DOI: 10.1007/s10198-017-0891-9 PMID: 28439750

Attallah, O., Al-Kabbany, A., Zaghlool, S. B., & Kholief, M. (2024). Immersive technology and ambient intelligence for assistive living, medical, and healthcare solutions. [). Frontiers Media SA.]. *Frontiers in Human Neuroscience*, *18*, 1376959. DOI: 10.3389/fnhum.2024.1376959 PMID: 38450225

Buttar, A. M., Shahid, M. A., Naz, S., & Akbar, M. A. (2025). MedTech Fusion in the Metaverse using business intelligence through AIoTBc: artificial intelligence, Internet of Things, blockchain. In *Healthcare Frontiers in the Metaverse* (pp. 19–54). Elsevier. DOI: 10.1016/B978-0-443-32998-2.00005-6

Faisal, S. M., Ishrat, M., & Khan, W. (2025). Digital Twins in Healthcare: Revolutionizing Patient Care and Medical Operations. In *Digital Twins for Smart Cities and Urban Planning* (pp. 69–89). CRC Press.

Faisal, S. M., Khan, W., & Ishrat, M. (2026). AI-Enhanced Collaboration and Teamwork in Virtual Learning Environments. In *Intelligent Learning Tools, Enhancing Student Skills, and Career Preparedness* (pp. 149–176). IGI Global Scientific Publishing. DOI: 10.4018/979-8-3373-9225-7.ch006

Faisal, S. M., Muniyandy, E., Lokesh, S., & Jayanthi, M. G. (2025). A Random Graph Diffusion Attention Network with Great Wall Construction and Clinical Metadata for Improved Kidney Cancer Diagnosis and Surgical Planning. *Biomedical Materials & Devices*, •••, 1–20. DOI: 10.1007/s44174-025-00447-6

Haque, S. A., Aziz, S. M., & Rahman, M. (2014). Review of cyber-physical system in healthcare. *International Journal of Distributed Sensor Networks*, *10*(4), 217415. DOI: 10.1155/2014/217415

Ishrat, M., Khan, W., Faisal, S. M., & Al Farsi, M. M. (2025). Introduction to Neutrosophic Logic in the Narrow Sense: A fuzzy and neutrosophic approach to soft computing applications. In *Soft Computing and Machine Learning* (pp. 83–101). CRC Press.

Ishrat, M., Khan, W., Faisal, S. M., Al Farsi, M. M., & Farooqui, N. A. (2025). Digital Twins Future Prospects in Smart Cities: Challenges of Urban Planning. In *Digital Twins for Smart Cities and Urban Planning* (pp. 53–68). CRC Press.

Islam[1], N., Ezcurra, V., Rader[1], J., Margondai, A., Willox, S., Von Ahlefeldt, C., & Mouloua, M. (2026). Transparency for Trust: Enhancing Acceptance and System Integration of Intelligent AI in Healthcare. *Intelligent Human Systems Integration: Disruptive and Innovative Technologies*, 285.

Lăzăroiu, G., Gedeon, T., Halicka, K., & Szpilko, D. (2025). Generative artificial intelligence-driven medical digital twin technologies in blockchain Internet of Things wearable sensor and computer vision-based extended reality healthcare metaverse. *Engineering Management in Production and Services, 17*(3).

Lisetti, C., Amini, R., & Yasavur, U. (2015). Now all together: Overview of virtual health assistants emulating face-to-face health interview experience. *Künstliche Intelligenz*, *29*(2), 161–172. DOI: 10.1007/s13218-015-0357-0

Mahajan, N., & Malpe, K. (2026). Interoperability and Standardization in Healthcare System Integration: Interfacing Wearable Devices with Electronic Health Records. *Artificial Intelligence and Machine Learning in Neurology*, *1*, 243–281. DOI: 10.1002/9781394389131.ch10

Manojkumar, K., Sengar, A. S., Jyothi, A. P., & Faisal, S. M. (2025). Energy-efficient routing and predictive sink mobility in mobile wireless sensor networks using reflection equivariant quantum neural network and star fish optimization algorithms. *Sustainable Computing : Informatics and Systems*, *48*, 101231. DOI: 10.1016/j.suscom.2025.101231

Maza, S., & Megouas, O. (2021). Framework for trustworthiness in software development. *International Journal of Performability Engineering*, *17*(2), 241. DOI: 10.23940/ijpe.21.02.p8.241252

Mohammadzadeh, Z., Shokri, M., Saeidnia, H. R., Kozak, M., Marengo, A., Lund, B. D., Ausloos, M., & Ghiasi, N. (2024). Principles of digital professionalism for the metaverse in healthcare. *BMC Medical Informatics and Decision Making*, *24*(1), 201. DOI: 10.1186/s12911-024-02607-y PMID: 39039522

Rajawat, A. S., Arora, R. K., Muqeem, M., Faisal, S. M., & Jamal, M. K. (2025). Enhancing IoT Efficiency by Minimizing Latency and Boosting Real-Time Processing with Edge Computing. *SN Computer Science*, *6*(6), 715. DOI: 10.1007/s42979-025-04192-x

Sabile, J. M. G., Zhang, P., Parwani, A. V., Chobrutsiky, B., Gandhi, A. P., & Srisuwananukorn, A. (2025). Toward Clinically Actionable Machine Learning and Artificial Intelligence Algorithms in Acute Leukemia: A Systematic Narrative Review. *Acta Haematologica*, *148*(5), 587–603. DOI: 10.1159/000547532 PMID: 40706562

Shafik, W. (2025). Patient-Centered Healthcare: Trust and Transparency Through Technology. In *AI and Blockchain Applications for Privacy and Security in Smart Medical Systems* (pp. 309–338). IGI Global Scientific Publishing.

Sowan, B. I., Qattous, H., Fasha, M., & Altarawneh, A. (2025). Enhanced Healthcare Through Metaverse Integration: Explainable AI and Blockchain for Trust, Security, and Immersive Experiences. *2025 1st International Conference on Computational Intelligence Approaches and Applications (ICCIAA)*, 1–7.

Tabassum, A., Ghaznavi, I., Abd-Alrazaq, A., & Qadir, J. (2025). Exploring the application of AI and extended reality technologies in metaverse-driven mental health solutions: Scoping review. *Journal of Medical Internet Research*, *27*, e72400. DOI: 10.2196/72400 PMID: 40829151

Viswanadham, N. (2021). Ecosystem model for healthcare platform. *Sadhana*, *46*(4), 188. DOI: 10.1007/s12046-021-01708-y

Compilation of References

Aarthi, S., Ravikumar, R. N., Balakrishnan, R., Pavithra, K., Jumaniyozov, F., & Praveen, V. M. (2025). Blockchain for seamless and transparent smart hospitality operations. In *Smart Operations and Enhancing Guest Experience in the Hospitality Industry* (pp. 187–218). IGI Global., DOI: 10.4018/979-8-3373-2145-5.ch007

Abbas, J. R., Meschtscherjakov, A., & Tscheligi, M. (2023). What is virtual reality? A healthcare-focused systematic review of definitions. *Journal of Biomedical Informatics*, *141*, 104356.

Abbas, J. R., O'Connor, A., Ganapathy, E., Isba, R., Payton, A., McGrath, B., Tolley, N., & Bruce, I. A. (2023). What is virtual reality? A healthcare-focused systematic review of definitions. *Health Policy and Technology*, *12*(2), 100741. DOI: 10.1016/j.hlpt.2023.100741

Abbas, S. R., Abbas, Z., Zahir, A., & Lee, S. W. (2024). Federated learning in smart healthcare: A comprehensive review on privacy, security, and predictive analytics with IoT integration. *Healthcare (Basel)*, *12*(24), 2587. DOI: 10.3390/healthcare12242587 PMID: 39766014

Abdallah, M., Abdallah, Q., Abukhalil, A., & Barqawi, L. (2025, April). *AI in Healthcare: Ethical and Regulatory Challenges*. In *2025 International Conference on New Trends in Computing Sciences (ICTCS)* (pp. 517–521). IEEE. DOI: 10.1109/ICTCS65341.2025.10989298

Abhishek, V., Binny, S., Johan, T., Raj, N., & Thomas, V. (n.d.). *Federated Learning: Collaborative Machine Learning without.*

Abhishek, V. A., Binny, S., Johan, T. R., Raj, N., & Thomas, V. (2022). Federated learning: Collaborative machine learning without centralized training data. *International Journal of Engineering Technology and Management Sciences*, *355–359*, 355–359. Advance online publication. DOI: 10.46647/ijetms.2022.v06i05.052

Abughazalah, M., Alsaggaf, W., Saifuddin, S., & Sarhan, S. (2024). Centralized vs. decentralized cloud computing in healthcare. *Applied Sciences (Basel, Switzerland)*, *14*(17), 7765. DOI: 10.3390/app14177765

Adil, M., Song, H., Khan, M. K., Mastorakis, S., Farouk, A., & Jin, Z. (2025). Metaverse in health care: Security challenges and pathways for future research. *IEEE Systems, Man, and Cybernetics Magazine*, *11*(1), 95–106. DOI: 10.1109/MSMC.2024.3368201

Adnan, M., Yi, Y., Wani, N. A., Alsenan, S., Khan, M. A., & Anwar, M. S. (2025). Neurosymbolic digital twin for cardiovascular disease prediction and personalized modeling. *IEEE Journal of Biomedical and Health Informatics*, 1–8. Advance online publication. DOI: 10.1109/JBHI.2025.3647298 PMID: 41433178

Afroogh, S., Akbari, A., Malone, E., Kargar, M., & Alambeigi, H. (2024). Trust in AI: Progress, challenges, and future directions. *Humanities & Social Sciences Communications*, *11*(1), 1–30. DOI: 10.1057/s41599-024-04044-8

Ahamed, S. I. (2018). The role of the Internet of Things (IoT) in personalised healthcare. *Journal of Ambient Intelligence and Humanized Computing*, *9*(5), 1433–1445.

Ahmed, A., Shahzad, A., Naseem, A., Ali, S., & Ahmad, I. (2025). Evaluating the effectiveness of data governance frameworks in ensuring security and privacy of healthcare data. *PLoS One*, *20*(5), e0324285. DOI: 10.1371/journal.pone.0324285 PMID: 40408373

Ahn, J. S., Ebrahimian, S., McDermott, S., Lee, S., Naccarato, L., Di Capua, J. F., Wu, M. Y., Zhang, E. W., Muse, V., Miller, B., Sabzalipour, F., Bizzo, B. C., Dreyer, K. J., Kaviani, P., Digumarthy, S. R., & Kalra, M. K. (2022). Association of artificial intelligence-aided chest radiograph interpretation with reader performance and efficiency. *JAMA Network Open*, *5*(8), e2229289. DOI: 10.1001/jamanetworkopen.2022.29289 PMID: 36044215

Akhmetov, A., Latif, Z., Tyler, B., & Yazici, A. (2025). Enhancing healthcare data privacy and interoperability with federated learning. *PeerJ. Computer Science*, *11*, e2870. DOI: 10.7717/peerj-cs.2870 PMID: 40567682

Akinola, S., & Telukdarie, A. (2023). Sustainable digital transformation in healthcare. *Sustainability (Basel)*, *15*(13), 10417. DOI: 10.3390/su151310417

Akter, M., Moustafa, N., & Turnbull, B. (2024). SPEI-FL: Serverless privacy edge intelligence-enabled federated learning in smart healthcare systems. *Cognitive Computation*, *16*(5), 2626–2641. DOI: 10.1007/s12559-024-10310-3 al Dhairyashil Patil, E. (2024). Federated learning in real-time medical IoT: Optimizing privacy and accuracy for chronic disease monitoring. *Journal of Electrical Systems*, *19*(3), 32–42. DOI: 10.52783/jes.649

Al Omar, A., Bhuiyan, M. Z. A., Basu, A., Kiyomoto, S., & Rahman, M. S. (2021). A systematic review of blockchain for consent management and privacy in healthcare: healthcare, *9*(2), 137.

Al, E. 'mari, S., Sanjalawe, Y., Fataftah, F., & Fataftah, F. (2026). Digital Twins and BI: Synchronizing Virtual Models With Real-Time Business Processes. In *Strategic AI Integration in Business Intelligence* (pp. 135-154). IGI Global Scientific Publishing.

Alabdulqader, E. A., Umer, M., Alnowaiser, K., Wang, H., Alarfaj, A. A., & Ashraf, I. (2024). Image Processing-based Resource-Efficient Transfer Learning Approach for Cancer Detection Employing Local Binary Pattern Features. *Mobile Networks and Applications*, *29*(4), 1–17. DOI: 10.1007/s11036-024-02331-x

Al-E'mari, S., Sanjalawe, Y., Kurdi, G., & Allehyani, B. (2025, April). Detection of ARP Spoofing Attack in Healthcare Networks Using a LSTM Model. In *2025 1st International Conference on Computational Intelligence Approaches and Applications (ICCIAA)* (pp. 1-7). IEEE. DOI: 10.1109/ICCIAA65327.2025.11012965

Alghamdi, A., Zhu, J., Yin, G., Shorfuzzaman, M., Alsufyani, N., Alyami, S., & Biswas, S. (2022). Blockchain Empowered Federated Learning Ecosystem for Securing Consumer IoT Features. *Analysis & Sensing*, *22*(18), 6786. Advance online publication. DOI: 10.3390/s22186786 PMID: 36146134

Ali, M., Naeem, F., Tariq, M., & Kaddoum, G. (2022). Federated learning for privacy preservation in smart healthcare systems: A comprehensive survey. *IEEE Journal of Biomedical and Health Informatics*, *27*(2), 778–789. DOI: 10.1109/JBHI.2022.3181823 PMID: 35696470

Ali, M., Salehnejad, R., & Mansur, M. (2018). Hospital heterogeneity: What drives the quality of health care. *The European Journal of Health Economics : HEPAC : Health Economics in Prevention and Care*, *19*(3), 385–408. DOI: 10.1007/s10198-017-0891-9 PMID: 28439750

Ali, S., Abdullah, , Armand, T. P. T., Athar, A., Hussain, A., Ali, M., Yaseen, M., Joo, M.-I., & Kim, H.-C. (2023). Metaverse in healthcare integrated with explainable AI and blockchain. *Sensors (Basel)*, *23*(2), 565. DOI: 10.3390/s23020565 PMID: 36679361

Aljawarneh, S. A., & Al-Quraan, R. (2023). Pneumonia detection using enhanced convolutional neural network model on chest x-ray images. *Big Data*. PMID: 37074075

Almogadwy, B., & Alqarafi, A. (2025). Fused federated learning framework for secure and decentralized patient monitoring in healthcare 5.0 using IoMT. *Scientific Reports, 15*(1), 24263. DOI: 10.1038/s41598-025-06574-w PMID: 40624105

Aloqaily, M., Bouachir, O., Karray, F., Al Ridhawi, I., & Saddik, A. E. (2023, November 1). Integrating Digital Twin and Advanced Intelligent Technologies to Realize the Metaverse. *IEEE Consumer Electronics Magazine, 12*(6), 47–55. DOI: 10.1109/MCE.2022.3212570

Al-Qaness, M. A., Zhu, J., Al-Alimi, D., Dahou, A., Alsamhi, S. H., Elaziz, M. A., & Ewees, A. A. (2024). Chest x-ray images for lung disease detection using Deep Learning techniques: A Comprehensive survey. *Archives of Computational Methods in Engineering, 31*(6), 3267–3301. DOI: 10.1007/s11831-024-10081-y

Alsalami, Z. A., Chandra Sekhar Reddy, L., Saritha, K., Ranitha, I. B., Nageshwari, R., & Govindaram, A. (2025), "Advancing Zero-Shot Spatio-Temporal Learning: A Novel Framework for AI-Generated Synthetic Intelligence Systems," 2025 International Conference on Metaverse and Current Trends in Computing (ICMCTC), Subang Jaya, Malaysia, 2025, pp. 1-4. DOI: 10.1109/ICMCTC62214.2025.11196460

Alshanketi, F., Alharbi, A., Kuruvilla, M., Mahzoon, V., Siddiqui, S. T., Rana, N., & Tahir, A. (2024). *Pneumonia Detection from Chest X-Ray Images Using Deep Learning and Transfer Learning for Imbalanced Datasets*. Deleted Journal., DOI: 10.1007/s10278-024-01334-0

Amann, J., Blasimme, A., Vayena, E., Frey, D., & Madai, V. I. (2020). Explainability for artificial intelligence in healthcare: A multidisciplinary perspective. *BMC Medical Informatics and Decision Making, 20*(1), 310. DOI: 10.1186/s12911-020-01332-6 PMID: 33256715

Amershi, S., Weld, D., Vorvoreanu, M., Fourney, A., Nushi, B., Collisson, P., Suh, J., Iqbal, S., Bennett, P. N., Inkpen, K., Teevan, J., Kikin-Gil, R., & Horvitz, E. (2019). Guidelines for human-AI interaction. *Proceedings of the 2019 CHI Conference on Human Factors in Computing Systems*, Article 3. DOI: 10.1145/3290605.3300233

Aminizadeh, S., Heidari, A., Dehghan, M., Toumaj, S., Rezaei, M., Navimipour, N. J., & Unal, M. (2024). Opportunities and challenges of artificial intelligence and distributed systems. *Artificial Intelligence in Medicine, 149*, 102779. DOI: 10.1016/j.artmed.2024.102779 PMID: 38462281

An, Q., Chen, W., & Shao, W. (2024). A Deep Convolutional Neural Network for Pneumonia Detection in X-ray Images with Attention Ensemble. *Diagnostics (Basel), 14*(4), 390. DOI: 10.3390/diagnostics14040390 PMID: 38396430

Antunes, R. S., André da Costa, C., Küderle, A., Yari, I. A., & Eskofier, B. (2022). Federated learning for healthcare: Systematic review and architecture proposal. [TIST]. *ACM Transactions on Intelligent Systems and Technology*, *13*(4), 1–23. DOI: 10.1145/3501813

Arikumar, K. S., Prathiba, S. B., Alazab, M., Gadekallu, T. R., Pandya, S., Khan, J. M., & Moorthy, R. S. (2022). FL-PMI: Federated Learning-Based Person Movement Identification through Wearable Devices in Smart Healthcare Systems. *Sensors (Basel)*, *22*(4), 1377. Advance online publication. DOI: 10.3390/s22041377 PMID: 35214282

Arpaia, P., De Benedetto, E., De Paolis, L., D'Errico, G., Donato, N., & Duraccio, L. (2022). Performance and usability evaluation of an extended reality platform to monitor patient's health during surgical procedures. *Sensors (Basel)*, *22*(10), 3908. DOI: 10.3390/s22103908 PMID: 35632317

Arrieta, A. B., Díaz-Rodríguez, N., Ser, J. D., Bennetot, A., Tabik, S., Barbado, A., & Herrera, F. (2020). Explainable Artificial Intelligence (XAI): Concepts, taxonomies, opportunities and challenges toward responsible AI. *Information Fusion*, *58*, 82–115. DOI: 10.1016/j.inffus.2019.12.012

Attallah, O., Al-Kabbany, A., Zaghlool, S. B., & Kholief, M. (2024). Immersive technology and ambient intelligence for assistive living, medical, and healthcare solutions. [). Frontiers Media SA.]. *Frontiers in Human Neuroscience*, *18*, 1376959. DOI: 10.3389/fnhum.2024.1376959 PMID: 38450225

Aziz, R., Banerjee, S., Bouzefrane, S., & Le Vinh, T. (2023). Exploring homomorphic encryption and differential privacy techniques towards secure federated learning paradigm. *Future Internet*, *15*(9), 310. DOI: 10.3390/fi15090310

Bagdasaryan, E., Veit, A., Hua, Y., Estrin, D., & Shmatikov, V. (2020). How to backdoor federated learning. *Proceedings of the 23rd International Conference on Artificial Intelligence and Statistics (AISTATS)*, 2938–2948.

Bagdasaryan, E., Veit, A., Hua, Y., Estrin, D., & Shmatikov, V. (2020). How to backdoor federated learning. *Proceedings of the 23rd International Conference on Artificial Intelligence and Statistics*, 2938–2948.

Balasubramanyam, A., Ramesh, R., Sudheer, R., & Honnavalli, P. B. (2024). Revolutionizing healthcare: A review unveiling the transformative power of digital twins. *IEEE Access : Practical Innovations, Open Solutions*, *12*, 69650–69678. DOI: 10.1109/ACCESS.2024.3399744

Band, S. (2020). Interpretability of machine learning in healthcare: Techniques and applications. *Health Informatics Journal, 26*(4), 2649–2664.

Bansal, G., Rajgopal, K., Chamola, V., Xiong, Z., & Niyato, D. (2022). Healthcare in metaverse: A survey on current metaverse applications in healthcare. *IEEE Access : Practical Innovations, Open Solutions, 10*, 119914–119946. DOI: 10.1109/ACCESS.2022.3219845

Baroud, S. Y. (2025), "AI-Powered Multi-Agent System for Type 2 Diabetes Care: IoT, Federated Learning and Mobile Health Integration," 2025 International Conference on Metaverse and Current Trends in Computing (ICMCTC), Subang Jaya, Malaysia, 2025, pp. 1-5. DOI: 10.1109/ICMCTC62214.2025.11196336

Barsom, E. Z., Graafland, M., & Schijven, M. P. (2016). Systematic review on the effectiveness of augmented reality applications in medical training. *Surgical Endoscopy, 30*(10), 4174–4183. DOI: 10.1007/s00464-016-4800-6 PMID: 26905573

Bashir, A. K., Victor, N., Bhattacharya, S., Huynh-The, T., Chengoden, R., Yenduri, G., Maddikunta, P. K. R., Pham, Q.-V., Gadekallu, T. R., & Liyanage, M. (2023, December 15). Federated Learning for the Healthcare Metaverse: Concepts, Applications, Challenges, and Future Directions. *IEEE Internet of Things Journal, 10*(24), 21873–21891. DOI: 10.1109/JIOT.2023.3304790

Bhardwaj, A. (2024). Revolutionize healthcare using Metaverse virtual worlds and augmented reality. In *Beyond the Realms: Navigating the Metaverse* (pp. 157–200). BENTHAM SCIENCE PUBLISHERS. DOI: 10.2174/9789815238457124010009

Bhatia, M., & Kumar, R. (2025). Digital twin technology in wireless communication: A comprehensive engineering survey. *IEEE Internet of Things Journal, 12*(12), 19144–19166. Advance online publication. DOI: 10.1109/JIOT.2025.3565843

Bhattacharya, P., Obaidat, M. S., Savaliya, D., Sanghavi, S., Tanwar, S., & Sadaun, B. (2022), "Metaverse Assisted Telesurgery in Healthcare 5.0: An Interplay of Blockchain and Explainable AI," *2022 International Conference on Computer, Information and Telecommunication Systems (CITS)*, Piraeus, Greece, 2022, pp. 1-5. DOI: 10.1109/CITS55221.2022.9832978

Bhuria, R., & Gupta, S. (2024, November). Innovative AI Solutions for Pneumonia Detection: Exploring DenseNet-161 in Medical Imaging. In 2024 5th International Conference on Data Intelligence and Cognitive Informatics (ICDICI) (pp. 638-643). IEEE.

Björnsson, B., Borrebaeck, C., Elander, N., Gasslander, T., Gawel, D. R., Gustafsson, M., Jörnsten, R., Lee, E. J., Li, X., Lilja, S., Martínez-Enguita, D., Matussek, A., Sandström, P., Schäfer, S., Stenmarker, M., Sun, X. F., Sysoev, O., Zhang, H., & Benson, M. (2020). Digital twins to personalise medicine. *Genome Medicine*, *12*(1), 4. DOI: 10.1186/s13073-019-0701-3 PMID: 31892363

Bommasani, R., Hudson, D. A., Adeli, E., Altman, R., Arora, S., von Arx, S., . . . Liang, P. (2021). On the opportunities and risks of foundation models. *arXiv preprint arXiv:2108.07258*.

Bonawitz, K., Ivanov, V., Kreuter, B., Marcedone, A., McMahan, H. B., Patel, S., & Seth, K. (2019). Practical secure aggregation for privacy-preserving machine learning. *Proceedings of the 2017 ACM SIGSAC Conference on Computer and Communications Security*, 1175–1191. https://doi.org/DOI: 10.1145/3133956.3133982

Bozkaya, E., Erel-Özçevik, M., Bilen, T., & Özçevik, Y. (2023). Proof of evaluation-based energy and delay aware computation offloading for digital twin edge network. *Ad Hoc Networks*, *149*, 103254. DOI: 10.1016/j.adhoc.2023.103254

Bozkurt, A., & Sharma, R. C. (2024). Trust, credibility and transparency in human-AI interaction: Why we need explainable and trustworthy AI and why we need it now. *Asian Journal of Distance Education*, *19*(2).

Brisimi, T. S., Chen, R., Mela, T., Olshevsky, A., Paschalidis, I. C., & Shi, W. (2018). Federated learning of predictive models from federated Electronic Health Records. *International Journal of Medical Informatics*, *112*, 59–67. DOI: 10.1016/j.ijmedinf.2018.01.007 PMID: 29500022

Bruynseels, K., Santoni de Sio, F., & Van den Hoven, J. (2018). Digital twins in health care: Ethical implications of an emerging engineering paradigm. *Frontiers in Genetics*, *9*, 31. DOI: 10.3389/fgene.2018.00031 PMID: 29487613

Burian, B. K., Harari, R. E., Robertson, J. M., Musson, D., Pozner, C. N., Doyle, T., & Dias, R. D. (2023). Using XR for medical training. *Applied Ergonomics*, *106*, 103902. DOI: 10.1016/j.apergo.2022.103902 PMID: 36162274

Buttar, A. M., Shahid, M. A., Naz, S., & Akbar, M. A. (2025). MedTech Fusion in the Metaverse using business intelligence through AIoTBc: artificial intelligence, Internet of Things, blockchain. In *Healthcare Frontiers in the Metaverse* (pp. 19–54). Elsevier. DOI: 10.1016/B978-0-443-32998-2.00005-6

Cabanillas-Carbonell, M., Pérez-Martínez, J., & Yáñez, J. A. (2023). 5G technology in the digital transformation of healthcare. *Sustainability*, *15*(4), 3178. DOI: 10.3390/su15043178

Cabrero-Holgueras, J., & Pastrana, S. (2023). Privacy-preserving deep learning over encrypted medical data. *Frontiers in Cardiovascular Medicine*, *10*, 1117360. DOI: 10.3389/fcvm.2023.1117360 PMID: 37187785

Cai, C. J., Winter, S., Steiner, D., Wilcox, L., & Terry, M. (2022). "Hello AI": Uncovering the onboarding needs of medical practitioners for human–AI collaborative decision-making. *Proceedings of the ACM on Human-Computer Interaction*, *6*(CSCW2), 1–24. https://doi.org/DOI: 10.1145/3555220

Carlini, N., Tramer, F., Wallace, E., Jagielski, M., Herbert-Voss, A., Lee, K., Roberts, A., Brown, T., Song, D., Erlingsson, Ú., Oprea, A., & Raffel, C. (2021). Extracting training data from large language models. Proceedings of the 30th USENIX Security Symposium (USENIX Security '21), 2633–2650.

Cavoukian, A. (2009). *Privacy by design: The 7 foundational principles*. Information and Privacy Commissioner of Ontario.

Chaddad, A., Wu, Y., & Desrosiers, C. (2023). Federated learning for healthcare applications. *IEEE Internet of Things Journal*, *11*(5), 7339–7358. DOI: 10.1109/JIOT.2023.3325822

Chaddad, A., Wu, Y., & Kateb, R. (2023), "Building a Better Metaverse: How Federated Learning is Revolutionizing Virtual Worlds," *2023 IEEE International Conference on E-health Networking, Application & Services (Healthcom)*, Chongqing, China, 2023, pp. 205-209. DOI: 10.1109/Healthcom56612.2023.10472354

Channa, A., Popescu, N., Skibinska, J., & Burget, R. (2021). The rise of wearable devices during the COVID-19 pandemic: A systematic review. *Sensors (Basel)*, *21*(17), 5787. DOI: 10.3390/s21175787 PMID: 34502679

Chauhan, H., Rawat, K., Kaur, G. K., Kumar, P., Joshi, N., & Singla, S. (2025), "Web of Science-Based Bibliometric Analysis of AI on Healthcare," 2025 6th International Conference on Intelligent Communication Technologies and Virtual Mobile Networks (ICICV), Tirunelveli, India, 2025, pp. 297-304. DOI: 10.1109/ICICV64824.2025.11085565

Chelani, N., Tripathy, S., Kumhar, M., Bhatia, J., Saxena, V., Tanwar, S., & Nayyar, A. (2024). Federated Learning for Internet of medical healthcare: Issues and challenges. *Scalable Computing Practice and Experience*, *25*(5), 4442–4455. DOI: 10.12694/scpe.v25i5.2905

Chengoden, R., Victor, N., Huynh-The, T., Yenduri, G., Jhaveri, R. H., Alazab, M., Bhattacharya, S., Hegde, P., Maddikunta, P. K. R., & Gadekallu, T. R. (2023). Metaverse for Healthcare: A Survey on Potential Applications, Challenges and Future Directions. *IEEE Access : Practical Innovations, Open Solutions*, *11*, 12765–12795. DOI: 10.1109/ACCESS.2023.3241628

Chen, J., Wang, W., Fang, B., Liu, Y., Yu, K., Leung, V. C. M., & Hu, X. (2023). Digital twin empowered wireless healthcare monitoring for smart home. *IEEE Journal on Selected Areas in Communications*, *41*(11), 3662–3676. Advance online publication. DOI: 10.1109/JSAC.2023.3310097

Chen, J., Yi, C., Okegbile, S. D., Cai, J., & Shen, X. (2024). Networking architecture and key supporting technologies for digital twin in personalized healthcare: A comprehensive survey. *IEEE Communications Surveys and Tutorials*, *26*(1), 706–746. Advance online publication. DOI: 10.1109/COMST.2023.3308717

Chen, K., & Liu, Y. (2025). Toward privacy-preserving AI standards for federated learning in 6G-enabled digital twin environments. *IEEE Communications Standards Magazine*, 1–8. Advance online publication. DOI: 10.1109/MCOMSTD.2025.3623142

Chen, M., Hao, Y., Cai, Y., Wang, Y., & Zhang, Y. (2021). Artificial intelligence in healthcare: Past, present and future. *Journal of Medical Systems*, *45*(9), 102–115.

Chokshi, K. (2025), "Enhancing User Immersion: AI-Driven Real-Time Interactions in Augmented and Virtual Reality Systems," *2025 International Conference on Sustainable Communication Networks and Application (ICSCN)*, Theni, India, 2025, pp. 507-512. DOI: 10.1109/ICSCN67106.2025.11308554

Choudhury, A., & Shamszare, H. (2023). Investigating the impact of user trust on the adoption and use of ChatGPT: Survey analysis. *Journal of Medical Internet Research*, *25*, e47184. DOI: 10.2196/47184 PMID: 37314848

Choudhury, A., Volmer, L., Martin, F., Fijten, R., Wee, L., Dekker, A., & van Soest, J. (2025). Advancing privacy-preserving health care analytics and implementation of the Personal Health Train: Federated deep learning study. *JMIR AI*, *4*, e60847. DOI: 10.2196/60847 PMID: 39912580

Chowdhury, S., & Kaur, A., B, S., Kanmani Prince, P. G., Agarwal, T., and Vashisht, N. (2025), "Advancements in IoT and Sensor-Enabled Wearable Devices for Healthcare Applications," 2025 International Conference on Automation and Computation (AUTOCOM), Dehradun, India, 2025, pp. 500-505. DOI: 10.1109/AUTOCOM64127.2025.10957159

Ciecierski-Holmes, T., Singh, R., Axt, M., Brenner, S., & Barteit, S. (2022). Artificial intelligence for strengthening healthcare systems in low- and middle-income countries: A systematic scoping review. *NPJ Digital Medicine*, *5*(1), 162. Advance online publication. DOI: 10.1038/s41746-022-00700-y PMID: 36307479

Corral-Acero, J., Margara, F., Marciniak, M., Rodero, C., Loncaric, F., Feng, Y., Gilbert, A., Fernandes, J. F., Bukhari, H. A., Wajdan, A., Martinez, M. V., Santos, M. S., Shamohammdi, M., Luo, H., Westphal, P., Leeson, P., DiAchille, P., Gurev, V., Mayr, M., & Lamata, P. (2020). The 'Digital Twin'to enable the vision of precision cardiology. *European Heart Journal*, *41*(48), 4556–4564. DOI: 10.1093/eurheartj/ehaa159 PMID: 32128588

Dal Mas, F., Massaro, M., Rippa, P., & Secundo, G. (2023). The challenges of digital transformation in healthcare. *Technovation*, *123*, 102716. DOI: 10.1016/j.technovation.2023.102716

Dankar, F. K., & El Emam, K. (2012). The application of differential privacy to health data. *Proceedings of the Joint EDBT/ICDT Workshops*, 158–166. DOI: 10.1145/2320765.2320816

Das, B. C., Zahid, R., Roy, P., & Ahmad, M. (2025). Spatial Data Governance for Healthcare Metaverse. In *Advances in Computer and Electrical Engineering* (pp. 305–330). IGI Global. DOI: 10.4018/979-8-3693-4373-9.ch013

Dayan, I., Roth, H. R., Zhong, A., Harouni, A., Gentili, A., Abidin, A. Z., & Kalpathy-Cramer, J. (2021). Federated learning for predicting clinical outcomes in patients with COVID-19. *Nature Medicine*, *27*(10), 1735–1743. DOI: 10.1038/s41591-021-01506-3 PMID: 34526699

De Alwis, C., Pham, Q.-V., & Liyanage, M. (2023). *"6G for Healthcare," in 6G Frontiers: Towards Future Wireless Systems*. IEEE.

Denecke, K., & Baudoin, C. R. (2022). AI and robotics in transformed health ecosystems. *Frontiers in Medicine*, *9*, 795957. DOI: 10.3389/fmed.2022.795957 PMID: 35872767

Dhanushya, J., Ruba, M., Ponkarthika, M., Soundarya, B., Sakthi Priya, V., Dhanushri, S., & Harikrishnan, S. (2025, April). AI-Powered Multipurpose Agrobot for Precision Farming: Crop Health Management, Fertilizer Recommendation and Yield Prediction. In *2025 International Conference on Recent Advances in Electrical, Electronics, Ubiquitous Communication, and Computational Intelligence (RAEEUCCI)* (pp. 1-6). IEEE.

Dhinakaran, D., Kumar, N. J., Ponnuviji, N. P., & Praveen Kumar, B. (2025). Safeguarding confidentiality and privacy in cloud-enabled healthcare systems with Spectrasafe encryption and dynamic k-anonymity algorithm. *Expert Systems with Applications*, *279*, 127584. DOI: 10.1016/j.eswa.2025.127584

Dhinakaran, D., Ramani, R., Edwin Raja, S., & Selvaraj, D. (2026). Enhancing clinical data security with the contextual polynomial-based data protection model (CPDPM). *Biomedical Signal Processing and Control*, *111*, 108329. DOI: 10.1016/j.bspc.2025.108329

Dhinakaran, D., Selvaraj, D., Dharini, N., Raja, S. E., & Priya, C. S. L. (2023). Towards a novel privacy-preserving distributed multiparty data outsourcing scheme for cloud computing with quantum key distribution. *International Journal of Intelligent Systems and Applications in Engineering*, *12*(2), 286–300.

Dhinakaran, D., Srinivasan, L., Gopalakrishnan, S., & Anish, T. P. (2025). An efficient data mining technique and privacy preservation model for healthcare data using improved darts game optimizer-based weighted deep neural network and hybrid encryption. *Biomedical Signal Processing and Control*, *100*(Part C), 107168. DOI: 10.1016/j.bspc.2024.107168

Diokadan, J., Divine, I. A., Emma, S., Makiwa, R. S., Celine, U., Nicholus, L., & Pasupula, R. (2025). Lupeol acetate from *Cleome viscosa* as a therapeutic candidate for myocardial infarction. *In Silico Pharmacology*, *13*(2), 1–14. DOI: 10.1007/s40203-025-00383-9 PMID: 40620913

Dionisio, J. D. N., Burns, W. G., & Gilbert, R. (2013). 3D virtual worlds and the metaverse: Current status and future possibilities. *ACM Computing Surveys*, *45*(3), 1–38. DOI: 10.1145/2480741.2480751

Divyashree, K. S. (2024). Blockchain Application on Healthcare Services in Metaverse. In *Advances in Medical Education, Research, and Ethics* (pp. 141–158). IGI Global. DOI: 10.4018/979-8-3693-5493-3.ch009

Diwan, S. A. (2025). Federated learning-enhanced sensor fusion for IoT-based distributed health systems: Prioritizing privacy and rapid medical intervention. *Intelligent Decision Technologies*, *19*(6), 4310–4327. DOI: 10.1177/18724981251370441

Domínguez-Rodríguez, S., Liz-López, H., Panizo-LLedot, A., Ballesteros, Á., Dagan, R., Greenberg, D., Gutiérrez, L., Rojo, P., Otheo, E., Galán, J. C., Villanueva, S., García, S., Mosquera, P., Tagarro, A., Moraleda, C., & Camacho, D. (2023). Testing the performance, adequacy, and applicability of an artificial intelligence model for pediatric pneumonia diagnosis. *Computer Methods and Programs in Biomedicine*, *242*, 107765. DOI: 10.1016/j.cmpb.2023.107765 PMID: 37704545

Doshi-Velez, F., & Kim, B. (2017). Towards a rigorous science of interpretable machine learning. *arXiv preprint arXiv:1702.08608.*

Dwork, C., & Roth, A. (2014). The algorithmic foundations of differential privacy. *Foundations and Trends® in Theoretical Computer Science, 9*(3–4), 211–407.

Dwork, C. (2006). Differential privacy. In *Proceedings of the 33rd International Colloquium on Automata, Languages and Programming* (pp. 1–12). DOI: 10.1007/11787006_1

El Rifai, O., Biotteau, M., de Boissezon, X., Megdiche, I., Ravat, F., & Teste, O. (2020). Blockchain-based federated learning in medicine. In *Artificial Intelligence in Medicine* (pp. 214–224). Springer International Publishing., DOI: 10.1007/978-3-030-59137-3_20

ElBedoui, K., Barhoumi, W., & Cho, J. (2025). SoK: Federated Learning and unlearning for medical image analysis. *Expert Systems: International Journal of Knowledge Engineering and Neural Networks, 42*(6), e70063. Advance online publication. DOI: 10.1111/exsy.70063

El-Saleh, A. A., Sheikh, A. M., Albreem, M. A., & Honnurvali, M. S. (2025). The internet of medical things (IoMT): Opportunities and challenges. *Wireless Networks, 31*(1), 327–344. DOI: 10.1007/s11276-024-03764-8

Esteva, A., Robicquet, A., Ramsundar, B., Kuleshov, V., DePristo, M., Chou, K., Cui, C., Corrado, G., Thrun, S., & Dean, J. (2019). A guide to deep learning in healthcare. *Nature Medicine, 25*(1), 24–29. DOI: 10.1038/s41591-018-0316-z PMID: 30617335

European Commission. (2021). *Ethics guidelines for trustworthy AI.* Publications Office of the European Union.

European Commission. (2021). *Proposal for a Regulation laying down harmonised rules on artificial intelligence.* AI Act.

European Commission. (2022). *European Health Data Space: Impact assessment report.*

European Commission. (2022). *Proposal for a regulation laying down harmonised rules on artificial intelligence.* AI Act.

European Health Data Space. (2025). *Regulation (EU) 2025/327 on the use and exchange of electronic health data.*

Faisal, S. M., Ishrat, M., & Khan, W. (2025). Digital Twins in Healthcare: Revolutionizing Patient Care and Medical Operations. In *Digital Twins for Smart Cities and Urban Planning* (pp. 69–89). CRC Press.

Faisal, S. M., Khan, W., & Ishrat, M. (2026). AI-Enhanced Collaboration and Teamwork in Virtual Learning Environments. In *Intelligent Learning Tools, Enhancing Student Skills, and Career Preparedness* (pp. 149–176). IGI Global Scientific Publishing. DOI: 10.4018/979-8-3373-9225-7.ch006

Faisal, S. M., Muniyandy, E., Lokesh, S., & Jayanthi, M. G. (2025). A Random Graph Diffusion Attention Network with Great Wall Construction and Clinical Metadata for Improved Kidney Cancer Diagnosis and Surgical Planning. *Biomedical Materials & Devices*, •••, 1–20. DOI: 10.1007/s44174-025-00447-6

Faridoon, A., & Kechadi, M. T. (2024). *Healthcare data governance, privacy, and security*. In *EAI International Conference on Body Area Networks* (pp. 261–271).

FDA. (2022). *Augmented and virtual reality in medical devices: Regulatory considerations.*

Feng, P., Xi, N., Jin, J., Zhang, J., & Ma, J. (2025). FLASH: Federated graph learning-based malicious bash script detection for industrial cyber–physical systems. *IEEE Transactions on Industrial Informatics*, *21*(6), 4979–4989. Advance online publication. DOI: 10.1109/TII.2025.3552649

Feretzakis, G., Papaspyridis, K., Gkoulalas-Divanis, A., & Verykios, V. S. (2024). Privacy-preserving techniques in generative AI and large language models: A narrative review. *Information (Basel)*, *15*(11), 697. DOI: 10.3390/info15110697

Finlayson, S. G., Subbaswamy, A., Singh, K., Bowers, J., Kupke, A., Zittrain, J., Kohane, I. S., & Saria, S. (2021). The clinician and dataset shift in artificial intelligence. *The New England Journal of Medicine*, *385*(3), 283–286. DOI: 10.1056/NEJMc2104626 PMID: 34260843

Fitzpatrick, K. (2023). Digital literacy, health literacy, and patient safety in AI-supported care. *Journal of Medical Internet Research*, •••, 25.

Fitzpatrick, P. J. (2023). Improving health literacy using the power of digital communications to achieve better health outcomes for patients and practitioners. *Frontiers in Digital Health*, *5*, 1264780. DOI: 10.3389/fdgth.2023.1264780 PMID: 38046643

Floridi, L., & Cowls, J. (2019). A unified framework of five principles for AI in society. *Harvard Data Science Review*, *1*(1).

Floridi, L., Cowls, J., Beltrametti, M., Chatila, R., Chazerand, P., Dignum, V., Luetge, C., Madelin, R., Pagallo, U., Rossi, F., Schafer, B., Valcke, P., & Vayena, E. (2018). AI4People—An ethical framework for a good AI society: Opportunities, risks, principles, and recommendations. *Minds and Machines*, *28*(4), 689–707. DOI: 10.1007/s11023-018-9482-5 PMID: 30930541

Food and Drug Administration. (2023). *Artificial intelligence and machine learning in software as a medical device: Action plan.*

Fuller, A., Fan, Z., Day, C., & Barlow, C. (2020). Digital twin: Enabling technologies, challenges and open research. *IEEE Access : Practical Innovations, Open Solutions*, *8*, 108952–108971. DOI: 10.1109/ACCESS.2020.2998358

G, A., S, A. D., Loganathan, V., Padma, E., Ilavarasan, S., and A, S. (2025), "Federated Learning and Edge AI for Privacy-Preserving Diabetes Prediction in Healthcare," 2025 3rd International Conference on Self Sustainable Artificial Intelligence Systems (ICSSAS), Erode, India, 2025, pp. 1116-1121.

Gade, K., Geyik, S. C., Kenthapadi, K., Mithal, V., & Taly, A. (2019). Explainable AI in Industry. *Proceedings of the 25th ACM SIGKDD International Conference on Knowledge Discovery & Data Mining*, 3203–3204. New York, NY, USA: ACM. DOI: 10.1145/3292500.3332281

Gadekallu, T. R.. (2023). Federated learning for the healthcare metaverse: Concepts, applications, challenges, and future directions. *IEEE Network*, *37*(1), 176–183. DOI: 10.1109/MNET.001.2200227

Gao, X., He, P., Zhou, Y., & Qin, X. (2024). Artificial intelligence applications in smart healthcare. *Future Internet*, *16*(9), 308. DOI: 10.3390/fi16090308

Garbagnati, A., & Wu, L. (2021). Creating Competitive Advantage: Privacy and Security by Design in mHealth and Digital Health Products. *Health Law.*, *34*, 9.

Garg, S., Dev, R., Singh, A. K., Sahani, S., Kumari, K., & Bandyopadhyay, A. (2025), "Edu-Metaverse: A Structured Architecture and Workflow Model for Digital and Blended Learning," 2025 3rd International Conference on Intelligent Systems, Advanced Computing and Communication (ISACC), Silchar, India, 2025, pp. 514-519. DOI: 10.1109/ISACC65211.2025.10969320

Garg, S., Singh, R., & Kaur, K. (2022). Cloud-edge collaboration for healthcare IoT: Challenges and future directions. *Future Generation Computer Systems*, *129*, 1–12.

Gatla, T. R. (2024). Revolutionizing healthcare with AI. *International Journal of Advanced Research and Interdisciplinary Scientific Endeavours*, *1*(2), 61–70.

Gawer, A. (2021). Digital platforms' boundaries: The interplay of firm scope, platform sides, and digital interfaces. *Long Range Planning*, *54*(5), 102045. DOI: 10.1016/j.lrp.2020.102045

Geels, F. W. (2002). Technological transitions as evolutionary reconfiguration processes. *Research Policy*, *31*(8–9), 1257–1274. DOI: 10.1016/S0048-7333(02)00062-8

George, S., Naveen, G., Saifullah, S., & Joe, I. P. (2022, June). An efficient neural network model for pneumonia detection. In 2022 International Conference on Computing, Communication, Security and Intelligent Systems (IC3SIS) (pp. 1-7). IEEE. DOI: 10.1109/IC3SIS54991.2022.9885488

Geyer, R. C., Klein, T., & Nabi, M. (2017). Differentially private federated learning: A client level perspective. *arXiv preprint arXiv:1712.07557.*

Ghatti, S., Yurish, L. A., Shen, H., Rheuban, K., Enfield, K. B., Facteau, N. R., & Dowdell, K. (2023). Digital twins in healthcare: A survey of current methods. *Archives of Clinical and Biomedical Research*, *7*(3), 365–381. DOI: 10.26502/acbr.50170352

Ghosh, S., Bhuniya, T., and Sona, D. R. (2025), "MediNet: An Optimized Networking Architecture for Secure and Efficient Healthcare Data Traffic Management," 2025 Innovations in Power and Advanced Computing Technologies (i-PACT), Surabaya, Indonesia, 2025, pp. 1-8.

Godbin, A. B., & Jasmine, S. G. (2024, July). Pediatric Pneumonia Detection in Chest X-ray Images: A Deep Feature Analysis Approach Enhanced with LightGBM. In *2024 IEEE International Conference on Electronics, Computing and Communication Technologies (CONECCT)* (pp. 1-6). IEEE. DOI: 10.1109/CONECCT62155.2024.10677083

Goktas, P., & Grzybowski, A. (2025). Ethical clinical challenges and trustworthy AI. *Journal of Clinical Medicine*, *14*(5), 1605. DOI: 10.3390/jcm14051605 PMID: 40095575

Gómez Bergin, A. D., & Craven, M. P. (2023). Virtual, augmented, mixed, and extended reality interventions in healthcare: A systematic review of health economic evaluations and cost-effectiveness. *BMC Digital Health*, *1*(1), 53. DOI: 10.1186/s44247-023-00054-9

Gopal, G., Suter-Crazzolara, C., Toldo, L., & Eberhardt, W. (2019). Digital transformation in healthcare–architectures of present and future information technologies. [CCLM]. *Clinical Chemistry and Laboratory Medicine*, *57*(3), 328–335. DOI: 10.1515/cclm-2018-0658 PMID: 30530878

Gor, J., Shah, H., Patel, J., Gupta, R., & Tanwar, S., and Mupaat (2025), "Explainable ML-based Secure Communication Framework for Robotic Telesurgery in Healthcare," 2025 International Conference on Metaverse and Current Trends in Computing (ICMCTC), Subang Jaya, Malaysia, 2025, pp. 1-7. DOI: 10.1109/ICMCTC62214.2025.11196540

Gowthaman, N., Ruba, M., Aswath, S., Hemavarshni, S. N., Bragadeshwaran, R., & Nithish, S. J. (2025, November). Iot Integrated Solution For Smart Vertical Crop Cultivation. In 2025 IEEE 7th International Conference on Computing, Communication and Automation (ICCCA) (pp. 1-6). IEEE.

Grieves, M., & Vickers, J. (2017). Digital twin: Mitigating unpredictable, undesirable emergent behavior in complex systems. In *Transdisciplinary perspectives on complex systems* (pp. 85–113). Springer. DOI: 10.1007/978-3-319-38756-7_4

Grote, T., & Berens, P. (2020). On the ethics of algorithmic decision-making in healthcare. *Journal of Medical Ethics*, *46*(3), 205–211. DOI: 10.1136/medethics-2019-105586 PMID: 31748206

Guerra-Manzanares, A., Lopez, L. J. L., Maniatakos, M., & Shamout, F. E. (2023). *Privacy-preserving machine learning for healthcare*. In Trustworthy ML for Healthcare (pp. 25–40).

Guidotti, R., Monreale, A., Ruggieri, S., Turini, F., Giannotti, F., & Pedreschi, D. (2018). A survey of methods for explaining black box models. *ACM Computing Surveys*, *51*(5), 1–42. DOI: 10.1145/3236009

Güler, O., & Polat, K. (2022). Classification performance of deep transfer learning methods for pneumonia detection from chest x-ray images. *Journal of Artificial Intelligence and Systems*, *4*(1), 107–126.

Gundu, L., Ramachandran, V., Butchi Raju, K., Hossain, R. R., Sreekanth, D., & Putta, P. (2025), "Blockchain-Enabled Decentralized Data Lakes for Secure and Transparent AI-Ready Data Storage," 2025 International Conference on Metaverse and Current Trends in Computing (ICMCTC), Subang Jaya, Malaysia, 2025, pp. 1-4. DOI: 10.1109/ICMCTC62214.2025.11196459

Gupta, R., Patil, M. R., & Thapa, R., Prachi, and Nathani, S. (2025), "AI Driven Nursing Assistant," 2025 International Conference on Electronics, Computing, Communication and Control Technology (ICECCC), Bengaluru, India, 2025, pp. 1-6.

Gupta, S., Sehgal, M., Makkar, R., Jain, S., & Rani, K. (2025), "Next Generation Smart Hospitals: AI, 6G, and IoT Integration," 2025 2nd International Conference on Computational Intelligence and Computing Applications (ICCICA), Samalkha, India, 2025, pp. 1-6. DOI: 10.1109/ICCICA67008.2025.11337707

Gupta, L., Salman, T., Ghubaish, A., Unal, D., Al-Ali, A. K., & Jain, R. (2022). Cybersecurity of multi-cloud healthcare systems. *Applied Soft Computing*, *118*, 108439. DOI: 10.1016/j.asoc.2022.108439

Gupta, M. (2021). Blockchain and artificial intelligence integration for secure 5G healthcare networks. *Computer Communications*, *171*, 137–145.

Gupta, P., Babbar, H., & Rani, S. (2023). Impact of Metaverse in Healthcare. In *SIBF 2023* (pp. 112–118). IEEE.

Habbal, A., Ali, M. K., & Abuzaraida, M. A. (2024). Artificial Intelligence Trust, Risk and Security Management (AI TRiSM): Frameworks, applications, challenges and future research directions. *Expert Systems with Applications*, *240*(122442), 122442. DOI: 10.1016/j.eswa.2023.122442

Haleem, A., Javaid, M., Singh, R. P., & Suman, R. (2023). Digital twin technology in healthcare. *Biomedical Technology*, *4*, 28–38. DOI: 10.1016/j.bmt.2023.02.001

Han, S., Ding, H., Zhao, S., Ren, S., Wang, Z., Lin, J., & Zhou, S. (2024). Practical and robust federated learning with highly scalable regression training. *IEEE Transactions on Neural Networks and Learning Systems*, *35*(10), 13801–13815. DOI: 10.1109/TNNLS.2023.3271859 PMID: 37289609

Ha, P. N., Doucet, A., & Tran, G. S. (2023, February). Vision Transformer for Pneumonia Classification in X-ray Images. In *Proceedings of the 2023 8th International Conference on Intelligent Information Technology* (pp. 185-192). DOI: 10.1145/3591569.3591602

Haque, S. A., Aziz, S. M., & Rahman, M. (2014). Review of cyber-physical system in healthcare. *International Journal of Distributed Sensor Networks*, *10*(4), 217415. DOI: 10.1155/2014/217415

Hasan, M. K., Ghazal, T. M., Saeed, R. A., Pandey, B., Gohel, H., Eshmawi, A. A., Abdel-Khalek, S., & Alkhassawneh, H. M. (2022). A review on security threats, vulnerabilities, and counter measures of 5G enabled Internet-of-Medical-Things. *IET Communications*, *16*(5), 421–432. DOI: 10.1049/cmu2.12301

Hasan, M. R., Ullah, S. M. A., & Islam, S. M. R. (2024). Recent advancement of deep learning techniques for pneumonia prediction from chest X-ray image. *Medica-Report*, *7*, 100106. DOI: 10.1016/j.hmedic.2024.100106

Hollan, J., Hutchins, E., & Kirsh, D. (2000). Distributed cognition: Toward a new foundation for human–computer interaction research. *ACM Transactions on Computer-Human Interaction*, *7*(2), 174–196. DOI: 10.1145/353485.353487

Horgan, D., Pesapane, F., Van der Buckle, M., De Maria, R., Dube, F., Singh, J., & Subbiah, V. (2024). Next-generation sequencing in healthcare systems. *Critical Reviews in Oncology/Hematology*, *201*, 104433. DOI: 10.1016/j.critrevonc.2024.104433 PMID: 38955310

Hosseini Mirmahaleh, S. Y., & Rahmani, A. M. (2025). Federated Learning in Smart Cities. In *Model Optimization Methods for Efficient and Edge AI: Federated Learning Architectures, Frameworks, and Applications* (pp. 351–389). IEEE. DOI: 10.1002/9781394219230.ch18

Huang, S.-C., Pareek, A., Seyyedi, S., Banerjee, I., & Lungren, M. P. (2022). Fusion of medical imaging and electronic health records using deep learning: A systematic review and implementation guidelines. *NPJ Digital Medicine*, *5*(1), 136. DOI: 10.1038/s41746-020-00341-z PMID: 33083571

Huang, Y., Li, Y. J., & Cai, Z. (2023). Security and privacy in metaverse: A comprehensive survey. *Big Data Mining and Analytics*, *6*(2), 234–247. DOI: 10.26599/BDMA.2022.9020047

Hulsen, T. (2023). Applications of the metaverse in medicine and healthcare. *Journal of Laboratory and Precision Medicine*. PMID: 38939198

Hùng, N. V., & Quân, T. M. (2023). Enterprise Data-Governance Operating Models for Scalable, High-Trust Healthcare Analytics and Decision Support Programs. *Orient Journal of Emerging Paradigms in Artificial Intelligence and Autonomous Systems*, *13*(12), 1–11.

Hussain, S. F. M., Karthikeyan, R., Ramamoorthi, S., Arafat, I. S., & Asif, N. A. H. (2024), "Security Enhanced Smart Hospital Management System Achieved through SELSTM Technique," 2024 2nd International Conference on Artificial Intelligence Trends and Pattern Recognition (ICAITPR), Hyderabad, India, 2024, pp. 1-11. DOI: 10.1109/ICAITPR63242.2024.10960016

Hwang, S. O., & Majeed, A. (2024). Analysis of federated learning paradigm in medical domain: Taking COVID-19 as an application use case. *Applied Sciences (Basel, Switzerland)*, *14*(10), 4100. Advance online publication. DOI: 10.3390/app14104100

International Organisation for Standardisation. (2023). *ISO/IEC 23894:2023—Information technology—Artificial intelligence—Guidance on risk management*.

Iqbal, A. I., Aamir, A., Hammad, A., Hafsa, H., Basit, A., Oduoye, M. O., Anis, M. W., Ahmed, S., Younus, M. I., & Jabeen, S. (2024). Immersive technologies in healthcare. *Journal of Primary Care & Community Health*, *15*, 21501319241293311. DOI: 10.1177/21501319241293311 PMID: 39439304

Ishrat, M., Khan, W., Faisal, S. M., & Al Farsi, M. M. (2025). Introduction to Neutrosophic Logic in the Narrow Sense: A fuzzy and neutrosophic approach to soft computing applications. In *Soft Computing and Machine Learning* (pp. 83–101). CRC Press.

Ishrat, M., Khan, W., Faisal, S. M., Al Farsi, M. M., & Farooqui, N. A. (2025). Digital Twins Future Prospects in Smart Cities: Challenges of Urban Planning. In *Digital Twins for Smart Cities and Urban Planning* (pp. 53–68). CRC Press.

Islam[1], N., Ezcurra, V., Rader[1], J., Margondai, A., Willox, S., Von Ahlefeldt, C., & Mouloua, M. (2026). Transparency for Trust: Enhancing Acceptance and System Integration of Intelligent AI in Healthcare. *Intelligent Human Systems Integration: Disruptive and Innovative Technologies*, 285.

Islam, S. M. R., Kwak, D., Kabir, M. H., Hossain, M., & Kwak, K. S. (2022). The Internet of Things for health care: A comprehensive survey. *IEEE Access : Practical Innovations, Open Solutions*, *3*, 678–708. DOI: 10.1109/ACCESS.2015.2437951

Islam, T. U., Mohammed, N., & Alhadidi, D. (2024). Privacy preserving vertical distributed learning for health data. *Journal of Surveillance. Security and Safety*, *5*(1), 1–18. DOI: 10.20517/jsss.2023.28

Ivanovic, M., & Macos, D. (2023), "Applications of Artificial Intelligence Methods in Medicine," *2023 International Conference on Information Technology (ICIT)*, Amman, Jordan, 2023, pp. 349-354. DOI: 10.1109/ICIT58056.2023.10226107

Jain, P., & Chawla, P. (2021), "A Novel Smart Healthcare System Design for Internet of Health Things," *2021 International Conference on Innovative Computing, Intelligent Communication and Smart Electrical Systems (ICSES)*, Chennai, India, 2021, pp. 1-8. DOI: 10.1109/ICSES52305.2021.9633869

Jalnnavar, A., Kanakareddi, S. G., Handur, V. S., Chikaraddi, A., & Giraddi, S. (2023, September). Disease Prediction Model Using Deep Transfer Learning. In International Conference on Intelligent Computing Systems and Applications (pp. 13-29). Singapore: Springer Nature Singapore.

Jamshidi, M., Hoang, D. T., & Nguyen, D. N. (2024). CNN-FL for biotechnology industry empowered by Internet-of-BioNano Things and digital twins. *IEEE Internet of Things Magazine*, *7*(5), 54–63. Advance online publication. DOI: 10.1109/IOTM.001.2400081

Jaszcz, A., Połap, D., & Srivastava, G. (2025). MultiMOORA-guided federated learning with knowledge-distillation stabilization for health monitoring devices as protection against poisoning attacks. *IEEE Internet of Things Journal*. Advance online publication. DOI: 10.1109/JIOT.2025.3638263

Javed, L., Anjum, A., Yakubu, B. M., Iqbal, M., Moqurrab, S. A., & Srivastava, G. (2023). ShareChain: Blockchain-enabled model for sharing patient data using federated learning and differential privacy. *Expert Systems: International Journal of Knowledge Engineering and Neural Networks*, *40*(5), e13131. Advance online publication. DOI: 10.1111/exsy.13131

Jayapradha, J., Boovaneswari, S., Sabarivadivelan, S., Uvarajan, D., & Sarathi, S. (2023), "A Telehealth System Driven by Artificial Intelligence for Effective Patient Consultation and Diagnosis in Hospitals," *2023 International Conference on System, Computation, Automation and Networking (ICSCAN)*, Puducherry, India, 2023, pp. 1-6. DOI: 10.1109/ICSCAN58655.2023.10395119

Jayasree, A., Gayatri, T., Vaishnavi, L., Jyothi, N. V. S. K. A., & Pujitha, M., and S. I. S. P. (2025), "Investing in the Virtual World: Why Digital Twins are the Next Big Opportunity," *2025 International Conference on Emerging Technologies in Computing and Communication (ETCC)*, Bangalore, India, 2025, pp. 1-7. DOI: 10.1109/ETCC65847.2025.11108421

Jayaweera, R., Agrawal, H., & Karie, N. M. (2025). Federated security for privacy preservation of healthcare data in edge-cloud environments. *Sensors (Basel)*, *25*(16), 5108. DOI: 10.3390/s25165108 PMID: 40871971

Jin, Q., Chen, Z., Xia, J., & Luo, J. (2023). Large language models for medical diagnosis tasks. *Nature Machine Intelligence*, *5*, 1–12.

Jones, D., Galvez, R., Evans, D., Hazelton, M., Rossiter, R., Irwin, P., & Fealy, S. (2023). XR technologies in primary medical care. *Virtual Worlds*, *2*(4), 359–373. DOI: 10.3390/virtualworlds2040021

Joshi, M., Pal, A., & Sankarasubbu, M. (2022). Federated learning for healthcare domain—Pipeline, applications and challenges. *ACM Transactions on Computing for Healthcare*, *3*(4), 40. Advance online publication. DOI: 10.1145/3533708

Kahalkar, K., & Vyas, U. (2024), "AI for Personalized Nutrition and Healthcare Management," 2024 2nd DMIHER International Conference on Artificial Intelligence in Healthcare, Education and Industry (IDICAIEI), Wardha, India, 2024, pp. 1-6. DOI: 10.1109/IDICAIEI61867.2024.10842744

Kairouz, P., McMahan, H. B., Avent, B., Bellet, A., Bennis, M., Bhagoji, A. N., ... & Zhao, S. (2021). Advances and open problems in federated learning. Foundations and trends® in machine learning, 14(1–2), 1-210.

Kairouz, P., McMahan, H. B., Avent, B., Bellet, A., Bennis, M., Bhagoji, A. N., … Zhao, S. (2021). Advances and open problems in federated learning. *Foundations and Trends® in Machine Learning, 14*(1–2), 1–210.

Kairouz, P., McMahan, H. B., Avent, B., Bellet, A., Bennis, M., Bhagoji, A. N., & Zhao, S. (2021). Advances and open problems in federated learning. *Foundations and Trends in Machine Learning*, *14*(1–2), 1–210. DOI: 10.1561/2200000083

Kameswaran, A., Nanthakumar, K., & Ruba, M. (2017). High performance pre-computation based self-controlled precharge-free content-addressable memory. *Journal of Electronics and Communication Systems*, *2*, 1–9.

Kang, J., Wen, J., Ye, D., Lai, B., Wu, T., Xiong, Z., Nie, J., Niyato, D., Zhang, Y., & Xie, S. (2024, February). Blockchain-Empowered Federated Learning for Healthcare Metaverses: User-Centric Incentive Mechanism With Optimal Data Freshness. *IEEE Transactions on Cognitive Communications and Networking*, *10*(1), 348–362. DOI: 10.1109/TCCN.2023.3316643

Karaca, C., & Aslan, H. (2021). A readiness model for artificial intelligence in healthcare institutions. *International Journal of Medical Informatics*, •••, 148.

Kaur, R., Singh, B., & Kumar, R. (2025), "Smart Disease Management: AI-Driven Approaches for Surveillance, Prediction, and Public Health Mitigation," 2025 7th International Symposium on Advanced Electrical and Communication Technologies (ISAECT), Mohali, Punjab, India, 2025, pp. 1-6. DOI: 10.1109/ISAECT68904.2025.11318794

Kausar, S., Naqvi, N., Akbar, S., Ratan Shah, S., Abbas, K., & Alam, M.. (2025). Socioeconomic indicators and their influence on mental health: A data-driven approach utilizing Python and R. *International Journal of Epidemiology and Health Sciences*, *6*, e92. Advance online publication. DOI: 10.51757/IJEHS.6.2025.720978

Kermany, D., Zhang, K., & Goldbaum, M. (2018), "Labeled Optical Coherence Tomography (OCT) and Chest X-Ray Images for Classification", Mendeley Data, V2, dataset description ma eslai cite grnuDOI: 10.17632/rscbjbr9sj.2

Khan, L. U., Han, Z., Saad, W., Hossain, E., Guizani, M., & Hong, C. S. (2022). Digital twin of wireless systems: Overview, taxonomy, challenges, and opportunities. *IEEE Communications Surveys and Tutorials*, *24*(4), 2230–2254. Advance online publication. DOI: 10.1109/COMST.2022.3198273

Kharbas, V. K., Raghu, N., & Choudhury, P. "Enhancing Rule-Based Methods for Pulmonary Effusion Diagnosis," *2024 15th International Conference on Computing Communication and Networking Technologies (ICCCNT)*, Kamand, India, 2024, pp. 1-5, DOI: 10.1109/ICCCNT61001.2024.10724858

Kohan, A., Xu, J., Xiao, L., Wu, X., Kukkar, A., Hussain, S., ... & Acharya, U. R. (2026). Human-Centered Pathways to Trustworthy AI in Healthcare: A Comparative Analysis of Explainable AI, Human-in-the-Loop, Hybrid AI, and Uncertainty Quantification Techniques.

Kompa, B., Snoek, J., & Beam, A. L. (2021). Second opinion needed: Communicating uncertainty in medical machine learning. *NPJ Digital Medicine*, *4*(1), 4. DOI: 10.1038/s41746-020-00367-3 PMID: 33402680

Kosanam, S., & Pasupula, R. (2024). Artificial intelligence approach in identification of differentially expressed genes of methyl glycoside against myocardial infarction. *Advances in Traditional Medicine*, *24*(1), 243–252. DOI: 10.1007/s13596-023-00691-5

Krithika, S., Jayachandran, T., Raghapriya, N. R., Ruba, M., Janani, C., & Sathiyavathi, S. (2025, April). An Effective Denial of Service Texture Features from Malware Grayscale Image. In 2025 3rd International Conference on Artificial Intelligence and Machine Learning Applications Theme: Healthcare and Internet of Things (AIMLA) (pp. 1-7). IEEE. DOI: 10.1109/AIMLA63829.2025.11041501

Kul, S., Celtek, S. A., & Balci, S. (2025). AI-enhanced power management strategies for next-generation hybrid electric vehicles: Deep reinforcement learning and predictive analytics. *2025 14th International Symposium on Advanced Topics in Electrical Engineering (ATEE)*, 1–6. DOI: 10.1109/ATEE66006.2025.11299906

Kumar, R. Kishore, Pandidurai, M., and Senthil Kamalesh, M. S. C. (2023), "Design of IoT-Based Rural Health Helper using Natural Language Processing," 2023 4th International Conference on Electronics and Sustainable Communication Systems (ICESC), Coimbatore, India, 2023, pp. 328-333.

Kumar, A., Kalpana, V., & Hariram, V. (2023), "Artificial Intelligence-Based Health Monitoring System on IoT Platform," *2023 Second International Conference on Augmented Intelligence and Sustainable Systems (ICAISS)*, Trichy, India, 2023, pp. 1458-1463.

Lakhan, A., Mohammed, M. A., Nedoma, J., Martinek, R., Tiwari, P., Vidyarthi, A., Alkhayyat, A., & Wang, W. (2023). Federated-learning based privacy preservation and fraud-enabled blockchain IoMT system for healthcare. *IEEE Journal of Biomedical and Health Informatics*, *27*(2), 664–672. DOI: 10.1109/JBHI.2022.3165945 PMID: 35394919

Lakshmi, D., Kondurkar, I., Kumar, R., & Banerjee, R. (2024). *Intelligent Healthcare Systems in the Metaverse*. In The Metaverse for the Healthcare Industry (pp. 17–32).

Lăzăroiu, G., Gedeon, T., Halicka, K., & Szpilko, D. (2025). Generative artificial intelligence-driven medical digital twin technologies in blockchain Internet of Things wearable sensor and computer vision-based extended reality healthcare metaverse. *Engineering Management in Production and Services, 17*(3).

Lazaros, K., Koumadorakis, D. E., Vrahatis, A. G., & Kotsiantis, S. (2024). Federated learning: Navigating the landscape of collaborative intelligence. *Electronics (Basel), 13*(23), 4744. Advance online publication. DOI: 10.3390/electronics13234744

Lehne, M., Luijten, S., Vom Felde Genannt Imbusch, P., & Thun, S. (2019). The use of FHIR in digital health - A review of the scientific literature. *Studies in Health Technology and Informatics*, *267*, 52–58. PMID: 31483254

Letafati, M., & Otoum, S. (2023), "Global Differential Privacy for Distributed Metaverse Healthcare Systems," 2023 International Conference on Intelligent Metaverse Technologies & Applications (iMETA), Tartu, Estonia, 2023, pp. 01-08. DOI: 10.1109/iMETA59369.2023.10294469

Letafati, M.. (2023). Digital healthcare in the metaverse: Insights into privacy and security. *IEEE Consumer Electronics Magazine*, *12*(4), 80–90. DOI: 10.1109/MCE.2023.3267412

Letafati, M., & Otoum, S. (2024, May). Digital Healthcare in the Metaverse: Insights into Privacy and Security. *IEEE Consumer Electronics Magazine*, *13*(3), 80–89. DOI: 10.1109/MCE.2023.3334494

Lian, Z., Yang, Q., Wang, W., Zeng, Q., Alazab, M., Zhao, H., & Su, C. (2022). DEEP-FEL: Decentralized, efficient and privacy-enhanced federated edge learning for healthcare cyber physical systems. *IEEE Transactions on Network Science and Engineering*, *9*(5), 3558–3569. Advance online publication. DOI: 10.1109/TNSE.2022.3175945

Li, K., Lau, B. P. L., Yuan, X., Ni, W., Guizani, M., & Yuen, C. (2023, December 15). Toward Ubiquitous Semantic Metaverse: Challenges, Approaches, and Opportunities. *IEEE Internet of Things Journal, 10*(24), 21855–21872. DOI: 10.1109/JIOT.2023.3302159

Lisetti, C., Amini, R., & Yasavur, U. (2015). Now all together: Overview of virtual health assistants emulating face-to-face health interview experience. *Künstliche Intelligenz, 29*(2), 161–172. DOI: 10.1007/s13218-015-0357-0

Li, T., Sahu, A. K., Talwalkar, A., & Smith, V. (2020). Federated learning: Challenges, methods, and future directions. *IEEE Signal Processing Magazine, 37*(3), 50–60. DOI: 10.1109/MSP.2020.2975749

Li, T., Sahu, A. K., Zaheer, M., Sanjabi, M., Talwalkar, A., & Smith, V. (2020). Federated optimization in heterogeneous networks. *Proceedings of Machine Learning and Systems, 2*, 429–450.

Liu, X., Yu, J., Liu, Y., Gao, Y., Mahmoodi, T., Lambotharan, S., & Tsang, D. H. K. (2023). Distributed intelligence in wireless networks. *IEEE Open Journal of the Communications Society, 4*, 1001–1039. DOI: 10.1109/OJCOMS.2023.3265425

Liu, X., Zhang, Y., Chen, H., & Xie, T. (2023). Secure and governed AI systems: Challenges and opportunities. *ACM Computing Surveys, 56*(2), 1–36.

Li, X., Gu, Y., Dvornek, N., Staib, L. H., Ventola, P., & Duncan, J. S. (2020). Multi-site fMRI analysis using privacy-preserving federated learning and domain adaptation: ABIDE results. *Medical Image Analysis, 65*(101765), 101765. DOI: 10.1016/j.media.2020.101765 PMID: 32679533

Li, Y.. (2024). The next generation of healthcare ecosystem in metaverse: Concept, framework, and challenges. [ScienceDirect journal article]. *Digital Health.*

Loftus, T. J., Ruppert, M. M., Shickel, B., Ozrazgat-Baslanti, T., Balch, J. A., Efron, P. A., Upchurch, G. R.Jr, Rashidi, P., Tignanelli, C., Bian, J., & Bihorac, A. (2022). Federated learning for preserving data privacy in collaborative healthcare research. *Digital Health, 8*, 20552076221134456. DOI: 10.1177/20552076221134455 PMID: 36325438

Longoni, C., Bonezzi, A., & Morewedge, C. K. (2019). Resistance to medical Artificial intelligence. *The Journal of Consumer Research, 46*(4), 629–650. DOI: 10.1093/jcr/ucz013

Lundberg, S. M., & Lee, S. I. (2017). A unified approach to interpreting model predictions. *Advances in Neural Information Processing Systems*, •••, 4765–4774.

Lu, T., Ji, S., Jin, W., Yang, Q., Luo, Q., & Ren, T. L. (2023). Biocompatible biosensors. *Sensors (Basel)*, *23*(6), 2991. DOI: 10.3390/s23062991 PMID: 36991702

Lyell, D., & Coiera, E. (2017). Automation bias and verification complexity: A systematic review. *Journal of the American Medical Informatics Association : JAMIA*, *24*(2), 423–431. DOI: 10.1093/jamia/ocw105 PMID: 27516495

Magalhães, R., et al. (2024). Mixed reality in the operating room: A systematic review. *Journal/venue as indexed in PMC.*

Mahajan, N., & Malpe, K. (2026). Interoperability and Standardization in Healthcare System Integration: Interfacing Wearable Devices with Electronic Health Records. *Artificial Intelligence and Machine Learning in Neurology*, *1*, 243–281. DOI: 10.1002/9781394389131.ch10

Malviya, R., Verma, S., Sundram, S., & Shah, H. (2025), "Chapter 13: Future Trends and Innovations of AI in Healthcare," in *Digital Blockchain: Big Data, Artificial Intelligence, and Virtual Reality in Healthcare Ecosystem*, De Gruyter, 2025, pp. 237-252. DOI: 10.1515/9783111574288-013

Mandel, J. C.. (2021). SMART on FHIR: A standards-based, interoperable apps platform for electronic health records. *Journal of the American Medical Informatics Association : JAMIA*, *28*(7), 1278–1287. DOI: 10.1093/jamia/ocab061 PMID: 26911829

Manojkumar, K., Sengar, A. S., Jyothi, A. P., & Faisal, S. M. (2025). Energy-efficient routing and predictive sink mobility in mobile wireless sensor networks using reflection equivariant quantum neural network and star fish optimization algorithms. *Sustainable Computing : Informatics and Systems*, *48*, 101231. DOI: 10.1016/j.suscom.2025.101231

Marzano, L., Bardill, A., Fields, B., Herd, K., Veale, D., Grey, N., & Moran, P. (2015). The application of mHealth to mental health: Opportunities and challenges. *The Lancet. Psychiatry*, *2*(10), 942–948. DOI: 10.1016/S2215-0366(15)00268-0 PMID: 26462228

Matta, S. S., & Bolli, M. (2025). Federated learning for privacy-preserving healthcare data sharing: Enabling global AI collaboration. *American Journal of Scholarly Research and Innovation*, *4*(1), 320–351. DOI: 10.63125/jga18304

Mayer, R. C., Davis, J. H., & Schoorman, F. D. (1995). An integrative model of organisational trust. *Academy of Management Review*, *20*(3), 709–734. DOI: 10.2307/258792

Maza, S., & Megouas, O. (2021). Framework for trustworthiness in software development. *International Journal of Performability Engineering*, *17*(2), 241. DOI: 10.23940/ijpe.21.02.p8.241252

Mazzocca, C., Romandini, N., Colajanni, M., & Montanari, R. (2023). FRAMH: A federated learning risk-based authorization middleware for healthcare. *IEEE Transactions on Computational Social Systems*, *10*(4), 1679–1690. DOI: 10.1109/TCSS.2022.3210372

Mbunge, E., Jiyane, S. E., & Muchemwa, B. (2022). Emotive sensory web in virtual healthcare. *Sensors International*, *3*, 100134. DOI: 10.1016/j.sintl.2021.100134

McCradden, M. D., Baba, A., Saha, A., Ahmad, S., Boparai, K., Fadaiefard, P., & Cusimano, M. D. (2020). Ethical concerns around use of artificial intelligence in health care research from the perspective of patients with meningioma, caregivers and health care providers: A qualitative study. *CMAJ Open*, *8*(1), E90–E95. DOI: 10.9778/cmajo.20190151 PMID: 32071143

McMahan, B.. (2017). Communication-efficient learning of deep networks from decentralised data. *Proceedings of AISTATS*.

McMahan, B., Moore, E., Ramage, D., Hampson, S., & Arcas, B. A. (2017, April). Communication-efficient learning of deep networks from decentralized data. In *Artificial intelligence and statistics* (pp. 1273–1282). PMLR.

McMahan, H. B., Moore, E., Ramage, D., Hampson, S., & Arcas, B. A. (2017). Communication-efficient learning of deep networks from decentralized data. *Proceedings of AISTATS*, 1273–1282.

Mehra, S., Singh, S. K., Kumar, S., Dubey, H., Arya, V., & Gupta, B. B. (2024). Transformative Approach for Prediction of Lung Disease Using Lung X-ray Images.

Melis, L., Song, C., De Cristofaro, E., & Shmatikov, V. (2019). Exploiting unintended feature leakage in collaborative learning. *Proceedings of the 2019 IEEE Symposium on Security and Privacy*, 691–706. https://doi.org/DOI: 10.1109/SP.2019.00029

Mennella, C., Maniscalco, U., De Pietro, G., & Esposito, M. (2024). Ethical and regulatory challenges of AI. *Heliyon*, *10*(4), e26297. DOI: 10.1016/j.heliyon.2024.e26297 PMID: 38384518

Mesko, B., & Győrffy, Z. (2023). The rise of the empowered physician in the digital health era: Viewpoint. *Journal of Medical Internet Research*, *25*, e40616. DOI: 10.2196/40616 PMID: 30912758

Meskó, B., & Topol, E. J. (2023). The imperative for regulatory oversight of large language models (or generative AI) in healthcare. *NPJ Digital Medicine*, *6*(1), 120. DOI: 10.1038/s41746-023-00873-0 PMID: 37414860

Messaoud, S., Bouaafia, S., Maraoui, A., Khriji, L., Ammari, A. C., & Machhout, M. (2022). AI-based virtual healthcare center. *The Canadian Journal of Infectious Diseases & Medical Microbiology*, *2022*, 6786203. PMID: 35069953

Misal, S. R., Mohan, L., Sundararajan, S. K., Bathala, B., Majumdar, S., & Sivakumar, C. (2025), "Telemedicine and Remote Patient Monitoring: Enhancing Access to Healthcare Through IoT and AI Technologies," 2025 First International Conference on Advances in Computer Science, Electrical, Electronics, and Communication Technologies (CE2CT), Bhimtal, Nainital, India, 2025, pp. 306-310. DOI: 10.1109/CE2CT64011.2025.10941287

Moassefi, M., Rouzrokh, P., Conte, G. M., Vahdati, S., Fu, T., Tahmasebi, A., Younis, M., Farahani, K., Gentili, A., Kline, T., Kitamura, F. C., Huo, Y., Kuanar, S., Younis, K., Erickson, B. J., & Faghani, S. (2023). Reproducibility of deep learning algorithms developed for medical imaging analysis: A systematic review. *Journal of Digital Imaging*, *36*(5), 2306–2312. DOI: 10.1007/s10278-023-00870-5 PMID: 37407841

Mohammadzadeh, Z., Shokri, M., Saeidnia, H. R., Kozak, M., Marengo, A., Lund, B. D., Ausloos, M., & Ghiasi, N. (2024). Principles of digital professionalism for the metaverse in healthcare. *BMC Medical Informatics and Decision Making*, *24*(1), 201. DOI: 10.1186/s12911-024-02607-y PMID: 39039522

Muinga, N., Magare, S., Monda, J., English, M., Fraser, H., Powell, J., & Paton, C. (2020). Digital health Systems in Kenyan Public Hospitals: A mixed-methods survey. *BMC Medical Informatics and Decision Making*, *20*(1), 2. DOI: 10.1186/s12911-019-1005-7 PMID: 31906932

Murmu, A., Kumar, P., Namasudra, S., & Reddy, M. R. (2025). GAN-based federated adversarial learning for enhancing security towards consumer digital ecosystems. *IEEE Transactions on Consumer Electronics*, *71*(1), 1102–1114. Advance online publication. DOI: 10.1109/TCE.2024.3522018

Musamih, A., Yaqoob, I., Salah, K., Jayaraman, R., Al-Hammadi, Y., Omar, M., & Ellahham, S. (2022). Metaverse in healthcare. *IEEE Consumer Electronics Magazine*, *12*(4), 33–46. DOI: 10.1109/MCE.2022.3223522

Myrzashova, R., Alsamhi, S. H., Shvetsov, A. V., Hawbani, A., & Wei, X. (2023). Blockchain meets federated learning. *IEEE Internet of Things Journal*, *10*(16), 14418–14437. DOI: 10.1109/JIOT.2023.3263598

Mystakidis, S. (2022). Metaverse. *Encyclopedia*, *2*(1), 486–497. DOI: 10.3390/encyclopedia2010031

Nambiar, R., & Nanjundegowda, R. (2024) "Harnessing Medical Imaging Applications: Survey on 3D Deep Learning Models for Image Segmentation," *2024 International Conference on Communication, Control, and Intelligent Systems (CCIS)*, Mathura, India, 2024, pp. 1-6, DOI: 10.1109/CCIS63231.2024.10932049

Nambiar, R., & Nanjundegowda, R. (2024, September). A Comprehensive Review of AI and Deep Learning Applications in Dentistry: From Image Segmentation to Treatment Planning [JRC]. *J Robot Control*, *5*(6), 1744–1752.

Nambiar, R., & Nanjundegowda, R. (2025, October). Detection of Missing Tooth Regions Using Deep Learning in Panoramic Radiographs for Dental Implant Planning. *Eng. Technol. Appl. Sci. Res.*, *15*(5), 28071–28076. DOI: 10.48084/etasr.13101

Naresh, V. S., Thamarai, M., & Allavarpu, V. D. (2023). Privacy-preserving deep learning in medical informatics. *Artificial Intelligence Review*, *56*(S1, Suppl 1), 1199–1241. DOI: 10.1007/s10462-023-10556-7

Nasra, P. (2024, August). Convolution Neural Network: A Proposed Method for Detecting Pneumonia from X-Ray Images. In *2024 Second International Conference on Intelligent Cyber Physical Systems and Internet of Things (ICoICI)* (pp. 1692-1697). IEEE. DOI: 10.1109/ICoICI62503.2024.10696221

National Institute of Standards and Technology. (2023). *Artificial Intelligence Risk Management Framework (AI RMF 1.0).*

National Institute of Standards and Technology. (2024). *Artificial Intelligence Risk Management Framework: Generative Artificial Intelligence Profile (NIST-AI-600-1).*

Nazi, Z. A., & Peng, W. (2024). Large language models in healthcare and medical domain: A review. [). MDPI.]. *Informatics (MDPI)*, *11*(3), 57. DOI: 10.3390/informatics11030057

Nelson, C. A., Pérez-Chada, L. M., Creadore, A., Li, S. J., Lo, K., Manjaly, P., Pournamdari, A. B., Tkachenko, E., Barbieri, J. S., Ko, J. M., Menon, A. V., Hartman, R. I., & Mostaghimi, A. (2020). Patient perspectives on the use of artificial intelligence for skin cancer screening: A qualitative study: A qualitative study. *JAMA Dermatology*, *156*(5), 501–512. DOI: 10.1001/jamadermatol.2019.5014 PMID: 32159733

Neshat, M., Ahmed, M., Askari, H., Thilakaratne, M., & Mirjalili, S. (2024). Hybrid Inception Architecture with Residual Connection: Fine-tuned Inception-ResNet Deep Learning Model for Lung Inflammation Diagnosis from Chest Radiographs. *Procedia Computer Science*, *235*, 1841–1850. DOI: 10.1016/j.procs.2024.04.175

Newitt, D. C., Zhang, Z., Gibbs, J. E., Partridge, S. C., Chenevert, T. L., Rosen, M. A., Bolan, P. J., Marques, H. S., Aliu, S., Li, W., Cimino, L., Joe, B. N., Umphrey, H., Ojeda-Fournier, H., Dogan, B., Oh, K., Abe, H., Drukteinis, J., Esserman, L. J., & Hylton, N. M. (2019). Test-retest repeatability and reproducibility of ADC measures by breast DWI: Results from the ACRIN 6698 trial: Test-Retest Repeatability of Breast DWI. *Journal of Magnetic Resonance Imaging*, *49*(6), 1617–1628. DOI: 10.1002/jmri.26539 PMID: 30350329

Nguyen, D. C., Ding, M., Pathirana, P. N., Seneviratne, A., Li, J., & Vincent Poor, H. (2021). Federated learning for internet of things: A comprehensive survey. *IEEE Communications Surveys and Tutorials*, *23*(3), 1622–1658. DOI: 10.1109/COMST.2021.3075439

Nguyen, D. C., Pham, Q. V., Pathirana, P. N., Ding, M., Seneviratne, A., Lin, Z., Dobre, O., & Hwang, W. J. (2022). Federated learning for smart healthcare. *ACM Computing Surveys*, *55*(3), 1–37. DOI: 10.1145/3501296

Nivedhitha, D. P., Madhumitha, G., Janani Sri, J., Jayashree, S., Surya, J., & Divya, D. M. (2024), "Conversational AI for Healthcare to Improve Member Efficiency," *2024 International Conference on Science Technology Engineering and Management (ICSTEM)*, Coimbatore, India, 2024, pp. 1-6. DOI: 10.1109/ICSTEM61137.2024.10561046

OECD. (2024). *AI in health: Huge potential, huge risks*. OECD Publishing.

OECD. (2024). *AI in Health: Huge potential, huge risks*. OECD Publishing.

Okegbile, S. D., Cai, J., Niyato, D., & Yi, C. (2022). Human digital twin for personalized healthcare: Vision, architecture and future directions. *IEEE Network*, *37*(2), 262–269. DOI: 10.1109/MNET.118.2200071

Okegbile, S. D., Cai, J., Zheng, H., Chen, J., & Yi, C. (2023). Differentially private federated multi-task learning framework for enhancing human-to-virtual connectivity in human digital twin. *IEEE Journal on Selected Areas in Communications*, *41*(11), 3533–3547. DOI: 10.1109/JSAC.2023.3310106

Ostrom, E. (2010). Polycentric systems for coping with collective action and global environmental change. *Global Environmental Change*, *20*(4), 550–557. DOI: 10.1016/j.gloenvcha.2010.07.004

Othman, S. B., Chakraborty, C., Singh, S., & Frikha, M. A. (2025). Federated learning-enabled digital twins for privacy-preserving cardiovascular disease detection in consumer electronics. *IEEE Transactions on Consumer Electronics*, 1. Advance online publication. DOI: 10.1109/TCE.2025.3634581

Ouchani, S., Boudouaia, M. A., & Tasidou, A. (2025). PRISM: A privacy safeguard for smart multiservices. *IEEE Software*, *42*(5), 107–115. Advance online publication. DOI: 10.1109/MS.2025.3542853

Oulefki, A., Amira, A., & Foufou, S. (2025). Digital twins and AI transforming healthcare systems through innovation and data-driven decision making. *Health Technology (Hong Kong)*, •••, 1–23.

Oyekan, B. (2024). Developing privacy-preserving federated learning models for collaborative health data analysis across multiple institutions without compromising data security. *Journal of Knowledge Learning and Science Technology ISSN: 2959-6386 (Online)*, *3*(3), 139–164. DOI: 10.60087/jklst.vol3.n3.p139-164

Palacholla, R. S., Fischer, N., Coleman, A., Agboola, S., Kirley, K., Felsted, J., Katz, C., Lloyd, S., & Jethwani, K. (2019). Provider-and patient-related barriers to and facilitators of digital health technology adoption for hypertension management: Scoping review. *JMIR Cardio*, *3*(1), e11951. DOI: 10.2196/11951 PMID: 31758771

Panwar, A., & Gupta, S. (2022). Deep learning models for early detection of pneumonia using chest X-ray images. In Proceedings of the International Conference on Paradigms of Communication, Computing and Data Sciences: PCCDS 2021 (pp. 701-709). Springer Singapore. DOI: 10.1007/978-981-16-5747-4_60

Pan, Z., Wang, H., Wan, J., Zhang, L., Huang, J., & Shen, Y. (2024). Efficient federated learning for pediatric pneumonia on chest X-ray classification. *Scientific Reports*, *14*(1), 23272. Advance online publication. DOI: 10.1038/s41598-024-74491-5 PMID: 39375440

Papadimitriou, O., Kanavos, A., & Maragoudakis, M. (2023, July). Automated pneumonia detection from chest x-ray images using deep convolutional neural networks. In 2023 14th International Conference on Information, Intelligence, Systems & Applications (IISA) (pp. 1-4). IEEE. DOI: 10.1109/IISA59645.2023.10345859

Paparova, D., Aanestad, M., Vassilakopoulou, P., & Bahus, M. K. (2023). Data governance spaces. *Information and Organization*, *33*(1), 100451. DOI: 10.1016/j.infoandorg.2023.100451

Park, C. W., Seo, S. W., Kang, N., Ko, B., Choi, B. W., Park, C. M., Chang, D. K., Kim, H., Kim, H., Lee, H., Jang, J., Ye, J. C., Jeon, J. H., Seo, J. B., Kim, K. J., Jung, K.-H., Kim, N., Paek, S., Shin, S.-Y., & Yoon, H. J. (2020). Artificial intelligence in health care: Current applications and issues. *Journal of Korean Medical Science*, *35*(42), e379. DOI: 10.3346/jkms.2020.35.e379 PMID: 33140591

Park, S. M., & Kim, Y. G. (2022). A metaverse: Taxonomy, components, applications, and open challenges. *IEEE Access : Practical Innovations, Open Solutions, 10*, 4209–4251. DOI: 10.1109/ACCESS.2021.3140175

Park, S., & Kim, Y. (2023). Virtual hospitals and metaverse healthcare services: Policy and practice implications. *Health Policy and Technology, 12*(1), 100721. PMID: 36683761

Pasupuleti, M. K., & Services, N. E. (2025). *Next-generation extended Reality (XR): A unified framework for integrating AR, VR, and AI-driven immersive technologies.* DOI: 10.62311/nesx/rrv325

Patel, M., Dayan, I., Fishman, E. K., Flores, M., Gilbert, F. J., Guindy, M., Koay, E. J., Rosenthal, M., Roth, H. R., & Linguraru, M. G. (2023). Accelerating artificial intelligence: How federated learning can protect privacy, facilitate collaboration, and improve outcomes. *Health Informatics Journal, 29*(4), 14604582231207744. DOI: 10.1177/14604582231207744 PMID: 37864543

Patel, P., & Hiriyanna, G. S. (2022). Pneumonia detection in x-ray chest images based on cnn and data augmentation. *International Journal for Research in Applied Science and Engineering Technology, 10*(7), 4639–4654. DOI: 10.22214/ijraset.2022.46031

Patidar, M., Pandey, G., & Koolagudi, S. G., S, K. K., & Chandra, V. (2024). Enhancing Paediatric Healthcare: Deep Learning-Based Pneumonia Diagnosis from Children's Chest X-rays. *IC3-2024: Proceedings of the 2024 Sixteenth International Conference on Contemporary Computing*, 128–135. https://doi.org/DOI: 10.1145/3675888.3676041

Pati, S., Baid, U., Edwards, B., Sheller, M., Wang, S.-H., Reina, G. A., Foley, P., Gruzdev, A., Karkada, D., Davatzikos, C., Sako, C., Ghodasara, S., Bilello, M., Mohan, S., Vollmuth, P., Brugnara, G., Preetha, C. J., Sahm, F., Maier-Hein, K., & Bakas, S. (2022). Federated learning enables the use of big data for rare cancer boundary detection. *Nature Communications, 13*(1), 7346. DOI: 10.1038/s41467-022-33407-5 PMID: 36470898

Pawassar, C. M., & Tiberius, V. (2021). Virtual reality in health care: Bibliometric analysis. *JMIR Serious Games, 9*(4), e32721. DOI: 10.2196/32721 PMID: 34855606

Pimentel, D., Gonçalves, J., & Nunes, N. J. (2022). Immersive virtual reality for medical training and education: A systematic review. *Journal of Medical Systems, 46*(5), 1–15.

Piwek, L., Ellis, D. A., Andrews, S., & Joinson, A. (2016). The rise of consumer health wearables: Promises and barriers. *PLoS Medicine*, *13*(2), e1001953. DOI: 10.1371/journal.pmed.1001953 PMID: 26836780

Plsek, P. E., & Greenhalgh, T. (2001). Complexity science: The challenge of complexity in health care. *BMJ (Clinical Research Ed.)*, *323*(7313), 625–628. DOI: 10.1136/bmj.323.7313.625 PMID: 11557716

Poovithaa, M., Ruba, M., Ponkarthika, M., Ragul, N., Ragul, V., & Sangeetha, K. (2025, November). IoT Smart Traffic Control System for Hill Roads with Emergency Vehicle Priority. In 2025 IEEE 7th International Conference on Computing, Communication and Automation (ICCCA) (pp. 1-6). IEEE.

Powell, R. A., Singh, S., & Torous, J. (2022). Patient trust and engagement in AI-based healthcare: A cross-sectional survey. *Digital Health*, •••, 8.

Pratap, A., Patel, Y. S., Yadav, R. N., Ahmadian, A., & Yadav, A. K. (2025). Containerized Internet of Medical Things and Serverless Computing for Smart Healthcare Systems. In *AI-Driven Smart Healthcare: Powered by Hyperscale Computing and Next Generation Networks* (pp. 49–60). IEEE. DOI: 10.1002/9781394297061.ch03

Protection, F. D. (2018). General data protection regulation (GDPR). *Intersoft Consulting, Accessed in October, 24*(1).

Punukollu, M. (2022). AI-driven genomic sequencing. *Los Angeles Journal of Intelligent Systems and Pattern Recognition*, *2*, 293–329.

Qayyum, A., Ahmad, K., Ahsan, M. A., Al-Fuqaha, A., & Qadir, J. (2021). Collaborative federated learning for healthcare: Multi-modal COVID-19 diagnosis at the edge. arXiv. https://arxiv.org/abs/2101.07511

Quan, X., Wang, K., Pan, J., & Fang, Z. (2026). Artificial intelligence in outpatient management: A simulation-based study in a Chinese tertiary hospital. *Frontiers in Artificial Intelligence*, *8*, 1696586. Advance online publication. DOI: 10.3389/frai.2025.1696586 PMID: 41561186

Quinn, T. P., Jacobs, S., Senadeera, M., Le, V., & Coghlan, S. (2022). The three ghosts of medical AI: Can the black-box present deliver? *Artificial Intelligence in Medicine*, *124*(102158), 102158. DOI: 10.1016/j.artmed.2021.102158 PMID: 34511267

Qu, Z., Li, Y., Liu, B., Gupta, D., & Tiwari, P. (2023). DTQFL: A digital twin-assisted quantum federated learning framework for intelligent diagnosis in healthcare. *IEEE Journal of Biomedical and Health Informatics*, *27*(12). Advance online publication. DOI: 10.1109/JBHI.2023.3303401 PMID: 37552590

Radianti, J., Majchrzak, T. A., Fromm, J., & Wohlgenannt, I. (2020). A systematic review of immersive virtual reality applications for higher education: Design elements, lessons learned, and research agenda. *Computers & Education*, *147*, 103778. DOI: 10.1016/j.compedu.2019.103778

Raghu, N.. (2025). Blockchain-Enhanced GAN Image Encryption Scheme for Cloud Computing. In Joshi, H. (Eds.), *Intelligent Systems and IoT Applications in Clinical Health* (pp. 367–392). IGI Global Scientific Publishing., DOI: 10.4018/979-8-3693-8990-4.ch016

Raghupathi, W., & Raghupathi, V. (2014). Big data analytics in healthcare: Promise and potential. *Health Information Science and Systems*, *2*(1), 3. DOI: 10.1186/2047-2501-2-3 PMID: 25825667

Rahman, M. A., & Al-Hazzaa, S. (2024), "Next-Generation Virtual Hospital: Integrating Discriminative and Large Multi-Modal Generative AI for Personalized Healthcare," GLOBECOM 2024 - 2024 IEEE Global Communications Conference, Cape Town, South Africa, 2024, pp. 3509-3514. DOI: 10.1109/GLOBECOM52923.2024.10901624

Rahman, M. A., Hossain, M. S., & Alrajeh, N. A. (2022). Securing IoT-based healthcare systems: Ransomware, privacy, and resilience challenges. *Future Generation Computer Systems*, *129*, 307–321.

Rajawat, A. S., Arora, R. K., Muqeem, M., Faisal, S. M., & Jamal, M. K. (2025). Enhancing IoT Efficiency by Minimizing Latency and Boosting Real-Time Processing with Edge Computing. *SN Computer Science*, *6*(6), 715. DOI: 10.1007/s42979-025-04192-x

Raji, I. D., Smart, A., White, R. N., Mitchell, M., Gebru, T., Hutchinson, B., & Barnes, P. (2020). Closing the AI accountability gap: Defining an end-to-end framework for internal algorithmic auditing. *Proceedings of FAT*. DOI: 10.1145/3351095.3372873

Rajkomar, A., Dean, J., & Kohane, I. (2019). Machine learning in medicine. *The New England Journal of Medicine*, *380*(14), 1347–1358. DOI: 10.1056/NEJMra1814259 PMID: 30943338

Rajkomar, A., Hardt, M., Howell, M. D., Corrado, G., & Chin, M. H. (2022). Ensuring fairness in machine learning to advance health equity. *Annals of Internal Medicine*, *175*(6), 866–872. DOI: 10.7326/M21-2749 PMID: 30508424

Raju, V. V. R., Ranaveer, I., Alabdeli, H. M., Selvaprasanth, P., & Raghatate, K. S., and S, L. S. (2025), "AI-Powered Real-Time Medical Diagnosis for Low-Resource Settings: A CNN-Based Edge AI and Blockchain-Integrated Solution," 2025 International Conference on Metaverse and Current Trends in Computing (ICMCTC), Subang Jaya, Malaysia, 2025, pp. 1-4. DOI: 10.1109/ICMCTC62214.2025.11196500

Ramani, R., Edwin Raja, S., Dhinakaran, D., Jagan, S., & Prabaharan, G. (2025). MapReduce-based big data framework using associative Kruskal poly kernel classifier for diabetic disease prediction. *MethodsX*, *14*, 103210. DOI: 10.1016/j.mex.2025.103210 PMID: 40026593

Rameez, M., & Logashree, M. J. (2024, October). Pneumonia Detection using Machine Learning Techniques. In 2024 8th International Conference on I-SMAC (IoT in Social, Mobile, Analytics and Cloud)(I-SMAC) (pp. 1803-1808). IEEE. DOI: 10.1109/I-SMAC61858.2024.10714803

Rani, S., Chauhan, M., Kataria, A., & Khang, A. (2023). *IoT equipped intelligent distributed framework*. In Springer Nature Singapore (pp. 97–114).

Rao, D. T. V. Dharmajee, Vidyadhari, C., Barathy, R., Afzal, M., Sargari, S., and Anakath, A. S. (2025), "Neuro-Symbolic AI-Driven Data Warehouses: Self-Learning Architectures for Dynamic Schema Evolution and Adaptive Query Optimization," 2025 International Conference on Metaverse and Current Trends in Computing (ICMCTC), Subang Jaya, Malaysia, 2025, pp. 1-5.

Rasouli, H., & Valmohammadi, C. (2020). Proposing a conceptual framework for customer identity and access management: A qualitative approach. *Global Knowledge, Memory and Communication*, *69*(1/2), 94–116. DOI: 10.1108/GKMC-02-2019-0014

Ratcliffe, J., Soave, F., Bryan-Kinns, N., Tokarchuk, L., & Farkhatdinov, I. (2021, May). Extended reality (XR) remote research: A survey of drawbacks and opportunities. In *Proceedings of the 2021 CHI conference on human factors in computing systems* (pp. 1-13). DOI: 10.1145/3411764.3445170

Rauniyar, A., Hagos, D. H., Jha, D., Håkegård, J. E., Bagci, U., Rawat, D. B., & Vlassov, V. (2024). Federated learning for medical applications: A taxonomy, current trends, challenges, and future research directions. *IEEE Internet of Things Journal*, *11*(5), 7374–7398. DOI: 10.1109/JIOT.2023.3329061

Ravikumar, A. S., Atamuratova, Z., Ashirova, A., Jurayev, K., & Hayitova, M. (2025). Comprehensive evaluation of AI-driven systems in modern hospital environments. In *Advances in Computational Intelligence and Robotics* (pp. 61–88). IGI Global Scientific Publishing. DOI: 10.4018/979-8-3373-2787-7.ch003

Ravikumar, R. S., Manujakshi, Aarthi, S., Urazbaeva, Y., & Tamilselvi, S. (2025). Navigating data privacy, security, and regulatory challenges in healthcare AI ensuring fairness, bias mitigation, interpretability, and trust. In *Transformative Role of Transformer Models in Healthcare* (pp. 25–54). IGI Global Scientific Publishing. DOI: 10.4018/979-8-3373-2038-0.ch002

Ravikumar, R. N., & Aarthi, S. (2025). AI-powered synergistic robotics and IoT ecosystems for predictive and preventive healthcare. In *Robotics and IoT Synergy in Next-Generation Healthcare* (pp. 1–32). IGI Global Scientific Publishing., DOI: 10.4018/979-8-3373-5447-7.ch001

Ravikumar, R. N., Aarthi, S., Dilshodbek, A., Satheesh Kumar, A., Eshkaraev, S., & Shanmugam, K. B. (2025). Integrating blockchain, smart contracts, and AI for decentralized healthcare in the metaverse. In *Blockchain-Based Healthcare Management in the Metaverse* (pp. 261–294). IGI Global Scientific Publishing., DOI: 10.4018/979-8-3373-1225-5.ch010

Ravikumar, R. N., Aarthi, S., Masharipova, G., Niyazova, N., Salaeva, N., & Buriyeva, D. (2025). Enhancing clinical decision-making and operational efficiency in healthcare using edge computing. In *Building Data-Driven Edge Systems for Business Success* (pp. 191–224). IGI Global Scientific Publishing., DOI: 10.4018/979-8-3373-1147-0.ch008

Ribeiro, M. T., Singh, S., & Guestrin, C. (2016). "Why should I trust you?" Explaining the predictions of any classifier. *Proceedings of the 22nd ACM SIGKDD International Conference on Knowledge Discovery and Data Mining*, 1135–1144.

Ribino, P., Ciampi, M., Islam, S., & Papastergiou, S. (2022). Swarm intelligence model for securing healthcare. *Procedia Computer Science*, *210*, 149–156. DOI: 10.1016/j.procs.2022.10.131

Rieke, N., Hancox, J., Li, W., Milletari, F., Roth, H. R., Albarqouni, S., Bakas, S., Galtier, M. N., Landman, B. A., Maier-Hein, K., Ourselin, S., Sheller, M., Summers, R. M., Trask, A., Xu, D., Baust, M., & Cardoso, M. J. (2020). The future of digital health with federated learning. *NPJ Digital Medicine*, *3*(1), 119. DOI: 10.1038/s41746-020-00323-1 PMID: 33015372

Rieke, N., Hancox, J., Li, W., Milletarì, F., Roth, H. R., Albarqouni, S., Bakas, S., Galtier, M. N., Landman, B. A., Maier-Hein, K., Ourselin, S., Sheller, M., Summers, R. M., Trask, A., Xu, D., Baust, M., & Cardoso, M. J. (2020). The future of digital health with federated learning. *npj. Digital Medicine*, *3*, 119. PMID: 33015372

Riva, G., Wiederhold, B. K., & Mantovani, F. (2022). Virtual reality in mental health: Advances and challenges. *Cyberpsychology, Behavior and Social Networking, 25*(1), 1–6. PMID: 34964667

Roehrs, A., Da Costa, C. A., & da Rosa Righi, R. (2017). OmniPHR: A distributed architecture model to integrate personal health records. *Journal of Biomedical Informatics, 71*, 70–81. DOI: 10.1016/j.jbi.2017.05.012 PMID: 28545835

Roychowdhury, S.. (2023). Hallucination-minimized data-to-answer framework for financial decision-makers. *2023 IEEE International Conference on Big Data (BigData)*, 4693–4702. DOI: 10.1109/BigData59044.2023.10386232

Ruba, M., Ponkarthika, M., Parameshwari, V., Girinath, V. P., Soundarya, B., Janani, M., & Santhini, C. (2025, February). Enhancing underwater tunnel safety through smart inspection: An ROV-based system with AI-powered crack detection using Canny edge detection. In Proceedings of the 2025 3rd International Conference on Intelligent Systems, Advanced Computing and Communication (ISACC) (pp. 1067–1072). IEEE. DOI: 10.1109/ISACC.2025

Ruba, M., Preetha, D. S., Ponkarthika, M., Gomathi, V., Sudha, E., & Pratheeba, C. (2026c). Smart Pedagogies and Intelligent Campuses: Reimagining Higher Education in the Digital Age. In Harnessing Geospatial Information Systems for Sustainable Economic and Regional Development (pp. 29-54). IGI Global Scientific Publishing.

Ruba, M., Ashwin Prabhu, G., Deka, J., Kavitha, D., Sathiya, S., & Pavithra, S. (2026a). Empowering learners and educators: The transformative role of conversational AI in personalized education and student support. In Assayed, S. (Ed.), *Enhancing student support and learning through conversational AI* (pp. 163–190). IGI Global Scientific Publishing., DOI: 10.4018/979-8-3373-3316-8.ch007

Ruba, M., Ashwin Prabhu, G., Robinson Joel, M., Vishnu Priya, K., Dharshani, L., & Dharani, R. (2026b). Integrating emerging technologies for organizational agility: An interdisciplinary approach to digital transformation. In Roache, D. (Ed.), *High performance leadership for organizational excellence: Innovation, technology, and resilience* (pp. 63–92). IGI Global Scientific Publishing., DOI: 10.4018/979-8-3373-6207-6.ch003

Ruba, M., Girinath, V. P., Ponkarthika, M., Santhini, C., Sakthi Priya, V., & Hemalatha, R. (2023, December). Design and implementation of smart internet-based real-time control of rover with artificial intelligence. In *2023 International Conference on Energy, Materials and Communication Engineering (ICEMCE)* (pp. 1–5). IEEE. DOI: 10.1109/ICEMCE2023

Rudin, C. (2019). Stop explaining black box machine learning models for high stakes decisions and use interpretable models instead. *Nature Machine Intelligence*, *1*(5), 206–215. DOI: 10.1038/s42256-019-0048-x PMID: 35603010

Saadat, H., Aboumadi, A., Mohamed, A., Erbad, A., & Guizani, M. (2021, June). Hierarchical federated learning for collaborative IDS in IoT applications. In *2021 10th Mediterranean Conference on Embedded Computing (MECO)* (pp. 1-6). IEEE. DOI: 10.1109/MECO52532.2021.9460304

Sabile, J. M. G., Zhang, P., Parwani, A. V., Chobrutsiky, B., Gandhi, A. P., & Srisuwananukorn, A. (2025). Toward Clinically Actionable Machine Learning and Artificial Intelligence Algorithms in Acute Leukemia: A Systematic Narrative Review. *Acta Haematologica, 148*(5), 587–603. DOI: 10.1159/000547532 PMID: 40706562

Sadilek, A., Liu, L., Nguyen, D., Kamruzzaman, M., Serghiou, S., Rader, B., Ingerman, A., Mellem, S., Kairouz, P., Nsoesie, E. O., MacFarlane, J., Vullikanti, A., Marathe, M., Eastham, P., Brownstein, J. S., Arcas, B. A. Y., Howell, M. D., & Hernandez, J. (2021). Privacy-first health research with federated learning. *NPJ Digital Medicine*, *4*(1), 132. DOI: 10.1038/s41746-021-00489-2 PMID: 34493770

Sai, S., Chamola, V., Choo, K.-K. R., Sikdar, B., & Rodrigues, J. J. (2024). Federated learning and NFT-based privacy-preserving medical-data-sharing scheme for intelligent diagnosis in smart healthcare. *IEEE Internet of Things Journal*, *11*(4), 5568–5577. Advance online publication. DOI: 10.1109/JIOT.2023.3308991

Sajed, S., Sanati, A., Garcia, J. E., Rostami, H., Keshavarz, A., & Teixeira, A. (2023). The effectiveness of deep learning vs. traditional methods for lung disease diagnosis using chest X-ray images: A systematic review. *Applied Soft Computing*, *147*, 110817. DOI: 10.1016/j.asoc.2023.110817

Sakharwade, V. R., Urkude, O. P., Thakur, S., Lokulwar, P., & Dasarwar, P. (2025), "Cloud-Based Healthcare Monitoring System," 2025 3rd International Conference on Intelligent Data Communication Technologies and Internet of Things (IDCIoT), Bengaluru, India, 2025, pp. 218-223. DOI: 10.1109/IDCIOT64235.2025.10915056

Salim, M. M., & Park, J. H. (2023). Federated learning-based secure electronic health record sharing scheme in medical informatics. *IEEE Journal of Biomedical and Health Informatics*, *27*(2), 617–624. Advance online publication. DOI: 10.1109/JBHI.2022.3174823 PMID: 35560105

Samek, W., Montavon, G., Vedaldi, A., Hansen, L. K., & Müller, K. R. (2019). *Explainable AI: Interpreting, explaining and visualizing deep learning*. Springer. DOI: 10.1007/978-3-030-28954-6

Sanjalawe, Y., Alqurashi, T., Alharbi, Z. H., Makhadmeh, S. N., & Alsharaiah, M. (2025). Adaptive graph attention-based federated learning for IoT intrusion detection: Mitigating poisoning attacks. *PeerJ. Computer Science*, *11*, e3281. DOI: 10.7717/peerj-cs.3281

Sanjaya, F. N., Balakrishnan, S., Sindiramutty, S. R., & Narputro, P. (2025), "XAI Technology in EEG Signal-Based Disease Detection Models," 2025 International Conference on Metaverse and Current Trends in Computing (ICMCTC), Subang Jaya, Malaysia, 2025, pp. 1-7. DOI: 10.1109/ICMCTC62214.2025.11196271

Santarsiero, F., Schiuma, G., Carlucci, D., & Helander, N. (2023). Role of innovation labs. *Technovation*, *122*, 102640. DOI: 10.1016/j.technovation.2022.102640

Santhini, C., Ruba, M., Sakthi Priya, V., & Hemalatha, R. (2025). Intercultural communication and assessment practices in the integration of AI with education. In *Generative AI Approaches to Sustainable Development in Higher Education*. IGI Global. DOI: 10.4018/979-8-3693-5623-4.ch010

Satav, S. D., Hasan, D. S., Pitchai, R., Mohanaprakash, T. A., Sultanuddin, S. J., & Boopathi, S. (2023). NGIoT in healthcare systems. In Global, I. G. I. (Ed.), (pp. 307–330).

Satyanarayanan, M. (2017). The emergence of edge computing. *Computer*, *50*(1), 30–39. DOI: 10.1109/MC.2017.9

Schmidt-Erfurth, U., Sadeghipour, A., Gerendas, B. S., Waldstein, S. M., & Bogunović, H. (2018). Artificial intelligence in retina. *Progress in Retinal and Eye Research*, *67*, 1–29. DOI: 10.1016/j.preteyeres.2018.07.004 PMID: 30076935

Seah, J. C. Y. (2021). Effect of a comprehensive deep-learning model on the accuracy of chest x-ray interpretation: A multi-reader, multi-case study. The Lancet Digital Health.

Sedlmair, M., Meyer, M., & Munzner, T. (2020). Criteria for rigor in visualization design study. *IEEE Transactions on Visualization and Computer Graphics*, *26*(1), 87–97. DOI: 10.1109/TVCG.2019.2934539

Selvaraj, D., Jeno, J., Ramani, R., Dhinakaran, D., & Prabaharan, G. (2025). AFCP data security model for EHR data using blockchain. *Journal of Cybersecurity and Information Management*, *15*(1), 22–33. DOI: 10.54216/JCIM.150103

Selvaraj, P., Kanmani, P., Naga Malleswari, Y. J., Burugari, V. K., & Mangalampalli, S. S. (2024). Infrastructural data visualization and improved user interfaces of energy consumption in smart cities. In Sagar, S., Poongodi, T., Dhanaraj, R. K., & Padmanaban, S. (Eds.), *Cyber physical energy systems* (pp. 357–397). Wiley., DOI: 10.1002/9781394173006.ch11

Seyhan, A. A., & Carini, C. (2019). Are innovation and new technologies in precision medicine paving a new era in patients centric care? *Journal of Translational Medicine*, *17*(1), 114. Advance online publication. DOI: 10.1186/s12967-019-1864-9 PMID: 30953518

Seymour, N. E., Gallagher, A. G., Roman, S. A., O'brien, M. K., Bansal, V. K., Andersen, D. K., & Satava, R. M. (2002). Virtual reality training improves operating room performance: Results of a randomized, double-blinded study. *Annals of Surgery*, *236*(4), 458–464. DOI: 10.1097/00000658-200210000-00008 PMID: 12368674

Shafik, W. (2025). Patient-Centered Healthcare: Trust and Transparency Through Technology. In *AI and Blockchain Applications for Privacy and Security in Smart Medical Systems* (pp. 309–338). IGI Global Scientific Publishing.

Shafique, A., Farea, A. A., & Qureshi, K. N. (2025). AI as a new paradigm for distributed healthcare networks. In *Artificial Intelligence-Based Smart Healthcare Systems* (pp. 97–118). Academic Press. DOI: 10.1016/B978-0-443-26476-4.00012-5

Shaheen, M., Farooq, M. S., Umer, T., & Kim, B. S. (2022). Applications of federated learning: Taxonomy, challenges, and research trends. *Electronics (Basel)*, *11*(4), 670. Advance online publication. DOI: 10.3390/electronics11040670

Shah, N. D., Steyerberg, E. W., & Kent, D. M. (2021). Big data and predictive analytics: Recalibrating expectations. *Journal of the American Medical Association*, *320*(1), 27–28. DOI: 10.1001/jama.2018.5602 PMID: 29813156

Shanmugaraja, T., Ruba, M., Priya, V. S., Venkatesh, T., Supriya, M., & Nallamuthu, M. (2023, September). ECG noise elimination using an FPGA version of a modified error normalized LMS adaptive filter. In AIP Conference Proceedings (Vol. 2764, No. 1, p. 060033). AIP Publishing LLC. DOI: 10.1063/5.0144367

Sheller, M. J., Edwards, B., Reina, G. A., Martin, J., Pati, S., Kotrotsou, A., Milchenko, M., Xu, W., Marcus, D., Colen, R. R., & Bakas, S. (2020). Federated learning in medicine: Facilitating multi-institutional collaborations without sharing patient data. *Scientific Reports*, *10*(1), 12598. DOI: 10.1038/s41598-020-69250-1 PMID: 32724046

Shickel, B., Tighe, P. J., Bihorac, A., & Rashidi, P. (2018). Deep EHR: A survey of recent advances in deep learning techniques for electronic health record analysis. *IEEE Journal of Biomedical and Health Informatics*, *22*(5), 1589–1604. DOI: 10.1109/JBHI.2017.2767063 PMID: 29989977

Shi, W., Cao, J., Zhang, Q., Li, Y., & Xu, L. (2016). Edge computing: Vision and challenges. *IEEE Internet of Things Journal*, *3*(5), 637–646. DOI: 10.1109/JIOT.2016.2579198

Shi, Y., Yu, H., & Leung, C. (2023). Towards fairness-aware federated learning. *IEEE Transactions on Neural Networks and Learning Systems*, *35*(9), 11922–11938. DOI: 10.1109/TNNLS.2023.3263594 PMID: 37037249

Shokri, R., Stronati, M., Song, C., & Shmatikov, V. (2017). Membership inference attacks against machine learning models. *Proceedings of the IEEE Symposium on Security and Privacy (SP)*, 3–18. DOI: 10.1109/SP.2017.41

Siau, K., & Wang, W. (2020). Building trust in artificial intelligence, machine learning, and robotics. *Cutting-Edge Technologies for Enterprise Systems*, 109–132.

Siddiqi, R., & Javaid, S. (2024). Deep learning for pneumonia detection in chest x-ray images: A comprehensive survey. *Journal of Imaging*, *10*(8), 176. DOI: 10.3390/jimaging10080176 PMID: 39194965

Singhal, K., Tu, T., Gottweis, J., Sayres, R., Wulczyn, E., Hou, L., & Natarajan, V. (2023). Towards expert-level medical question answering with large language models. *Nature*, *620*, 187–193.

Singh, Y., Farrelly, C. M., Hathaway, Q. A., Leiner, T., Jagtap, J., Carlsson, G. E., & Erickson, B. J. (2023). Topological data analysis in medical imaging: Current state of the art. *Insights Into Imaging*, *14*(1), 58. Advance online publication. DOI: 10.1186/s13244-023-01413-w PMID: 37005938

Slater, M., & Sanchez-Vives, M. V. (2016). Enhancing our lives with immersive virtual reality. *Frontiers in Robotics and AI*, *3*, 74. DOI: 10.3389/frobt.2016.00074

Sodero, S., Dhungana, N., & Sandoe, F. (2025). Vital mobilities of medical oxygen: Theorising oxygen justice. *Social Science & Medicine*, *364*, 117464. DOI: 10.1016/j.socscimed.2024.117464 PMID: 39579440

Song, C., Ristenpart, T., & Shmatikov, V. (2017). Machine learning models that remember too much. *ACM CCS*, 587–601.

Sowan, B. I., Qattous, H., Fasha, M., & Altarawneh, A. (2025). Enhanced Healthcare Through Metaverse Integration: Explainable AI and Blockchain for Trust, Security, and Immersive Experiences. *2025 1st International Conference on Computational Intelligence Approaches and Applications (ICCIAA)*, 1–7.

Sravanthi, G., Karuna, G., Selvi, S., Mohamed, H., & Jenifer, S., and K, V. (2025), "Ethical AI for Data Governance: A Fairness-Centric Approach to Responsible Decision-Making in Enterprise Systems," 2025 International Conference on Metaverse and Current Trends in Computing (ICMCTC), Subang Jaya, Malaysia, 2025, pp. 1-5. DOI: 10.1109/ICMCTC62214.2025.11196531

Steinhubl, S. R., Muse, E. D., & Topol, E. J. (2015). The emerging field of mobile health. *Science Translational Medicine*, *7*(283), 283rv3. Advance online publication. DOI: 10.1126/scitranslmed.aaa3487 PMID: 25877894

Stephanie, V., Khalil, I., & Atiquzzaman, M. (2023). Digital twin enabled asynchronous SplitFed learning in e-healthcare systems. *IEEE Journal on Selected Areas in Communications*, *41*(11), 3650–3661. DOI: 10.1109/JSAC.2023.3310103

Stephanie, V., Khalil, I., & Atiquzzaman, M. (2024, February). DSFL: A Decentralized SplitFed Learning Approach for Healthcare Consumers in the Metaverse. *IEEE Transactions on Consumer Electronics*, *70*(1), 2107–2115. DOI: 10.1109/TCE.2024.3360994

Stoumpos, A. I., Kitsios, F., & Talias, M. A. (2023). Technology acceptance in healthcare. *International Journal of Environmental Research and Public Health*, *20*(4), 3407. DOI: 10.3390/ijerph20043407 PMID: 36834105

Strubell, E., Ganesh, A., & McCallum, A. (2019). Energy and policy considerations for deep learning in NLP. *Proceedings of the 57th Annual Meeting of the ACL*, 3645–3650. DOI: 10.18653/v1/P19-1355

Subbaswamy, A., & Saria, S. (2020). From development to deployment: Dataset shift, causality, and shift-stable models in health AI. *Biostatistics (Oxford, England)*, *21*(2), 345–352. DOI: 10.1093/biostatistics/kxz041 PMID: 31742354

Sung, H., Kim, M., Park, J., Shin, N., & Han, Y. (2024). Effectiveness of virtual reality in healthcare education: A systematic literature review and meta-analysis. *Sustainability (Basel)*, *16*(19), 8520. DOI: 10.3390/su16198520

Sun, L., Tian, J., & Muhammad, G. (2023). FedKC: Personalized federated learning with robustness against model poisoning attacks in the metaverse for consumer health. *IEEE Journal of Biomedical and Health Informatics*, *27*(11), 5643–5654. DOI: 10.1109/JBHI.2023.3304128

Sun, T., He, X., & Li, Z. (2023). Digital twin in healthcare. *Digital Health*, *9*, 20552076221149651. DOI: 10.1177/20552076221149651 PMID: 36636729

Sun, Z., Kairouz, P., Suresh, A. T., & McMahan, H. B. (2022). Can you really backdoor federated learning? *Proceedings of the 35th Conference on Neural Information Processing Systems (NeurIPS)*.

Su, X., An, L., Cheng, Z., & Weng, Y. (2023). Cloud–edge collaboration-based bi-level optimal scheduling for intelligent healthcare systems. *Future Generation Computer Systems*, *141*, 28–39. DOI: 10.1016/j.future.2022.11.005

Swarup, L. P. D. R, R. Jain, R. N, L. A. Bewoor and V. M. Kumar, "MRI-Based Epilepsy Seizure Detection Using Combined Approach of CNN With SVM Networks," *2024 IEEE 4th International Conference on ICT in Business Industry & Government (ICTBIG)*, Indore, India, 2024, pp. 1-6, DOI: 10.1109/ICTBIG64922.2024.10911487

Tabassum, A., Ghaznavi, I., Abd-Alrazaq, A., & Qadir, J. (2025). Exploring the application of AI and extended reality technologies in metaverse-driven mental health solutions: Scoping review. *Journal of Medical Internet Research*, *27*, e72400. DOI: 10.2196/72400 PMID: 40829151

Taimoor, N., & Rehman, S. (2022). Reliable and resilient AI and IoT-based personalised healthcare services: A survey. Retrieved from https://arxiv.org/abs/2209.05457

Tanenbaum, A. S., & Van Steen, M. (2017). *Distributed systems: Principles and paradigms* (2nd ed.). Pearson.

Tang, P.. (2025). The efficacy of virtual reality on the rehabilitation of musculoskeletal disorders: An umbrella review. *Journal of Clinical Medicine*, *14*(3), 623. DOI: 10.3390/jcm14030623

Tang, Y., Pan, D., Qin, P., & Lv, L. (2023). Lattice-based group signature with message recovery for federal learning. *Applied Sciences (Basel, Switzerland)*, *13*(15), 9007. DOI: 10.3390/app13159007

Tan, T. F., Li, Y., Lim, J. S., Gunasekeran, D. V., Teo, Z. L., Ng, W. Y., & Ting, D. S. (2022). Metaverse and virtual healthcare in ophthalmology. *Asia-Pacific Journal of Ophthalmology*, *11*(3), 237–246. DOI: 10.1097/APO.0000000000000537 PMID: 35772084

Tanveer, F., Iradat, F., Iqbal, W., Alsagri, H. S., Alhakbani, H. A. A., Ahmad, A., & Khan, F. A. (2025). Balancing privacy and performance in healthcare: A federated learning framework for sensitive data. *Digital Health*, *11*(20552076251381770), 20552076251381770. DOI: 10.1177/20552076251381769 PMID: 41018509

Thangalakshmi, S., Mohankumar, N., Jayanthi, L. N., Blessy, Y. M., Meenakshi, R., & Rajmohan, M. (2025), "Telemedicine Platforms with Cloud-Based AI-Driven Diagnostics in Hospitals," *2025 International Conference on Visual Analytics and Data Visualization (ICVADV)*, Tirunelveli, India, 2025, pp. 137-143. DOI: 10.1109/ICVADV63329.2025.10961133

Tjoa, E., & Guan, C. (2020). A survey on explainable artificial intelligence (XAI): Toward medical XAI. *IEEE Transactions on Neural Networks and Learning Systems, 32*(11), 4793–4813. DOI: 10.1109/TNNLS.2020.3027314 PMID: 33079674

Tonekaboni, S., Joshi, S., McCradden, M. D., & Goldenberg, A. (2019). What clinicians want: Contextualizing explainable machine learning for clinical end use. Retrieved from https://arxiv.org/abs/1905.05134

Tonekaboni, S., Joshi, S., McCradden, M. D., & Goldenberg, A. (2023). What clinicians want: Contextualizing explainable machine learning for clinical end use. *Proceedings of Machine Learning Research, 126*, 1–21.

Topol, E. (2019). *Deep medicine: How artificial intelligence can make healthcare human again*—basic Books.

Topol, E. (2023). *Deep medicine: How artificial intelligence can make healthcare human again* (updated perspectives). Basic Books.

Topol, E. (2019). *Deep medicine: how artificial intelligence can make healthcare human again.*

Topol, E. (2019). *Deep medicine: How artificial intelligence can make healthcare human again.* Basic Books.

Topol, E. J. (2019). High-performance medicine: The convergence of human and artificial intelligence. *Nature Medicine, 25*(1), 44–56. DOI: 10.1038/s41591-018-0300-7 PMID: 30617339

Torkzadehmahani, R., Nasirigerdeh, R., Blumenthal, D. B., Kacprowski, T., List, M., Matschinske, J., Spaeth, J., Wenke, N. K., & Baumbach, J. (2022). Privacy-preserving artificial intelligence techniques in biomedicine. *Methods of Information in Medicine, 61*(S 01), e12–e27. DOI: 10.1055/s-0041-1740630

Trivedi, J., Tahir, M., & Isoaho, J. (2025). AI-enhanced threat intelligence in remote patient monitoring: A survey on recent advances, challenges and future research directions. *IEEE Access : Practical Innovations, Open Solutions, 13*, 106465–106488. Advance online publication. DOI: 10.1109/ACCESS.2025.3572626

Tyagi, R. K. R. N and R. Kumar, "An Innovative Deep Learning Method for Enhancing Image Resolution," *2024 2nd World Conference on Communication & Computing (WCONF)*, RAIPUR, India, 2024, pp. 1-6, DOI: 10.1109/WCONF61366.2024.10692190

U.S. Food and Drug Administration. (2022). (2021–2024). *Good machine learning practice for medical device development: Guiding principles* (FDA/Health Canada/MHRA).

Ula, M., Muhathir, M., & Sahputra, I. (2022). Optimization of multilayer perceptron hyperparameter in classifying pneumonia disease through X-Ray images with speeded-up robust features extraction method. IJACSA). *International Journal of Advanced Computer Science and Applications*, *13*(10). Advance online publication. DOI: 10.14569/IJACSA.2022.0131025

Ullah, H., Manickam, S., Obaidat, M., Laghari, S. U. A., & Uddin, M. (2023). Metaverse technology in healthcare. *IEEE Access : Practical Innovations, Open Solutions*, *11*, 69686–69707. DOI: 10.1109/ACCESS.2023.3286696

Upreti, D., Yang, E., Kim, H., & Seo, C. (2024). A comprehensive survey on federated learning in the healthcare area: Concept and applications. *Computer Modeling in Engineering & Sciences*, *140*(3), 2239–2274. DOI: 10.32604/cmes.2024.048932

V. M S. S. S, T. Krishnamurthy, Chaithra, R. N and S. G, "Advanced Encryption Strategies for Protecting Patient Data in IoMT Applications," *2025 6th International Conference for Emerging Technology (INCET)*, BELGAUM, India, 2025, pp. 1-6, DOI: 10.1109/INCET64471.2025.11139937

Vaidhehi, M., Malathy, C., Sudhakaran, P., Cherian, A. K., Geetha, R., & And Kumar, G. M. (2025). Toward Smart Healthcare in Digital Twin for 6G-Powered Sustainable Ultra-Smart Cities. In *Driving Innovation through AI and Digital Twin for 6G Powered Sustainable Ultra Smart Cities* (pp. 183–210). Wiley. DOI: 10.1002/9781394411320.ch8

Vallée, A. (2023). Digital twin for healthcare systems. *Frontiers in Digital Health*, *5*, 1253050. DOI: 10.3389/fdgth.2023.1253050 PMID: 37744683

Vanmathi, C.. (2024). Blockchain integration in healthcare: A comprehensive review of applications, challenges, and solutions. *Frontiers in Digital Health.*

Vashisht, S., & Rani, S. (2025). AI-standardized secure digital twins for smart home ecosystems. *IEEE Communications Standards Magazine*, 1–5. Advance online publication. DOI: 10.1109/MCOMSTD.2025.3619536

Vayena, E., Blasimme, A., & Cohen, I. G. (2020). Machine learning in medicine: Addressing ethical challenges. *PLoS Medicine*, *17*(11), e1002689. DOI: 10.1371/journal.pmed.1002689 PMID: 30399149

Vayena, E., Dzenowagis, J., Brownstein, J. S., & Sheikh, A. (2020). Policy implications of big data in the health sector. *Bulletin of the World Health Organization*, *98*(1), 66–68. DOI: 10.2471/BLT.17.197426 PMID: 29403102

Veale, M., & Borgesius, F. Z. (2021). Demystifying the draft EU Artificial Intelligence Act. *Computer Law Review International*, *22*(4), 97–112. DOI: 10.9785/cri-2021-220402

Vemuri, S. S., Kotha, S., Voruganti, S., Kunam, P. R., Nandini, A., & Kumar Mishra, T. (2024, September). Pneumonia Detection from X-Ray Images Using Deep Transfer Learning. In International Conference on Computing, Communication and Learning (pp. 205-219). Cham: Springer Nature Switzerland.

Viswanadham, N. (2021). Ecosystem model for healthcare platform. *Sadhana*, *46*(4), 188. DOI: 10.1007/s12046-021-01708-y

Wamema, J., Alunyu, A., Amiyo, M., & Nabukenya, J. (2023). Enterprise architecture requirements for standardising digital health in Uganda's health system. *Health Policy and Technology*, *12*(4), 100805. DOI: 10.1016/j.hlpt.2023.100805

Wang, C., Liu, S., Yang, H., Guo, J., Wu, Y., & Liu, J. (2023). Ethical considerations of using ChatGPT in health care. *Journal of medical Internet research, 25*, e48009.
WHO guidance. (2021). *World Health Organization*. Ethics and governance of artificial intelligence for health

Wang, G., Badal, A., Jia, X., Maltz, J. S., Mueller, K., Myers, K. J., Niu, C., Vannier, M., Yan, P., Yu, Z., & Zeng, R. (2022). Development of metaverse for intelligent healthcare. *Nature Machine Intelligence*, *4*(11), 922–929. DOI: 10.1038/s42256-022-00549-6 PMID: 36935774

Wang, Q., Cheng, H., & Wang, W. (2025). Video-PSG: An intelligent contactless monitoring system for sleep staging. *IEEE Transactions on Bio-Medical Engineering*, *72*(3), 965–977. DOI: 10.1109/TBME.2024.3480813 PMID: 39405136

Wang, Q., Chen, S., Wu, M., & Li, X. (2025). Digital twin-empowered federated incremental learning for non-IID privacy data. *IEEE Transactions on Mobile Computing*, *24*(5), 3860–3877. Advance online publication. DOI: 10.1109/TMC.2024.3517592

Wang, Y., Li, C., Qu, L., Cai, H., & Ge, Y. (2023). Application and challenges of a metaverse in medicine. *Frontiers in Robotics and AI, 10*, 1291199. DOI: 10.3389/frobt.2023.1291199 PMID: 38152305

Wang, Y., Su, Z., Zhang, N., Xing, R., Liu, D., Luan, T. H., & Shen, X. (2022). A survey on metaverse: Fundamentals, security, and privacy. *IEEE Communications Surveys and Tutorials*, *25*(1), 319–352. DOI: 10.1109/COMST.2022.3202047

Wang, Z., Wei, H., Huang, Y., Wei, Y., & Chen, J. (2023). Naturally sourced hydrogels. *Chemical Society Reviews*, *52*(9), 2992–3034. DOI: 10.1039/D2CS00813K PMID: 37017633

Wassan, S., Liudajun, , Ying, H., Dongyan, H., & Fei, P. (2025). Federated learning and differential privacy: Machine learning and deep learning for biomedical image data classification. *Digital Health*, *11*, 20552076251358532. DOI: 10.1177/20552076251358531 PMID: 40949674

Weber, P., Carl, K. V., & Hinz, O. (2023). Applications of explainable artificial intelligence in finance—A systematic review of finance, information systems, and computer science literature. *Management Review Quarterly*, *74*(2), 867–907. DOI: 10.1007/s11301-023-00320-0

Wen, B.. (2025), "Voice-based AI Agents: Filling the Economic Gaps in Digital Health Delivery," *2025 IEEE International Conference on Digital Health (ICDH)*, Helsinki, Finland, 2025, pp. 220-232. DOI: 10.1109/ICDH67620.2025.00040

WHO. (2023). *Global strategy on digital health 2020–2025: Progress report.*

Wiederhold, B. K. (2022). Metaverse meets medicine. *Cyberpsychology, Behavior and Social Networking*, *25*(1), 1–2. DOI: 10.1089/cyber.2021.29234.editorial PMID: 34964667

Williamson, O. E. (1985). *The economic institutions of capitalism: Firms, markets, relational contracting*. Free Press.

World Health Organisation. (2023). *Global strategy on digital health 2020–2025: Progress report.*

Wosik, J., Fudim, M., Cameron, B., Gellad, Z. F., Cho, A., Phinney, D., & Katz, J. N. (2020). Telehealth transformation: COVID-19 and the rise of virtual care. *Journal of the American Medical Informatics Association : JAMIA*, *27*(6), 957–962. DOI: 10.1093/jamia/ocaa067 PMID: 32311034

Wu, B., Huang, J., & Duan, Q. (2025). Real-time intelligent healthcare enabled by federated digital twins with AoI optimization. *IEEE Network*. Advance online publication. DOI: 10.1109/MNET.2025.3565977

Wu, J. T., Wong, K. C. L., Gur, Y., Ansari, N., Karargyris, A., Sharma, A., Morris, M., Saboury, B., Ahmad, H., Boyko, O., Syed, A., Jadhav, A., Wang, H., Pillai, A., Kashyap, S., Moradi, M., & Syeda-Mahmood, T. (2020). Comparison of chest radiograph interpretations by artificial intelligence algorithm vs radiology residents. *JAMA Network Open, 3*(10), e2022779. DOI: 10.1001/jamanetworkopen.2020.22779 PMID: 33034642

Xu, J., Glicksberg, B. S., Su, C., Walker, P., Bian, J., & Wang, F. (2021). Federated learning for healthcare informatics. *Journal of Healthcare Informatics Research, 5*(1), 1–19. DOI: 10.1007/s41666-020-00082-4 PMID: 33204939

Xu, M., Yoon, S., Fuentes, A., & Park, D. S. (2023). A comprehensive survey of image augmentation techniques for deep learning. *Pattern Recognition, 137*, 109347. DOI: 10.1016/j.patcog.2023.109347

Xu, X., Sun, Y., Liu, Q., & Wang, Z. (2023). Digital twin-driven smart healthcare: Framework and applications. *IEEE Journal of Biomedical and Health Informatics.*

Yamuna, V., Babu, G. S., Raju, V. A. G., Manchala, Y., Ramakrishna, G., & Savalapurapu, K. (2024), "AI-Based eHealth Care Framework with IoT," 2024 2nd International Conference on Signal Processing, Communication, Power and Embedded System (SCOPES), Paralakhemundi Campus, Centurion University of Technology and Management, Odisha, India, 2024, pp. 1-6. DOI: 10.1109/SCOPES64467.2024.10990919

Yang, E. (2023). Immersive technologies in healthcare built environments. *Frontiers in Medical Technology, 5*, 1184925. DOI: 10.3389/fmedt.2023.1184925 PMID: 37799269

Yang, G. (2022). From black-box to explainable AI in healthcare: Existing approaches, challenges and future directions. *Computational and Structural Biotechnology Journal, 20*, 1234–1250.

Yang, Q., Liao, H., Zhang, Z., & Ding, Y. (2023). Metaverse-enabled digital twins for healthcare: Opportunities and challenges. *IEEE Internet of Things Journal.*

Yang, W., Xiang, W., Yang, Y., & Cheng, P. (2023). Optimizing federated learning with deep reinforcement learning for digital twin empowered industrial IoT. *IEEE Transactions on Industrial Informatics, 19*(2), 1884–1893. DOI: 10.1109/TII.2022.3183465

Yang, Y.. (2023). Metaverse for healthcare: Technologies, challenges, and opportunities. *International Journal of Crowd Science*. Agbo, C. C., Mahmoud, Q. H., & Eklund, J. M. (2019, April). Blockchain technology in healthcare: a systematic review. []. MDPI.]. *Health Care*, *7*(2), 56.

Yang, Y., & Mei, G. (2022). Pneumonia recognition by deep learning: A comparative investigation. *Applied Sciences (Basel, Switzerland)*, *12*(9), 4334. DOI: 10.3390/app12094334

Yao, D., Xu, Z., Lin, Y., & Zhan, Y. (2023). Accurate and intelligent diagnosis of pediatric pneumonia using X-ray images and blood testing data. *Frontiers in Bioengineering and Biotechnology*, *11*, 1058888. Advance online publication. DOI: 10.3389/fbioe.2023.1058888 PMID: 37292095

Yenduri, G., ... (2023), "Federated Learning for the Metaverse: A Short Survey," 2023 International Conference on Intelligent Metaverse Technologies & Applications (iMETA), Tartu, Estonia, 2023, pp. 1-10. DOI: 10.1109/iMETA59369.2023.10294796

Ye, T., Xue, J., He, M., Gu, J., Lin, H., Xu, B., & Cheng, Y. (2019). Psychosocial factors affecting artificial intelligence adoption in health care in China: Cross-sectional study. *Journal of Medical Internet Research*, *21*(10), e14316. DOI: 10.2196/14316 PMID: 31625950

Yildirim, A. E., & Canayaz, M. (2023). A novel deep learning-based approach for prediction of neonatal respiratory disorders from chest X-ray images. *Biocybernetics and Biomedical Engineering*, *43*(4), 635–655. DOI: 10.1016/j.bbe.2023.08.004

Zaman Wani, R. U., & Can, O. (2025). FED-EHR: A privacy-preserving federated learning framework for decentralized healthcare analytics. *Electronics (Basel)*, *14*(16), 3261. Advance online publication. DOI: 10.3390/electronics14163261

Zhang, Y., ... (2025). Federated transfer learning for digital twin-based CT medical imaging analysis. arXiv preprint arXiv:2509.08018. https://arxiv.org/abs/2509.08018

Zhang, J.. (2023). Metaverse-based healthcare: A systematic review. *Journal of Medical Internet Research*, *25*, e45352.

Zhang, J., Zhu, H., Wang, F., Zhao, J., Xu, Q., & Li, H. (2022). Security and privacy threats to federated learning: Issues, methods, and challenges. *Security and Communication Networks*, *2022*, 1–24. DOI: 10.1155/2022/2886795

Zhang, P., & Kamel Boulos, M. N. (2022). Privacy-by-design environments for large-scale health research and federated learning from data. *International Journal of Environmental Research and Public Health*, *19*(19), 11876. Advance online publication. DOI: 10.3390/ijerph191911876 PMID: 36231175

Zhang, P., & Kamel Boulos, M. N. (2023). Generative AI in medicine and healthcare: Promises, opportunities and challenges. *Future Internet*, *15*(9), 286. DOI: 10.3390/fi15090286

Zhang, Y., Lu, Y., & Liu, F. (2023). A systematic survey for differential privacy techniques in federated learning. *Journal of Information Security*, *14*(02), 111–135. DOI: 10.4236/jis.2023.142008

Zhang, Y., & Zhao, L. (2025). Resilient multi-layer LSTM digital twin framework for athlete logistics and safety in 6G. *IEEE Communications Standards Magazine*, 1–8. Advance online publication. DOI: 10.1109/MCOMSTD.2025.3630497

Zhu, H., Han, G., Hou, J., Liu, X., & Ma, Y. (2023). Knowledge sharing for pulmonary nodule detection in medical cyber-physical systems. *IEEE Journal of Biomedical and Health Informatics*, *27*(2), 625–635. Advance online publication. DOI: 10.1109/JBHI.2022.3220430 PMID: 36346863

Zou, J., & Schiebinger, L. (2018). AI can be sexist and racist—It is time to make it fair. *Nature*, *559*(7714), 324–326. DOI: 10.1038/d41586-018-05707-8 PMID: 30018439

Zuboff, S. (2019). *The age of surveillance capitalism*. PublicAffairs.

About the Contributors

Soufiene Ben Othman is an Assistant Professor of computer science at the Applied College, King Faisal University, Saudi Arabia from 2025. He received his Ph.D. degree in computer science from Manouba University in 2016 for his dissertation on "Secure data aggregation in wireless sensor networks. He also holds M.S. degrees from the Monastir University in 2012. My research interests focus on the Internet of Medical Things, Wireless Body Sensor Networks, Wireless Networks, Artificial Intelligence, Machine Learning and Big Data. Dr. Ben Othman has published more than 120 papers at reputed international journals, conferences, and book chapters. He is an Editorial Board Member in the different Journals and Conferences. He serves as an associate editor/academic editor for international journals including IEEE Access, IEEE Sensors, IEEE Internet of Things, Elsevier, Springer, Taylor & Francis, IGI, IET, Telecommunication Computing Electronics and Control, and Wiley. Dr. Ben Othman is a Technical Program Committee Member for more than a dozen of international conferences.

***

Salam Al-E'mari earned her Ph.D. in Cybersecurity from Universiti Sains Malaysia (USM) in 2022. She is the Chair of the Information Security Department and an Assistant Professor at the University of Petra (UoP). With expertise in Blockchain, Deep Learning, and Network Security, she has contributed significantly to cybersecurity research. She previously earned her Bachelor's and Master's in Computer Science from Yarmouk University, Jordan, shaping her strong foundation in security and technology.

Adinarayana Andy is a licensed pharmacist and research scientist with over sixteen years of experience bridging clinical pharmacy practice, pharmaceutical innovation, and operations management. A multidisciplinary expert, Dr. Andy holds a unique combination of credentials: a PhD in Biotechnology, an MBA in Project Management, and active licensure as a pharmacist. Served as Pharmacist-in-Charge at Weatherwax Family Pharmacy in Michigan, Dr. Andy directs clinical operations with a focus on medication therapy management (MTM), immunization initiatives, and public health outreach. His leadership is grounded in extensive industry experience with global pharmaceutical organizations, including BMS-Biocon, Cadila Pharmaceuticals, and Dr. Reddy's Laboratories. In these roles, he contributed significantly to drug development, regulatory affairs, and quality assurance frameworks. Andy earned his PhD in Biotechnology from Acharya Nagarjuna University and an MBA from the University of the Cumberlands, USA. He also holds a Master of Pharmacy in Pharmaceutical Analysis & Quality Assurance from Biju Patnaik University of Technology and a Bachelor of Pharmacy from Andhra University.

Aravind Kumar B is a final-year Mechanical Engineering student with a growing interest in advanced technologies including Artificial Intelligence, digital systems, and interdisciplinary research applications. His academic background provides a strong foundation in analytical thinking, problem-solving, and system design. He is particularly interested in the convergence of engineering principles with emerging digital technologies such as AI, federated learning, and immersive systems

Muralidhar B is a professionally qualified dental surgeon. He holds Ph.D. from Canara Bank School of Management Studies, Bangalore University after his MBA from Christ University. He has 18 years of total teaching experience spanning across dental education, healthcare management and general management and 4 years of corporate experience. He has worked as research associate in Institute for Social and Economic Change, Bangalore in a project entitled as "Management By and For Common Man: An Exploration of the Concept and Direction for Future"post Ph.D. He had secured 28th rank in S.S.L.C (10th Standard) examination for Karnataka State in 1993. His 31 patents have been published and 2 design patents have been granted. He has 41 research publications to his credit out of which 33 are Scopus-indexed and 5 are ABDC indexed. He has co-authored 13 books. He is currently working as Assistant Professor (Grade-3) in Department of Business Management Studies, School of Commerce, Jain Deemed to be University, Bangalore.

Anmol Budhewar serves as an Assistant Professor in Computer Engineering, with research interests spanning artificial intelligence, machine learning, blockchain-enabled systems, and secure computing architectures. In the previous academic year, he published one Scopus-indexed research article and one IEEE international conference paper, demonstrating his commitment to high-quality scholarly dissemination. He contributes extensively to the academic peer-review ecosystem, serving as a reviewer for multiple international journals and edited books, and earning several Certificates of Excellence for review quality. Notably, he reviewed four research articles for SN Computer Science (Springer Nature) on topics including blockchain security, medical image analysis, fraud detection, and authentication systems. His academic work emphasizes integrating intelligent computational models with real-world applications in healthcare, cybersecurity, and data-driven decision systems. Through research, reviewing, and teaching, he strengthens methodological rigor and interdisciplinary innovation in computer science scholarship.

Dhinakaran Damodaran, is an Associate Professor in the Department of Computer Science and Engineering at Vel Tech Rangarajan Dr. Sagunthala R&D Institute of Science and Technology, Chennai. He holds a B.E., M.E., and Ph.D. in Computer Science from Anna University. His research expertise includes Privacy-Preserving Data Mining, Artificial Intelligence, Internet of Things (IoT), MANETs, Cloud Computing, and Image Processing. A prolific researcher, he has presented over 30 papers at international conferences, published more than 60 articles in reputed international journals, and filed three patents. He has been honoured as one of the Top 2% Scientists globally by Elsevier and Stanford University. He is actively supervising Ph.D. scholars and serves as a reviewer for reputed international journals and conferences, reflecting his strong commitment to academic excellence and research advancement. His innovative contributions and dedication to academia have made a significant impact on the evolving fields of Computer Science and Engineering.

Selvaraj Damodaran is working as a professor in the Department of Electronics and Communication Engineering at Panimalar Engineering College. He obtained his B.E Degree from Madras University, ME degree from Anna University and Ph.D. from Sathyabama University. He has a vast teaching experience of 21 years. He has published more than 75 papers at various refereed journals and conferences. His area of interest is in the field of signal processing, image processing, Biomedical Instrumentation, wireless communication, Artificial Intelligence, Machine learning, Data Mining and Antenna Design. He is a member of IEEE and life member of IETE.

Darshan Devaraju received his Ph.D. degree from Visvesvaraya Technological University (VTU). He obtained his M.Tech. degree in Digital Electronics and Communication Systems from Visvesvaraya Technological University, India, in 2011, and his B.E. degree in Electronics and Communication Engineering from Visvesvaraya Technological University, Belgaum, in 2008. He is currently serving as an Assistant Professor in the Department of Electronics and Communication Engineering at S J B Institute of Technology, Kengeri, Bengaluru–560060, Karnataka, India. His research interests include Computer Networking, Communication Engineering, Wireless Sensor Networks, and the Internet of Things (IoT). He has published several papers in national and international journals and conferences.

Jaypalsinh A. Gohil is a distinguished academic and researcher with over 18 years of experience in computer science education. Currently serving as Associate Professor at Faculty of Computer Applications, Marwadi University, Rajkot, he specializes in artificial intelligence, blockchain technology, database management systems, and system development methodologies. An accomplished Ph.D. supervisor at Marwadi University, Dr. Gohil has guided multiple research scholars, authored books on system analysis and design, published extensively in international journals and conferences, and contributed as a technical program committee member in numerous esteemed events. He is also recognized for his leadership roles, professional achievements, and his mentoring excellence, which has been acknowledged institutionally. His patented innovations include advancements in waste disposal management and wireless communication systems, reflecting his contributions to the technological and academic landscape in India.

Swapna H R holds two Ph.D. degrees in Management — one from CMR University, Bangalore, and another from Rayalaseema University, Kurnool. She is an MBA in Finance from VTU University. She has over 18 years of teaching experience in the areas of Finance, Analytics, Statistics, Entrepreneurship, and Human Resource Management, along with 4 years of industry experience. Her research expertise spans Statistics, Behavioural Finance, Employee Engagement, Artificial Intelligence, Entrepreneurship, research on millennials, customer engagement, social media, and the health sector. She has published over 100 research articles in National and International Journals, of which 46 have been indexed in Scopus, Web of Science (WoS), Emerald, Springer, and ABDC. She has presented papers at National and International Conferences, including in the USA, Malaysia, and Spain, and has received several Best Paper Presenter Awards. She has authored over 25 textbooks in the fields of Statistics, Entrepreneurship, Business Analytics, Healthcare, and Event Management. Her book Business Analytics received the Golden Book Award of 2022. She also received the Excellence Researcher Award on May 30, 2025. Another feather in her cap is her achievement in the field of Intellectual Property Rights, with 14 patents published, 2 granted, and 4 more filed. She has also curated and developed a SWAYAM course titled "Microfinance and Self-Help Groups," contributing to the promotion of inclusive education and financial literacy at the national level. She serves as an editor for several Scopus-indexed journals under

IGI Global, Public Administration and Policy (Emerald Publishing), and PubMed-indexed medical journals. She is an active member of ENACTUS, an international social entrepreneurship forum linked with several NGOs, where she contributes to sustainability initiatives and drives impactful community projects. She passionately mentors students to develop sustainable business solutions and promotes social innovation and environmental responsibility. Dr. Swapna has also been at the forefront of social service initiatives such as organizing blood donation camps in association with the Rotary Club and TTK, supporting the Ministry of Education's One-on-One COVID-19 emotional support drive, and leading environmental awareness campaigns like "One Earth."

Krishna Inala has received his Ph.D. degree from the Electronics and Electrical Engineering Department, Indian Institute of Technology, Guwahati, Assam, India in August 2020. The title of his thesis is "Impact of Communication Systems on Distributed Node Voltage and Vehicle to Grid Controller in a Smart Grid Scenario". He received his M.E. degree in Communication and Networking from Anna University, Chennai, India in 2011. He obtained his B.Tech. degree in Electronics and Communication Engineering from JNTU, Hyderabad, India in 2008. Dr. Krishna Pavan Inala's current research applies Artificial Intelligence and Machine Learning to make Smart Grids more efficient and secure. His work mainly focuses on Vehicle-to-Grid (V2G) systems, communication networks, and Advanced Metering Infrastructure (AMI) security. He studies how communication affects grid performance and develops intelligent algorithms for safe and efficient energy exchange. His ongoing work includes IoT-based smart metering and reinforcement learning for grid optimization. Overall, his research connects Smart Grids, AI, and communication to build smarter and more reliable energy networks

Rampelli Manojkumar received his Ph.D. in Power Engineering from the Indian Institute of Technology Guwahati in 2023. He obtained his Master of Technology in Power and Energy Systems from the National Institute of Technology Karnataka, Surathkal, India, in 2015. He is currently an Assistant Professor in the Department of Electrical and Electronics Engineering at BVRIT Hyderabad College of Engineering for Women. He is currently the Editorial Board Member of Scientific Reports, Early Career Editor for the International Journal of Ambient Energy and the Guest Editor for PLOS ONE. Additionally, he is an active reviewer for around 30 SCI journals. He has been a speaker at the IEEE Smart Grid webinar series and has contributed to multiple funded research projects on smart transformer-based microgrid systems and distributed generation management. He has published 10 Q1 journal papers, including articles in IEEE Transactions on Power Systems, IEEE Transactions on Industrial Informatics, and Sustainable Cities and Society. His research expertise spans energy management, hybrid AC/DC distribution systems, energy storage, and power electronics applications in modern distribution systems.

Pratiksha Meshram is working as Assistant professor in Department of IT at SVKM's NMIMS MPSTME Shirpur campus. She has passion towards development in the field of AI, Machine learning & deep learning for the applications in health care. She has organized & conducted several workshops & guest lectures for students & faculties. She has guided several projects of undergraduate students including inter disciplinary projects. She has filed one patent & published more than 12 research articles in emerging technologies

Arindam Mitra, an Assistant Professor in the Department of Electrical Engineering at NIT Rourkela, has been advancing power systems research with a focus on machine learning, system identification, and predictive maintenance since his Ph.D. at IIT Kanpur. His innovative work earned him the Karandikar Best Ph.D. Thesis Award (2024), POSOCO Power System Award (2023), and SIIC Student Innovation Award (2024). With high-impact publications and three patents, he bridges research and practical energy solutions. Dr. Mitra has presented globally at conferences and leads research on applying machine learning to enhance power system reliability and efficiency at NIT Rourkela.

Raghu N has Ten years of experience in Academic and Research. He received the Ph.D. (2020) in Electronics Engineering from Jain University, and B.E. in Electronics and Telecommunications Engineering from VTU University, Karnataka. His research interests were in RF Communication and Image Processing. He has published his research findings in various Scopus indexed Journals and International conferences. He is a member of various professional bodies.

Suganthi N received the bachelor's degree in Electrical and Electronics Engineering from Bharathiyar University in 2001, the master's degree in Electrical Power and Energy System from Uttar Pradesh Technical University in 2013, and Ph.D. in Electrical Engineering from Visvesvaraya University respectively. She is currently working as an Assistant Professor at the Department of Electrical and Electronics Engineering, Dayananda Sagar College of Engineering. Her research areas include microgrid, renewable energy systems, energy storage systems. She can be contacted at email: suganthi_neelagiri@yahoo.com.

Reshma PH is a distinguished academician and counselor with extensive qualifications, including an M.COM, PG Diploma in Accounting & Taxation, MBA from Bharathiar University, and a Ph.D. in GHRM (Green Human Resource Management) from JJTU University, Rajasthan. With 8.5 years of academic experience, she has held roles as research coordinator, In-charge HOD, and participated in various research programs and conferences, Presented research articles in national and international conferences and published articles in UGC CARE journal, WOS and Scopus. She has designed course curriculums for Undergraduate programmes at Jain (Deemed -to-be University). Authored books on CRM, financial accounting, Corporate Administration for Bangalore university. Dr. Reshma, an member & Associate Editor in Association of Global Academicians and Researchers (AGAR) and Project Guide for national and international students, she has received appreciation awards for organizing national-level FDPs, webinars, Conferences. She is currently an Assistant Professor at Jain (Deemed-to-be University), contributing to course curriculum design, and serving as a member of the research team and MOOC developer. Her diverse areas of interest include HR, Accounts and other management subjects, reflecting her expertise and passion for all aspects of academia.

Ramesh Pittala is a seasoned academic professional with over 20 years of experience in teaching, research, and academic administration. He specializes in Data Mining and Information Retrieval, holding a Ph.D. in Geo-Spatial Data Mining from Rayalaseema University and an M.Tech in Software Engineering from JNTUK, where he secured a university gold medal. As an Associate Professor at Anurag University, he has previously held key positions at KL Deemed to be University and KLR College of Engineering and Technology, serving as Vice Principal and Head of the Department. His research focuses on artificial intelligence, machine learning, cloud computing, and geospatial data mining, with numerous publications in SCOPUS and SCI-indexed journals. He is also a reviewer for prestigious journals like the *Journal of Big Data*. Dr. Babu possesses expertise in AWS, Linux, DevOps tools, and machine learning, with certifications including IBM DB2 and Enterprise Design Thinking Practitioner. His contributions extend to patents in natural language processing and intelligent systems, demonstrating his commitment to technological innovation. Recognized for academic excellence, he has received accolades such as a gold medal for his M.Tech performance and a Letter of Appreciation for his long-standing contributions to academia. His administrative experience includes NBA accreditation and curriculum design, further reinforcing his leadership in higher education.

Aarthi S is a dedicated Assistant Professor in Computer Science with over six years of teaching experience. She is currently pursuing her Ph.D. at Marwadi University, Gujarat, and holds an M.Phil. and MCA from Bharathiar University, Tamil Nadu. Throughout her academic career, Aarthi has specialized in programming languages such as C++, Java, and C, and contributed to research in recommender systems and AI-related data privacy. She has published journal articles, contributed to book chapters, and actively participated in technical workshops. Known for her student mentorship and engagement in academic events, Aarthi remains committed to fostering innovation and excellence in computer science education.

Edwin Raja S, Associate Professor, Department of Computer Science and Engineering in Vel Tech Rangarajan Dr.Sagunthala R&D Institute of Science and Technology, Chennai. He has completed his Ph.D. in Information and Communication Engineering from Anna University-chennai in the year 2021. He obtained his M.Tech. (Network Engineering) in the year 2010 from Kalasalingam University, Krishnan kovil and B.E. (Computer Science and Engineering) in the year 2006 from C.S.I Institute of Technology, Thovalai. He has more than thirteen plus years of teaching experience and his area of interests are Cyber Security, Big Data Analytics, Machine Learning & Computer Networks. He has published more than 4 research articles in various journals and conferences. Also, he has published 3 patents, acted as reviewer in reputed journals.

Madhu S has 32+ years of experience in academia and industry. A prolific author and researcher, he has authored 100+ books, holds 2⅞ design patent, 5 utility patent published, published 30+ articles and book chapters, and has won multiple awards. He serves as a consultant, keynote speaker, jury member, resource person, and academic mentor, guiding hundreds of students and contributing widely to research and innovation. BoS and BoE member for various universities.

Shashikala S V received her B.E degree in Computer Science from Mysore University, Karnataka in 1990 and M. Tech in Computer Science and Engineering from Visvesvaraya Technological University in 2005, Ph.D. degree from VTU. She is a Professor and Head in the department of computer science at B.G.S Institute of Technology; B.G.Nagar, Mandya and having totally 25 years of teaching experience. She has presented many papers in National level conferences and also presented many papers in international conferences; she has published 5 papers in International Journals. Her main research interests include computer networks, big data and data mining. She can be contacted at email: shashisv7@gmail.com

T. Aditya Sai Srinivas is an accomplished academician currently serving as an Associate Professor in the Department of Computer Science and Engineering at Ravindra College of Engineering for Women, Kurnool. He holds a Ph.D. in Internet of Things (IoT) from the prestigious VIT University, Vellore, where he specialized in cutting-edge IoT frameworks and intelligent systems. With a strong research orientation, he has published over 50 research papers in reputed international journals. His academic contributions extend beyond research, having authored multiple textbooks in computer science and engineering. Dr. Srinivas is actively involved in mentoring students and guiding innovative projects in emerging technologies like ML, IoT, and FL. He is also a regular contributor to academic conferences and technical symposiums. His work reflects a commitment to both scholarly excellence and practical application in the evolving tech landscape. .

Yousef Sanjalawe is an Assistant Professor specializing in Cybersecurity and Cloud Computing at the University of Jordan (JU), Jordan. He earned his PhD in Cloud Computing from Universiti Sains Malaysia (USM) in 2020, where his research focused on enhancing cloud service broker selection using optimization algorithms. Dr. Sanjalawe has extensive experience in academia, research, and professional training. He has supervised Ph.D. students in Cybersecurity, Cloud Computing, IoT, Fog Computing, Optimization, and Artificial Intelligence (AI). From 2023 to 2024, he served as the Chair of the Cybersecurity Department at the American University of Madaba (AUM), Jordan, and from 2022 to 2024, he was an Assistant Professor in Cybersecurity at AUM.

Manasha Saqib is an accomplished academician and researcher in the field of Computer Science and Engineering, with specialized expertise in Internet of Things (IoT), network security, cryptography, wireless sensor networks, and authentication protocols. She earned her Ph.D. in Computer Science & Engineering (2023) from the Islamic University of Science and Technology, Awantipora, where her doctoral research focused on developing a lightweight security authentication framework for IoT environments. She completed her M.Tech in Computer Science & Engineering with distinction from Jamia Hamdard, New Delhi, and her B.E. in Computer Science & Engineering with distinction from SSM College of Engineering and Technology, University of Kashmir. Dr. Saqib has demonstrated consistent academic excellence, qualifying the UGC National Eligibility Test (NET) and receiving prestigious fellowships including the Maulana Azad National Fellowship (JRF & SRF) from UGC. She is also a recipient of the Merit-cum-Minority Scholarship awarded by the Government of India. Her research contributions have been widely recognized, including a Best Paper Award at the 4th International Conference on Innovations in Data Analytics (ICIDA 2025). She currently serves as an Assistant Professor in the Department of Computer Science & Engineering at the University of People. Previously, she has held teaching and academic positions at esteemed institutions such as National Institute of Technology Srinagar, University of Kashmir, and Central University of Kashmir. With a strong commitment to teaching and mentorship, she has taught a wide range of undergraduate and postgraduate courses, including Database Management Systems, Computer Networks, Operating Systems, Data Structures, and Information & Network Security.

Swapnali Somwanshi is a dedicated microbiology graduate with strong academic and teaching experience. She completed her M.Sc. in Microbiology from SRTM University, Nanded, with 86.92% and holds a B.Sc. degree from the same university. Her research project focused on the isolation and identification of lactic acid bacteria from raw cow milk. She also holds a PG Diploma in Clinical Research (2023) and has qualified the PhD entrance examination in 2024. She has professional experience as an Assistant Professor at Yeshwant Mahavidyalaya, Nanded, and as an HR Executive at iPlace Consultancy. Her interests include research, teaching, reading, writing, and continuous learning.

Aman Suresh Tharayil is an Assistant Professor in Pharmacy Practice, currently serving at the Faculty of Pharmacy, Dr. M.G.R. Educational and Research Institute, Chennai. With a Pharm.D and ongoing PhD in Pharmacy Practice from SIMATS, he brings academic depth and clinical insight to his teaching and research. His teaching repertoire includes subjects such as pharmacotherapeutics, biostatistics, and pharmacoepidemiology for undergraduate and doctoral pharmacy programs. Dr. Aman is an active contributor to scholarly literature with multiple publications in Scopus and Web of Science-indexed journals, including research on diabetes, nephrology, and pharmacovigilance. His work has earned recognition such as subject-wise ranks at RGUHS and a prestigious ASCPT LMIC Travel Grant. Beyond academia, Dr. Aman has reviewed over 200 manuscripts and serves on editorial boards of reputed journals like Acta Scientific Pharmaceutical Sciences, PLOS ONE, and Cureus. He is also a frequent workshop resource person and guest lecturer on clinical pharmacy and regulatory topics. With strong skills in academic mentorship, interdisciplinary collaboration, and public health education, he actively bridges classroom instruction with real-world clinical practice.

Venkataramana Vemana is a Lead AI and Data Engineer with over a decade of experience in designing and implementing enterprise-scale Generative AI and Big Data solutions. His expertise spans AI system architecture, cloud-native data pipelines, and LLM operationalization, enabling organizations to deploy intelligent and efficient AI-driven systems at scale. At Elevance Health, Venkat worked as Engineer Lead Sr and led initiatives that reduced enterprise LLM costs by nearly 80% and designed retrieval-augmented generation (RAG) frameworks that transformed customer service efficiency. He has extensive hands-on experience with AWS, Azure, Databricks, and Snowflake, and deep technical proficiency in Python, Scala, and JavaScript. Venkat's professional focus lies in bridging the gap between data engineering and applied AI, with proven success in optimizing ETL pipelines, automating AI workflows, and benchmarking large language models such as GPT-4o, Claude 3, and LLaMA 3. His leadership in AI operationalization has accelerated digital transformation across enterprise environments. He holds a Master's degree in Computer Science from Virginia International University, USA, and a Bachelor's degree in Computer Science and Engineering from JNT University, India. Certified in AWS and Azure AI technologies, Venkat continues to drive innovation through scalable, secure, and high-impact AI solutions.

Index

A

B

C

D

E

F

G

H

R

S

T

V